DYNAMICS OF NUTRITION SUPPORT

Assessment, Implementation, Evaluation

DYNAMICS OF NUTRITION SUPPORT

Assessment, Implementation, Evaluation

Editor

Susanna H. Krey, R.D., M.Ed.
Vice President, Health Promotion
Saint Vincent Charity Hospital and Health Center
Cleveland, Ohio

Coeditor

Rebecca L. Murray, R.D.
Senior Dietitian
The Department of Dietetics
The Ohio State University Hospitals
Columbus, Ohio

APPLETON-CENTURY-CROFTS/Norwalk, Connecticut

0-8385-1890-7

Notice: The author(s) and publisher of this volume have taken care that the information and recommendations contained herein are accurate and compatible with the standards generally accepted at the time of publication.

86 87 88 89 / 10 9 8 7 6 5 4 3 2 1

Prentice-Hall of Australia, Pty. Ltd., Sydney
Prentice-Hall Canada, Inc.
Prentice-Hall Hispanoamericana, S.A., Mexico
Prentice-Hall of India Private Limited, New Delhi
Prentice-Hall International (UK) Limited, London
Prentice-Hall of Japan, Inc., Tokyo
Prentice-Hall of Southeast Asia (Pte.) Ltd., Singapore
Whitehall Books Ltd., Wellington, New Zealand
Editora Prentice-Hall do Brasil Ltda., Rio de Janeiro

Library of Congress Cataloging-in-Publication Data

Dynamics of nutrition support.

Includes index.
1. Parenteral feeding.   2. Nutrition—Evaluation.
3. Nutrition—Requirements.   4. Enteral feeding.
I. Krey, Susanna H.   II. Murray, Rebecca L. [DNLM:
1. Enteral Feeding.   2. Nutrition.   3. Nutritional
Requirements.   4. Parenteral Feeding. WB 400 D997]
RM224.D96 1986   615.8′55   85–30802
ISBN 0–8385–1890–7

Design: Lynn M. Luchetti

PRINTED IN THE UNITED STATES OF AMERICA

For I was hungry and you gave me food,
I was thirsty and you gave me drink, . . .
I was sick and you looked after me, . . .

Matt. 25:35, 36

To our parents with love
and
To Chuck . . . megathanks!!

Contributors

Molly Aalyson, M.S., R.D.
Clinical Nutritionist
Clinical Nutrition Unit
University Hospital
Boston, Massachusetts

Shana Bader, R.D.
Nutrition Consultant
Division Adolescent Medicine
Montefiore Medical Center
Bronx, New York
Formerly, Nutrition Support Dietitian
Nutritional Support Service
Hackensack Medical Center
Hackensack, New Jersey

Emma Cataldi-Betcher, R.D., M.S.
Student, UMDNJ-Rutgers Medical School
Camden, New Jersey
Formerly, Nutrition Support Dietitan
Nutrition Support Service
St. Barnabas Hospital Medical Center
Livingston, New Jersey

Nathaniel Clark, M.S.
Student, Worcester Medical School
University of Massachusetts
Worcester, Massachusetts
Formerly, Clinical Dietitian in
  Hyperalimentation and Research
  Associate in Nutrition/Metabolism
New England Deaconess Hospital
Boston, Massachusetts

Charlette Gallagher-Allred, R.D., Ph.D.
Former Faculty Member
Medical Dietetics Division
College of Medicine
The Ohio State University
Columbus, Ohio

Ruth Hooley, M.B.A., R.D.
Director, AMI Medical Choice Plan/
Contracting Manager, Sierra Pacific Region
American Medical International, Inc.
Brea, California
Formerly, Clinical Nutrition Specialist,
Nutritional Assessment
The Cleveland Clinic Foundation
Cleveland, Ohio

Anne Marie Hunter, M.S., R.D.
Director, Clinical Nutrition Services
St. John's Regional Medical Center
Joplin, Missouri

Terry Jensen, R.D.
Nutrition Consultant
Houston, Texas

Susanna H. Krey, R.D., M.Ed.
Vice President, Health Promotion
Saint Vincent Charity Hospital and Health
  Center
Cleveland, Ohio

Grace M. Lockett, M.P.H., R.D.
Research Assistant
Case Western Reserve University
School of Medicine
Cleveland, Ohio

Lucinda K. Lysen, R.D., R.N., B.S.N.
Clinical Dietitian
Oncology and Surgery Units
Christ Hospital
Oak Lawn, Illinois;
Research Associate in Nutritional Support
Northwestern Memorial Hospital
Chicago, Illinois

Laura E. Matarese, M.S., R.D.
Clinical Nutrition Specialist,
Nutritional Assessment
The Cleveland Clinic Foundation
Cleveland, Ohio

Michelle Mosner, R.D.
Nutrition Consultant
Middletown, New York

Rebecca L. Murray, R.D.
Senior Dietitian
The Department of Dietetics
The Ohio State University Hospitals
Columbus, Ohio
Formerly, Clinical Specialist in Nutrition
  Support
Akron General Medical Center
Akron, Ohio

Regina O'Shea, R.D., M.S.
Nutritional Support Dietitian
Boston, Massachusetts
Formerly, Nutrition Support Dietitian
Boston City Hospital
Boston, Massachusetts

Karen A. Porcelli, R.D., M.S.
Director, Clinical Nutrition Center
Saint Vincent Charity Hospital and Health
  Center
Cleveland, Ohio

Mary Rajala, M.S., R.D.
Student, Mayo Medical School
Rochester, Minnesota
Formerly, Nutrition Support Dietitian
Lahey Clinic Medical Center
Burlington, Massachusetts

Eva Shronts, R.D.
Nutrition Support Resource Specialist
University of Minnesota Hospitals &
  Clinics
Minneapolis, Minnesota

Joanne Wade, M.S., R.D.
Director, Department of Dietetics
New England Deaconess Hospital
Boston, Massachusetts;
Adjunct Assistant Professor of Nutrition
Sargent College of Allied Health
  Professions
Boston University
Boston, Massachusetts

Connie Stone Williams, R.D.
Clinical Assessment Supervisor
St. John's Regional Health Center
Biomedical Services
Springfield, Missouri

Lorraine See Young, R.D., M.S.
Clinical Dietitian
Nutrition Support Service
Brigham and Womens Hospital
Boston, Massachusetts

Contents

Foreword

The introduction of our ability to intervene nutritionally by the intravenous route in the late 1960s has stimulated the entire field of nutrition care in clinical medicine. The use of the enteral route, which has been an accepted mode of nourishing patients for decades, was primarily the responsibility of clinical dietitians. The technological advancements of the 1960s propelled both our awareness of hospital-based malnutrition and our abilities to intervene nutritionally to new highs. *The Dynamics of Nutrition Support* provides an in-depth and comprehensive review of these principles of nutrition support.

Unprecedented in clinical medicine, the growth of clinical nutrition has stimulated an interdisciplanary approach to medical care unrivaled in any other arena. It has become firmly established that a unified effort combining skills of physician, dietitian, nurse, and pharmacist (the nutrition support team) is the ideal way to deliver nutrition support to critically ill patients. The fully operational team demands from all of its members a commitment to knowledge and to quality clinical care that transcends the traditional roles played by its individual participants in past decades. Therefore, a comprehensive book such as this, written to provide additional knowledge and expertise to the dietitian, is to be applauded.

As a physician who has taken it upon himself to acquire advanced training in the field of nutrition, and as one who has been fortunate enough to have a pharmacist, a nurse, and a dietitian (who is the editor of this book), I realize that despite all the advances, especially in TPN and the rebirth of enteral hyperalimentation, in the majority of hospitals in the United States this type of multidisciplinary nutrition support expertise has not been available. In most situations, it is the dietitian who still has the full-time interest in and responsibility for the nutritional needs of the hospitalized patient. Frequently the clinical dietitian functions as a generalist and therefore, when asked to provide expertise in aggressive nutrition support, has a need for a reference, such as this book, to solve the nutritional problems of patients. *The Dynamics of Nutrition Support* focuses on the role of the dietitian as a hands-on clinically involved professional and has been written by dietitians to assist dietitians in acquiring the necessary knowledge to provide more effective patient care. However, its content, though written for dietitians, will be of value to all other disciplines involved in nutrition support.

I congratulate the editors, Susanna Krey and Rebecca Murray, who are responsible for providing this book, which I believe will become the standard for clinical dietitians involved in nutrition support for years to come

and which will raise the profession to new levels of excellence.

William P. Steffee, M.D., Ph.D.
Director, Department of Medicine
Saint Vincent Charity Hospital and Health
  Center
Cleveland, Ohio

Preface

A better understanding of the metabolic response to stress, the refinement of nutritional requirements in certain disease states, along with the advancement in the technology of enteral and parenteral nutrition, has led to an increasing need for continued education for the practitioner. *The Dynamics of Nutrition Support,* written by dietitians specializing in nutrition support from across the country, is designed to provide both the theoretical framework and practical application for the clinical dietitian who provides nutrition care to patients requiring aggressive nutrition support.

There are many practicing clinical dietitians who do not have the luxury of Nutrition Support Teams or the close association with other health care providers who have expertise in clinical nutrition. Frequently they are the sole persons responsible for all nutrition services for the patient and therefore require the support of this book, written by their colleagues who have had both formalized training and years of experience in nutrition support at large medical centers. With the aid of this book and its emphasis on the clinical application of the subject, the clinical dietitian will become more knowledgeable and effective in delivering nutrition services to patients requiring such aggressive nutrition intervention.

In addition to dietitians, there are many other professionals that can benefit from this reference manual. Physicians, residents, nurses, pharmacists, and students in each of these disciplines will find this comprehensive discussion of nutrition support extremely practical and helpful. Since nutrition support is frequently not addressed in undergraduate or graduate nutrition education, *The Dynamics of Nutrition Support* will become a useful text for these courses. As there are few books currently available that discuss nutrition support as comprehensively, nutrition/dietetic interns will find this reference invaluable during their clinical rotations.

The practical perspective of the book is enhanced by its organization. Its contents are organized according to a systems approach. The major sections take the reader through the necessary clinical steps to implement appropriate nutritional therapy. The reader is taken through the process of assessment, development of a nutrition care plan, implementation of the plan, and then evaluation ultimately to reassess appropriateness and effectiveness of therapy. Due to the importance of this focus, the Editors recognize the existence of repetition of certain important concepts. These have not been deleted as the Editors expect this book to be used as a reference and therefore not read sequentially.

The *Dynamics of Nutrition Support* consists of six major sections that discuss the most important principles of nutrition support for the practioner. Part I, introducing nutrition support, gives an excellent overview of the scope of the problem of hospital malnutrition, general assessment parameters used, indications for intervention, and an overview of the effectiveness of the current treatment modalities. Chapter 2 discusses the need for the multidisciplanary approach to effective implementation of nutrition support whereas Chapter 3 focuses on the unique role and contribution of the clinical dietitian in providing nutrition support.

Part II discusses in depth the major components and tools used to evaluate nutritional status, i.e., the nutrition history and physical assessment, laboratory values, anthropometry, and immune function tests. Recognizing the importance of understanding the strengths and weaknesses of assessment tools, Chapter 8 discusses these tools and helps the reader appropriately interpret the data to meaningfully determine nutritional status. Chapter 9 is an often overlooked topic that is vitally important to the discussion of nutritional risk because it focuses on the need to establish systems to identify patients at risk so that the problem of hospital malnutrition can be prevented.

Once nutritional status is determined, Part III discusses both the theoretical and practical aspects of determining nutritional requirements: protein and energy, vitamin and mineral, and fluid and electrolyte, all of which are essential to formulate the nutrition care plan. The authors of this section have done a superb job in presenting much of this information in tabular form, making this information always readily available and accessible. Frequently, this is data which nor-

mally has to be looked up in numerous other texts.

Part IV discusses the implementation of enteral therapy, indications, formula composition and selection, current delivery equipment, complications and administration guidelines, and a practical perspective on home enteral therapy. Of special significance is the discussion of modular formulas and the extensive critique of enteral tubes, pumps, and bags that are available today.

Paralleling the enteral section, a comprehensive review of the implementation of the parenteral nutrition care plan is accomplished in Part V. Of special interest in this section is the comprehensive analysis of parenteral solution substrates, formulation principles and procedures, and the in-depth discussion of altering parenteral support for specific disease states.

Part VI is a section often overlooked, as it focuses on the continued need for reassessment of treatment plans to assure appropriateness and effectiveness of treatment regimes. Additionally, the last chapter is dedicated to a discussion of parenteral and enteral transition techniques because from the dietitian's perspective aggressive nutrition support, in most cases, is a temporary measure that leads ultimately to transition to an oral diet, which is the goal to which this profession strives.

Lastly, the Editors hope that all nutrition support clinicians will find this book a valuable contribution to the discipline of clinical nutrition and that through it, better nutrition care will be provided to all patients, which will have made this effort worthwhile.

Susanna H. Krey
Rebecca L. Murray

Acknowledgments

We wish to express our gratitude for being given the opportunity to write and edit this textbook. We are deeply appreciative to our families, friends, instructors, professional colleagues, students, and patients for the support, example, encouragement, instruction, insight, and ideas that they provided. In particular, we wish to recognize Dr. William Steffee, M.D., Ph.D. and Dr. Calvin L. Long, Ph.D., who gave us the benefit of their experience and who helped us to shape our own professional growth.

We wish to thank Ronnie Chernoff, Ph.D., R.D., who saw the need for dietitians to publish a reference on nutrition support. We are also grateful to the officers of the Dietitians in Critical Care Dietetic Practice Group who supported us in our initial ventures.

Thanks belong to the editors at Appleton-Century-Crofts who made this book possible. We especially thank Terri Sternberg, the developmental editor for her initial development effort, and Marion Kalstein-Welch, acquisitions editor, whose encouragement, support, and patience kept us going.

We acknowledge the authors who contributed to this work for their enthusiasm, assistance, and willingness to rewrite. Special thanks go to Mary Iles, M.S., R.D. and Margarita Nagy, M.S., R.D. for their perspectives, assistance and advice. We wish also to acknowledge the authors of *The Dynamics of Clinical Dietetics,* Marion Mason, Burness G. Wenberg, and P. Kay Welsch, who stimulated our thinking in the system's approach to nutritional care.

Diane Stocker, Ruth Prebel, Inge Koenig, and Ginny Highfill deserve recognition for their secretarial support. We also wish to remember with gratitude Barbara Rankin, Medical Illustrator, who gave us her best and last works.

Becky wishes to thank Laura Knapp, M.S., R.D., Ellen Sours, R.D., and Donald W. Moorman, M.D. for their support and encouragement.

Sue especially would like to thank her nutritional colleagues at Saint Vincent—Karen, Maria, Cora, Mary, Veronica, Ann, Karin, Sue, Marlene, Fran and, of course, Kathy—for their support and contribution to her understanding of their critical roles in patient care.

Lastly, but most importantly, we would like to thank Chuck Miller, whose help and patience "was awesome" and whose pepperoni pizza helped us make it through the nights. "You're a good man Charlie Miller."

DYNAMICS OF NUTRITION SUPPORT

Assessment, Implementation, Evaluation

Part I. INTRODUCING NUTRITION SUPPORT

1. Rationale for Nutrition Support

Michele Mosner
Shana Bader

This chapter focuses on the incidence of hospital malnutrition, the factors involved in its metabolic onset, the tools used to detect malnutrition, and the modes used to intervene nutritionally in order to reverse malnutrition. Nutrition support refers to the maintenance or repletion of nutrition status by provision of required nutrients, often by other than conventional means. The effectiveness of nutrition support in the reversal of malnutrition and the outcome of illness will be presented.

THE INCIDENCE OF MALNUTRITION

Protein–calorie malnutrition (PCM) is usually considered a disease common to children from underdeveloped countries. Investigators, however, have reported comparable states in hospitalized American patients. In 1955, Rhoads and Alexander[1] observed cases of starvation in U.S. hospitals induced by nutrient losses from illness and injury rather than food deprivation. In 1974, Dr. Charles Butterworth[2] exposed "The Skeleton in the Hospital Closet," iatrogenic malnutrition, and evoked nationwide attention to the prevalence and causes of PCM in U.S. hospitals. Butterworth[2] surveyed the medical records of 80 medical–surgical patients hospitalized 2 weeks or more. He detailed many undesirable practices that affected the nutritional health of hospitalized patients (Table 1–1). Butterworth's exposition of malnutrition triggered a series of evaluations documenting the incidence of PCM (Table 1–2).[3–7] These surveys show the incidence of malnutrition in hospitalized patients ranges between 30 and 50 percent. The prevalence appears relatively constant despite the various types of hospitals, different types of illnesses, and socioeconomic status of the patients. Using anthropometric parameters, Bistrian et al. reported the striking finding of 50 percent prevalence of PCM among surgical patients of an urban municipal hospital.[3] A later study indicated 45 percent of patients on the general medical service of the same institution exhibited symptoms of PCM.[4] Mullen's group[5] studied the incidence of malnutrition in elective surgical patients admitted to an urban Veterans Administration hospital. Thirty-five percent of these patients demonstrated 3 or more abnormal nutritional and immunologic measurements.[5] Weisner et al.[6] evaluated the nutrition status of consecutive medical patients upon admission to a teaching hospital and throughout hospitalization. The 48 percent likelihood of malnutrition upon

TABLE 1–1. UNDESIRABLE PRACTICES THAT AFFECT THE NUTRITION HEALTH OF HOSPITALIZED PATIENTS

1. Failure to record height and weight routinely.
2. Prolonged use of glucose and saline intravenously. Maintaining NPO for prolonged periods.
3. Failure to observe patient's food intake.
4. Withholding meals for diagnostic tests.
5. Ignorance about the composition of vitamins and other nutritional products.
6. Failure to recognize increased metabolic needs due to injury or illness.
7. Failure to evaluate nutrition status before surgery.
8. Failure to administer nutrition support after surgery.
9. Delay of nutrition support until presence of advanced depletion.
10. Failure to realize the role of nutrition in prevention and recovery from infection; the unwarranted reliance on antibiotics.
11. Ignorance about the composition and proper administration of tube feedings.

admission increased to 69 percent 2 or more weeks later. Nutrition status worsened in over 75 percent of patients with normal values upon admission. This prospective study indicated malnutrition was hospital-related and not a mere reflection of the nutrition status of patients upon admission. A downward trend of nutrition status during hospitalization was associated with increased mortality rate and lengthened hospital stay.[6] Willard's recent findings revealed a 32 percent incidence of malnutrition in patients admitted by family practitioners to a private community hospital.[7] Studies detailing the incidence of malnutrition specific to patient age[8] and disease[9,10] are increasing in availability.

We need to update rather than accept statistics quantifying the incidence of malnutrition in diversified hospital settings and in specific disease states. Updated knowledge about the incidence of PCM in rural, community, and urban hospitals helps plan staffing, tools, and educational needs for nutrition intervention. Realization of those diseases associated with the greatest incidence of PCM provides a screening tool for early identification of high-risk patients.

TABLE 1–2. THE INCIDENCE OF MALNUTRITION

Investigator	Date	% Malnutrition	Criteria	Type Patient	Type Hospital
Bistrian et al.[3]	1974	50	AMC, wt for ht, TSF, albumin	General surgical	Urban municipal
Bistrian et al.[4]	1976	44 or more	AMC, wt for ht, TSF, albumin, lymphocyte count	General medical	Urban municipal
Mullen et al.[5]	1979	35	3 abnormal measurements of 16 nutritional and immunologic factors	Elective surgical	Urban VA
Weisner et al.[6]	1979	On admission—48 After 2 weeks—69	Scoring system based on serum folate, wt for ht, TSF, AMC, lymphocyte count, albumin, Hct, and serum vitamin C	General medical	Teaching hospital
Willard et al.[7]	1980	31.5	Wt for ht, TSF, AMC, albumin, and lymphocyte count	General medical or surgical	Private community

Now that the extensive incidence of malnutrition in hospitals has been documented, the role of the dietitian in this historic process needs mention. If the dietitian is the expert in nutrition services, why was hospital malnutrition so rampant? Historically, dietary department structure has not allowed dietitians across the country to be an integral part of the health care team. Dietitians were long considered food service personnel and not part of the clinical division of the hospital. The dietitian's role did not involve screening or identifying patients who were at high risk for malnutrition. Traditionally, the education of most dietitians lacked concentration on the tools used to assess and treat malnutrition. Today's clinical dietitian works in a dramatically new era. Now nutrition refers less to food service and more to the nutrition support of the patient. The hospital-based dietitian is well aware of the altered metabolism in illness and the major role nutrition plays in recovery. This book was created based on the concept that education about nutrition assessment techniques, data interpretation, and nutrition intervention is the first step toward the critical involvement of dietitians in a team effort to prevent hospital malnutrition.

Concern about the poor nutrition status of hospitalized patients led to the advent of nutrition support, that is, the means to provide nutrients for the prevention or treatment of malnutrition. Nutrition support teams surfaced. These teams of hospital-based health professionals with specialized training were organized for the purpose of treating patients with nutritional problems, particularly PCM. Chapter 2 extensively discusses the multidisciplinary approach to nutrition support.

HOW MALNUTRITION DEVELOPS: THE METABOLIC ONSET

To understand the development of malnutrition in the hospitalized patient, the reader must understand the metabolic response to starvation and stress (Table 1–3). Endocrine status and metabolism interact to determine the onset and extent of malnutrition.

During starvation, in the absense of exogenous glucose, glucagon is stimulated. Glucagon is the hormone of nutritional mobilization that promotes utilization of energy reserves. There is little stored carbohydrate. The 80 kcal available from blood glucose and the 250 to 300 kcal stored as glycogen are utilized within a 12-hour fasting period (Fig. 1–1).[11] The body's other potential source of glucose is protein. Glucagon stimulates gluconeogenesis from amino acids. Gluconeogenesis ensures glucose for obligatory users: the brain, blood cells, and renal medulla. The rest of the body adapts to use of free fatty acids (from adipose stores) and ketones (the byproducts of fat metabolism) for energy. The nonobese person has approximately 135,000 kcal stored as dispensable triglycerides in adipose tissue.

Although body proteins potentially constitute a fairly large energy source, their conservation is crucial to host survival. Little, if any, "storage protein" exists. Therefore, use of body proteins as fuel results in deterioration of body functions. Thus, in prolonged starvation, metabolic adaptations occur with the net result that the body progressively uses more free fatty acids, ketones, and keto-acids and less glucose. Consequently, body protein mass is preserved. By 30 days of total starvation, free fatty acids and ketones are the major fuel utilized by the brain and body.[12]

Stress due to trauma, sepsis, or infectious disease increases the catabolism of glycogen and protein. Gluconeogenesis is maintained despite elevated insulin levels and high plasma glucose concentrations. This enables the stressed individual to meet requirements for obligatory glucose users and to supply increased energy for repair of wounded tissues. Proteolysis occurs with a redistribution of body protein from the muscle, gut, and skin to meet amino acid requirements for synthesis of viscera and plasma proteins crucial for recovery (Fig. 1–2). Impaired ketone body adaptation is observed since insulin reduces

TABLE 1–3. METABOLIC RESPONSE TO STRESS

Hormonal Change	Physiologic Impact	Effect on Tissue Substrate	Net Result
↑ Glucocorticoids ↑ Catecholamines	↑ Glycogenolysis	↑ Glucose for energy	Hyperglycemia with insulin resistance
↑ Glucagon	↑ Lipolysis	↑ Free fatty acids and ketones for energy	Marked wasting body protein mass
	↑ Proteolysis	↑ Gluconeogenesis and synthesis of acute phase proteins	
↑ Insulin	↑ Glucose utilization	↑ Glucose and amino acids needed for energy	No ketoadaptation
	↓ Fat mobilization	↓ Use FFA and ketones as source energy	
↑ Glucocorticoids ↑ Catecholamines	↑ Glycogenolysis	↑ Glucose (but rate of utilization greater than production)	Hypoglycemia
↑ Glucagon	↑ Lipolysis ↑ Proteolysis	↑ FFA, ↑ Ketones	Moderate wasting body protein mass to preserve visceral protein status
↓ Insulin	↓ Glucose utilization ↓ Proteolysis ↑ Fat mobilization	↓ Glucose for obligatory users only ↑ Use FFA and ketones as energy source	Ketoadaptation

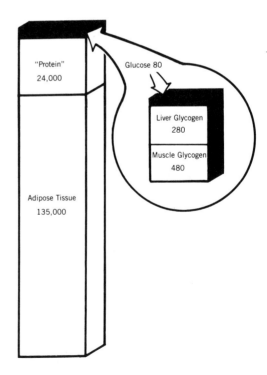

Figure 1–1. Energy reserves of 70-kg man, expressed in kilocalories. Note relatively small amount of available carbohydrate. Body protein, which can readily be converted to glucose, is not stored for any reason, since all proteins are functional. *(From Steffee WP: Malnutrition in hospitalized patients. JAMA 244(23):2631, 1980.)*

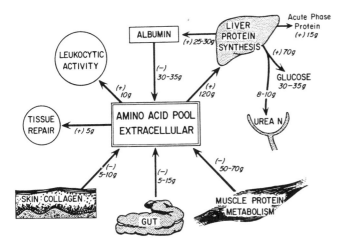

Figure 1–2. Alterations in protein metabolism with injury. Protein reserves from muscle, gut, and skin are released to support biosynthesis in areas more critical for recovery. Provision of exogenous protein and energy will fortify amino acid pools and support this metabolic response. *(From Benotti P, Blackburn GL: Protein and calorie or macronutrient metabolic management of the critically ill patient. Critical Care Medicine 7(12):521, 1979.)*

lipolysis in adipose tissue. The constant need for glucose via gluconeogenesis and amino acids via proteolysis results in a rapid wasting of body protein during stress.

In summary, in the starved state, the breakdown of body protein is slow, spared by progressive fat oxidation to meet energy needs. Clinically, wasting of body fat and moderate lysis of skeletal protein allow preservation of visceral protein status. In severe stress, conversely, marked wasting of body protein mass occurs rapidly without ketone body adaptation. In Chapter 10 there is a more detailed discussion of the metabolic response to stress and starvation.

Many physiologic changes occur in PCM as a result of alterations in body composition and function. To reiterate, most energy derived from endogenous sources during starvation comes from proteolysis of skeletal muscle and lipolysis of body fat. Protein from all body organs, however, is mobilized and utilized as well. The loss of organ mass and protein has a major impact on organ function. Consider respiratory function in PCM. As intercostal and diaphragmatic muscles waste, progressive deterioration of respiratory effort and lessened ventilatory response to hypoxic stimuli result, explaining the frequency of pneumonia and bronchitis among malnourished patients.[13] Renal function deterio-

rates as well. Decreased urea concentration in the renal medulla induces loss of kidney concentrating ability. Diuresis occurs despite progressive dehydration.[14] The gastrointestinal tract wastes with loss of muscular function, resulting in decreased gastric mobility and early satiety. Atrophy of gut mucosa is well reported in patients undergoing protein malnutrition. Plicae circulares disappear and villi shorten, flatten, and fuse. The microvilli, where the final act of digestion and absorption occurs, disappear.[15] The circle is vicious. Malnutrition causes reduced digestive capacity, increased transit time, and malabsorption, which then compound to escalate malnutrition. The devastating clinical picture of liver dysfunction occurs as a late finding in PCM. Subclinical changes, however, include depletion of microsomal enzymes necessary to metabolize drugs and depressed protein synthesis.[16] Cardiac mass decreases as starvation progresses. Cardiac output drops since demands are less from a diminished body cell mass. Refeeding must be started cautiously and slowly. The increased basal metabolic rate associated with substrate administration often precipitates cardiac overload. Skeletal function is impaired by the muscle-wasting effects of malnutrition. Its critical importance for ambulation contributes to complications associated with prolonged bedrest and consequently slows rehabilitation.

THE TOOLS USED TO DETECT MALNUTRITION

The identification of an obviously starving patient requires no special investigation other than a careful history and physical examination. Since the effects of severe malnutrition may be life threatening or irreversible, however, detection of early malnutrition is critical. This early identification enables orchestration of nutrition support in an effective, preventive, and economic fashion.

The nutrition assessment is a tool to measure nutrition status as reflected by changes in body composition and function. Figure 1–3 summarizes the nutrition assessment techniques to be discussed and the body component each measures. This section presents the nutrition assessment tools routinely used to diagnose malnutrition and highlights their strengths and weaknesses.

Weight for height is the most commonly used tool to assess nutrition status. Individuals with body weight less than 80 percent ideal often present with PCM, particularly if the weight loss occurred rapidly. Weight for height, however, has limited validity as an assessment tool, particularly in edematous states.

Anthropometry is a science which describes body composition through measurements of its external morphology (Fig. 1–3). Measurement of triceps skinfold (TSF) gives an indirect estimate of subcutaneous fat stores. The TSF refers to a double fold of skin and the fat between it on the posterior aspect of the nondominant arm midway between the acromial process of the scapula and the olecranon process of the ulna. The triceps area is universally accessible in men and women and refractory to edema.

During stress and starvation, skeletal muscle protein reserves are mobilized to meet the demands for synthesis of acute phase and secretory proteins, leading to a progressive depletion of this compartment. Arm muscle circumference (AMC) and creatinine–height index (CHI) assess skeletal muscle mass. AMC is mathematically derived using measurements of midupper arm circumference (MAC) and TSF. CHI requires 24-hour consecutive urine collections to measure creatinine excretion. Creatinine is a secretory protein excreted from muscle at a constant rate in proportion to the amount of lean body mass of a given individual. Obviously, creatinine excretion would be lower than standard in a protein-depleted patient. It is important to note that inaccuracy of the consecutive urine collections, the presence of renal disease, and ascites invalidate CHI as an accurate indicator of lean body mass.

Lack of valid statistical standards of comparison limit the interpretation of anthropometric findings. The usefulness of the Jelliffe standards for the U.S. population is questionable since measurements were derived from different nationality groups by various investigators at different times.[18] Gray and Gray[19] found the commonly used

Figure 1–3. Body composition can be simply estimated by anthropometrics or secretory protein levels. *(From Bistrian, B.R: Nutritional assessment and therapy of protein–calorie malnutrition in the hospital. JADA 71:394, 1977.)*

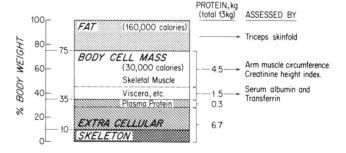

Jelliffe anthropometric standards varied dramatically from U.S. population averages reported in the Health and Nutrition Examination Study (HANES)[21] and the U.S. Ten-State Survey.[20] The authors suggest interpretation of anthropometric data for the U.S. population in percentiles derived from the U.S. Ten-State Survey. The HANES[21] 71–74 survey provided good standards of comparison for both ethnic and elderly populations. The reader may refer to Chapter 6 for further discussion about the use and interpretation of anthropometric findings.

The ability to synthesize secretory proteins, serum albumin, and transferrin, is used to assess functional capacity of the visceral compartment. Mitchell and Lipschitz[22] found serum albumin the best predictor of malnutrition in both young and old healthy subjects. Albumin below 4 g/dl was unusual.[22] Conversely, depressed hepatic protein synthesis with albumin production only 50 percent normal is well recognized during protein deprivation. Seltzer and associates[23] revealed a fourfold increase in complications and a sixfold increase in mortality in patients with serum albumin concentrations below 2.5 g/dl. Unfortunately, serum albumin lacks specificity in that hepatic disease or nephrosis often reduces levels in normally nourished patients. Courtrey et al.[24] found serum albumin tends to overdiagnose malnutrition in hospitalized patients. The routine postural changes from upright to recumbent positions during hospitalization resulted in a rapid decline in serum albumin levels.[24] To further confuse matters, dehydration, clinically common upon admission, abnormally elevates albumin levels. Clearly, albumin is not reliable as a sole determinant of visceral protein status.

For cost and time efficiency, transferrin is often extrapolated mathematically from total iron-binding capacity (TIBC), that is, transferrin (mg/dl) = (TIBC × 0.8) − 43. Mitchell and Lipschitz[22] ascertained TIBC was a good indicator of malnutrition in males of all ages. In contrast, in females, iron stores rather than nutrition status exerted a major

influence on the measurement. In addition to invalidity in iron deficiency, elevated values occur in pregnancy, hypoxia, and chronic blood loss. Decreased values occur in chronic infection, pernicious anemia, liver damage, iron overload and protein-losing enteropathies as well as PCM.[25] Transferrin is a more sensitive indicator of PCM than serum albumin. Its shorter half-life of 8 to 10.5 days compared to 20 days for albumin allows better detection of changing nutrition status since transferrin levels are restored with refeeding.[26]

The relationship between nutrition status and immune function has long been the subject of interest and controversy. Cannon et al.[27] reported depression of visceral protein status causes a decrease in antibody production and opsin formation. This leads to the theoretical assumption that malnutrition decreases immunocompetence. In support of this theory, Rhoads and Alexander[28] correlated an increased number of infectious complications in protein-depleted patients as compared to those with normal protein levels.

How can immunodeficiency be ascertained? Immune function and response may be detected by delayed hypersensitivity (DH) skin test response. Delayed hypersensitivity simply measures reactivity to intradermal injections of common recall antigens.

Many investigators have demonstrated that anergy, the lack of response to skin testing, predicts poor outcome following operation or injury. Meakins et al.[29] reported a 36 percent mortality and a 52 percent infectious complication rate in anergic patients. Reactive patients experienced only a 4 percent mortality and 10 percent infectious complication rate. Upon reassessment, anergic patients whose skin tests failed to improve suffered a mortality of 74 percent. In contrast, those patients who maintained a normal skin test response demonstrated only a 2 percent mortality rate.[29] Meakins' data failed to establish nutrition status as a determinant factor influencing immune function; 84 percent of anergic patients converted to reactivity by surgical intervention and less than 20 percent converted secondary to nutrition support and immunostimulants.[30]

Blackburn et al.[31] hypothesize that nutrition status is a predominant factor associated with immune function; 229 patients studied serially received aggressive nutrition support. Seventy-eight percent of initially anergic patients regained immunocompetence after 2 to 3 weeks of intensive nutrition support. Those who responded to nutrition support exhibited lower mortality than those who failed to respond. The authors noted only a prospective randomized study could demonstrate a causative relationship between improved nutrition status, skin test responsiveness, and improved prognosis. Such prospective randomized studies would need to compare the immune function status of anergic patients after intensive nutrition support with that of anergic patients provided only conventional nutritional management. Clearly, the ethical justification of such a controlled study is questionable.

Difficulties in the interpretation of skin test responsiveness as a measure of nutrition status in the hospitalized patient stems from the potential for other factors such as advancing age,[32] malignant disease,[33] drugs, sepsis, and trauma to influence reactivity. Researchers note immune suppression, infection,[34] or zinc deficiency[35] may make DH an unreliable index of nutritional status.

An ideal assessment tool for detection of malnutrition would meet the following four criteria:

1. High sensitivity (low false-negatives)—consistently positive in patients with malnutrition
2. Nutrition sensitivity—showing normal values after nutritional repletion
3. High specificity (low false-positives)—consistently negative in patients without malnutrition
4. Nutrition specificity—unaffected by nonnutrition factors

No single assessment tool meets all of these criteria, therefore, clinicians need to in-terpret isolated indicators of malnutrition with great caution. To overcome the weaknesses of any single tool, nutrition assessment using all available parameters is widely practiced.

Recently, investigators have focused on the predictive power of nutrition assessments. The predictive value of any assessment tool is judged by the degree to which a high-risk or low-risk classification changes the likelihood of morbidity. The Prognostic Nutrition Index (PNI) is a correlation of several measurements (i.e., albumin, TSF, transferrin, and DH) used to quantitate operative complication risk (as a percentage) for an individual patient. Ongoing research at the University of Pennsylvania by Mullen and associates continues to provide strong evidence that PNI can identify patients at high risk for operative morbidity and mortality.[36,37] Use of PNI is controversial. Baker et al.[38] found no single assessment parameter separated patients at high risk from those at low risk of morbidity. They contend that combining objective measurements individually of low predictive power into a statistically derived index does not produce a predictive assessment technique to identify high-risk patients.

In summary, nutrition assessment based on all available parameters is our best means to diagnose malnutrition. Prediction of nutritionally-based morbidity and mortality in a clinically relevant manner, however, remains controversial.

THE DEFINITION OF MALNUTRITION

The nutrition assessment diagnoses the type and extent of malnutrition. Malnutrition is commonly described in three categories: marasmus, kwashiorkor, and marasmus-kwashiorkor mix (refer to Table 1–4 for a comparison of the three types of malnutrition).

Marasmus is characterized by depressed anthropometric measurements with preservation of visceral protein status and immu-

TABLE 1–4. CLASSIFICATION OF MALNUTRITION

Type of Malnutrition	Assessment Parameters		Onset	Nutritional Deficiency
	Depressed	*Preserved*		
Kwashkiorkor	Albumin Transferrin DH	Weight for height TSF AMC CHI	Acute, severe catabolism	Protein
Marasmus	Weight for height TSF AMC CHI	Albumin Transferrin DH	Chronic, moderate catabolism	Protein and calories
Marasmus–kwashkiorkor mix	Albumin Transferrin DH Weight for height TSF AMC CHI	None	Acute, severe catabolism superimposed on chronic, moderate catabolism	Protein and calories

nocompetence. An intake of inadequate protein and kilocalories, often in association with chronic illness, results in this gradual wasting of skeletal muscle and subcutaneous fat.

In kwashiorkor, anthropometric measurements are preserved with depression of visceral proteins and decline in immunologic competence. The onset of kwashiorkor is rapid in the well-nourished individual who suffers acute, severe catabolic stress coupled with substandard nutrient intake. This state is often observed during the course of severe illness when low protein, hypocaloric diets are provided to patients.

Marasmus-kwashiorkor mix presents with depressed anthropometric measurements, depressed visceral protein status, and rapid impairment of cellular immunity. A typical patient is one who has mobilized fat and skeletal muscle while sparing protein for a considerable time. Inevitably, either the reserves are exhausted or additional catabolic stress occurs. A consequent rapid decline in visceral protein synthesis ensues. Clinically, poor immunologic competence, edema, and vital organ dysfunction necessitate immediate, vigorous nutrition support. The classifi-

cation of malnutrition is discussed in further detail in Chapter 8.

MODES OF NUTRITION SUPPORT

With the assessment techniques and information now available, hospital malnutrition or risk for malnutrition can be identified and prevented. Nutrition support is indicated for those patients who cannot eat, should not eat, will not eat, or cannot eat enough.

There are two forms of nutrition support: enteral and parenteral. Enteral therapy is always the preferred route for those patients who have a functional gastrointestinal tract. This route makes use of the patient's own digestive and absorptive capacity, thereby increasing efficiency of nutrient utilization. Access to the enteral route may be gained via a nasogastric tube, a nasoduodenal tube, a feeding gastrostomy, or jejunostomy. Parenteral therapy via a peripheral or central vein is indicated for the patient whose alimentary tract is dysfunctional secondary to gastrointestinal disease, injury or surgery. Parts 4 and 5 discuss in depth both the indications and implementation of the various modes of nutrition support.

THE EFFECTIVENESS OF NUTRITION SUPPORT

As clinicians, we believe in the effectiveness of nutrition support. A review of the existing literature, however, does not prove it unequivocally beneficial in most disease entities. Unfortunately, most research is largely uncontrolled and mainly testimonial in nature. To prove the effectiveness of nutrition support, a well-devised study will demonstrate that nutritional intervention improves the outcome of illness above and beyond the restoration of nutrition status, in a controlled manner. What are the clinical criteria that concretely quantify the improved outcome of an illness? Reduced morbidity and mortality, decreased complications, and shortened length of hospital stay are such criteria. In view of escalating medical care costs, hospital budgetary restraints, federal spending cutbacks, and the implementation of prospective reimbursement, justification of the expenditures for nutrition support services is inevitable. Limited economic resources necessitate the need to quantify the benefits of nutrition support.

In only a few disease states have randomized, controlled studies been conducted which document nutrition support as having dramatically altered the course of illness. These include acute renal failure and pediatric respiratory distress syndrome. Improved survival and decreased complications from acute renal failure were demonstrated with the use of nutrition support by Abel et al.[39] A population of 53 adult patients was adequately randomized for age, renal diagnosis, and renal dysfunction. Twenty-one of 28 patients who received renal failure fluid containing essential L-amino acids and hypertonic glucose recovered from their renal failure while only 11 of 25 given glucose alone recovered. Abel et al. observed that glucose combined with essential amino acids seemed to alleviate some early causes of death, that is, from electrolyte imbalances. With the shortening of the time span of renal failure, reversal of azotemia, and its atten-

dant catabolic state (as observed in the experimental group), the later complications of sepsis, central nervous impairment, hemorrhage, and congestive heart failure might be precluded. Indeed, complications during the period of acute renal failure were handled significantly better by the group that received renal failure fluid than by Abel's control group.

Gunn and associates[40] studied 40 premature infants in whom respiratory distress prevented oral feedings. Two groups of infants were formed that included infants of comparable age, birth weight, gestational age, and severity of respiratory distress syndrome. Both groups contained equal numbers of infants with weights of less than 1500 g. The experimental group received total nutrition needs via peripheral vein. The control group received 10 percent glucose and electrolytes until oral feedings could be established. For the majority of infants over 1500 g, the period for either regimen was too short to affect mortality. In the group of infants under 1500 g, however, a long period of time was necessary before complete oral nutrition was possible. For infants weighing less than 1500 g, the survival rate of 71 percent (5/7) for the alimented group compared favorably with the 37 percent (3/8) survival rate for the glucose group. A controlled study with larger numbers is needed to corroborate Gunn's results. Based on the findings reported, however, ethical justification will be a deterrent to confirmatory studies.

When certain illnesses have historically high mortality rates, case studies demonstrating improved quality and quantity of life related to the use of nutrition support convince us of its effectiveness. History, then, serves as the control group. Illnesses with historically high mortality rates include short bowel syndrome, intractable diarrhea in infancy, and gastrointestinal fistulas.

Broviac and Scribner[41] studied six patients with various degrees of massive small bowel resection whom we would have expected to develop incapacitating malnutrition. All benefited enormously from parenteral nutrition

(PN) as an adjunct to oral intake. Similarly, MacFayden[42] followed 40 patients with short bowel syndrome during a 3-month treatment regime that combined PN and oral nutrition support. Ninety percent of the patients maintained their nutrition status with oral diet alone. Only 10 percent required prolonged home PN. Obviously, nutrition support improved quality of life by enabling patients to go home and resume individual lifestyles.

There are no randomized, controlled studies to prove the effectiveness of nutrition support in intractable diarrhea in infancy. However, Hyman et al.[43] and Keating and Ternberg[44] reported two studies in which 100 percent of infants survived this illness with a known 40 percent mortality rate.[45]

In the past, the treatment of gastrointestinal fistulas has been associated with a 40 to 60 percent morbidity and mortality rate.[46] With bowel rest and conventional intravenous therapy, a typical patient became severely catabolic, septic, often with renal failure inducing severe morbidity or even fatal consequences. MacFayden et al.[47] evaluated the combined benefits of PN and complete bowel rest in 62 patients who had 78 gastrointestinal fistulas. Spontaneous fistula closure was documented in 70.5 percent of all patients. The mortality was only 6.67 percent in the total study group. Dietal[48] also reported a low 9.3 percent mortality in a series of 100 patients receiving PN and bowel rest for the management of gastrointestinal fistulas. Importantly, the investigators documented that, compared with patients who received inadequate nutrition, the duration of hospitalization was only half as long for patients who received intensive nutrition support.[48]

Numerous uncontrolled, nonrandomized studies and testimonials demonstrate the beneficial impact of nutrition support on the outcome of disease and surgery. The following is a review of the more convincing studies. Based on admission nutrition assessment and PNI, Mullen et al.[49] identified a high-risk group of operative candidates. In this high-risk group, nutrition support produced a 2.5-fold reduction in postoperative complications, a 6-fold reduction in major sepsis, and a 5-fold reduction in mortality.[49] Copeland and associates[50] reported the effect of PN as an adjunct to radiation therapy in cancer patients. Nutrition support allowed 95 percent of the poor-risk, nutritionally depleted patients to complete radiation therapy without complaints of anorexia, nausea, or vomiting; 54 percent of the patients responded with a greater than 50 percent reduction in tumor size. Remarkably, reduction in tumor size was positively correlated with improved indices of nutrition status.[50]

The salubrious effects of nutrition support reported in uncontrolled studies raises the question of whether controlled prospective studies could be ethically justified. In essence, in the absence of definitive trials, acceptance and practice of nutrition support in many illnesses and in the perioperative period remain open to critical evaluation.

REFERENCES

1. Rhoads JE, Alexander CE: Nutritional problems of surgical patients. Ann NY Acad Sci 63:268, 1955
2. Butterworth CE: The skeleton in the hospital closet. Nutr Today March/April:8, 1974
3. Bistrian BR, Blackburn GL, Hallowell E, Heddle R: Protein status of general surgical patients. JAMA 230(6):858, 1974
4. Bistrian BR, Blackburn GL, Vitale J, et al.: Prevalence of malnutrition in general medical patients. JAMA 235(15):1567, 1976
5. Mullen JL, Gertner MH, Buzby GP, et al.: Implications of malnutrition in the surgical patient. Arch Surg 114:121, 1979
6. Weisner RL, Hunker EM, Krumdieck CL, Butterworth CE: Hospital malnutrition: A prospective evaluation of general medical patients during the course of hospitalization. Am J Clin Nutr 32:418, 1979
7. Willard MD, Gilsdorf RB, Price RA: Protein–calorie malnutrition in a community hospital. JAMA 243(17):1720, 1980
8. Brenia R, Ratcliff S, Barbour GL, Krummer M: Malnutrition in the hospitalized geriatric patient. J Am Geriatrics Soc 30(7):432, 1982

9. Newmark SR, Sublett D, Blake J, Geller R: Nutritional assessment in a rehabilitation unit. Arch Phys Med Rehabil 62:279, 1981

10. Tomaiolo PP, Kraus V: Nutritional status of hospitalized alcoholic patients. JPEN 4(1):1, 1980

11. Steffee WP: Malnutrition in hospitalized patients. JAMA 244(23):2630, 1980

12. Meguid MM, Collier MD, Howard LJ: Uncomplicated and stressed starvation. Surg Clin North Am 61:1529, 1981

13. Doekel RL, Zwillich CW, Scoggin CH: Clinical semistarvation: Depression of the hypoxic ventilatory response. N Engl J Med 295:358, 1976

14. Klahr S, Alleyne GAO: Effects of chronic protein–calorie malnutrition on the kidney. Kidney Int 3:129, 1973

15. Levine GM, Deren JJ, Steifer E: Role of oral intake in maintenance of gut mass and disaccharidase activity. Gastroenterology 67:975, 1974

16. Krishnaswamy K, Naidu AN: Microsomal enzymes in malnutrition as determined by plasma half-life of antipyrine. Br Med J 1:538, 1977

17. Grant JP: Current practices of nutritional assessment–functional assessment. In Levenson SM (ed): Nutritional Assessment: Present Status, Future Directions and Prospects. Columbus, Ohio: Ross Laboratories, 1981, pp 137–141

18. Jelliffe D: The Assessment of the Nutritional Status of the Community. World Health Organization Monograph No. 53, Geneva, 1966

19. Gray GE, Gray LK: Validity of anthropometric norms used in assessment of hospitalized patients. JPEN 3(5):366, 1979

20. Ten-State Nutrition Survey. DHEW pub. no. (HSM) 72–8130 through 72–8134. U.S. Department of Health, Education and Welfare, Health Services and Mental Health Administration Centers for Disease Control, Vol I–V 1968–70

21. Abraham S: Preliminary findings of the first health and nutrition examination survey. United States. 1971–74: Anthropometrics and clinical findings. DHEW pub. no. (HRA) 75–1229, 1975

22. Mitchell C, Lipschitz DA: The effect of age and sex on the routinely used measurements to assess the nutritional status of hospitalized patients. Am J Clin Nutr 36:340, 1982

23. Seltzer MH, Cooper DN, Inger P: Instant nutritional assessment. JPEN 3:157, 1979

24. Courtrey M, Greene H, Folk C, et al.: Rapidly declining serum albumin values in newly hospitalized patients: Prevalence, severity and contributing factors. JPEN 6(2):143, 1982

25. Grant A: Nutritional Assessment Guidelines, 2nd ed. Berkeley, Calif.: Cutter Laboratories, 1979, p 37

26. Bistrian BR: Cellular immunity in semistarved states in hospitalized adults. Am J Clin Nutr 28:1148, 1975

27. Cannon PR, Wissler RW, Woolride RL: Relationship of protein deficiency to surgical infections. Ann Surg 120:514, 1944

28. Rhoads FE, Alexander CE: Nutritional problems of surgical patients. Ann NY Acad Sci 63:268, 1955

29. Meakins JL, Dietsch JB, Bubenick O: Delayed hypersensitivity. Indicator of acquired failure of host defenses in sepsis and trauma. Ann Surg 186:241, 1977

30. Meakins JL, Christou NV, Shizgal HM: Therapeutic approaches to anergy in surgical populations. Ann Surg 190:286, 1979

31. Blackburn GL, Bistrian BR, Harvey K: Indices of PCM as predictors of survival. In Levenson SM (ed): Nutritional Assessment: Present Status, Future Directions and Prospects. Columbus, Ohio: Ross Laboratories. 1981, pp 131–137

32. Johnson WC, Ulrich F, Mequid MM: The role of delayed hypersensitivity in predicting postoperative morbidity and mortality. Am J Surg 137:536, 1979

33. Ohnuma T, Holland JF: Nutritional consequences of cancer, chemotherapy, and immunotherapy. Cancer Res 37:2395, 1977

34. Nimberg F, Manniel JA: Correlation between energy and circulating immune suppressive factor following major surgical trauma. Ann Surg 190:297, 1979

35. Golden MHN, Harland PSEG, Golden BE, Jackson AA: Zinc and immunocompetence in protein–energy malnutrition. Lancet 1:1226, 1978

36. Mullen JL, Buzby GP, Matthews DC, et al.: Reduction of operative morbidity and mortality by combined preoperative and postoperative nutritional support. Ann Surg 192(5):604, 1980

37. Smale BF, Mullen JL, Buzby GP, Rosato EF: The efficacy of nutritional assessment and support in cancer surgery. Cancer 47:2375, 1981

38. Baker JP, Detsky AS, Whitwell J, et al.: A comparison of the predictive value of nutri-

tional assessment techniques. Hum Nutr: Clin Nutr 36C:233, 1982

39. Abel RM, Beck CH Jr, Abbott WM, et al.: Improved survival from acute renal failure following treatment with intravenous essential L -amino acids and glucose. N Engl J Med 288:695, 1973

40. Gunn T, Reaman G, Outerbridge EW, Colle E: Peripheral total parenteral nutrition for premature infants with respiratory distress syndrome: A controlled study. J Pediatr 92:608, 1978

41. Broviac JW, Scribner BH: Prolonged parenteral nutrition in the home. Surg Gynecol Obstet 139:24, 1974

42. MacFayden BV Jr: The management of intestinal fistulas. In Miller TA, Dudrick SJ (eds): The Management of Difficult Surgical Problems. Austin, Texas: University of Texas Press, 1981, pp 216–224

43. Hyman CJ, Reiter J, Rodman J, Drash AL: Parenteral and oral alimentation in the treatment of the nonspecific protracted diarrheal syndrome of infancy. J Pediatr 78:17, 1981

44. Keating JP, Ternberg JL: Amino acid hypertonic glucose treatment for intractable diarrhea in infants. Am J Dis Child 122:226, 1971

45. Avery GB, Villavicencio O, Lilly JR, Randolph JG: Intractable diarrhea in early infancy. Pediatrics 41:712, 1968

46. Edmunds LH, Williams GM, Welch CE: External fistulas arising from the gastrointestinal tract. Ann Surg 152:445, 1960

47. MacFayden BV Jr, Dudrick SJ, Ruburg RC: Management of gastrointestinal fistulas with parenteral hyperalimentation. Surgery 74:100, 1973

48. Dietal M: Nutritional management of external small bowel fistulas. Can J Surg 19:505, 1976

49. Mullen JL, Buzby GP, Matthews DC, et al.: Reduction of operative morbidity and mortality by combined preoperative and postoperative nutritional support. Ann Surg 192(5):604, 1980.

50. Copeland EM, Souchon EA, MacFayden BV Jr, et al.: Intravenous hyperalimentation as an adjunct to radiation therapy. Cancer 39:607, 1977

2. Introduction to the Multidisciplinary Approach to Nutrition Support

Emma Cataldi-Betcher
Eva Shronts

HISTORIC BACKGROUND ON THE NUTRITION SUPPORT TEAM

The advent of total parenteral nutrition (TPN) in the mid-1960s, as a means of nutritionally supporting patients in whom the gastrointestinal (GI) tract was not usable, ushered in a new era of medical practice.[1] Almost simultaneously with the advent of this new therapeutic modality came the realization that just as the benefits of the therapy could be life saving to the critically ill patient, the potential complications could be fatal. There were several causes of TPN-associated complications. First and foremost, the primary provider of medical care, the physician, has historically received little or no nutrition education in medical schools. Second, the appropriate compounding of safe and sterile TPN solutions necessitated the acquisition of new skills by the pharmacist, including a knowledge of incompatibilities. Third, the most easily identified major TPN-associated complication was sepsis, secondary to prolonged intravenous cannulation. Inadequate site preparation and contamina-tion at the time of line insertion or inadequate follow-up site care were to blame. Physicians and nurses shared the responsibility for the high incidence of catheter-related sepsis.[2] Therefore, logic dictated that a collaborative effort between the physician, pharmacist, and nurse was needed for the safe and efficacious use of TPN. As the approach to TPN became more organized and sophisticated, the skills of a dietitian were needed to evaluate pretherapy nutrition history and to facilitate patient transition from TPN to oral or enteral therapy. Thus the first nutrition support "teams" were organized. They were organized because of the recognition that the complexities of this new therapy require a multidisciplinary approach in order to be carried out safely and effectively.

THE NUTRITION SUPPORT SERVICE

Prevalence in U.S. Hospitals

According to a recently published Nutrition Support Team Directory,[3] 46 of the 50 states report having nutrition support teams. According to this survey, the heaviest concentration of teams is found in Pennsylvania (45), California (40), Illinois (39), Ohio (35), and New York (33). There are a total of approximately 600 teams throughout the United States, constituting approximately 8.6 percent of all hospitals. These numbers are quite impressive, especially in view of the fact that the first organized teams were not formed until the early 1970s.

Rationale for Nutrition Support Services (NSS)

The prevalence of malnutrition in hospitalized patients has been well documented in the past.[4-6] Malnutrition has been associated with increased morbidity and mortality.[7-8] Therefore, it would seem prudent that within the realm of good medical practice, we would seek to provide high quality nutrition support, prevent and correct malnutrition where identified, prevent and reduce morbidity in an effort to reduce hospital stays, and lower mortality rates.

The provision of high-quality nutrition support requires a multidisciplinary team approach. To justify the need for a "team," it is necessary to demonstrate its cost effectiveness. Only by documenting a reduction in morbidity and mortality directly attributable to the "team" intervention in malnutrition or inappropriate use of TPN can we expect support from hospital administrations in these times of prospective reimbursement characterized by intense pressure for cost containment. In recent years several articles have been published describing this process.

A 2-year prospective study was conducted by Nehme in 1980 comparing two groups of patients receiving TPN therapy.[9] The "team" patients were managed by the nutrition support team and the "nonteam" patients were managed by their individual physicians. The complication rates of both groups were compared. The "nonteam" group had a much higher incidence of mechanical, septic, and metabolic complications.

Rombeau et al. noted results similar to Nehme's.[10] A retrospective study was conducted on a group of patients that received TPN. The group was divided into three categories: patients who received TPN prior to the formation of the team (pre-NSS), during the transition period in which the team was being formed (trans-NSS), and following the formation of the team (post-NSS). The results indicated that increased involvement of the nutrition support team in patient management resulted in a decreased incidence of TPN-associated complications and improved documentation of the indications for TPN, nutritional requirements, and catheter care. Similar data were obtained by Ditmer-Schutz and Egging.[11] In addition, they were able to document improvement in nutrition status based on serum albumin and weight gain.

Friedman et al. were able to document substantial cost savings to their institution as a result of their "team" intervention.[12] The accomplishments directly attributable to the "team" were more appropriate utilization of TPN, decreased patient days on TPN, decreased number of bottles of TPN solution given to each patient, and decreased amounts of TPN solutions wasted.

Further documentation of the benefits of a "team" is provided by Seltzer et al.[13] A savings in cost to their institution was documented as a result of education provided to the physicians and health team members, development of standardized protocols for the use of nutrition support and team management of patients.

The above data leave little doubt that a multidisciplinary team approach is indicated for optimal nutrition support. The cost effectiveness of a "team" in terms of reduced TPN-associated morbidity and mortality and cost savings as a result of standardized protocols and decreased solution wastage are readily apparent. At this point, however, we are still lacking good documentation regarding the effects of improved nutrition status on clinical outcome.

Administrative/Organizational Alternatives

The overall objectives of a particular institution will determine the administrative/organizational structure of a particular nutrition support service. Most medical institutions are dedicated to three principal activities: patient care, education, and research. The priority assigned to each of these issues is determined by many factors. Institutions vary in size, they may be for-profit or nonprofit, public or private, university affiliated or not, and provide differing levels of care (i.e., primary, secondary, tertiary). All of these factors will influence how a nutrition support service will fit in and what role it will play (Table 2–1). In general, four basic types of administrative/organizational structures may be identified (Table 2–2).[2,13–17] For any given institution a particular type of nutrition support service will be appropriate. For example, a small primary care community hospital may require only an informal committee of interested health professionals who meet regularly to evaluate the appropriateness of the use of nutrition support relative to accepted standards of practice. In contrast, a large teaching institution may begin by forming a committee with representatives from interested departments and progress gradually to a formal nutrition support service as interest in and utilization of the service grow.

Functions and Responsibilities of Team Members—The Process of Team Decision Making

Team-work as defined by Webster[18] is: joint action by a group of people, in which each person subordinates his individual interest and opinions to the unity and efficiency of the group.

As the above definition implies, a successful "team" is dependent on cooperation among team members along with a mutual respect for each other's unique contribution to the team effort.

TABLE 2–1. AN EXAMPLE OF NUTRITION SUPPORT TEAM FUNCTIONS AND ACTIVITIES

A. Inpatient Consultation
   Nutritional and metabolic assessment and management of patients requiring enteral or parenteral nutrition
   Elective
   Daily monitoring; daily team rounds

B. Home Nutrition Support Program
   Patient education and training for home parenteral and enteral nutrition
   Discharge planning
   Nutrition Support Service Clinic

C. Education Program
   Clinical rotations for surgery residents, pharmacy students, and dietary interns
   Lectures to medical, nursing, dietary, and pharmacy staffs
   Development and maintenance of educational materials for health professional use
   Development and maintenance of educational materials for patient use

D. Quality Assurance
   Development of hospital guidelines, policies and procedures, standing orders, and monitoring forms for the management of parenteral and enteral nutrition

E. Research
   Development and evaluation of new products for nutrition and metabolic support
   Development and evaluation of parameters for the assessment of metabolic and nutrition status
   Provide access to patients for interested biomedical professionals in the institution community

F. Visitation Program
   Inhouse program for the education of interested health professionals, which includes clinical experience in the diagnosis and management of nutrition and metabolic disease, instruction in establishing a Nutrition Support Service, and written educational materials

TABLE 2–2. ADMINISTATIVE/ORGANIZATIONAL ALTERNATIVES FOR A NUTRITION SUPPORT SERVICE

Type I *Metabolic/Nutrition Support Committee*	Type II *Metabolic/Nutrition Support Team (Informal)*	Type III *Metabolic/Nutrition Support Team (Formal)*	Type IV *Metabolic/Nutrition Support Service (NSS)*
Members are interested individuals or representatives of interested departments who volunteer their time on a part-time basis. Meet regularly to address nutrition support issues and develop policies and procedures. Do not function as a consult service.	Members are interested individuals or representatives of interested departments. Members are funded by parent departments to participate on the "team" on a part-time basis. Meet regularly for patient rounds. Develop policies and procedures. May develop and provide educational programs. Function as a consult service.	Members are individuals of differing disciplines indentified as permanent "team" members. Members are funded by parent departments to participate on the "team" on a full-time basis. Meet regularly for patient rounds. Develop policies and procedures. Develop and provide educational programs. May engage in research. Function as a consult service and/or may be responsible for all patients receiving nutrition support therapy (enteral/parenteral).	Members are individuals of differing disciplines identified as permanent full-time "team" members. The "team" is funded via a separate cost center, may be a subset of an existing department (i.e., pharmacy, surgery). Meet regularly for patient rounds. Develop policies and procedures. Develop and provide education programs. Actively participate in research. Function as a consult service and/or may be responsible for all patients receiving nutrition support therapy (enteral/parenteral).

In a nutrition support team, the physician, dietitian, pharmacist, nurse, and other health professionals contribute their unique abilities in the areas of patient care, education, quality assurance, and research.

The daily functions of a particular team and the responsibilities of the various team members vary from institution to institution. In general, however, certain standard activities are usually associated with each discipline represented on the team.

The Physician. The physician as the leader of the team is in charge of the overall ac-

tivities of the team. In some settings the physician may be involved in direct patient care by performing all invasive procedures (e.g., central line placement for TPN) and writing orders for nutrition support therapy. In other settings, the physician may only oversee the nutrition support provided and direct the team in the care of the patients requiring nutrition support. In addition, the physician acts as a resource to the team and other health team members on the effects of disease, surgical procedures, and medications on nutrition status. Finally, a critical part of the physicians's role is to represent the nutrition support team to the medical staff on a peer level (Table 2–3).[14–15,19–21]

The Dietitian. No nutrition support team is complete without the services of a competent clinical dietitian. The dietitian on the team is the principal resource on nutrition assessment tools, techniques, and data interpretation. In addition, the dietitian designs and implements specialized enteral nutrition regimens and transitional feedings from parenteral to enteral nutrition therapy. In many settings, the dietitian may also participate in

TABLE 2–3. AN EXAMPLE OF THE PHYSICIAN'S ROLE ON A NUTRITION SUPPORT TEAM

To provide the theoretical, practical, and medical insight within which the service functions

To act as a resource for the medical staff in the care of patients receiving nutrition support

To assess the impact of disease, pathology, and medical condition on the need for, route of, and formulation of appropriate nutrition support

To help prevent complications; to provide care and insight into the management of complications

To make team rounds on all patients and be available on a 24-hour basis

To assist in protocol and guideline development and implementation

To evaluate appropriateness of therapy in its indications and applications

To assist in patient education, training, and communication

To promote an atmosphere of care, cooperation, and interaction

To act as liaison between the service, hospital staff, and administration

To promote, establish, and maintain active research in clinical nutrition

To organize and participate in education programs for students, residents, and medical and hospital pharmacy, nursing and dietetic staffs

To establish, promote, and participate in a program of community, local, and national education

To promote an atmosphere of professional growth for the service members

designing and implementing parenteral nutrition regimens. A wise dietitian, however, will always collaborate with a knowledgeable pharmacist to determine unique compounding considerations when working with parenteral nutrition. The dietitian is a resource on enteral nutrition delivery systems (feeding tubes, containers, and pumps) and educates patients and health team members on their use. Patient education especially as related to home enteral feedings is a major component of the dietitian's responsibility. Finally, the dietitian acts as a liaison between the staff clinical dietitians and the nutrition support team, facilitating communication on patient progress and transfer of nutrition therapy from the team to the staff dietitian (Table 2–4).[19,21–23]

The Nurse. A nurse well versed in the tools and techniques associated with administering nutrition support therapy is of inestimable value to a nutrition support team. In most settings the nurse's role will include assisting with central line placement, catheter site care, and administering skin test recall antigens. In addition, the nurse has a close relationship with the staff nurses and works with them to monitor the overall quality of nursing care provided to patients receiving parenteral or enteral nutrition and assists them in solving any problems relative to the technical functioning of the equipment. The nurse also participates in discharge planning of patients receiving nutrition support and assists in patient as well as health team education. Finally, the nurse utilizes her unique training in providing educational and emotional support to patients and their families prior to initiation of and during nutrition support therapy (Table 2–5).[15,19–21,24–25]

The Pharmacist. In some institutions, the Department of Pharmacy is the leader in nutrition support. Training programs in nutrition support are now available for pharmacists throughout the United States. The pharmacist's experience with drug delivery systems is easily adaptable to nutrition sup-

TABLE 2–4. AN EXAMPLE OF THE DIETITIAN'S ROLE ON A NUTRITION SUPPORT TEAM

I. Patient Care
 A. Inpatient
  Perform initial and follow-up nutrition assessments based on pertinent medical, laboratory, and patient interview data
  Plan, implement, and evaluate enteral and parenteral nutrition prescriptions specific to individual patient nutrition and metabolic requirements
  Participate in daily patient rounds and health care team rounds as appropriate. Provide input relevant to patient's nutrition support
  Maintain daily monitoring records of patient's nutritional intake and nutrition/metabolic status. Facilitate necessary changes in nutrition support therapy
  Provide continuity of care between Nutrition Support Service (NSS) and primary ward dietitian by continued communication regarding patient progress
  Provide psychological support for the patient (and family) prior to, throughout, and at the termination of nutrition support therapy
 B. Outpatient (NSS Clinic)
  Perform (initial and follow-up nutrition assessments based on pertinent medical, laboratory, and patient interview data
  Plan and implement nutrition support therapy or necessary changes in nutrition support therapy
  Contact HEN provider to communicate any changes in the medical/HEN supplies used for the patient
  Review the patient's medications for drug-nutrient interactions with recommendations for changes as indicated in conjunction with all NSS team members
  Schedule next clinic visit including laboratory data to be obtained at the next clinic visit in conjunction with all NSS team members
  Telephone contact as needed with the patient and/or local public health nurse to monitor the patient's progress on weeks the patient does not visit the NSS Clinic
II. Education
 A. Patient
  Educate patient (and family) regarding the rationale and various aspects (i.e., necessary equipment, type of formula) of nutrition support therapy
  Review, update, and develop appropriate educational material for inpatient and outpatient use
 B. Health Team (Physicans, Dietitians, Nurses, Pharmacists)
  Serve as a resource on nutrition support products, materials, and techniques especially as related to enteral nutrition
  Participate in workshops, inservices, and other educational programs to facilitate proper management of patients receiving nutrition support
  Review, update, and develop appropriate educational materials
  Provide education on nutrition support products, materials and techniques as well as the management of the diseases of nutrition and metabolism to surgery residents, pharmacy students, and dietetic interns rotating through the NSS
  Serve as a liaison between the NSS and Nutrition Department
  Participate in the orientation of new employees to the care of patients receiving nutrition support
 C. Other
  Participate in local, regional, and national programs on nutrition support
  Provide classes in the Dietetic Internship Program on Nutrition Support
  Provide classes on Enteral Nutrition in the Pharm.D. Residency Program and Undergraduate Pharmacy Program as requested
  Provide classes in the Undergraduate Nursing Program as requested
  Provide education to other health professionals through the NSS Visitation Program
III. Quality Assurance
  Participate in reviewing, updating and developing policies and procedures regarding enteral nutrition administration

TABLE 2–4. *(Continued)*

Develop guidelines for the initiation, advancement, discontinuation (transition feeding or diet), and monitoring of enteral nutrition therapy

Develop standardized methods (e.g., routine physician's order forms, monitoring flow sheets) to facilitate the proper use and management of enteral nutrition

Participate in Nutrition Department Formulary Committee as a standing committee member in evaluation of new enteral formulas

IV. Research

Participate in nutrition and metabolic research conducted by the NSS

Assist in data collection especially as related to nutrition status

Monitor patients participating in research projects and record data necessary for product evaluation

V. Home Enteral Nutrition (HEN) Program

Assess the patient's medical/nutritional problem as an indication for home enteral nutrition, considering alternative methods (e.g., oral or parenteral nutrition) of providing nutrition support

Assist in evaluating HEN candidates' ability to manage enteral nutrition administration in the home

Coordinate HEN Program as follows:

Assess patient's health benefits status to determine extent of coverage for HEN

Contact HEN provider chosen for the patient or other facility (e.g., nursing home, local hospital) to establish long-term availability of HEN supplies

Provide nursing staff and/or primary care dietitian with guidelines and teaching materials to be used in training patients and family members; assist in training nursing staff/primary care dietitian/patient as needed

Plan and implement appropriate feeding schedule for home, if needed

Assist in completing prescriptions, insurance forms, statement of medical necessity, etc., as needed

Develop and maintain written patient education materials to be used in conjunction with inhospital training

Assist in contacting Home Health Department to arrange for home nursing visitation, as needed

Arrange for patient follow-up in NSS Clinic to include frequency of clinic visits and laboratory evaluation

VI. Professional Activities

Maintain an up-to-date base of knowledge regarding nutrition support by reading appropriate professional journals, attending local, regional and national meetings or conferences

Prepare and submit materials for publication

Actively participate in professional organizations on the local, regional, and/or national level not only as related to Nutrition Support, but also as related to Nutrition/Dietetics in general

---

port delivery systems. Of particular value to the nutrition support team is the pharmacist's knowledge of parenteral solution incompatability, admixture of drugs, and aseptic solution preparation. In addition, the pharmacist is a resource on the tools and techniques associated with parenteral nutrition administration. The pharmacist can also be of value to the dietitian in several areas. As the enteral system is frequently utilized for drug administration, the pharmacist may assist in evaluating possible drug formula incompatibilities, drug dosage form altera-tions, and drug-induced feeding intolerance. Like the dietitian and nurse, the pharmacist is involved in discharge planning of patients receiving nutrition support and assists in the training of patients, families, and health team members (Table 2–6).[19–20,26–27]

Other Health Professionals. Other health professionals such as respiratory therapists, occupational therapists, physical therapists, and social workers play an important role in the nutrition support of patients. In many institutions one or more of these health pro-

TABLE 2–5. AN EXAMPLE OF THE NURSE'S ROLE ON A NUTRITION SUPPORT TEAM

A. Patient Care

Assist in initial patient assessment of patients receiving nutrition support; provide nursing input into multidisciplinary health care plan to meet total needs of patient

Provide psychological support for the patients (and their family) receiving nutrition support

Make patient rounds to evaluate the quality of patient care delivered and the level of technical expertise and theoretical knowledge of various nursing staffs

Consult with nursing management staff, medical staff, and members of hospital administration to implement changes to improve patient care

Promote continuity of care especially in planning posthospital nursing follow-up

Participate in Nutrition Support Team outpatient clinic to meet nursing needs of patients on home nutrition support

B. Patient Education

Incorporate patient education in plan of care

Interpret to patients, family, and staff the rationale of various aspects of nutrition support

Develop appropriate patient education tools

Review, revise, and develop teaching forms and records to be utilized by patients and nursing staff

Evaluate the primary nurse education of patient regarding home training for enteral and parenteral nutrition support assisting as indicated

Provide bedside patient education

C. Quality Assurance

Identify need for quality standards of nursing care and implement current standards in area of nutrition and metabolism

Identify need and assist in writing policies and procedures as related to nutrition and metabolism

Serve on appropriate task forces

D. Staff Education

Identify learning needs regarding nutrition support and provide appropriate learning experiences in formal and informal groups

Collaborate with head nurse, station instructor, and primary nurse in assessing and evaluating the patient's nursing needs; make recommendations for patient care and posthospital care as related to nutrition support

Participate in workshops and other appropriate staff programs

Participate in bedside staff education

Participate in unit care conferences as appropriate

Participate in orientation of new employees to the care of patients receiving nutrition support

Assist in developing of clinical expertise, technical competence, and assessment skills of staff nurses

Assist nursing staff in learning new procedures regarding nutrition and metabolism

E. Professional Growth

Maintain current knowledge of trends in nursing especially related to nutrition support

Attend appropriate conferences

F. Research

Assist in research projects related to patient care

Collect and record data and prepare materials for publication

Identify need for initiation and participation in nursing studies and research projects

Participate in the evaluation of nutrition support products

TABLE 2-6. AN EXAMPLE OF THE PHARMACIST'S ROLE ON A NUTRITION SUPPORT TEAM

A. Inpatient Service

Participation in daily patient rounds providing input on and maintaining monitoring records of patient's metabolic status

Formulation of parenteral nutrition regimen specific to individual patient requirements and considering cost of the solutions availble (e.g., compounded versus standard)

Liaison between NSS and the IV Admixture Area

Team resource on commercially available and investigational parenteral nutrition products including technical apparatus such as filters, infusion pumps

Education of patients about their parenteral nutrition therapy

Minimize waste of solutions by assisting in appropriate selection of TPN solutions and close monitoring of patients to minimize complications necessitating acute changes in TPN formulation

Monitoring patient's daily drug therapy for drug-nutrient interactions

B. Quality Assurance

Develop policies and procedures in collaboration with the IV supervisor for the proper compounding, labeling, and sterility testing of all parenteral nutrition products

Develop guidelines for the initiation, monitoring, and discontinuation of parenteral nutrition

Develop standardized methods, e.g., solution order forms, TPN monitoring flow sheet, to facilitate the proper use and management of parenteral nutrition

C. Education

Precept clinical rotations for Pharm.D., undergraduate, and graduate pharmacy students to provide them with experience in the management of diseases of nutrition and metabolism

Provide staff pharmacists with clinical experience in the management of diseases of nutrition and metabolism through participation in daily patient evaluation and monitoring

Provide lectures to the pharmacy staff, pharmacy students, and the hospital staff in general on the proper management of patients requiring parenteral nutrition

Provide education to surgery residents rotating through the Nutrition Support Service

Provide education to dietary interns rotating through the Nutrition Support Service

Provide education to other health professionals through the Nutrition Support Service's visitation program

D. Research

Conduct original research on the pharmaceutical aspects of parenteral nutrition, e.g., defining electrolyte compatability limits, evaluating drug-TPN solution compatability, defining stability of parenteral nutrition solutions

Participate in nutrition and metabolic research conducted by the NSS; assure that experimental products used in this research are appropriately handled and dispensed and that all records for the FDA, etc., are correctly maintained; monitor patients participating in this research and record data necessary for product evaluation

E. Home Parenteral Nutrition Program

Provide nursing staff with guidelines and teaching flow sheets to be used in training the patient in catheter care and solution administration

Obtain an IV infusion pump for patient to learn the use of in the hospital and have available for use at home

Assess patient's health benefits status to determine the extent of coverage for Home Parenteral Nutrition

Contact local hospital or private Home TPN service to establish long-term availability of TPN supplies and solutions

Complete prescriptions, insurance forms, statement of medical necessity, and other paper work necessary for discharge of patient on Home TPN

Evaluate patient's ability to compound TPN solutions at home. If the patient is a candidate, instruct patient in the proper aseptic technique and procedures for compounding Home TPN solutions. If patient is using premixed Home TPN solutions from a private Home TPN service, instruct patient in the proper aseptic technique and procedures for adding vitamins

Develop and maintain written patient education materials to be used in conjunction with inhospital training

Contact Home Health Department to arrange for home nursing visitation as needed

Arrange mechanism and schedule for following patient at home to include frequency of clinical visits and laboratory evaluation

Evaluate patients who return for clinic visits

fessionals may be incorporated into nutrition support teams as permanent full-time members.

ESTABLISHING A NUTRITION SUPPORT TEAM

Administrative Support

Today's health care administrators are faced with many critical challenges. Advances in health care technology have led to earlier diagnosis and treatment of disease and prolonging death; however, there remains a limited amount of financial resources available to support the system. The cost of health care and restrictive governmental regulations continue to escalate in direct proportion. The prospective reimbursement payment system for Medicare patients comes as a direct result of these escalating costs.

Since hospital administration is consistently being confronted with funding cutbacks, why would they then be interested in establishing a nutrition support team?[28]

An effective nutrition support team can assure quality nutrition care, which is an obligation of all hospitals and medical centers. As discussed earlier, complications of malnutrition can be prevented by adequate means of nutrition support, which can lead to reduced lengths of hospital stay.

To effectively gain administrative support, members of a potential nutrition support team must convince administration of the importance of specialized sophisticated nutritional care. One approach may be to document the current incidence of malnutrition within the medical center utilizing supportive literature describing the prevention of complications and deaths secondary to the appropriate use of nutrition support therapies.[14] Administration must be assured that the nutrition support team is dedicated to quality assurance such that it will continually strive to provide quality nutrition support at the least cost. The team may assume responsibility for the selection of nutrition products that are available for use in the hospital as a part of cost containment. This

may include developing an enteral product formulary and standardized parenteral solutions with guidelines for appropriate usage of these products.[29] A well-organized team may also qualify for research grants, which not only expands the team's clinical data base but will provide recognition to the hospital.

Physician Support

A dietitian's chief interest is the nutritional care of the patient. Among physicians, the patient's nutritional care is not always a high priority. It often becomes necessary for a dietitian to generate the interest of the medical staff in nutrition support. Several options are available to generate such an interest. A personal appointment can be made with the Chairman of the Department of Medicine or Surgery to discuss institutional needs. A committee can be formed with appropriate medical staff members to further discuss the issues. Information can be presented at medical grand rounds on nutrition assessment and specialized nutrition support solutions. It may be beneficial to approach the newest members of the medical and surgical staff as well as the residents. Frequently, this group of physicians is more acquainted with nutrition support, expresses an interest in new knowledge, and perhaps has more time to donate to committees.

In addition to lectures and inservices presented by the dietetic staff, arrangements can be made to invite medical experts to the institution to stimulate physician interest. Pharmaceutical companies maintain speaker's bureaus and can offer enlightening suggestions as well as financial support.

Patient Selection and Referral Systems

Total Care Versus Consult Service. The first variable to consider is which type of nutrition support team will best meet the needs of the institution. Do the resources and personnel to develop an informal team currently exist? Have provisions been allocated to establish a separate department or extension under a present department? Titles such as "TPN Committee," "Nutrition Support Service," and "Surgical Nutrition Team" may be insignificant if the members are devoted to patient care. Conceptually, health care professionals available for consultation, assessment, and/or implementation of nutrition support therapies are identified as a "team."

Team structure will vary with the type of care rendered (see section "Administrative/ Organizational Alternatives" and Table 2–2). One such concept is the total care team, usually existing as a separate department or under the department of medicine or surgery. This department's employees may include, but are not limited to, physicians, dietitians, nurses, pharmacists, secretary, physical therapist, social worker, and researcher. Guidelines, protocols, and quality of nutritional care are assured by such a team. Total specialized nutrition support and monitoring is provided by this department. Attending physicians would then refer their patients for nutritional management.

Another trend in nutritional care is the referral or consult service. Members may be employed under one department such as medicine, surgery, or pharmacy, or employed interdepartmentally. Specific job functions may vary (Tables 2–4 through 2–6). Similar to the total care team, guidelines, protocols, and quality assurance will be maintained, in addition to inhouse staff development. The primary differences are that attending physicians continue to care for their own patients but are able to consult with the nutrition support team for assistance.

Regardless of the team format, an experienced registered clinical dietitian is mandatory. Assessing past and present nutrition status, recognizing normal and abnormal nutrition requirements and knowledge of enteral nutrition cannot be accomplished without an experienced dietitian's input.

Protocol Development

Protocols are designed to deliver consistency in the manner of care. They can also be re-garded as a work model for patient care. Any nutrition support team will require protocols ranging from assessment procedures through monitoring results of therapy.[30] Protocols, or policies and procedures, must be specific and indicate a sequence for indentification, implementation, and follow-up processes.

Policies and procedures that govern your institution will set preliminary guidelines. Any protocol already in existence pertaining to nutrition support should be reviewed by the nutrition support team for acceptance or revisions. Any new or revised protocols must be submitted for review by the executive or medical staff, according to institutional policy. Newly developed forms that will be entered in the patient's medical record will also require prior approval before utilization. It is imperative to observe preexisting hospital policies, especially those related to chart entries.

Once protocols are established and approved by the medical staff and administration, they must be adhered to. Deviations from set procedures should be discouraged in an effort to maintain quality care. Methods to assure compliance of the new protocols must be developed by the nutrition support team.[30] Some examples of such methods are staff education, administrative support, and newsletter updates. Protocols should then be revised as trends change or as institutional situations warrant.

In the same manner as institutions and personnel vary, so will protocols and policies and procedures. It is suggested to contact area institutions with already existing policies and refer to those when establishing your own. Many references are also available.

Billing Mechanisms

Mechanisms for billing and generating income by nutrition support services are still in their infancy. There are not any set guidelines for reimbursement of hospital-based nutrition support teams. As with varying protocols, billing mechanisms also vary from team to team.

Fees for services rendered are a chargeable item by some teams. Once a cost center is established for the team, they may then charge a separate fee-for-services such as a nutritional assessment or consultation. Fees for products (i.e., solutions or equipment rental) can be inflated to help defray the costs of noncharged services provided by the team.[31,32] For example, the daily rental charge for a feeding pump can be inflated by a few dollars to help cover the cost of the more expensive enteral formulas.

Many nutrition support teams are faced with justifying their costs to hospital administrators. This is especially true now with the introduction of the Medicare Diagnosis Related Group (DRG) Payment System, introduced in 1984. Under this new prospective reimbursement system, both the nutrition support modalities and nutrition support teams have received much attention as to how these products and services are reimbursed under the DRG structure.

Many claim that costs of nutrition support have been calculated and therefore included in the averages which make up the DRG rates. Such people maintain that the average length of stay for a DRG assumes nutritional therapy has been provided. If this therapy were not provided, it is hypothesized that length of stay would increase due to patient complications that would arise secondary to inadequate nutrition status.[33] Others claim that there is no scientific evidence that nutrition support will decrease length of stay and therefore question the cost justification for the service.[33]

In a seminar in 1984, Hull contended that nutrition support is indeed cost effective in the DRG era.[34] He reported two main reasons for this cost effectiveness: (1) increased reimbursement from identification of patients with the diagnosis of malnutrition and (2) lower hospital costs due to the treatment of hospital malnutrition rather than allowing complications to ensue. Hull has demonstrated, as shown in Table 2–7, that in certain diagnoses malnutrition can be considered a "comorbidity or complicating condition," thereby resulting in increased revenue for the hospital.

Many centers have instituted an organized approach to the assessment and identification of malnutrition and have set up the necessary systems with their medical records departments to facilitate coding this information on to the physician's discharge summary for those DRGs for which a complicating condition is acceptable. This process requires establishment of objective criteria for the identification of malnutrition, in most cases acceptance of the criteria by the medical staff, implementation of a screening mechanism by the hospital clinical dietetics or nu-

TABLE 2–7. EFFECT OF COMORBIDITY OR COMPLICATION (CC) ON REIMBURSEMENT FOR MAJOR LARGE BOWEL SURGICAL PROCEDURE (AGE UNDER 70)

		Relative Weight		Standard Rate[a]		Reimbursement
DRG without CC	149	2.2154	×	$3021.35	=	$6693.50
DRG with CC	148	2.5493	×	$3021.35	=	$7702.33
		Incremental Reimbursement			=	$1008.83[b]

[a]Ohio urban hospital

[b]Not all CCs cause these dramatic incremental incomes. Most surgical procedures have a 10 to 25 percent associated increase, but most medical DRGs have a 5 to 9 percent increase and a lower relative weight.

Reprinted with permission from Hull, SF: Nutrition support is profitable and cost-effective in the DRG era. Columbus, Ohio: Ross Laboratories, 1984.[34]

trition support team staff, and coordination with the hospital's medical records department to consider and list malnutrition as one of the secondary diagnoses in the appropriate patient cases.

Much additional research needs to be done in this area to continue to document the effect of malnutrition on length of stay and morbidity as well as the overall cost effectiveness of the various modes of nutrition support in this new cost-conscious environment.

Job Descriptions of Members

See "Functions and Responsibilities of Team Members—The Process of Team Decision Making" section and also Tables 2–4 through 2–6.

Quality Assurance

Standards of performance are not unique to business and industry. Quality assurance programs and patient care audits measure accuracy levels and analyze job functions for evaluation. Health professionals began using managerial techniques in the 1960s. The 1970s brought further definition to these procedures. The American Dietetic Association (ADA) developed a "Professional Standards Review Procedure Manual"[35] and "Guidelines for Evaluating Dietetic Practice"[36] which clearly define Professional Standards Review Organization (PSRO) and the dietitian's role. The Joint Committee on the Accreditation of Hospital (JCAH)[37] 1980 edition of the Accreditation Manual contains a new standard on quality assurance for the entire hospital. Only dietetic departments are specified, however, not separate nutrition support services.

Active participation by nutrition support team members is necessary to improve patient care. To meet this objective, process criteria need to be identified. Process criteria refer to specific team members functions and actions that should be taken dependent on,

for example, nutrition support therapies and diagnosis. A quality assurance program for the entire nutrition support program, from cost analysis to tube feeding preparation, is beyond the scope of this text. Concentration will therefore be devoted to dietetic performance specific to specialized nutrition care.

Refer to your own institution's Quality Assurance Committee when defining criteria. Another ADA manual entitled "Patient Care Audit: A Quality Assurance Audit Procedures Manual for Dietitians" will also serve as a helpful reference.[38]

Because nutrition support dietitians' roles will vary with team structure, the complexity of your quality assurance program will be influenced. Refer to the suggested protocol/process criteria for enteral tube feeding and parenteral nutrition support care (Table 2–8).

Criteria for process audits need verification and clarification. RUMBA is the acronym that represents the desired characteristics of measured criteria. The initials represent:

• Relevant
• Understandable
• Measurable
• Behavioral
• Achievable

Procedures for patient care audits are outlined in Figure 2–1.

Two types of audit systems exist. It will be necessary to define your goals when selecting a system, although both systems may become interrelated.

The retrospective or patient care audit is designed to improve patient care from preexisting data. This system utilizes completed medical records and is applicable to groups of patients. Specific treatments, outcomes, nutrition intervention, and so forth determine the process criteria for evaluation. Duration of parenteral and enteral treatments, complications, dietitian's assessment, and so forth can all be measured by retrospective or patient care audits. Examples of process cri-

TABLE 2–8. PROCESS CRITERIA FOR ENTERAL TUBE FEEDING AND PARENTERAL NUTRITION SUPPORT CARE

A. Process Criteria: Nutrition Support Dietitian
   TOPIC: Enteral Tube Feedings
   Objective: To ensure nutrition adequacy of selected formula; to provide optimal enteral support through adequate delivery techniques, assure patient tolerance and nutrition requirements; plan, implement and evaluate enteral care.

   I. Confirmation
As soon as order is received into department, clerk will transcribe orders. Delivery of product will occur no later than 1½ hours.

  II. Contact
Dietitian will make initial patient contact within 1 working day.

 III. Assessment
Dietitian will obtain and document pertinent nutritional evaluation data:
1. Nutrition history
   a. Weight/appetite changes
   b. Food aversions, intolerance
   c. Past dietary modifications
2. Review medical chart
   a. Diagnosis
   b. Pertinent laboratory data related to nutrition
   c. Medications, previous surgery, long-term treatments affecting nutrition status

 IV. Planning/Implementation
Dietitian will assure nutrition adequacy of formula selected.
1. Determine nutrition requirement, include stress factors for kcals, protein, fluids, etc.
2. Determine present nutrients received, i.e., formula, volume, kcal/cc, route, etc.
3. Recommend formula/level to achieve nutrient needs
4. Discuss with physician, nursing as needed

  V. Evaluation
Dietitian will evelute progress of modes of therapies.
1. Monitor tolerance of formula and delivery route
2. Evaluate patient status via pertinent lab data
3. Recommend necessary modification to therapy
4. Reenter in progress notes biweekly, in long-term patient (greater than 3 weeks) bimonthly

 VI. Transitional Feedings
Weaning from tube feedings to a p.o. diet will be the staff dietitian's responsibility upon physician's orders.
1. Evaluate with biweekly calorie count or as necessary to assure optimal nutrient intakes

B. Process Criteria: Nutrition Support Dietitian
   TOPIC: Parenteral Nutrition Support
   Objective: To ensure nutrition adequacy of selected formula; to assess present nutritional status; to plan, implement and evaluate weaning regimen

   I. Contact
Dietitian will make initial patient contact within 1 working day to begin assessment.

  II. Assessment
Dietitian will obtain and document pertinent nutritional evaluation data:
1. Nutrition history
   a. Weight/appetite changes
   b. Food aversions, intolerance
   c. Past dietary modifications

TABLE 2–8. (Continued)

    2. Review medical chart
      a. Diagnosis
      b. Pertinent laboratory data related to nutrition status
      c. Medications, previous surgery, long-term treatments affecting nutrition status

III. Planning/Implementation
Dietitian will:
    1. Determine nutrition requirements including stress factors for kcals, protein, etc.
    2. Determine present nutrients received via current solution orders
    3. Set up calorie count on designated days per protocol orders

IV. Evaluation
Dietitian will evaluate patient progress to mode of selected parenteral therapy:
    1. 24-hour calorie count to be done simultaneously with a 24-hour urine collection for urea nitrogen
    2. Calculate nitrogen balance from UUN and determine nitrogen
    3. Evaluate patient status via pertinent nutrition lab data
    4. Recommend necessary modifications to therapy
    5. Reenter in progress notes biweekly, in long-term patient (greater than 3 weeks) enter and evaluate bimonthly

V. Transitional Feedings
Weaning from parenteral nutrition support to enteral nutrition support to oral feedings will be planned and evaluated by the nutrition support dietitian at the physician's discretion.
    1. Evaluate with biweekly calorie counts or as necessary to assure optimal nutrient intakes

teria for patients receiving enteral tube feedings may be:

- Percent of patients assessed by dietitian within 1 working day
- Percent of patients receiving nasogastric tube feedings via Levin or small Silastic feeding tube
- Percent of patients experiencing diarrhea and formula intolerances
- Percent of patients receiving simultaneous parenteral nutrition support and duration
- Percent of weight/heights unrecorded
- Percent of patients gaining +10 percent body weight and documented

Criteria selected will vary according to selected patient audit topics grouped by treatment or diagnosis. Results of patient care audits are very important both inter- and intradepartmentally. Retrospective audits provide a feedback mechanism to the nutrition support team. Results may indicate the need for reorganization, more accurate monitoring systems, redefining policies and resources, and providing expanded staff. Action may be taken to develop expanded programs due to observed deficiencies. Although timely, retrospective audits are necessary to provide hospital administration with updated standards and practices of patient care.

The second type of patient audit is the prospective or concurrent audit. An ongoing, up-to-date audit modality is created by reviewing active patients' medical records on an individual basis. Monitoring forms serve as a data collection resource. Action is individualized and patient oriented, as opposed to the administratively oriented action of the retrospective patient care audit. Nutrition assessment parameters and support treatments delivery techniques used are pertinent concurrent audit data.

Figure 2–2 provides examples of a monitoring form that can also serve as a prospective patient audit data collection sheet. Problems and changes can be identified and implementation can begin immediately. Effects of treatment on patient progress and

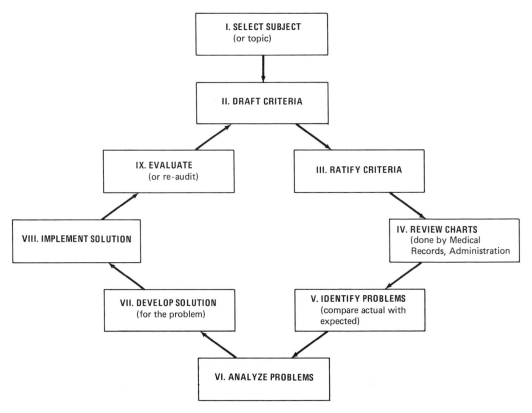

Figure 2–1. Procedure for patient care audit. *(Adapted from Walters F, Crumley SJ (eds): Patient Care Audit: A Quality Assurance Manual for Dietitians. Chicago: ADA, 1978.)*

outcomes are shown by prospective audits. Quality of services delivered is evaluated and thus serves as a quality assurance mechanism.

At present, federal regulations specific to the dietitian's role within a nutrition support service or to a nutrition support service as a separate entity do not exist.

The ADA has continuing contact and input with the Joint Commission on Accreditation of Hospitals (JCAH). Appointed dietitians from ADA serve as liaisons to JCAH and contribute to the accomplishments of the Progressional and Technical Advisory Committees. In this capacity, ADA can review JCAH regulations with regard to nutrition care and

dietetic services. Because of this interaction, the 1980 JCAH Accreditation Manual[37] places increased emphasis on the nutritional care of the patient.

Prior to these efforts, certain standards and interpretations were not present. Now, documentation of nutrition assessments, policies, and procedures for enteral and TPN are expected. The extent of nutritional assessment and required involvement of the dietitian, however, is not interpreted. Excerpts from the 1980 JCAH Manual, Dietetic Services Section, are as follows:

Standard I. *Interpretation line 5–10.*

A qualified dietitian shall assure that the

provision of high quality nutritional care to patients is maintained. . . . The on-site time commitment must be sufficient to provide at least the following: . . . any required *nutritional assessments.*

(Usually dependent on state and local standards.)

Standard III. Dietetic Services shall be guided by written policies and procedures. *Interpretation line 44–48.*
* Nutritional assessment and counseling and diet instruction.
* The role, as appropriate, of the dietetic department/service in the preparation, storage, distribution and administration of *enteric tube feedings* and *total parenteral nutrition programs.*

(The Pharmaceutical Services section of the JCAH Manual elaborates on the requirements of total parenteral nutrition policies and procedures.)

Standard V. Dietetic services shall be provided to patients in accordance with a written order by the responsible practitioner, and appropriate dietetic information shall be recorded in the patient's medical record.
Interpretation lines 22–25.
Summary of the dietary history and/or *nutritional assessment*, when the past dietary pattern is known to have a bearing on the patient's condition or treatment.
Standard VI. The quality and appropriateness of nutritional care provided by the dietetic service shall be frequently reviewed and evaluated.
Interpretation line 22.
Qualified dietitians participate in committee activities concerned with nutritional care.

Standard VI focuses on quality assurance, as does the entire 1980 edition of the Accreditation manual for the overall hospital. The participation of a dietitian on any nutrition committee clearly mandates the expertise of a dietitian to any parenteral/metabolic service. By doing so, the qualified dietitian is assured involvement on a TPN team, as well as assuring quality by a professional solely trained in nutritional care. Implementation of additional quality control mechanisms are suggested to evaluate the appropriateness of nutritional care rendered, such as evaluating menus for nutritional adequacy, possessing a means to identify patients not receiving oral intake, assess patients' nutrient intake, and patient or family understanding of dietary regimens. JCAH site evaluators assist directors of dietetic services to implement quality control mechanisms within their institutions. As of 1980, quality assurance programs are a standard to be met for JCAH Accreditation.

Training Programs for Current Staff

Ongoing staff education and training programs are a necessity to any organization or department. Team members will possess knowledge and skills from prior educational and work experiences. Institutional policies and techniques vary, however, rendering it necessary to develop and utilize orientation and staff-training programs. Clinical and technical knowledge of nutrition support application is an educational requirement dependent on the particular position and institution. New team members require an in-depth overview of all policies, procedures, and techniques used within the nutrition support department.

Current staff development necessitates continuing education in areas of expertise. Professional memberships—the American Dietetic Association (ADA) and the American Society for Parenteral and Enteral Nutrition (ASPEN)—provide educational materials through their myriad of publications. Industry also provides a wealth of information via tapes, booklets, and presentations. It is suggested to keep updated on industry's educational materials and utilize their resources.

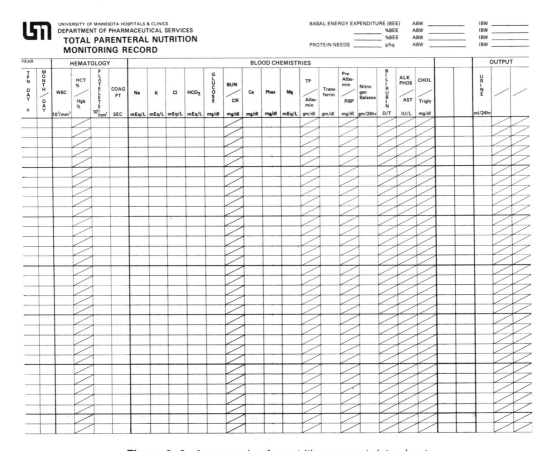

Figure 2–2. An example of a nutrition support data sheet.

Meetings and seminars specific to nutrition support are a common occurrence. As another means of self-continuing education, current staff members are urged to attend area seminars. Journal clubs within the team or invited guests are encouraged. Because a wealth of information exists between a physician, dietitian, nurse, and pharmacist, sharing knowledge will lead to beneficial results. To spotlight a journal club session on aseptic catheter care by the team nurse or compatible vitamin additives to TPN solutions by the pharmacist will enhance the learner's as well as the teacher's skills and knowledge bank. To extend an invitation to other inhouse experts on select topics will again contribute to current staff

continuing education. Suppose your nutrition support team delivered therapy to a primarily adult population. An information education hour with an experienced member of the neonatology staff would expand your knowledge of infant nutrition. Frequently, clinical dietitians manage cancer patients but are not experts on tumor response to therapy or particular antineoplastic drugs. An interested oncologist or nurse practitioner might be able to explain the kinesiology involved. By calling upon inhouse resources, promotion of your team or dietetic service will take place as well as the development or enhancement of rapport among those involved.

Visiting other institutions practicing nu-

AGE, YRS _____
SEX _____
HT, CM _____
USUAL WEIGHT, KG _____ ; IBW, KG _____

DO **NOT** FILE IN
MEDICAL RECORD —
RETURN TO PHARMACY —
BOX 611 MAYO

PATIENT IDENTIFICATION PLATE

INTAKE					TEMP	WT	TPN SOLUTION															TPN INTAKE		P O INTAKE		COMMENTS
P O Ent-eral	OTHER I.V. FLUIDS	TPN V O L U M E	I.V. LIPID conc vol	MAX. IN 24 HR	KG		AMINO ACID FINAL CONC.	DEX-TROSE FINAL CONC.	Na	K	Mg	P	Ca	Cl	A C E T A T E	Multi-vits.	Vit. K mg/24hr		P R O T E I N	CALO-RIES	P R O T E I N	CALO-RIES	
ml/24hr	ml/24hr	ml/24hr	ml/24hr	°F			%	%	mEq/L	mEq/L	mEq/L	mmols/ L	mEq/L	mEq/L	mEq/L	Trace Elem. Soln. ml/24hr	Reg Insulin units/L		gm/24hr	KCAL/ 24hr	g/24hr	KCAL/ 24hr	

trition support can be essential to staff development. ASPEN has a list of institutions willing to donate time and efforts to those seeking direction in procedures. For those planning to develop a team, visiting an already existing unit could set an example and answer many questions on techniques, promotion, and approval. Very often, another institution acquires new equipment (i.e., metabolic cart or computerized calorie counts); team members would then be advised to plan a visit to determine their needs.

When an existing team develops new policies and procedures or techniques, all team members and those directly involved should be thoroughly familiar with the procedure. As in the above-cited institutional visitation, all new techniques and machinery should be demonstrated clearly so all team members can be resourceful. By complying to standards developed for training your current staff specific to nutrition support, the service and team devotion will produce excellent results.

Training Hospital Staff

One can clearly state all registered dietitians should be knowledgeable in nutrition support techniques and nurses caring for patients should be knowledgeable in catheter care and tube-feeding delivery. Pharmacists require a working knowledge in specific parenteral nutrition support solutions; physicians require expertise in selecting therapies and calling upon the health care professionals to assist in the delivery of care, while everyone needs to recognize the undernourished, compromised, or hypermetabolic patient so implementation of nutrition support can begin.

House staff orientation programs should contain nutrition support lectures so that rotating residents and medical students can become familiar with the resources and techniques available. The responsibility will be upon the nutrition support team in cooperation with the medical or inservice education departments to provide this knowledge. In addition to the rotating physicians, all new employees associated with nutrition support techniques should receive education and review of policies and procedures.

New clinical dietitians, nurses, and pharmacists should be familiar with the service. In addition to improved knowledge of nutrition support, your audience will gain respect for your services. Programs should include all of the following:

- Recognizing nutrition deficiencies, assessments
- Nutrition support techniques
- Explanation of team members' roles
- Pertinent guidelines, policies, and procedures
- Outline team availability and resources
- Encourage consultation and utilization of monitoring

Promoting a nutrition support service or concept is a continual effort for effective results. Newsletters or routine update notices developed by the service can be a successful means of promotion and education. When new products are added to the formulary (i.e., tubings, formulas), a flash product update will be an effective introduction. Special nutritional topics should be highlighted in your circulatory newsletter or update. Cancer cachexia and indications for trace element therapy are examples of useful information that can be described. Physicians and other pertinent health care professionals will then be better educated regarding nutrition support therapies.

Medical grand rounds or special meetings for physicians should include an occasional spotlight on nutrition support. Either an interested well-versed physician or guest-physician/lecturer will gain their attention. Day-long seminars sponsored by your own institution, including guest speakers, will promote your service and provide house staff education.

There are many avenues open when developing and implementing educational programs on nutrition support therapies. Goals and behavioral objectives should be focused on the audience and their needs. Continuing education and training is a vital component to any successful unit.

SUMMARY

In the last decade, technologic and medical advances have made it possible to provide nutrition to patients who previously would have succumbed to death by starvation. This sophisticated mode of nutrition support therapy necessitated the collaborated efforts of a physician, dietitian, nurse, and pharmacist for safe and efficacious use. As cost containment has become a major issue in health care, however, the nutrition support team is faced with the burden of proving that its existence is not only beneficial to the patient, but that its activities can be cost effective and even revenue generating. Once the nutrition support team is formed, it must continually strive for optimal provision of nutritional care at minimum cost. The activities of the team have to be documented to evaluate its efficacy and to provide documentation to hospital administration if further support is needed in the future. A successful nutrition support team is one in which all team members have an appreciation of each other's unique talents and ability to contribute to the nutritional care of patients, has an ongoing quality assurance system, is cost effective, and is able to document that as a result of its intervention there is a reduction in morbidity and mortality.

REFERENCES

1. Dudrick SJ, Wilmore DW, Vars HM, et al.: Long-term parenteral nutrition with growth, development and positive nitrogen balance. Surgery 64:134–142, 1968
2. Kaminski MV, Burke WA: The establishment and function of a metabolic support service. J Surg Pract Sept/Oct:25–48, 1979
3. Nutrition Support Team Directory. Columbus, Ohio: Ross Laboratories, 1983
4. Butterworth CE: The skeleton in the hospital closet. Nutr Today March/April:4–8, 1974
5. Bistrian BR, Blackburn GL, Hallowell E, et al.: Protein status of general surgical patients. JAMA 230:858–860, 1974
6. Bistrian BR, Blackburn GL, Vitale J, et al.: Prevalence of malnutrition in general medical patients. JAMA 235:1567–1570, 1976
7. Weisier RL, Hunker EM, Krumdieck CL, et al.: Hospital malnutrition: A prospective evaluation of general medical patients during the course of hospitalization. Am J Clin Nutr 32:418–426, 1979
8. Seltzer MH, Bastidas JA, Cooper DM, et al.: Instant nutritional assessment. JPEN 1:25, 1977
9. Nehme AE: Nutritional support of the hospitalized patient—the team concept. JAMA 243:1906–1908, 1980
10. Rombeau JL, Settle RG, Melnik G: Contemporary nutritional support in VA medical centers. Nutr Supp Serv 2(2):12–15, 1982
11. Ditmer-Schutz D, Egging P: Quality assurance in TPN. Nutr Supp Serv 2(10):13–16, 1982
12. Friedman MH, Higa AM, Davis AJ: A unique team approach to optimal nutritional support with minimal cost. Nutr Supp Serv 3(3):27–28, 1983
13. Seltzer MH, Slocum BA, Cataldi-Betcher EL, et al.: Nutrition support: Team approach. Am J IV Ther Clin Nutr Feb:13–46, 1981
14. Shronts EP, Teasley KT: Development of a nutrition support service. Nutr Supp Serv 3(2):55–58, 1983
15. Secter R: Nutritional support services in a community hospital. Report of the Fourth Ross Roundtable on Medical Issues. Columbus, Ohio: Ross Laboratories, 1983, pp 35–36
16. Cataldi-Betcher E: An example of a nutrition support team. Report of the Fourth Ross Roundtable on Medical Issues. Columbus, Ohio: Ross Laboratories, 1983, pp 32–34
17. Niemiec PW: The nutrition support team structure at the Medical University of South Carolina. Report of the Fourth Ross Roundtable on Medical Issues. Columbus, Ohio: Ross Laboratories, 1983, p 31
18. Webster's New World Dictionary of the American Language. Cleveland and New York: The World Publishing Company, 1966
19. Blackburn GL, Bothe A, Lahey MA: Organization and administration of a nutrition support service. Surg Clin North Am 61:709–719, 1981
20. Skoutakis VA, Martinez DR, Miller WA, et al.: Team approach to total parenteral nutrition. Am J Hosp Pharm 32:693–697, 1975
21. Jensen TG, Dudrick SJ: Implementation of a multidisciplinary nutritional assessment program. J Am Diet Assoc 79:258–266, 1981
22. Chernoff R: The team concept: The dietitian's responsibility. JPEN 3(2):89–90, 1979
23. Wade JA: Role of a clinical dietitian specialist on a nutrition support service. J Am Diet Assoc 70:185–189, 1977
24. Linsley K: The concept of a parenteral nutrition support team from a nurse's viewpoint. Nutr Supp Serv 1(5):33–34, 1981
25. Rowan-Page P, Turnamian SL, et al.: Nutritional support: The role of the nurse-clinician. Nutr Supp Serv 1(1):36–37, 1981
26. Hopkins RJ: Expanding the pharmacist's role in nutritional support service. Nutr Supp Serv 1(8):20–23, 1981
27. Vanderveen TW: Future trends for pharmacy involvement in enteral nutrition. Report of the Fourth Ross Roundtable on Medical Issues. Columbus, Ohio: Ross Laboratories, 1983, pp 40–43
28. D'Eramo D: The hospital administrator's consideration of nutrition support teams. Report of the Fourth Ross Roundtable on Medical Issues. Columbus, Ohio: Ross Laboratories, 1983, pp 15–17
29. Seltzer MH, Asaadi M, Coco A, et al.: The use of a simplified standardized hyperalimentation formula. JPEN 2:28–30, 1978
30. Burke WA, Burkhart V, Pierpaoli PG: A

Guide for a Nutrition Support Service. Deerfield, Illinois: Travenol Laboratories, 1980

31. Final Report of the Task Force on Payment for Pharmacy Service. ASHP, October, 1979

32. Curtiss FR: Reimbursement for clinical pharmacy services. Topics in Hospital Pharmacy Management, May, 1982, pp. 6–21

33. Nathanson, M: Payment incentives feed controversy over advantages of nutritional support. Modern Healthcare, May 15:42–48, 1984

34. Hull, SF: Nutrition support is profitable and cost-effective in the DRG era. Presentation by Ross Laboratories Division of Abbott Laboratories at the Abbott Investor Seminar. Columbus, Ohio: Ross Laboratories, June 15, 1984, pp. 1–10

35. The American Dietetic Association, Professional Standards Review Procedure Manual. Chicago: ADA, 1976

36. The American Dietetic Association, Guidelines for Evaluating a Dietetic Practice: A Report of the Professional Standards Review Committee. Chicago: ADA, 1976

37. Joint Commission on Accreditation of Hospitals. Accreditation Manual for Hospitals. Chicago: JCAH, 1980

38. Walters F, Crumley SJ (eds): Patient Care Audit: A Quality Assurance Manual for Dietitians. Chicago: ADA, 1978

3. The Role of the Clinical Dietitian in Nutrition Support

Anne Marie Hunter

HISTORY AND TRADITION

"Feed a cold, starve a fever."

In 1883 dietary treatment in American hospitals was limited to basically four classifications: (1) full diet, (2) half diet, (3) low fever or spoon diet, and (4) special diet. Rice water and barley water were prescribed for fever based on the premise "the higher the fever, the thinner and more bland the food."[1]

One hundred years later, nutrition is recognized as an established science and its application in health and disease is based on scientific fact not folklore or happenstance. Few would argue, then, that the previously mentioned hypothesis is not only unfounded, but that the converse is true: the higher the fever the greater the energy requirements.

The facts and the science have evolved over a century of growth, challenge, and discovery in the medical and health care professions, and the function of the clinical dietitian has been substantially altered in this metamorphosis. Dietetics as a profession had its beginnings in the early part of the 20th century and focused on the procurement, preparation, and distribution of food.[2] From the inception of the profession, the fundamental responsibility of the dietitian has been that of monitoring the diet, and it remains so to this day.[3]

Dietetics branched into therapeutic adaptation of the diet with the discovery of insulin in the treatment of diabetes. Dietary modifications were identified and interrelated with other disease processes, and the application of clinical dietetics became an essential component of treatment.

CLINICAL DIETETICS DEFINED

Inclusive dietetic practice involves the application of nutrition science to the health care of people. When further delineated into the clinical component, "clinical dietetics is nutritional care, offered in an environment where clients and their needs, physical, socioemotional, and intellectual, are the primary foci of professional effort."[4]

The primary concern of the profession of dietetics is the nutritional health of people. As Huenemann states, dietitians are interpreters of nutrition science, which must be translated into not only the language but the lives of people.[5] Clinical dietetics is a health service profession, and assurance of optimal nourishment is the thrust of the professional.

EDUCATIONAL PREPARATION FOR DIETITIANS WITH A CLINICAL EMPHASIS

The minimum acceptable undergraduate requirements for an entry level clinical dietitian to attain membership in the American Dietetic Association (ADA) must adhere to the Plan IV Program as established by the association in 1973. Basic requirements include competencies in four general knowledge areas: physical and biologic sciences— chemistry, inorganic and organic, human physiology, and microbiology; behavioral and social sciences—sociology or psychology, economics; professional sciences—food composition, physical and chemical changes, quality, acceptability and aesthetics, nutrition, management theory, and principles; communication sciences—writing, creative or technical, mathematics, and learning theory or educational methods.

Additional competencies required for specialization in clinical dietetics include biochemistry and biochemical analysis, cultural anthropology or sociology, an additional nutrition course, nutrition in disease, statistics, and recommended anatomy or advanced physiology or genetics. A practicum for clinical experience must be evidenced either through an approved dietetic internship or a coordinated undergraduate program with a clinical component.

Upon completion of academic and clinical practicum requirements, registration as a dietitian is accomplished by successful performance on the written national examination administered by the ADA. Registered Dietitians are recognized by the initials R.D. after their name which identifies them as qualified professionals. To maintain active registration status, Registered Dietitians must meet established continuing education requirements in 5-year increments. Finally, although not presently a requirement for practice, an increasing number of Registered Dietitians have pursued advanced academic degrees or clinical practicums in their area of interest or specialization.

PROFESSIONALISM, ETHICS, AND THE CLINICAL DIETITIAN

When addressing the issue of the role of the clinical dietitian in modern health care, one must understand that what is inherently involved is an obligation. This obligation has as its core the adherence to two basic codes: professional and ethical.

Professionalism

A professional code deals with those criteria that describe the philosophy of a given profession and the responsibilities of the members. Health professions often are concerned with five major areas: (1) professional competence, (2) relationships with colleagues, (3) relationships with clients, (4) legal responsibilities, and (5) responsibilities to society.[6] Of these five tenets, professional competence is foremost, and all succeeding issues are continually affected by it.

Dietetics as a profession is at a crossroad. Competence, imagery, and projection are central and recurring themes in times of professional transition and specifically in terms of the clinical dietitian. Professional competence encircles the initial educational process, the ability to interpret theory into practice, the confidence to be an independent decision maker and change agent,[7] the fortitude to be creatively innovative, and the continual incorporation of new theory, knowledge, and skill into practice.

The clinical dietitian should be perceived as being knowledgeable, purposeful, consistent, and having presence.[8] Credibility and confidence are not intrinsic characteristics of the professional upon course completion but are earned through experience and accomplishment. "The development—

good or bad—of the professional continues as long as the profession is practiced."[8]

To attain the status of a clinician in dietetic practice, it is necessary to shed historic duties and mores of the dietitian, and to tenaciously embrace the challenges that lie before us. As the scope of dietetic practice becomes further delineated, the professional obligation of the clinical dietitian is to accept open accountability for clinical nutrition intervention, and to retreat from the comforts of the kitchen and the service of food.

Studies have shown that the clinical dietitian's self-image is often more negative than that perceived by other members of the health care team.[9–11] Feelings of subordination and subservience persist only as long as the perceiver allows them to. Eleanor Roosevelt expressed it succinctly when she stated, "No one can make you feel inferior without your consent."

Dietitians have a professional responsibility to project themselves and to demonstrate their expertise in an erudite manner. The intensity associated with effecting change must touch the center of each professional clinical dietitian's practice to ensure that the majority are trendsetters and to establish clinical dietetics as the speciality it is. Professional competence and professionalism are growth processes. They are ongoing, and they are achieved on a singular basis through the intellectual curiosity and vision of the professional.

Ethics

The professional code and professional competence focus on the minimal knowledge and skill required to perform the technical tasks of a profession. They do not ensure that, in terms of the patient's or client's care, ethics, in the philosophic sense, will be involved in treatment and outcome. Thomasma suggests that, in this age of increased specialization and professionalism, the need exists for ethical decision making—using reason in the analysis of values.[12] The basis for the ethical force of professional decisions is the patient's need, which can only be met by the opinion of the health expert.[13]

What then is "acting ethically"? Simply put, it means that one has analyzed one's decisions in light of one's standards of the right and the good. A health professional is virtually forced by current advances in technology and consequent ethical issues to analyze the impact of decisions on the aims of the many disciplines dealing with human health. . . . The challenge to act ethically is ruled by the values one "professes" as a professional. For nutritionists and dietitians, the primary value professed is health as a balance of nutritional forces.[12]

Therefore, as dietitians and health care professionals, we have the additional obligation to attend not only to the patient's needs but also to their values in decisions directly affecting their care.

RESPONSIBILITIES OF THE CLINICAL DIETITIAN

The ADA issued a Position Paper on Clinical Dietetics in March 1982.[14] The paper addresses the role and function of all registered dietitians involved in clinical dietetics. It does not define specific responsibilities of clinical dietetic specialists in advanced practice.

The responsibilities of the clinical dietitian are categorized into five conceptual levels though actual clinical practice involves a mixture of all classifications. The levels delineate responsibilities related to (1) direct care of patients/clients, (2) intraprofessional, (3) interprofessional, (4) intraorganizational, and (5) interorganizational.

Level I: Direct Care of Patients/Clients

The clinical dietitian is accountable for the management or delivery of nutrition services to individuals. These include responsibility for:

- Establishing assessment criteria, screening clients, developing a nutritionally relevant data base, and evaluating information to identify nutrition problems and assess food practices, nutrition status, and dietary needs of individual clients.
- Constructing a written nutrition care plan in consultation with the client and the health care team. This plan includes client-referenced long-range goals and short-term objectives, individualized nutrient requirements and appropriate food sources, methods of feeding, dietary modifications, food patterns, and the plan for diet counseling and nutrition education.
- Coordinating clinical nutrition services and implementing or establishing procedures to facilitate and monitor achievement of client goals and objectives.
- Evaluating and documenting the effectiveness of nutrition intervention; monitoring food acceptance; assessing response to nutrition care, including diet counseling and making appropriate revisions in the nutrition care plan.
- Providing for effective diet counseling of individuals and a program of relevant nutrition education for groups of clients.

Level II: Intraprofessional

The clinical dietitian is responsible for the promotion of the profession, and for the application of the art and the science of human nutrition toward the prevention and the treatment of disease. The responsibilities include:

- Providing leadership for the advancement of contemporary dietetic service in all aspects of nutrition care services.
- Developing and maintaining standards of quality dietetic practice in the clinical setting.
- Applying findings of current research and investigation to the practice of dietetics.

- Engaging in applied nutrition research to study problems related to dietetic practice and the delivery of nutrition care services.
- Participating in educational programs for dietetic students.

Level III: Interprofessional

The third conceptual level requires the clinical dietitian to coordinate and integrate nutrition care services with other facets of health care. The dietitian is accountable for:

- Contributing nutrition-related expertise to discussions regarding health care of patients/clients.
- Participating in decision-making processes related to nutrition care of patients/clients and delivery of nutrition care services.
- Coordinating clinical dietetic activities with functions of food service administration within the health care institution.
- Providing a program of inservice and nutrition education for health team members.
- Participating in interdisciplinary evaluation studies relevant to nutrition care services.

Level IV: Intraorganizational

The clinical dietitian in an institutional setting must participate in a quality assurance program to ensure that the food served is satisfactory to the patients/clients and meets nutrient needs. This encompasses:

- Assuring that patient master menus are nutritionally adequate and comply with established standards and criteria.
- Establishing specifications and procedures for the preparation and service of menu items, special food products, dietary supplements, and formulas.
- Establishing and maintaining standards

and procedures for an effective system of patient food services.

- Implementing the functions of management to provide for planning and goal setting, cost control, coordination of activities, communication, orientation, training, supervision and administration of clinical dietetic personnel; and evaluation of clinical nutrition and patient food services.
- Establishing criteria and implementing, monitoring, and evaluating nutrition care services to maintain standards of quality in dietetic practice in the institution.

Level V: Interorganizational

The clinical dietitian should identify and utilize external influences that affect the scope and quality of nutritional care. Responsibility is indicated for:

- Identifying sources and obtaining funds to support food and nutrition projects which may improve nutrition care services to individual patients/clients.
- Specifying policies and procedures to assure compliance with laws, regulations, and professional guidelines in the provision of nutrition care services.
- Consulting with elected representatives about legislation affecting nutrition care services.[14]

The criteria reflect the ideology of the parent organization of clinical dietetic practitioners in a period of acknowledged transition. The generalist clinical dietitian is charged with responsibilities that involve nutrition screening, assessment, method of feeding, product selection, monitoring, decision making, education, application of research to practice, and establishing standards and quality of practice. Many of these criteria provide the fundamental data base necessary for the clinical dietitian to be functional on the health care team and in nutrition support.

RELATIONSHIP TO THE HEALTH CARE TEAM

The delegation of routine tasks—making out patients' menus and diets, checking diet changes and trays, food tallying, confirming diet orders, supervising food preparation, and charting food intake—to dietetic assistants and technicians have freed the dietitian to assume an active role as a member of the health care team.

A health team is a group of health professionals with a variety of skills, knowledge, values and attitudes who work together to solve health problems. . . . What makes this group of people working together a team is that each member of the team needs the other team member to provide . . . services. . . . No one person has all of the skills and knowledge to manage these (patients') problems.[15]

As a member of the team, the dietitian has the responsibility to participate in decision making for treatment that requires expertise in the areas of nutritional assessment, implementation, manipulation, supplementation, acceptance, compliance, and follow-up.

The dietitian interacts as a colleague on an equal basis with each member of the health care team. Participation on the team affords dietitians the opportunity to clearly demonstrate their abilities as the resource for nutrition intervention. The visibility and involvement of clinical dietitians on the team enforce the importance of nutrition as an essential component of treatment, and their quality performances increase their credibility as practitioners and health care providers.

THE GENERALIST CLINICAL DIETITIAN AND NUTRITION SUPPORT

Butterworth, in his startling account "The Skeleton in the Hospital Closet," forced health care practitioners to acknowledge the overwhelming prevalence of protein–calorie malnutrition (PCM) in hospitalized patients.[16] This article was very timely, as the field of enteral and parenteral nutrition was in its infancy. Historically, enteral and parenteral nutrition, or specialized nutrition support, as it is often referred to, has enjoyed recognition as a specialty for only a decade.

Ideally, enteral and parenteral nutrition therapy is the function of an established and defined nutrition support team. Each member of the team has advanced training and experience in nutrition support. Minimal members of the team include a physician, a dietitian, a nurse, and a pharmacist. Because of its youth, however, it is estimated that only approximately 8.6 percent of the hospitals in the United States have nutrition support teams.[17,18]

In the facilities that have established teams, nutrition support generally is offered as a service by request-for-consultation. It is not mandatory for patients nutritionally at risk to be evaluated by the team, or for patients on hospital admission to be screened for actual or impending malnutrition. Therefore, either due to the absence of the service or the lack of referral, the detection of malnutrition and the recommendation for specialized nutrition support fall into the realm of responsibility of the generalist clinical dietitian.

Nutrition Screening

It is critical for the clinical dietitian to have an understanding of PCM and its effect on hospitalized patients in terms of morbidity and mortality prior to the initiation of any tasks related to enteral and parenteral nutrition. Prospective nutrition screening of patients on hospital admission by the clinical dietitian can alert the physician to individuals nutritionally at risk.

Nutrition screening should evaluate minimal parameters such as serum albumin, total lymphocyte count (TLC), weight changes (especially loss), and anthropometric measurements of triceps skinfold (TSF), mid-arm

muscle circumference (MAMC), and weight for height.[19] Standard values indicating abnormality of each parameter should be established prior to the screening, and the clinical dietitian must comprehend the relationship of each value to the interpretation. The clinical dietitian must be able to perform the mechanics, that is, anthropometric measurements, of a nutrition screening.

Nutrition Assessment

If a patient is found to be at risk nutritionally, the clinical dietitian should perform an indepth nutrition assessment. The assessment should include the evaluation of subjective and objective data. Subjective data are acquired through personal interviews with the patient regarding diet history, food intake, appetite changes, nausea, vomiting, difficulty chewing or swallowing, food allergies and intolerances, recent involuntary weight loss, constipation, diarrhea, medical history and diseases related to impaired nutrient absorption, and physical signs of malnutrition.[20–24]

Objective data evaluate anthropometric measurements, laboratory data, and skin test anergy. Anthropometric measurements include weight for height, ideal body weight, percent weight loss, TSF, MAC, and MAMC. Laboratory parameters reviewed are serum albumin, serum transferrin, TLC, creatinine–height index (CHI), and nitrogen balance. Skin test anergy is determined by challenge with at least three intradermal recall antigens.[20–24]

The dietitian should be aware of his or her patient population in terms of primary and secondary diagnoses, and adjust and adapt the nutrition assessment accordingly. Each assessment should be interpreted individually. Information extracted from the assessment criteria should indicate to the dietitian the need for monitoring caloric intake from food and/or whether enteral or parenteral nutrition therapy should be considered for the patient. Documentation of nutrition intake should be concise but inclusive, and indicate numerable changes in intake, weight, laboratory data, and any other factors that may alter nutrition therapy.

Formula Selection

The clinical dietitian has a working knowledge of supplemental, whole meal replacement, and modular enteral formulas to ensure an appropriate and intelligent selection of enteral nutrition therapy. The dietitian is well versed in nutrient content and indications for use of the various enteral and parenteral products and must be aware of administration techniques and procedures for both types of therapy and possible complications of each. Drug–nutrient reactions must be an additional concern and decision making must relate to current research and literature findings.

The Professional Challenge

Open communication and rapport with physicians and allied health personnel is central to recognition, participation, and effecting change. Clinical dietitians must act as spokespersons for their professional selves. They must maintain inquisitive personas, and present themselves in a scholarly manner—verbally and in writing.

Through the use of audits, standards, and quality assurance, the dietition can demonstrate in a nonthreatening way the prevalence of PCM, the need for nutrition therapy, and the positive effects for patients who have received nutrition intervention. Over and over again, the clinical dietitian must demonstrate and document to ensure that adequate nutrition is the standard for all individuals.

In these uncertain times of reimbursement for health services rendered, and with dwindling benefits payable by the federal government, it behooves clinical dietitians to fervently grasp this opportunity to indelibly establish themselves as the experts in nutritional care. Role usurpation by ill-qualified personnel and self-proclaimed "experts" can only occur if clinical dietitians fail to assert themselves and to demonstrate their abilities.

Specialized nutrition support is the standard of care for patients nutritionally at risk. When indicated, the provision of anything less is substandard treatment and raises issues of incompetent professional practice.[17] Recognition of the need for nutrition support is the responsibility of all health care professionals but particularly of the clinical dietitian whose professional training is channeled toward the nutrition assessment and nutrition care of patients.

Change requires courage and a confirmed dedication to an ultimate goal and the greater good. Enteral and parenteral nutrition therapy can provide the link necessary to substantially alter the professional role of the dietitian. The clinical dietitian is obligated to accept the challenge.

THE NUTRITION SUPPORT DIETITIAN SPECIALIST

Evolution of the Dietitian Specialist

As medical science has advanced, specialization in practice has become standard and clinical dietetics has necessarily become more diversified. Dietitians have restricted their clinical practice and declared specialization in such areas as renal, diabetes, cardiology, obesity, pediatrics, and enteral and parenteral nutrition. Specialists in dietetics function not only as resource persons for patients and clients but also as consultants to colleagues.

Professional preparation for dietetic specialities is ill defined, and standards of dietetic practice are either too broad in spectrum or nonexistent. Suffice it to say, however, that the clinical dietitian specialist in nutrition support should have a minimum of 1 year's experience as a generalist clinical dietitian and demonstrate evidence of advanced and continuous educational preparation. Previous experience should have included exposure to, familiarity with, and at least minimal participation in decision making for specialized nutrition support. The aspiration toward the completion of graduate academic education in clinical nutrition should be a strong consideration for the nutrition support dietitian specialists to ensure competent participation in the initiation of and contribution to clinical research projects, and to acquire a more sophisticated comprehension of metabolic processes.

Scope of Practice for the Nutrition Support Dietitian Specialist

The scope of practice for the dietitian specialist in nutrition support includes a working knowledge of nutrient requirements in health and disease, nutrition assessment techniques, enteral product formularies and parenteral solutions, equipment available for the delivery of enteral feedings, patient monitoring, transitional feedings, and patient follow-up. The dietitian specialist is also responsible for patient and professional education, and for participation in continuing education to update and improve knowledge and skills in specialized nutrition support.

The nutrition support dietitian specialist ideally practices in the environment of a nutrition care team.[25-29] The overriding responsibility of the specialist is the same as that of all dietitians in clinical practice, that is, the translation of the physician's diet order into practical, palatable, acceptable, and appropriate food, nutritional products, or formulas. The nutrition support dietitian specialist has the responsibility to inform and educate all members of the team as to indications for use, cost, nutrient source, and composition of enteral products, optimal methods of transitional feeding, and proper selection of products in the presence, absence, or return of gastrointestinal (GI) function.[27]

Evaluation of Nutrition Status

The specialist is charged with the ability to integrate biochemical and physiologic alterations that occur in disease or trauma with the appropriate nutrition therapy. He or she must be able to recognize the need for instituting or altering specialized nutrition support in actual or impending protein–calorie malnutrition, trauma, stress, hypermetabolic illness, impaired GI function, cancer, liver, renal or respiratory failure, chronic diseases, and preparation for surgical procedures.[26]

Nutrition assessment techniques and determination of nutrient requirements based on age, sex, weight for height, activity level, and the presence or absence of fever are the initial tasks of the nutrition support specialist. The interpretation of this objective data, the patient's ability to tolerate food by mouth or in another form via GI tract, and the medical condition of the patient are major determining factors in the choice or combination of nutrition therapies prescribed.

The dietitian specialist must be well versed in previously mentioned nutrition assessment methods and incorporate more sophisticated assessment parameters such as the Prognostic Nutrition Index (PNI)[30] and indirect calorimetry[31] when appropriate and available. Assessment criteria and standards must be adjusted, deleted, or altered based on current scientific evidence and research. The dietitian specialist must be aware of significant alterations present in standard assessment data as a result of underlying disease process or metabolic conditions and not due to depleted nutrition status.

When nutrition status has been evaluated, the entire team determines the individual nutrition support care plan. If parenteral nutrition is the therapy of choice, the dietitian specialist may recommend specific volumes of solution, determine parenteral solution composition, and assess daily intake of nutrients in the formulary.[29]

Responsibilities of the Nutrition Support Dietitian Specialist for Selection, Implementation, and Monitoring of Nutrition Therapy

If enteral therapy is indicated, it is the dietitian specialist's responsibility to select the appropriate enteral product to satisfy nutrient requirements and GI absorptive capability, recommend enteral tubes and pumps, and establish volume, concentration, and rate of progression protocols for delivery.[25,26,29] The specialist is responsible for the successful implementation of the product for the patient. The overwhelming proliferation of enteral products and feeding modules must be continually reviewed and evaluated by the dietitian, and product usage must be adjusted to ensure appropriate product delivery and utilization.

The nutrition support specialist is responsible for observing and recording the patient's response to parenteral and enteral nutrition therapy. This involves daily monitoring of nutrient delivery, intake, and patient tolerance to therapy. Serial nutrition assessments of anthropometric and biochemical data must be performed to determine efficacy of therapy and patient improvement.

Transitional Feeding

As nutrition or metabolic status improves, the patient may be weaned from aggressive nutrition support. Transition may be sequential from parenteral to enteral tube to oral feeding or may be from any starting point to the next logical progression. The primary concern in this phase of nutrition therapy is to return the patient to the most normal method and route of feeding without sacrificing the delivery of required nutrients. It is often at this point that combination nutrition therapies are utilized. Parenteral therapy should be gradually deleted while enteral is introduced and tolerance is noted, and intake by mouth should begin while an enteral tube feeding is delivered concomitantly or supplementally.

The dietitian specialist is the key member of the nutrition care team involved in transitional feeding. It is his or her responsibility to coordinate the appropriate mode of transition by consultation with the team regarding medical progress and also through patient interview.

It is feasible to progress from intravenous nutrition therapy to oral intake bypassing enteral tube administration depending upon the individual patient's condition. The rule of thumb, however, in all transitional feeding techniques is a gradual decrease in the initial therapy with an attendant increase in and progression of the intermittent or end therapy. When nutrient intake has increased to acceptable levels either by mouth or via the selected end therapy, the initial feeding modality may be terminated.[32]

Rapport and Liaison Between the Nutrition Support Dietitian Specialist and the Staff Clinical Dietitians

The nutrition support dietitian specialist confers with the generalist clinical dietitian and other dietitian specialists who have been involved with the patient's nutrition care prior to the initiation of specialized nutrition support. The specialist and the generalist act as co-advisors to each other and follow the patient's course together.

Interaction of the Dietitian Specialist with the Patient and Family

It is important to stress that the patient be involved in the nutrition therapy, and that the nutrition team establish an open rapport with the patient from the time of the initial consultation. The dietitian specialist plays a vital role in the education of the patient in terms of the comprehension, initiation, and maintenance of the prescribed therapy. The family should be involved in the educational process as well to ensure consistency and continuity of the nutrition support, and adequacy of nutrient intake when the aggressive therapy has been discontinued.

The development of a positive relationship between the dietitian specialist and the patient and family while in the hospital is critical to ensure adherence to therapy after discharge to home. The dietitian is responsible for providing follow-up service to the patient either in the home or as an outpatient and is readily available to the patient and family for any concerns regarding the nutrition therapy.

Participation in Research

The practice area of nutrition support is an ideal environment for the generation of clinical nutrition research projects. Research design, the accumulation of valid data, and publication of results are responsibilities of the dietitian specialist.

The interpretation and incorporation of theoretical findings strengthen and update professional decision making and clinical practice. Visible involvement of the dietitian specialists in clinical research increases their credibility and professional image.

PROFESSIONAL PROGRESSION

The 1972 ADA Report "The Profession of Dietetics"[33] identified aspects of dietetic educational preparation, professional organization, and dietetic practice that required improvement or adaptation to adequately attend to the nutrition needs of the public and to sustain the livelihood of the profession. The Commission found that the basic educational process of the dietitian was deficient and recommended the attendant integration of didactic learning and clinical experience. The study also suggested that the ADA establish and operate through four basic councils. The report cited anticipated projections for the future of the profession including increased differentiation in the roles and functions of dietitians, increased specialization in dietetic practice, new and additional competencies necessary to practice effectively, and increased association with other health professionals.

A number of educational institutions responded to the suggestions of the Commission and either established coordinated undergraduate programs combining theory with practice or instituted competency-based education.[34] The association did establish the Councils on Practice, Education, and Research that, today, are viable components of the organization.

The Commission recommended that the ADA assume responsibility for the competency of the dietetic practitioner by registration and certification. Registration, in effect since 1969, ensured entry level competency through educational preparation and written examination. Dietitians either in specialized practice or through advanced professional education should be eligible for certification by written and oral examinations.

An Ad Hoc Committee on specialty Board Certification in Dietetics was formed in 1975 by the House of Delegates of the ADA to study the feasibility of establishing the American Board of Dietetic Specialties.[35] The proposal was submitted to the House of Delegates in October 1979 and was defeated. Since that time, the issue of specialty board certification has not been reintroduced to the House of Delegates.

Ten years have elapsed since the Commission published the report on the profession, and the issue of specialty board certification has been in limbo for the past 4 years. The aforementioned changes in dietetic education apply to the training of the generalist clinical dietitian. At the present time, definitive criteria have not been established for educational preparation or method of certification to legally identify dietitian specialists that includes those dietitians who have restricted their practice to nutrition support.

Specialized nutrition support has afforded the patient a viable option in nutrition care. Various health care disciplines are incorporating the use of this therapy into clinical practice and are developing guidelines and standards for certification as specialists in this field. The delivery of enteral and parenteral therapies solely by individuals with marginal education in nutrition is most disconcerting. Optimal nourishment of patients will suffer if the dietitian is not an active participant in nutritional care decision making. The exclusion of the involvement of the registered dietitian in specialized nutrition therapy can become a reality unless the profession restructures the educational process, identifies standards of dietetic practice, and institutes specialty board certification to assure competencies.

The future is now. The uniqueness of registered clinical dietitians in terms of training is factual. The contributions they are able to make must be perfected and exploited. The writings of Dag Hammarskjöld remind us "You have not done enough, you have never done enough so long as it is still possible that you have something of value to contribute. This is the answer when you are groaning under what you consider a burden and an uncertainty prolonged ad infinitum."[36]

REFERENCES

1. Franklin GS: Hygiene of low diet. JAMA 1:416, 1883
2. Schiller R: The challenge facing clinical dietitians today. Dietetic Currents 6:4, 1979
3. Ohlson MA: Diet therapy in the past 200 years. J Am Dietet Assoc 69:490, 1976
4. Mason M, Wenberg BG, Welsch PK: The clinical dietitian at work. In The Dynamics of Clinical Dietetics. New York: Wiley, 1977, pp 3–27
5. Huenemann RL: Leadership and quality in nutritional care: Our role in today's world. J Am Dietet Assoc 78:124, 1981
6. Wagstaff MA, DeMassa MV: Professional ethics: Reflection and anticipation. J Am Dietet Assoc 78:321, 1981
7. Peck EB: The "professional self" and its relation to change processes. J Am Dietet Assoc 69:534, 1976
8. DeMarco MR: Professionalism. J Am Dietet Assoc 72:579, 1978
9. Calvert S, Parish HY, Oliver K: Clinical dietetics: Forces shaping its future. J Am Dietet Assoc 80:350, 1982
10. Schiller R, Vivian VM: Role of the clinical dietitian—Part I. J Am Dietet Assoc 65:284, 1974
11. Schiller R, Vivian VM: Role of the clinical dietitian—Part II. J Am Dietet Assoc 65:287, 1974
12. Thomasma DC: Human values and ethics: Professional responsibility. J Am Dietet Assoc 75:533, 1979
13. Pellegrino ED: Ethics and the moment of truth. JAMA 239:960, 1978
14. The American Dietetic Association Position Paper on Clinical Dietetics. J Am Dietet Assoc 80:256, 1982
15. Seigel B: Organization of the primary care team. Pediatr Clin North Am 21:341, 1974
16. Butterworth CE: The skeleton in the hospital closet. Nutr Today March/April: 4, 1974
17. Seltzer MH: Specialized nutrition support: The standard of care. JPEN 6:185, 1982
18. Nutrition Support Team Directory. Columbus, Ohio: Ross Laboratories, 1983
19. Freed BA, Chase G, Kaminski MV: Initiation of an admission nutritional screening program in an urban community hospital. Nutritional Support Services 2:8:19, 1982
20. Maillet JO: Evaluating your assessment program. Nutritional Support Services 2:4:19, 1982
21. Jensen TG, Dudrick SJ: Implementation of a multidisciplinary nutritional assessment program. J Am Dietet Assoc 79:258, 1981
22. Winborn AL, Banaszek NK, Freed BA, et al.: A protocol for nutritional assessment in a community hospital. J Am Dietet Assoc 78:129, 1981
23. Hooley RA: Clinical nutritional assessment, a perspective. J Am Dietet Assoc 77:682, 1980
24. Seltzer MH: The clinical corner. JPEN 6:5:455, 1982
25. Johnson EQ: The therapeutic dietitian's role in the alimentation group. J Am Dietet Assoc 62:648, 1973
26. Wade JE: Role of a clinical dietitian specialist on a nutrition support service. J Am Dietet Assoc 70:185, 1977
27. Chernoff R: The team concept: The dietitian's responsibility. JPEN 3:2:89, 1979
28. Committee on Dietitians' Affairs. ASPEN monograph—role of the clinical dietitian on a nutrition care team, 1980
29. Hooley RA: The role of the registered dietitian on a nutrition support team. Nutritional Support Services 1:1:52, 1981
30. Buzby GP, Mullen JL, Matthews DC, et al.: Prognostic nutritional index in gastrointestinal surgery. Am J Surg 139:160, 1980
31. Feurer ID: Clinical application of indirect calorimetry. Clin Nutr Newsletter 1: April, 1983
32. Skipper A: Transitional feeding and the dietitian. Nutritional Support Services 2:8:45, 1982

33. Study Commission on Dietetics: The Profession of Dietetics. Chicago: ADA, 1972
34. Hart M: Competency-based education. J Am Dietet Assoc 69:616, 1976
35. Ad Hoc Committee: Certification in dietetic specialties: Proposed guidelines for establishing the American board of dietetic specialties. J Am Dietet Assoc 74:153, 1979
36. Hammarskjöld D: Markings. New York: Alfred A Knopf, 1968, p 198

Part II. IDENTIFYING THE PATIENT AT NUTRITION RISK

4. The Nutrition History and Physical Assessment
Ruth Hooley

Nutrition assessment consists of collecting and evaluating a number of types of information including patient history and physical examination, biochemical data, anthropometric measurements, and tests of immune function. From this data base (Fig. 4–1), the practitioner can:

1. Identify the patient at nutrition risk
2. Determine the nutrition care plan
3. Implement the nutrition care plan (via enteral or parenteral nutrition support)
4. Evaluate the efficency of the nutrition care plan (through sequential patient monitoring of nutrition status)

It is the purpose of this chapter to look at a portion of the nutrition assessment process, namely, the nutrition history and physical assessment.

MEDICAL RECORD REVIEW

The first step of any nutrition status evaluation is collection of preliminary data from the medical record. Ideally, this medical record review occurs before the initial patient interview as it provides clues for the practitioner to look for when screening for nutrition status. The initial medical record review serves a number of useful functions.

1. Identification of factors that increase a patient's risk of developing primary or secondary malnutrition
2. Identification of existing nutrient deficiency disease signs and symptoms
3. Identification of significant psychosocial factors with short- or long-term nutrition ramifications
4. Identification of co-existing disease states or treatments with nutrition ramifications
5. Identification of past nutrition problems and therapy

The Medical History

In general, malnutrition can be divided into two major etiologic categories—primary malnutrition and conditional or secondary malnutrition. The medical history can provide information relating to both types of malnutrition.

Primary malnutrition generally occurs because of inadequate diet, because of altered food supply, or because of a shift from a wide to a narrow choice of foods. It may also be due to overabundance of certain nutrients (e.g., calories, fluoride).

Normally, primary malnutrition is a socioeconomic phenomenon. High incidences of primary malnutrition are associated with

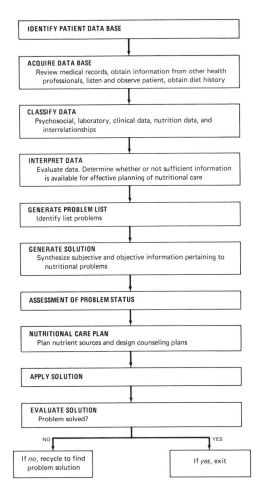

Figure 4–1. Steps in nutritional care plan formation. *(Adapted from Hunt SM, Groff JL, and Holbrook JM: Nutrition: Principles and Clinical Practice. New York: John Wiley, 1980, Figure 12–1, p 420.)*

factors such as age, sex, race, ethnic group, and economic background.

Secondary or conditional malnutrition occurs when the diet is potentially adequate but for various reasons the individual is unable to properly make use of available food. Conditional forms of malnutrition are much more prevalent in affluent societies and in hospitals or other health care settings. Eight general categories of conditional malnutrition have been identified:

1. Decreased appetite, change in eating patterns or bizarre eating habits (e.g., anorexia nervosa, alcoholism, food faddism)
2. Impaired ability to ingest foods (e.g., oropharyngeal disease, fracture or paralysis in the oral area, esophageal strictures)
3. Impaired ability to digest and absorb foods (e.g., intrinsic factor deficiency, Crohn's disease)
4. Faulty transport (e.g., abetalipoproteinemia, chyluria)
5. Impaired utilization (e.g., diabetes mellitus)
6. Excessive losses (e.g., Addison's disease, primary aldosteronism, exudate from burns, fistulas)
7. Increased requirements due to stress and catabolism (e.g., surgery, sepsis)
8. Drug-induced nutrient deficiencies (e.g., megaloblastic anemia from chronic administration of oral contraceptive agents)

Table 4–1 provides a list of conditions that exist frequently in hospital patients in which one or more of the above categories of primary or secondary malnutrition can occur.

DIET HISTORY

When indicated, the diet history patient interview usually comes after the medical record review. It assists the practitioner in a number of ways that include

1. Gaining further information about the quality and quantity of patient's fluid and food intake as well as factors that influence his or her choice of foods
2. Determining problem areas or possible nutrient deficiencies or toxicities in the patient's past and present diet
3. Indicating areas of special attention

TABLE 4–1. THE MEDICAL RECORD REVIEW: CONDITIONS COMMONLY ASSOCIATED WITH INCREASED RISK FOR MALNUTRITION

General Category	Clinical Examples	General Category	Clinical Examples
Body Weight Aberrations	Usual Body Weight 1. 20% over ideal 2. 10% under ideal Recent significant gain or loss (10% gain or loss of usual body weight in last 6 months) Voluntary? Involuntary? Recorded height and weight Children: Inappropriate weight for height Pregnancy: Deviation from normal weight gain	Chronic Diseases (General)	Diabetes mellitus Hypertension Hyperlipidemia Coronary artery disease Chronic lung disease Chronic renal disease Chronic liver disease Circulatory problems or heart failure Carcinoma Mental retardation Psychosis Epilepsy Rheumatoid arthritis Peptic ulcer disease Prolonged comatose state
Increased Metabolic Needs	Fever Infection Hyperthyroidism Burns Surgery or soft tissue trauma (within last 6 months) Skeletal trauma Growth (children, pregnancy) Cortiscosteroid therapy	Diseases or Surgery of the GI Tract	Congenital malformations Pancreatic insufficiency Malabsorption states Blind loop syndrome Severe diarrhea GI fistula Resection of stomach or small bowel Intestinal bypass
Increased Nutrient Losses	Draining fistulas Open Wounds Draining abscesses Effusions Chronic blood losses Chronic renal dialysis Exudative enteropathies Burns	Medications	Insulin or other hypoglycemic agents Vitamin–mineral supplements Corticosteroids Anticoagulants MAO inhibitors Diuretics Antacids Ethanol Oral contraceptive agents Tricyclic antidepressants Phenylhydantoin

that should be further evaluated as a part of the overall nutrition care plan

The depth of the diet history depends on the information that the dietitian has collected from the medical history and laboratory values regarding the nutrition status and relative nutritional risk at which the patient is placed, as in the following:

1. Patients who are obese, extremely overweight, or who have had a recent weight loss. Frequently malnutrition is not recognized in overweight persons

who may be protein depleted because their size fails to attract attention to their nutrient needs. Patients who are underweight are more vulnerable because the somatic and visceral proteins may be already wasted.

2. Patients who, for socioeconomic reasons, fail to ingest adequate amounts of food in their usual diet, who have suffered from severe to moderate maldigestion and/or malabsorption, or who are unable to consume food orally for more than 5 days because of recent surgery or trauma or physical impairment to the head/neck and upper gastrointestinal (UGI) tract.

3. Patients with increased metabolic requirements due to pregnancy, rapid growth, or a chronic disease.

4. Patients taking any medication (usually for long periods of time) that alters nutrient requirements and/or metabolism (e.g., Dilantin, Prednisone).

5. Patients with continual losses of body constituents, as from draining fistulas, emesis, diarrhea, chronic blood loss, and chronic renal dialysis. The dietary history may elicit the length of time over which these losses have occurred and the type of dietary measures taken in the past to treat them.

6. Patients who have selected dietary patterns and intake based on religious, health, or ecologic factors that may include restrictions or excessive intakes of nutrients (e.g., Zen-macrobiotic diet, vegan diet, or any weight reduction diet).

7. Patients with increased metabolic requirements due to burns, sepsis, or trauma. Such patients are difficult to obtain diet histories from when they are unstable and the diet history usually does not provide information on their present nutrient needs. It may be necessary, however, to obtain it after the patient begins to stabilize in order to plan nutrition care during the recuperative and restorative phase of convalescence.

The diet history may be the first contact that the dietetic practitioner has with the patient. Approach the patient in an unhurried, relaxed manner and explain the reason for the questions and body measurements (or other physical examination) and the type of information requested in the interview. Ask openended (Table 4–2) and nondirected questions (i.e., "What did you drink?" rather than "Did you drink any milk?") using verbal and nonverbal cues that focus the patient on the issues of concern. Body posture, eye contact, and careful recording of information are important nonverbal clues in conveying the importance of the interview. Convey a nonjudgmental acceptance of the patient and his or her responses during the dietary interview (e.g., an onion sandwich is just a matter of taste, economics, and environment).

Good listening is important. During the interview, think about the following questions:

1. What does the speaker mean?
2. How does the speaker know?
3. What is the speaker leaving out?
4. What themes or patterns is the speaker suggesting? Important themes to cue in on include attitudes toward food and eating concerns of health and disease, factors motivating lifestyle, strengths and assets of the individual, previous experiences with diet modification.

If there are any discrepancies or ambiguities in the data provided by the patient, confirm and clarify the data. For example, if an emaciated 60-year-old man with esophageal cancer, undergoing radiation therapy, states that his appetite is excellent, there may be a discrepancy. Ask further questions and observe his intake of food to clarify what he means by "excellent."

Proper record keeping facilitates analysis and retrieval of information. Record data obtained during the interview in a systematic, objective manner for later use. When entering this data on the medical record, use the subjective, objective, assessment, plan (SOAP) format.

TABLE 4–2. DIET HISTORY—INTERVIEWING TECHNIQUES

Question Type	Definition
Continuing	
Affective	Statement in which the helper (counselor) reflects a feeling the helpee has not yet labeled
Content	Statement which summarizes or reflects the content of the prior statement or statements
Self-referent	
Aside	Statement the helper makes to himself or herself
Self-disclosing	Statement of factual information on the part of the helper about himself or herself
Self-involving	Statement of the helper's personal response to helpee's statements
Leading	
Advice	Statement that provides an alternative mode of behavior (actions or thoughts) for the helpee
Closed questions	Questions that can be answered "Yes," or "No," or with one or two words
Influence	Statement used to change the attitudes, beliefs, and, indirectly, the behavior of the helpee
Open questions	Questions that cannot be answered "Yes," "No," or with one or two words
Teaching	Statement made to instruct the helpee on appropriate nutrition practices

Adapted from Danish S, Ginsberg MR, et al.: The anatomy of a dietetic counseling interview. J Am Diet Assoc 75:626, 1979.

Record the nutrition care plan generated by a nutrition support team or an individual dietetic practioner, either in the medical record or on a cardex. Include (1) a list of problems, (2) a plan of action for taking care of each problem, and (3) dated record of actions taken.

For further review of interviewing and diet history techniques, please refer to the bibliography.

Levels of Assessment of Dietary Intake

Assessment of dietary intake may be conducted at three levels of depth. The level selected should

1. Consider the mental status, clinical condition, and degree of under- or overnutrition of the patient under evaluation
2. Provide sufficient information to develop an adequate nutrition care plan

The diet history may include a family interview as well as the patient interview to provide sufficient reliable information to evaluate preadmission dietary adequacy.

Level 1: Nutrition Screening. Level 1 provides a minimal level diet history and is generally indicated when patient malnutrition is not a major clinical concern. It consists of the following components:

1. Determination of recent diet modifications, whether ordered by physician or self-imposed, and for what reason.
2. History of weight change:
   a. Preillness weight
   b. Present weight (should be directly measured)
   c. Desirable weight for height
   d. Time period over which weight change occurred (if applicable)
3. Changes in appetite, ability to taste and smell.
4. Eating patterns:
   a. Number of meals/snacks per day
   b. Changes in food tolerance
   c. Time period over which changes occurred (if applicable)
   d. Comparison of usual intake to

basic 4 food groups (Tables 4–3 and 4–4)

5. Assessment of mechanical feeding problems—Any difficulty in chewing or swallowing.
6. Presence of diarrhea or constipation. If present, how long?
7. Usage of vitamin/mineral supplements.

Level 1 screening should generate sufficient information to determine:

1. Whether the present diet order will provide enough nutrients in a form that the patient can digest and absorb
2. Whether there are any gross nutrient imbalances that need further physical, clinical, biochemical, and psychosocial evaluation

Level 2: Intermediate Level. Level 2 provides an intermediate level diet history, generally indicated when specific nutrient imbalances are suspected or as a routine component of a full nutrition assessment. Level 2 assessment consists of the Level 1 parameters with the following additions:

1. Completion of 24-hour recall of food intake and/or food frequency questionnaire to provide a semiquantitative determination of foods eaten. The 24-hour recall reflects eating patterns prior to hospitalization, which may or may not be usual for the patient. The accuracy of the recall of the amount and kind of food taken depends on the mental status of the patient. It is general at best, since several days may have elapsed since hospitalization. A description of a typical day with meal times and menu included often provides a less biased record of general intake than would a 24-hour recall. A food frequency record assists in obtaining a more detailed history and in identifying inadequate intake of specific nutrients. The patient is asked to indicate whether a food item is consumed daily, weekly, monthly, yearly, or never (Table 4–5).
2. A 3-day calorie and protein count may be useful in assessing the patient's current nutritional intake and compliance with diet.

Level 3: In-Depth Dietary History. Level 3 is frequently used in nutrition surveys and re-

---

TABLE 4–3. THE BASIC 4 FOOD GROUPS: RECOMMENDED NUMBER OF SERVINGS PER DAY (BY AGE GROUP)

Food Group	Recommended Number of Servings per Day				
	Child	*Adolescent*	*Adult*	*Pregnant Adult*	*Lactating Adult*
Bread and cereals	4	4	4	4	4
Vegetables and fruits					
Green leafy	1	1	1	1	1
Orange vegetable	1 at least every other day, if green leafy not used				
Citrus or other vitamin C rich	1	1	1	1	1
Potatoes and others	To achieve a total of 4 or more servings when added to above				
Milk and milk products	2–3	4	2	3–4	4
Meats, poultry, fish, eggs, legumes	2	2	2	3	2
Others	As needed to provide extra calories and make food palatable				

TABLE 4–4. THE BASIC 4 FOOD GROUPS: A SCREENING SYNOPSIS OF THEIR NUTRIENT CONTRIBUTION[a]

Food Group	Kcal	Protein	Niacin, Thiamin, Riboflavin, Pyridoxine	Folic Acid	Vitamin B_{12}	Vitamin C	Vitamin A and Carotene	Vitamin D	Vitamin E	Ca	P	Fe
Meat	+	+	+	−	+	−	−	−	+	−	+	+
Dairy	+	+	+	−	+	−	+	+	−	+	+	−
Bread/cereal	+	−	+	+	−	−	−	−	+	−	+	−
Fruit	+	−	−	±	−	+	+	−	−	−	−	−
Vegetable	+	−	+	+	−	+	+	−	−	+	−	+

[a]Some cereal products are enriched with iron. Liver is rich in vitamin A and folic acid. Fresh orange juice contains significant amounts of folic acid. Most vegetable oils contain abundant amounts of vitamin E.
Adapted from Van Itallie TB: Assessment of Nutritional Status. In Thorn GW, Adams RD (eds): Harrison's Principles of Internal Medicine, 7th ed. Table 75-2, p. 420. New York: McGraw-Hill, 1974.

search programs. This type of history may include keeping a diet diary and activity record for 1 week. Shopping habits and the social and ethnic influence on the diet may also be evaluated. Food is often weighed for a quantitative analysis. The information from this type of history can be particularly helpful in weight reduction or other programs with behavior modification components; however, given the complexity of data collection and evaluation, it is rarely used in the clinical setting.

PHYSICAL ASSESSMENT

In conjunction with the diet history, clinical or physical patient examination is an essential component of indepth nutrition assessment. Numerous structural and functional clinical findings are known to be associated with various states of malnutrition. Like any other clinical evaluation, however, physical patient examination for the purpose of ruling out clinical presentation of malnutrition has a number of limitations:

1. Sign nonspecificity: The fact that some early clinical signs of malnutrition lack specificity should be recognized. Common clinical signs of malnutrition (e.g., glossitis, cheilosis, angular stomatitis, follicular hyperkeratosis, and other skin lesions) can be caused by more than one nutrient deficiency and numerous other nonnutritional factors.
2. Deficiency states overlap: Malnutrition and the clinical presentation of various dietary deficiencies are generally not isolated to single nutrients. Single lesions are commonly caused by the lack of more than one nutrient (e.g., "glossitis" may be seen in riboflavin, niacin,

TABLE 4–5. FOOD FREQUENCY QUESTIONNAIRE

The following questionnaire is to help the dietitian determine frequency of food use. It should be used in conjunction with a 24-hour recall of food intake. Record as accurately as possible. Amounts should be recorded in measurable units (e.g., cups, pounds, teaspoons). Frequencies should be recorded in measurable units of time (e.g., 1/day, 3/mo, 2/week).

1. Do you drink milk? If so, what kind? _____ whole   How much? _____
   _____ 2%
   _____ skim
   _____ other

2. Do you use fats? If so, what kinds? _____ butter   How much? _____
   _____ margarine
   _____ oil
   _____ other

3. How often do you eat meat? _____ poultry? _____ fish? _____ eggs? _____
   cheese? _____ cold cuts? _____ peanut butter and dried beans? _____

4. Do you eat snack foods?   Which ones?   How often?   How much?
   _____   _____   _____
   _____   _____   _____
   _____   _____   _____

5. What vegetables do you eat? How often?
   (a) broccoli _____ green peppers _____ cooked greens _____ carrots _____
       sweet potatoes _____ winter squash _____
   (b) tomatoes _____ raw cabbage _____ white potatoes _____ other raw veg. _____
   (c) aspargus _____ beets _____ cauliflower _____ corn _____ cooked
       cabbage _____ celery _____ peas _____ green or yellow beans _____
       lettuce _____

6. What fruits do you eat? How often?
   (a) apples or applesauce _____ apricots _____ bananas _____ berries _____
       cherries _____ grapes or grape juice _____ peaches _____ pears _____
       pineapple _____ plums _____ prunes _____ raisins _____ other _____
   (b) oranges and orange juice _____ grapefruit and grapefruit juice _____

7. Bread and cereal products
   (a) How much bread do you eat with meals? _____ Between meals? _____
   (b) Do you eat cereal daily? _____ Weekly? _____ Cooked? _____ Dry? _____
   (c) How often do you eat foods such as rice, macaroni, spaghetti, etc? _____

8. Do you eat canned soup? _____ Homemade soup? _____ What kinds? _____
   How often? _____

9. Do you use salt? _____ Do you salt foods before tasting them? _____ Do you cook with salt?
   _____ Do you "crave" salt or salty foods? _____

10. How many teaspoons of sugar or honey do you use per day? _____ (Be sure to include sugar used in cereal, toast, fruit, and in coffee, tea, etc.)

11. Do you drink any of the following?

Beverage	How Often	How Much Each Day
Water	_____	_____
Coffee, tea, decaf, etc.	_____	_____
Carbonated beverages, punch	_____	_____
Beer, wine, liquor	_____	_____
Other	_____	_____

12. Are there any other foods not listed above that you eat frequently?
    _____
    _____

folic acid, and iron deficiencies). Clinical signs associated with biochemical and other tests help to identify specific nutrients responsible for a given clinical lesion. The simultaneous lack of multiple nutrients, however, can make a final diagnosis difficult.

3. Examiner bias: Lack of consistency in the observations of two or more examiners, and in those of the same examiner at different times are a constant source of error when clinically evaluating a patient. The less defined the physical criteria adopted, the more biased the assessment. Observer bias may be reduced by adopting uniform, well-defined physical assessment criteria.

4. Patient bias: Patient bias may affect the clinical examination. The questions designed to elicit presenting complaints and past medical history are likely to influence answers given by the patient. In general, complaints or observations volunteered by the patient tend to be less biased than responses to specific questions asked by practitioner. Use openended questions to obtain information whenever possible. Review the past medical history for areas on which to focus the clinical examination or further biochemical testing.

Keeping these limitations of physical patient examination in mind, the World Health Organization has developed a classification system for the most common physical findings. Tables 4–6 and 4–7 describe and define specific signs and symptoms associated and not associated with malnutrition. Table 4–8 uses a systems approach, listing:

1. Signs indicating probable deficiency of one or more nutrients at the present time or in the recent past
2. Signs indicating probable long-term malnutrition in combination with other factors
3. Signs not related to nutritional status

Interpretation of Clinical Signs. Because most physical signs are nonspecific, they are generally interpreted as part of a group of signs and symptoms common to a particular nutrient malnutrition state. The greater the number of signs within a specific group that the clinician observes, the greater the likelihood that the patient has a true nutrient deficiency. For example, glossitis may be seen in numerous deficiency states, but if glossitis occurs with other symptoms of iron deficiency, the likelihood of iron deficiency as an etiology for the glossitis is increased. Listed in Table 4–9 by nutrient are the major clinical signs and symptoms of malnutrition. The reader is cautioned that this table is merely a summary reference. Many of the listed signs and symptoms vary widely in sensitivity or specificity.

TABLE 4–6. DEFINITION AND DESCRIPTION OF PHYSICAL SIGNS COMMONLY ASSOCIATED WITH MALNUTRITION: BY SYSTEMS

General Appearance:

Apathy. Unreactive, unresponsive, inattentive, and disinterested to surroundings.

Irritability. Hyperresponsive, excessive or overreaction to minor stimuli, particularly manifested through crying or unusual indication of fear as a result of minor or relatively insignificant happenings.

Kwashiorkor. Pitting edema at least on the pretibial region. Underweight, undersized, undeveloped for age (in infants and children). Muscular wasting may be present but masked by edema. Apathy of some degree may be present. In children, changes in the hair are usually noted, such as thinning, easy pluckability with dyspigmentation or flag sign, and changes in texture to silken, sparse hair. Dermatosis with desquamation (flaky-paint) with or without hyperpigmentation may be present.

Marasmus. Evidence of pronounced wasting of subcutaneous fat without edema. Significant apathy may be present. Frequently the face and eyes may appear unusually bright due to the combination of wasting and eye prominence. In children, the child is usually considerably underdeveloped in relation to age. There may or may not be associated hair changes such as dyspigmentation, thinness, and easy pluckability. Signs of other nutrient deficiencies may be present.

Pallor. Paleness and loss of color of skin, nail beds, mucosa, and lips.

Eyes

Angular palpebritis. Excoriation and fissuring of the corners of the eyes. Often associated with angular stomatitis.

Bitot's spots. Well-demarcated, superficial, dry, grayish or chalky-white foamy lesions, triangular or irregular in shape, more often confined to the regions lateral to the cornea and never overlying it. Do not confuse with pterygium.

Blepharitis. Redness, crusting or ulceration of the margins of the eyelids.

Circumcorneal and scleral pigmentation. Unusual brownish coloring of the whites of the eyes. Common in dark-skinned people (nonnutritional). May also present as a pigmented ring around the cornea.

Conjunctival xerosis. Cloudiness, lack of luster; dryness and dullness confined to the conjunctiva (a few seconds' exposure by drawing back the eyelid will aid in its identification). Do not confuse with chemical or environmental irritation, or pterygium or pingueculae.

Corneal vascularization. Invasion of the cornea with capillaries and fine blood vessels, which can be more clearly defined by opthalmoscopic examination. Can occur in any inflammation or irritation of the cornea.

Corneal xerosis. Cornea becomes dull, milky, hazy, or opaque, especially the lower, central area.

Keratomalacia (xerophthalmia). Generally begins with the presence of Bitot's spots with progressive xerosis and keratinization of the corneal epithelium. The cornea eventually becomes opaque, soft, and even necrotic. The term "keratomalacia" usually applies to the advanced condition.

Hair

Dyspigmentation. Distinct lightening of the hair from its normal color. Do not confuse with dyed or bleached hair.

Easy pluckability. tufts of hair can easily be pulled out of the head, with moderate force and without pain. Generally occurs with other hair changes.

Flag sign. Characterized by alternating zones of lightness and darkness along length of hair. Uncommon.

Lack of luster. Dull, dry, brittle hair. Also consider other environmental and chemical causes.

Thin and sparse hair. Hair becomes thin and fine in texture, with a somewhat sparse distribution. Color changes of some degree are usually present.

Face

Malar and supraorbital hyperpigmentation. Hyperpigmented areas with or without skin cracking. Do not confuse with Addison's Disease, or vitiligo.

TABLE 4–6. (*Continued*)

Moonface. Rounded prominence of cheeks, which protrude over the general level of the nasolabial folds. The mouth presents a pursed-in appearance (usually found in preschool children with kwashiorkor).

Pallor; diffuse depigmentation. Present in skin and mucous membranes.

Nasolabial dyssebacea. Consists of greasy, thread-like projections, greyish, yellowish, or pale in color, most commonly located in the nasolabial folds and nostrils. It may also be seen on the bridge of the nose, eyebrows, and back of the ears. May also be due to poor hygiene.

Lips

Angular scars. Healed lesions of angular stomtitis that, dependent on the time elapsed, may appear pink or blanched.

Angular stomatitis. Sodden and excoriated lesions associated with fissuring of the angles of the mouth. The fissures may be shallow or deep and may be confined to a small area at the angles or may extend into the mouth on the inside and a few millimeters onto the skin outside. Milder lesions are seen more easily with the mouth half open. The lesion should be noted only if both angles of the mouth are involved. Angular stomatitis may also be caused by poor denture fit, herpes, and syphilis.

Cheilosis. A lesion characterized by vertical fissuring, later complicated by redness, swelling, and ulceration of areas of lips other than angles. May also occur with environmental exposure.

Chronic depigmentation of lower lip. Usually central. May be healed cheilosis.

Tongue

Atrophic papillae. The papillae (taste buds) have disappeared, giving the tongue an extremely smooth appearance. The condition may be central or marginal. May also occur in nonnutritional anemia.

Edema of the tongue. Edematous indentations along the edge of the tongue.

Fissures. Cracks on the surface of the tongue, with no papillae on their sides or floors. Definite break in epithelium.

Geographic tongue. Tongue with irregularly distributed patchy areas of denudation and atrophy. Sometimes also appears on the gums.

Hyperemic and hypertrophic papillae. Papillae are hypertrophic and red or pink and give the tongue a granular or pebbly appearance (red strawberry). Also consider dietary irritants.

Magenta tongue. The tongue is purplish-red in color; numerous morphologic changes may co-exist.

Pigmented tongue. Punctate or patchy areas of mucosal pigmentation.

Scarlet and raw tongue (glossitis). The tongue is bright red in color, usually normal size or slightly atrophic, denuded, and very painful.

Teeth

Attrition. The cutting borders of incisors and the cusp of the molars may be flattened.

Caries. Dental decay.

Enamel erosion. Sharply defined areas of erosion usually around the gum margin.

Enamel hypoplasia. Defective formation of the enamel, usually generalized over tooth surface. To be distinguished from enamel abrasion due to mechanical causes.

Fluorosis. Mottled discoloration of tooth enamel resulting from excessive fluorine ingestion during tooth development. Presents as opaque paper white areas in the tooth enamel, ranging in size from a few flecks to entire enamel surface (in which case a brown stain is frequently seen).

Mottled enamel. Mottled tooth with chalky white and brownish areas with or without erosion of the enamel. Do not confuse with enamel hypoplasia or staining from tetraclyines taken during tooth development.

Gums

Recession of gum. Gum tissue atrophy sometimes exposing the roots of the teeth; often secondary to pyorrhea.

(*continued*)

TABLE 4–6. (*Continued*)

Spongy, bleeding gums. Purplish, spongy, swelling of the interdental papillae and/or gum margins. May bleed easily on slight pressure. May also be caused by chronic fluorosis or hydantoinates (Dilantin, etc.), poor hygiene, and lymphoma.

Glands

Gynecomastia. Bilateral enlargement of the nipple and glandular breast tisse (in men).

Parotid enlargement. Chronic, visible, noninflammatory swelling of the parotids (glands just below the earlobes); significant only if bilateral.

Thyroid enlargement. The gland is visible and palpably enlarged. Enlargement may be diffuse or nodular. Inspection and palpation while the patient swallows may be helpful in the diagnosis. Also caused by cysts, tumors, and hyperthyroidism.

Skin

Ecchymoses. Relatively large areas of hemorrhage under the skin.

Flaky paint dermatosis. Resembles cracked enamel paint. Extensive, often bilateral hyperpigmented patches of skin or superficial ulceration. It can occur anywhere but is characteristically present on the buttocks, backs of thighs, and perineum. Peel off to leave hypopigmented skin or superficial ulcers.

Follicular hyperkeratosis. (1) Lesion consists of hyperkeratosis surrounding the mouth of the hair follicle and forming the plaque that resembles a spine. It is readily detected by the spiky feeling it gives when the palm is passed over the lesion and has a characteristic distribution—frequently confined to the buttocks, thighs, and, in general, extensor aspects of the extremities. The surrounding skin is dry and lacks the usual amount of moisture and oiliness. (2) Follicular lesion is morphologically similar, but the mouths of the hair follicles contain blood or pigment. The intervening skin is not dry. The condition is usually seen in adults. The distribution is usually over the abdomen and extensor aspects of the thighs.

Intertriginous lesions. Raw, red and macerated lesions in skin flexors prone to constant friction, such as groins, buttocks, axillary folds; often secondarily infected.

Mosaic dermatosis. Seen on the skin over the shins; always bilateral. Large mosaic plaques are firmly adherent in the center but show a tendency to peel off at the periphery.

Pellagrous dermatosis. Typical skin lesions are symmetrical, clearly demarcated, hyperpigmented areas with or without exfoliation. The latter, when present, starts in the center of the patch. Lesions are common in exposed areas; when they appear round the neck, the condition is called Casal's necklace. *Acute:* red swollen with itching, cracking, and exudate. *Chronic:* dry, rough, thickened and scaly with brown pigmentation. Consider thermal, sun, or chemical burns and Addison's disease.

Petechiae. Small hemorrhagic spots on the skin or mucous membranes. Application of the blood pressure tourniquet may sometimes bring about petechiae. Also occurs in hematologic disorders, trauma, liver disease, and anticoagulant overdose.

Scrotal and vulval dermatosis. Desquamating lesion of the skin, often highly irritant. Secondary infection may intervene. Consider fungus infection.

Thickening and pigmentation of pressure points. Diffuse thickening, with pigmentation, of the pressure points, such as knees, elbows, and front and back of the ankles. The knuckles may also be involved. Affected areas may be wrinkled, with or without fissuring.

Xerosis. Generalized dryness with brawny desquamation. Consider environmental and hygiene factors, aging, hypothyroidism, uremia, ichthyosis.

Nails

Koilonychia. Bilateral spoon-shaped deformity of the nails in older children and adults. Consider Plummer-Vinson's syndrome (koilonychia, dysphagia, glossitis, anemia) and clubbing.

Transverse ridging or grooving of nails. Recorded if present in nails of more than one extremity.

TABLE 4–6. (*Continued*)

Subcutaneous Tissue

Edema. Usually apparent over ankles and feet and may extend to other areas of extremities; it may involve genitals, face, and serous cavities. In early stages detected by firm pressure for a few seconds on the lower portion of the medial surface of the tibia. The sign is taken as positive if there is a visible and palpable pit that persists after the pressure is removed. Occurs in conditions of sodium and water retention, pregnancy, protein-losing enteropathy, varicose veins, and stasis.

Fat. Increase or decrease determined by palpation of skinfold.

Muscular and Skeletal Systems

Beading of ribs. Symmetrical nodular enlargement of the costochondral junctions. Consider renal rickets and malabsorption.

Craniotabes. Lesions consist of areas of softening of the skull, usually involving the occipital and parietal bones. The bones dent on pressure and recoil after the pressure is removed. The sign is positive only in infancy.

Epiphyseal enlargement. Enlargement of the epiphyseal ends of long bones, particularly of radius and ulna at the level of the wrist, and tibia and fibula at the level of the ankle. Consider trauma, congenital deformity, renal disease, and malabsorption.

Frontal and parietal bossing. Thickening of the frontal and parietal eminences of the skull.

Intramuscular hematoma. Usually of calf or thigh; bleeding into muscle.

Knock-knees or bowlegs. Legs curve outward at the knees; legs bowed outward; consider congenital deformity.

Muscular wasting. In early stages, the condition is most obvious in the area of the shoulder girdle and upper arm. Prominence of body skeleton.

Winged scapula. Shoulder blades protrude; may be a sign of loss of muscle tone and wasting.

Internal Systems

Cardiovascular

Blood pressure. Elevated.

Cardiac enlargement. Enlarged heart. Generally nonnutritional; may occur in anemia and beriberi.

Tachycardia. Rapid heart rate; may occur in anemia and beriberi.

Gastrointestinal

Hepatomegaly. Enlarged liver; liver edge palpable more than 2 cm below costal margin; occurs with numerous medical conditions.

Nervous System

Calf tenderness. Squeeze calf muscle firmly between thumb and forefinger; significant only if bilateral; consider deep vein thrombosis, and peripheral neuropathy of other causes.

Condition of ocular fundus. Abnormalities of back of eyes, visible through opthalmoscope.

Loss of ankle and knee jerks. Significant only if absolute and bilateral. Consider peripheral neuropathy of other causes.

Loss of position sense

Loss of vibratory sense. Tested with tuning fork; significant only if bilateral.

Mental confusion. Confusion and irritability.

Motor weakness. Inability to squat and then stand three to four times in a row.

Sensory loss

Psychomotor change. Listlessness, apathy.

TABLE 4–7. DEFINITION AND DESCRIPTION OF PHYSICAL SIGNS NOT RELATED TO MALNUTRITION

Hair

Alopecia. Baldness.

Artificial discoloration. Chemical or environmental.

Face

Acne rosacea. Chronic condition of skin or nose, forehead, and cheeks. Red coloration is due to dilated capillaries plus acne-like skin elevations.

Acne vulgaris. Common acne. Chronic inflammation of sebaceous glands that produce small pink skin elevations generally on the face, back, and/or chest.

Eyes

Follicular conjunctivitis. Round or pinkish bodies under the eyelids.

Pannus. A virus-caused infection; cornea is invaded with blood vessels that causes it to appear cloudy or opaque.

Pingueculae. Small yellow or pigmented raised spots on the exposed sclera, generally close to the cornea. Generally seen in older people.

Pterygium. Wing-shaped tissue extending from the corner of the eye to the cornea.

Lips

Chapping. Exposure to harsh climate.

Tongue

Aphthous ulcer. Small ulcers, especially the reddish or whitish spots in the mouth that characterize "canker sores."

Leukoplakia. Thickened white patches on mucous membranes of the mouth.

Teeth

Malocclusion. Faulty meeting of teeth or jaws.

Gums

Pyorrhea. Chronic gum inflammation around teeth with gums receding; gums are red and bleed easily; gums generally are not swollen.

Glands

Allergic or inflammatory enlargement of thyroid and parotid.

Skin

Acneiform eruptions. Skin eruptions resembling acne.

Epidermophytoses. Fungal infection.

Folliculosis. Prominence of hair follicles on thighs and extensor surfaces of forearms and over pressure points; the surrounding skin is healthy; commonly observed in adolescents.

Ichthyosis. Dry, rough, scaly skin due to hypertrophy of the horny layer.

Miliaria. Sweat retention by inner skin layers. Produces small, pale or red lesions in the skin; also known as heat rash or prickly heat.

Sunburn

Muscular and Skeletal Systems

Funnel chest. Funnel-shaped deformity of front of chest wall.

Kyphoscoliosis. Backward and lateral curvature of the spinal column.

Internal Systems

Gastrointestinal

Splenomegaly. Enlarged spleen; usually nonnutritional.

TABLE 4–8. SIGNS USED FOR CLINICAL EVALUATION OF NUTRITION STATUS: EXAMINATION BY SYSTEMS

	Signs Indicating Probable Deficiency of One or More Nutrients at the Present Time or in Recent Past	Signs Indicating Probable Long-Term Malnutrition in Combination with Other Factors	Signs Not Related to Nutrition Status
Hair	Dyspigmentation Easy pluckability Flag sign Lack of luster Thin, sparse, hair		Alopecia Artificial coloration
Face	Moonface Nasolabial dyssebacea Pallor/diffuse depigmentation	Malar/supraorbital hyperpigmentation	Acne rosacea Acne vulgaris
Eyes	Angular palpebritis Bitot's spots Xerophthalmia/keratomalacia Xerosis (conjunctival and corneal)	Circumcorneal injection Circumcorneal and scleral pigmentation Conjunctival injection Corneal opacities and scars Corneal injection Blepharitis	Follicular conjunctivitis Pannus Pingueculae Pterygium
Lips	Angular scars Angular stomatitis Cheilosis	Chronic depigmentation of lower lip	Chapped lips
Tongue	Atrophic papillae Edema Glossitis Magenta tongue	Fissures Geographic tongue Hyperemic and hypertrophic papillae Pigmented tongue	Aphthous ulcer Leukoplakia
Teeth	Mottled enamel	Attrition Caries Enamel erosion Enamel hypoplasia	Malocclusion
Gums	Spongy, bleeding gums	Gum recession	Pyorrhea
Glands	Parotid enlargement Thyroid enlargement	Gynecomastia	Allergic or inflammatory enlargement of thyroid/parotid
Skin	Ecchymosis Flaky paint dermatosis Follicular hyperkeratosis (Types I and II) Pellagrous dermatosis Petechiae	Intertriginous lesions Mosaic dermatosis Thickening and pigmentation of pressure points	Acneiform eruptions Epidermophytoses Folliculosis Ichthyosis Miliaria Sunburn

(continued)

TABLE 4–8. (*Continued*)

	Signs Indicating Probable Deficiency of One or More Nutrients at the Present Time or in Recent Past	Signs Indicating Probable Long-Term Malnutrition in Combination with Other Factors	Signs Not Related to Nutrition Status
	Scrotal and vulval dermatosis		
	Xerosis		
Nails	Koilonychia	Transverse ridging/grooving	
Subcutaneous Tissue	Edema		
	Fat		
Musculoskeletal System	Beading of ribs	Deformities of the thorax	Funnel chest
	Craniotabes	Winged scapula	Kyphoscoliosis
	Epiphyseal enlargement		
	Frontal and parietal bossing		
	Intramuscular of subperiosteal hematoma		
	Knock-knees or bowlegs		
	Muscular wasting		
	Diffuse or local skeletal deformities		
Internal Systems			
Cardiovascular	Cardiac enlargement	Blood pressure	
	Tachycardia		
Gastrointestinal	Ascites		Splenomegaly
	Hepatomegaly		
Nervous	Apathy	Condition of ocular fundus	
	Irritability		
	Calf tenderness		
	Loss of ankle and knee jerks		
	Loss of position sense		
	Loss of vibratory sense		
	Mental confusion		
	Motor weakness		
	Sensory loss		
	Psychomotor change		

TABLE 4-9. GENERAL GUIDE FOR INTERPRETATION OF CLINICAL SIGNS OF MALNUTRITION

Nutrient Abnormality Name	Clinical Sign Associated with Deficiency
General	
Obesity	Excessive weight in relation to height (or other skeletal indices)
	Excessive skinfolds
Undernutrition	Apathy/irritability
(Starvation)	Low weight for height (or other skeletal indices)
	Exaggerated skeletal prominences/subcutaneous fat loss
	Loss of skin elasticity
Protein/Calorie	General: Edema
	Muscle wasting
	Low body weight for height (or other skeletal indices)
	Psychomotor changes
	Hair—dyspigmentation
	—easy pluckability
	—thin, sparse
	—lack of luster
	—flag sign
	Moonface
	Flaky paint dermatosis
	Diffuse skin depigmentation
	Parotid enlargement
	Cheilosis
	Small heart, decreased cardiac output
	Hepatomegaly (fatty)
	Delayed wound healing and tissue repair
	[a]Kwashiorkor: Edema
	Normal (or excessive) subcutaneous fat with normal or decreased muscle mass
	Hair easily pluckable
	[a]Marasmus: "Starved" appearance
	Depressed weight/height
	Depressed triceps skinfold and arm muscle circumference
Essential Fatty Acids	
EFA Deficiency	Scaly skin lesions
	Thrombocytopenia
	Poor wound healing
EFA Toxicity	High P/S fatty acid ratio may promote:
	Gallstone formation
	Elevated lithogenicity of bile
	Elevated bile salt formation
Water-Soluble Vitamins	
B-Complex Vitamins	General: Blepharitis
	Perioral angular fissures, scars, cheilosis, oral glossitis, atrophic papillae, weakness, paresthesias of legs
Thiamin	General: Loss of ankle jerks and knee jerks
(Beriberi)	Sensory loss and motor weakness
	Calf muscle tenderness; weak thighs

(*continued*)

TABLE 4–9. (*Continued*)

Nutrient Abnormality Name	Clinical Sign Associated with Deficiency
	Cardiovascular dysfunction; heart enlargement, tachycardia, high output failure
	Edema
	Ophthalmoplegia (Wernicke's syndrome)
	Neurologic: Ophthalmoplegia footdrop (Wernicke's syndrome)
	Confabulation, disorientation (Korsakoff's psychosis)
	Dry (atrophic) beriberi: Loss of ankle, knee jerks
	Sensory loss (paresthesia, hyperthesia, anesthesia)
	Fatigue, decreased attention span
	Wet beriberi: Above neurologic manifestations
	Above cardiovascular dysfunctions prominent (tachycardia, right-sided cardiac failure with systolic hypertension, venous distention, peripheral cyanosis, pulmonary congestion)
	Wernicke's encephalopathy: Neurologic (mild confusion to coma with ophthalmoplegia with 6th nerve weakness and lateral or vertical nystagmus; cerebellar ataxia; confabulation; permanent impairment of retentive memory, cognitive function; death, if untreated)
	Infantile beriberi: Acute cardiac failure
	Aphonia (silent crying)
	Clinical signs suggestive of meningitis
Riboflavin (Ariboflavinosis)	Angular stomatitis; angular scars
	Cheilosis
	Central atrophy of lingual papillae
	Magenta tongue
	Angular palpebritis
	Corneal vascularization
	Nasolabial dyssebacea
	Scrotal and vulval dermatosis
	Glossitis (oral)
Niacin/Tryptophan (Pellagra)	Pellagrous dermatosis
	Anorexia
	Gastric achlorhydria
	Small bowel atrophy/inflammation
	Diarrhea
	Scarlet and raw tongue (glossitis)
	Tongue fissuring
	Atrophic lingual papillae (hypertrophic fungiform papillae)
	Malar and supraorbital pigmentation
	Cheilosis
	Neurologic: apathy, neurasthenia; "pain" in extremities; peripheral neuropathy, myelopathy, encephalopathy
	Dermatologic lesions, generally bilateral
	Thickened hyperkeratotic/hyperpigmented skin without inflammation over exposed skin surface and pressure points

TABLE 4–9. *(Continued)*

Nutrient Abnormality Name	Clinical Sign Associated with Deficiency
	Macerated, erythematous skin lesions in moist areas (e.g., scrotum, vulva)
	Amenorrhea, increased abortion rate
Pyridoxine/B_6[b]	Neurologic: Peripheral neuropathy (sensory)
	Irritability/nervousness
	Apathy/depression
	Somnolence
	Convulsive seizures with electroencephalographic abnormalities
	Filiform hypertrophy of lingual papillae
	Aphthous stomatitis
	Nasolabial seborrhea
	Acneiform papular rash (forehead)
	Increased excretion of urinary xanthurenic acid
Pantothenic Acid[b]	Gastrointestinal: Vomiting
	Malaise
	Abdominal distress, cramps
	Heel tenderness
	Neurologic: Personality changes
	Insomnia
	Weakness and cramps in legs
	Paresthesia in hands and feet
Folic Acid/Vitamin B_{12}	Weakness, tiredness, headache, palpitation
	Dyspnea, sore tongue (glossitis), anorexia
	Paresthesia (vitamin B_{12} only)
	Constipation (especially vitamin B_{12})
	Diarrhea (especially folate)
	Megaloblastic bone marrow
	Anemia, leukopenia, thrombocytopenia, with macrooxalocytes and hypersegmented polys
	Fever
	Icteris plus pallor
	Neurologic (proven in vitamin B_{12} deficiency):
	Diminished vibration sense
	Diminished position sense
	Ataxia
	Neurologic (seen in folate and B_{12} deficiency):
	Paranoid ideation
	Impaired mentation
	Malabsorption
	Achylia (gastria)—primary in B_{12} deficiency; secondary in folate deficiency
	Weight loss (especially folate deficiency)
	Pigmentation, vitiligo
	Postural hypotension (especially B_{12} deficiency)
Biotin[b]	Scaly, eczematoid dermatitis (arms, legs, feet)
	Atrophy of lingual papillae, cheilosis

(continued)

TABLE 4–9. (*Continued*)

Nutrient Abnormality Name	Clinical Sign Associated with Deficiency

Vitamin C/Ascorbic Acid (Scurvy)	"Graying" of mucous membranes
	Increased skin dryness
	Depression, lassitude, anorexia, nausea
	Muscle cramps, paresthesia
	Hypercholesteremia
	Electrocardiogram abnormalities
	Adults: Anorexia, weakness
	    Neurasthenia, joint/muscle aching
	    Increased prominence of hair follicles on thighs and buttocks (follicular hyperkeratosis)
	    Perifollicular hemorrhages
	    Skin hemorrhage (petechial, ecchymoses—spread from lower extremities to rest of body, especially in areas exposed to trauma)
	    Muscle hemorrhages, in and around joints
	    GI mucosa hemorrhage
	    Kidney hemorrhage
	    Pericardium hemorrhage
	    Gums (gingiva) hemorrhagic then necrotic (scorbutic gums)
	    Interdental papillae become swollen, bluish red in color, may become secondarily infected. With time, teeth fall out.
	    Impaired healing of new wounds, dehiscence of old wounds (old wounds open at scar site)
	    Anemia
	Infants: Failure to thrive, apprehension of infant when handled
	    Irritability, tender extremities, pseudoparalysis
	    Purpuric lesions
	    Hemorrhage of gum adjacent to erupting teeth
	    Hemorrhage: Epistaxis
	             Retrobulbar hemorrhage
	             Hematuria
	             Bloody diarrhea
	    X-ray examination shows "ground glass" bone appearance, thinning of cortex
	    Anemia

Choline (Signs of deficiency seen in animals)	Mammals: Fatty infiltration of liver, hemorrhagic kidney damage Poultry: Perosis (tendon defect resulting in leg deformity) Man: Clinical deficiency manifestations unknown
Inositol (Signs of deficiency seen in animals)	Female gerbils: Hypocholesteremia, fat deposition in intestinal mucosa, dermatitis; weight loss with eventual death Man: Clinical deficiency manifestations unknown

Fat-Soluble Vitamins
Vitamin A
	Hypovitaminosis A: Night blindness
	                       Conjunctival, corneal xerosis
	                       Keratomalacia
	                       Bitot's spots
	                       Follicular keratosis (Type I)

TABLE 4–9. *(Continued)*

Nutrient Abnormality Name	Clinical Sign Associated with Deficiency
	Hypervitaminosis A: (Acute): Transient hydrocephalus
	Vomiting
	(Chronic): Fatigue, lethargy, malaise
	Abdominal discomfort
	Bone/joint pain
	Severe, throbbing headaches
	Insomnia, night sweats
	Restlessness
	Loss of body hair, brittle nails
	Constipation
	Irregular menses
	Emotional lability
	Dry, scaly, rough skin
	Peripheral edema
	Mouth fissures
	Exophthalmus
	Hypercarotenosis: Yellow skin (usually paleness of hands and soles of feet)
Vitamin D (Rickets)	Occurs in children: "Saber-skin" deformity
	Knobby deformities at end of long bones
	Epiphyseal displacement/muscular hypotonia
	Rachitic rosary; knock-knees, bowed legs
	Delayed tooth eruption
	Craniotabes (in infants)
	Delayed closure of the fontanelles (in infants)
	Skull "bossing"
	Dorsolumbar kyphosis/lordosis
	Radiologic findings: Concave cupping of epiphysis with spreading of epiphysis-metaphysis junction; inner cup margin fringing and stippling. Coarse trabeculae and thin cortex.
(Osteomalacia)	Occurs in adults: Affects shafts of long bones and flat bones (e.g., pelvis)
	Radiologic findings: Asymmetric pelvic deformity with narrowing of outlet; minute ribbon-like fractures of long bones
	Refer also to calcium
(Vitamin D Toxicity)	Hypervitaminosis D: Anorexia, nausea, vomiting, polyuria, polydipsia, weakness, nervousness, pruritis
	Renal function impairment
	Metastatic calcification (especially in kidney)
	Localized osteoporosis
Vitamin E (Vitamin E Deficiency)	Neuropathy (cerebellar hemorrhage, small blood vessel proliferation; absent Purkinje cells)
	Myopathy and creatinuria
	Ceroid pigment deposition in smooth muscle
Vitamin K	Depressed blood coagultion factors (i.e., elevated prothrombin time)

(continued)

TABLE 4–9. (*Continued*)

Nutrient Abnormality Name	Clinical Sign Associated with Deficiency
Major Minerals	
Calcium	
(Hypocalcemia)	Bone demineralization
	Neurologic: Mild, diffuse encephalopathy, laryngospasm, convulsions (serum Ca below 7 mg/dl)
	Tetany: Paresthesias of lips, tongue, fingers, feet
	Carpopedal spasm
	Spasm to facial musculature
	Refer also to vitamin D
(Hypercalcemia)	Constipation
	Anorexia, nausea and vomiting
	Abdominal pain; ileus
	Polyuria, nocturia
	Neurologic: Emotional lability, confusion, delirium, psychosis, coma, stupor (serum Ca above 12 mg/dl)
	Skeletal muscle weakness
	Shock, renal failure, death (Ca above 18 mg/dl)
Phosphorus	
(Hypophosphotemia)	Weakness, paresthesia, confusion
	Malaise, anorexia
	Skeletal aches
	Convulsions, death
(Hyperphosphatemia)	When combined with hypocalcemia and exacerbated by phosphate feeding or infusion:
	Enhanced neuroexcitability, tetany, convulsions
Magnesium	Anorexia
(Hypomagnesemia)	Nausea, vomiting
	Lethargy, weakness, tremor
	Personality change
	Tetany (i.e., positive Trousseau or Chvostek sign or spontaneous cardopedal spasm)
	Muscle fasciculations
	Depression of deep tendon reflexes
	Hypotension
	Respiratory depression
	Deep anesthesia, cardiac arrest
Iron	
(Iron deficiency anemia)	Hypochromic, microcytic anemia
	Weakness, increased fatigability
	Pallor, dyspnea on exertion, palpitation
	Coldness, paresthesias of hands and feet
	Capricious appetite, flatulence
	Epigastric distress with eructation
	Constipation or diarrhea
	Nausea
	Pica (i.e., geophagia, starch-eating, pagophagia)
	Glossitis, angular stomatis
	Patterson-Kelly's syndrome (dysphagia, hypochromic anemia, postcricoid esophageal stricture)

TABLE 4–9. (*Continued*)

Nutrient Abnormality Name	Clinical Sign Associated with Deficiency
(Iron overload, hemochromatosis)	Lusterless, brittle, thin fingernails and toenails Koilonychia Cardiac dilation, vitiligo, dependent edema (Hgb less than 6 g/dl) Cirrhosis Diabetes, pituitary failure Hyperpigmentation of the skin (bronze) Cardiac failure (often preceded by atrial arrhythmias)
Sodium (Hyponatremia)	Change in mental status Lethargy, confusion If progressive: Stupor, neuromuscular hyperexcitability, convulsions, prolonged coma, death
(Hypernatremia)	CNS dysfunction characterized by: Confusion, neuromuscular hyperexcitability, seizures, coma
Potassium (Hypokalemia)	Muscular weakness, paralysis, respiratory failure Muscular malfunction, respiratory hypoventilation, paralytic ileus, hypotension, muscle twitches, tetany Premature atrial and ventricular contractions Ventricular and atrial tachycardia
(Hyperkalemia)	Nodal and ventricular arrhythmias
Chloride (Hypochloremia)	In infants: Vomiting, diarrhea, metabolic alkalosis, growth retardation NOTE: Changes in plasma chloride concentration generally follow those of plasma sodium concentration
Trace Minerals Iodine (Iodine deficiency)	Goiter
Copper (Copper deficiency)	Anemia, leukopenia, neutropenia Skeletal demineralization (osteoporosis), metaphyseal spur formation, soft tissue calcification Kinky (steely) hair Depigmentation of skin and hair Hypothermia Seizures and cerebral degeneration
(Copper intoxication)	Nausea, vomiting Epigastric pain, diarrhea, ptyalism Headache, dizziness Weakness, metallic taste Tachycardia, hypertension, coma Jaundice, hemolytic anemia, hemoglobinuria Uremia, death
Zinc (Zinc deficiency)	Anemia, depressed cell-mediated immunity, iron deficiency Hepatosplenomegaly, hypogonadism, poor growth Anorexia, hypogeusia Diarrhea

(*continued*)

TABLE 4–9. (*Continued*)

Nutrient Abnormality Name	Clinical Sign Associated with Deficiency
(Zinc toxicity)	Mental depression Alopecia Moist excemoid rash (paranasal, oral, perioral, groin) Geophagia Nausea, vomiting Stomach cramps Diarrhea, fever
Manganese (Manganese deficiency)	Weight loss Transient dermatitis Nausea and vomiting Changes in hair/beard color, slow hair growth Hypocholesterolemia
(Manganese toxicity)	Neurologic changes resembling Parkinson's and Wilson's diseases (i.e., cerebellar ataxia, tremor, progressive neuron destruction)
Cobalt (Cobalt deficiency)	See vitamin B_{12} deficiency
(Cobalt toxicity)	Congestive heart failure Polycythemia Pericardial effusion Thyroid hyperplasia Neurologic abnormalities
Chromium (Chromium deficiency)	Glucose intolerance Peripheral neuropathy (mental confusion) Weight loss
Molybdenum (Molybdenum deficiency)	Amino acid intolerance clinically characterized by tachycardia, tachypnea, central scotomas, night blindness, irritability, coma
Selenium (Selenium deficiency)	Muscle pain, tenderness (leg) Cardiomyopathy characterized by ventricular fibrillation, extrasystoles, tachycardia, pulmonary edema, cardiomegaly
(Selenium toxicity)	Skin: Burns, pruritic red papules, brittle nails Hair: Alopecia GI: Nausea, vomiting, gastrointestinal pain, "metallic taste" CNS: Weakness, depression
Fluoride (Fluoride deficiency)	Increased dental caries Bone thinning
(Fluoride toxicity)	Chronic edemic dental fluorosis: Mottled teeth

[a]Marasmus and kwashiorkor may co-exist in the same patient.
[b]Many clinical signs/symptoms experimentally seen by inducing dietary deficiency along with using vitamin antagonists.

BIBLIOGRAPHY

Medical History Review

Grant A: Nutritional Assessment Guidelines, 2nd ed. Berkeley, Calif: Cutter Medical, 1979

Van Itallie TB: Malnutrition: Concepts of pathogenesis and treatment. In Wintrobe MM, Thorn GW, Adams RD, et al. (eds): Harrison's Principles of Internal Medicine, 7th ed. New York: McGraw-Hill, 1974, pp 415–417

Diet History and Nutrition Care Plan

Becker BG, Indik BP, Beeuwkes AM: Dietary Intake Methodologies: A Review. Tech Rep 03188–2, T. Ann Arbor: University of Michigan School of Public Health, 1960

Burke BS: The dietary history as a tool in research. J Amer Diet Assoc 23:1041, 1947

Danish SJ, Guinsberg MR, Terrell A, et al.: The anatomy of a dietetic counseling interview. J Amer Diet Assoc 75:626–629, 1979

Forcier JI, Knight MA, Sheehan ET: Point of view: Acculturation in clinical dietetics. J Amer Diet Assoc 70:181, 1977

Foster JT: A hospital administratory view of the shared responsibility. J Amer Diet Assoc 76:539, 1975

The American Dietetic Association: Handbook of Clinical Dietetics. New Haven, Conn: Yale University Press, 1981, p 113

Van Itallie TB: Assessment of Nutritional Status. In Wintrobe MM, Thorn GW, Adams RD, et al.: Harrison's Principles of Internal Medicine, 7th ed. New York: McGraw-Hill, 1974, pp 418–422

Hayes-Bautista DE: Modifying the treatment: Patient compliance, patient control, and medical care. Soc Sci Med 10:233, 1976

Huenemann RL, Turner D: Methods of dietary investigation. J Amer Diet Assoc 18:562, 1942

Hunt SM, Groff JL, Holbrook JM: Nutrition: Principles and Clinical Practice. New York: John Wiley, 1980, Chapter 12

Krause MV, Mahan LK: Food Nutrition and Diet Therapy, 6th ed. Philadelphia: W.B. Saunders, 1979

Marr JW, Heady JA, Morris JN: Towards a method for large scale individual diet surveys. Proc 3rd Intl Cong Diet, 1961, p 85

Mason M, Wenberg BG, Welsh PK: The Dynamics of Clinical Dietetics, 2nd ed. New York: John Wiley, 1982

Suitor CW, Hunter MF: Nutrition: Principles and Application in Health Promotion. Philadelphia: J.B. Lippincott, 1980

Wade J: Role of a clinical dietitian specialist on a nutrition support service. J Amer Diet Assoc 70:185, 1977

Weise J: Dietary Interviewing (Cassette). Amer Diet Assoc, 1976

Young CM, Hagan CG, Tucker RE, Foster WD: A comparison of dietary study methods. J Amer Diet Assoc 35:677, 1959

Young CM: The interview itself. J Amer Diet Assoc 35:677, 1959

Zifferblatt SM, Wilbur CS: Dietary counseling: Some realistic expectations and guidelines. J Amer Diet Assoc 70:591, 1977

Physical Assessment

General References

Abraham S: Preliminary Findings of the First Health and Nutrition Examination Survey, United States, 1971–1972. Anthropometric and Clinical Findings. DHEW Publication No. (HRA) 75–1229, Rockville, Md, USDHEW, 1975

Berkow R (ed): The Merck Manual of Diagnosis and Therapy, 13th ed. Rahway, NJ: Merck & Co, 1977

Christakis G (ed): Nutritional assessment in health programs. Am J Public Health 63:part II, November, 1973

Dorlands' Illustrated Medical Dictionary, 25th Edition. Philadelphia: W.B. Saunders, 1974

Grant A: Clinical assessment. In Grant A (ed): Nutritional Assessment Guidelines. Berkeley: Cutter Laboratories, 1979

Isaksson B: Recommended methods used in nutritional status assessment: Clinical signs and symptoms. Bibl Nutrition Diet 20:52–61, 1974

Jellife DB: Direct nutritional assessment of human groups. In Jelliffe DB (ed): The Assessment of the Nutritional Status of the Community. WHO Monograph series No. 53. Geneva: World Health Organization, 1966, pp 10–96

Sandstead HH: Clinical manifestations of certain classical deficiency diseases. In Goodhart RS, Shils ME (eds): Modern Nutrition in Health and Disease, 6th ed. Philadelphia: Lea & Febiger, 1980

World Health Organization—Expert Committee on Medical Assessment of Nutritional Status. WHO Technical Report Series No. 258, Geneva: World Health Organization, 1963

Specific Nutrient Deficiencies

Calories and Proteins

Butterworth CE, Weinsier RL: Malnutrition in hospitalized patients: Assessment and treatment. In Goodhart RS, Shils ME (eds): Modern Nutrition in Health and Disease, 6th ed. Philadelphia: Lea & Febiger, 1980, pp 667–684

DeMaeyer EM: Protein-energy malnutrition. In Beaton GH, Bengoa JM (eds): Nutrition in Preventive Medicine. WHO Monograph Series No. 62. Geneva: World Health Organization, 1976, pp 23–54

Essential Fatty Acids

Grant A: Clinical Assessment. In Grant A (ed): Nutritional Assessment Guidelines. Berkeley: Cutter Laboratories, 1979

Viteri FE, Torún B: Protein-calorie malnutrition. In Goodhart RS, Shils ME (eds): Modern Nutrition in Health and Disease, 6th ed. Philadelphia: Lea & Febiger, 1980, pp 697–720

Faulkner WJ, Flint LM: Essential fatty acid deficiency associated with total parenteral nutrition. Surg Gynecol Obstet 144:665–667, 1977

Thiamin

Chang M, Gill T: Hypothermia, neurologic dysfunction, and sudden death in a man with carcinoma. South Med J 74(12):1509–13, 1981

Gardner TW, Rao K, Poticha S, Wertz R: Acute visual loss after gastroplasty (letter). Am J Ophthalmol 93(5):658–60, 1982

Gill GV, Bell DR: Persisting nutritional neuropathy amongst former war prisoners. J Neurol Neurosurg Psychiatry 45(10):861–5, 1982

Harper CG: Confusion, coma, and death from a preventable disease. Med J Aust 2(5):219–21, 1981

Kâtsura E, Oiso T: Beriberi. In Beaton GH, Bengoa, JM (eds): Nutrition in Preventive Medicine. WHO Monograph Series, No. 62. Geneva: World Health Organization, 1976, pp 136–145

MacLean JB: Wernicke's encephalopathy after gastric plication (letter). JAMA 248(11):1311, 1982

Milius G, Rose S, Owen DR, Schenken JR: Probable acute thiamine deficiency secondary to gastric partition for morbid obesity. Nebr Med J 67(6):147–50, 1982

Neal RA, Sauberlich HE: Thiamin. In Goodhart RS, Shils ME (eds): Modern Nutrition in Health and Disease, 6th ed. Philadelphia: Lea & Febiger, 1980, pp 197–204

Rothrock JF, Smith MS: Wernicke's disease complicating surgical therapy for morbid obesity. J Clin Neurol Ophthalmol 1(3):195–9, 1981

Tampi R, Alexander WS: Wernicke's encephalopathy with central pontine myelinolysis presenting with hypothermia. NZ Med J 95(708):342–4, 1982

Riboflavin

Horwitt MK: Riboflavin. In Goodhart RS, Shils ME (eds): Modern Nutrition in Health and Disease, 6th ed. Philadelphia: Lea & Febiger, 1980, pp 197–204

Niacin

Barakat MR: Pellagra. In Beaton GH, Bengoa JM (eds): Nutrition in Preventive Medicine, WHO Monograph Series No. 62. Geneva: World Health Organization, 1976, pp 126–135

dos Santos JR, Vannucchi H, Marchini JS, Dutra de Oliveira J: Nutritional care of hospitalized patients in Brazil with particular reference to pellagra and alcoholism as complicating factors. Prog Clin Biol Res 77:719–27, 1981

Horwitt MK: Niacin. In Goodhart RS, Shils ME (eds): Modern Nutrition in Health and Disease, 6th ed. Philadelphia: Lea & Febiger, 1980, pp 204–209

Vitamin B_6

Minns R: Vitamin B_6 deficiency and dependency. Dev Med Child Neurol 22(6):795–9, 1980

Sauberlich HE, Canham JE: Vitamin B_6. In Goodhart RS, Shils ME (eds): Modern Nutrition in Health and Disease, 6th ed. Philadelphia: Lea & Febiger, 1980, pp 216–229

Pantothenic Acid

Sauberlich HE: Pantothenic Acid. In Goodhart RS, Shils ME (eds): Modern Nutrition in Health and Disease, 6th ed. Philadelphia: Lea & Febiger, 1980, pp 209–216

Folic Acid and Vitamin B_{12}

Botez MI: Hypotonia and folate deficiency in children. (letter). J Pediatr 96(4):774, 1980

Dans CV: Tobacco-alcohol amblyopia: A proposed biochemical basis for pathogenesis. Med Hypotheses 7(11):1317–28, 1981

Herbert V, Colman N, Jacob E: Folic acid and vitamin B_{12}. In Goodhart RS, Shils ME (eds): Modern Nutrition in Health and Disease, 6th ed. Philadelphia: Lea & Febiger, 1980, pp 229–258

Kosik KS, Mullins TF, Bradley WG, et al.: Coma and axonal degeneration in vitamin B_{12} deficiency. Arch Neurol 37(9):590–2, 1980

Layrisse M, Roche M, Baker SJ: Nutritional anaemias. In Beaton GH, Bengoa JM (eds): Nutrition in Preventive Medicine. WHO Monograph Series No. 62. Geneva: World Health Organization, 1976, pp 55–82

Munoz-Garcia D, Del Ser T, Bermajo F, Portera A: Truncal ataxia in chronic anticonvulsant treatment. Association with drug-induced folate deficiency. J Neurol Sci 55(3):305–11, 1982

Semple CG, Williamson JM: Pernicious anaemia in a young man presenting with dyspepsia. Postgrad Med J 58(681)439–40, 1982

Zucker DK, Livingston RL, Nakra R, Clayton PJ: B_{12} deficiency and psychiatric disorders: Case report and literature review. Biol Psychiatry 16(2):197–205, 1981

Biotin

Appel JA, Briggs GM: Biotin. In Goodhart RS, Shils ME (eds): Modern Nutrition in Health and Disease, 6th ed. Philadelphia: Lea & Febiger, 1980, pp 274–279

Bozian RC, Moussavian N, Piepmeyer JL: Biotin deficiency during prolonged home total parenteral nutrition. Am J Clin Nutr 34:622, 1981

Ascorbic Acid

Connelly TJ, Becker A, McDonald JW: Bachelor scurvy. Int J Dermatol 21(4):209–11, 1982

Hodges RE: Ascorbic acid. In Goodhart RS, Shils ME (eds): Modern Nutrition in Health and Disease. Philadelphia: Lea & Febiger, 1980, pp 259–274

Hodges RE: Scurvy. In Beaton GH, Bengoa JM (eds): Nutrition in Preventive Medicine, WHO Monograph Series No. 62. Geneva: World Health Organization, 1976, pp 120–125

Choline

Appel JA, Briggs GM: Choline. In Goodhart RS, Shils ME (eds): Modern Nutrition in Health and Disease, 6th ed. Philadelphia: Lea & Febiger, 1980, pp 282–286

Inositol

Appel JA, Briggs GM: Inositol. In Goodhart RS, Shils ME (eds): Modern Nutrition in Health and Disease, 6th ed. Philadelphia: Lea & Febiger, 1980, pp 286–291

Vitamin A

Domen HAPC: Xerophthalmia. In Beaton GH, Bengoa JM (eds): Nutrition in Preventive Medicine. WHO Monograph Series No. 62. Geneva: World Health Organization, 1976, pp 94–110

Lui NST, Roels OA: Vitamin A and Carotene. In Goodhart RS, Shils ME (eds): Modern Nutrition in Health and Disease, 6th ed. Philadelphia: Lea & Febiger, 1980, pp 142–159

Menon K, Vijayarashavan K: Sequelae of severe xerophthalmia—a follow-up study. Am J Clin Nutr 33(2):218–20, 1980

Vitamin D

Danielsson A, Lorentzon R, Larsson SE: Normal hepatic vitamin-D metabolism in icteric primary biliary cirrhosis associated with pronounced vitamin-D deficiency symptoms. Hepatogastroenterology 29(1):6–8, 1982

DeLuca HF: Vitamin D. In Goodhart RS, Shils ME (eds): Modern Nutrition in Health and Disease, 6th ed. Philadelphia: Lea & Febiger, 1980, pp 160–169

Hey H, Lund B, Sirensen OH, Lund B: Delayed fracture healing following jejunoileal bypass surgery for obesity. Calcif Tissue Int 34(1):13–5, 1982

Paunler L: Rickets and osteomalacia. In Beaton GH, Bengoa JM (eds): Nutrition in Preventive Medicine. WHO Monograph Series No. 62. Geneva: World Health Organization, 1976, pp 111–119

Siegle RL, Rabinowitz JG: Radiographic findings resembling scurvy and rickets in prematures on hyperalimentation. Mt Sinai J Med (NY) 48(3):241–5, 1981

Toomey F, Hoag R, Batton D, Vain N: Rickets associated with cholestasis and parenteral nutrition in premature infants. Radiology 142(1):85–8, 1982

Watson RC, Grossman H, Meyers MA: Radiologic findings in nutritional disturbances. In Goodhart RS, Shils ME (eds): Modern Nutrition in Health and Disease, 6th ed. Philadelphia: Lea & Febiger, 1980, pp 641–666

Vitamin E

Drake JR, Fitch CD: Status of vitamin E as an erythropoietic factor. Am J Clin Nutr 33:2386–2393, 1980

Guggenheim MA, Rinsel SP, Silverman A, et al.: Progressive neuromuscular disease in children with chronic cholestasis and vitamin E deficiency: Clinical and muscle biopsy findings and treatment with alpha-tocopherol. Ann NY Acad Sci 393:84–95, 1982

Horwitt MK: Therapeutic uses of vitamin E in medicine. Nutrition Review 38:105–113, 1980

Horwitt MK: Vitamin E. In Goodhart RS, Shils

ME (eds): Modern Nutrition in Health and Disease, 6th ed. Philadelphia: Lea & Febiger, 1980, pp 181–190

Howard L, Ovesen L, Satya-Murti S, Chu R: Reversible neurological symptoms caused by vitamin E deficiency in a patient with short bowel syndrome. Am J Clin Nutr 36(6):1243–9, 1982

Lloyd BW, Dubowitz V: Progressive neurological disorder associated with obstructive jaundice and vitamin E deficiency. Neuropediatrics 13(3):155–7, 1982

Rosenblum JL, Keating JP, Prensky AL, Nelson JS: A progressive neurologic syndrome in children with chronic liver disease. N Engl J Med 304(9):503–8, 1981

Vitamin K

Olsen RE: Vitamin K. In Goodhart RS, Shils ME (eds): Modern Nutrition in Health and Disease, 6th ed. Philadelphia: Lea & Febiger, 1980, pp 170–180

Calcium, Phosphorus, Fluoride

Avioli LV: Calcium and Phosphorus. In Goodhart RS, Shils ME (eds): Modern Nutrition in Health and Disease, 6th ed. Philadelphia: Lea & Febiger, 1980, pp 294–310

Shaw JH, Sweeney EA: Nutrition in relation to dental medicine. In Goodhart RS, Shils ME (eds): Modern Nutrition in Health and Disease, 6th ed. Philadelphia: Lea & Febiger, 1980, pp 852–891

Magnesium

Shils ME: Magnesium. In Goodhart RS, Shils ME (eds): Modern Nutrition in Health and Disease, 6th ed. Philadelphia: Lea & Febiger, 1980, pp 310–324

Vincent JL, Buset M, Dufaye P, et al.: Circulatory shock associated with magnesium depletion. Intensive Care Med 8(3):149–52, 1982

Iron

Beutler E: Iron. In Goodhart RS, Shils ME (eds): Modern Nutrition in Health and Disease, 6th ed. Philadelphia: Lea & Febiger, 1980, pp 324–355

Sodium, Potassium, Chloride

Randall HT: Water, electrolytes and acid-base balance. In Goodhart RS, Shils ME (eds): Modern Nutrition in Health and Disease, 6th ed. Philadelphia: Lea & Febiger, 1980, pp 355–395

Simopoulos AP, Bartter FC: The metabolic consequences of chloride deficiency. Nutrition Review 38:201–205, 1980

Trace Minerals—General

Beaton GH: Some other nutritional deficiencies. In Beaton GH, Bengoa JM (eds): Nutrition in Preventive Medicine. WHO Monograph Series No. 62. Geneva: World Health Organization, 1976, pp 146–158

Sandstead HH, Burk RF, Booth GH, Darby WJ: Current concepts on trace minerals: Clinical considerations. Med Clin North Am 54:1509–1531, 1970

Burch RE, Sullivan JF: Diagnosis of zinc, copper, and maganese abnormalities in man. Med Clin North Am 60:655–660, 1976

Fleming CR, McGill DB, Hoffman HN, Nelson RA: Total parenteral nutrition. Mayo Clinic Proc 51:187–199, 1976

Li TK, Vallee BL: The biochemical and nutritional roles of other trace elements. In Goodhart RS, Shils ME (eds): Modern Nutrition in Health and Disease, 6th ed. Philadelphia: Lea & Febiger, 1980, pp 395–408

Iodine

Cavalieri RR: Iodine. In Goodhart RS, Shils ME (eds): Modern Nutrition in Health and Disease, 6th ed. Philadelphia: Lea & Febiger, 1980, pp 395–408

Clements FW: Endemic goiter. In Beaton GH, Bengoa JM (eds): Nutrition in Preventive Medicine. WHO Monograph Series No. 62. Geneva: World Health Organization, 1976, pp 83–93

Copper

Heller, RM, Kirchner SG, O'Neill JA, et al.: Skeletal changes of copper deficiency in infants receiving prolonged total parenteral nutrition. J Pediatr 92:947–949, 1978

Tanaka Y, Hatano S, Nishi Y, Usui T: Nutritional copper deficiency in a Japanese infant on formula. J Pediatr 96:255–256, 1980

Zinc

Burch RE, Sullivan JF: Clinical and nutritional aspects of zinc deficiency and excess. Med Clin North Am 60:675–685, 1976

Cavdar UH: Zinc deficiency and geophagia (letter). J Pediatr 100(6):1003–4, 1982

Kay RG, Tasman-Jones C, Rybus J, et al.: A syndrome of acute zinc deficiency during parenteral alimentation in man. Ann Surg 183:331–340, 1976

Michie DD, MacFarlane MD, Wirth FH: Zinc and total parenteral nutrition. South Med J 70:985–986, 1977

Pekarek RS, Sanstead HH, Jacob RA, Barcome DF: Abnormal cellular immune responses during acquired zinc deficiency. Am J Clin Nutr 32:1466–1471, 1979

Strobel CT, Byrne WJ, Abramovits W, et al.: A zinc-deficiency dermatitis in patients on total parenteral nutrition. Intern J Dermatol 17:575–581, 1978

Weber TR, Sears N, Davies B, Grosfeld JL: Clinical spectrum of zinc deficiency in pediatric patients receiving total parenteral nutrition (TPN). J Pediatr Surg 16(3):236–40, 1981

Manganese

Burch RE, Sullivan JF: Diagnosis of zinc, copper, and manganese abnormalities in man. Med Clin North Am 60:655–660, 1976

Chromium

Freund H, Atamian S, Fischer JE: Chromium deficiency during total parenteral nutrition. JAMA 241:496–498, 1979

Jeejeebhoy KN, Chu RC, Marliss EB, et al.: Chromium deficiency, glucose intolerance, and neuropathy reversed by chromium supplementation, in a patient receiving long-term total parenteral nutrition. Am J Clin Nutr 30:531–538, 1977

Molybdenum

Abumrad NN, Schneider AJ, Steele D, Rogers LS: Amino acid intolerance during prolonged total parenteral nutrition (TPN) reversed by molybdenum. Am J Clin Nutr 34:618, 1981

Selenium

Diskin CJ, Tomasso CL, Alper JC, et al.: Long-term selenium exposure. Arch Intern Med 139:824–826, 1979

Johnson RA, Baker SS, Fallon JT, et al.: An accidental case of cardiomyopathy and selenium deficiency. N Engl J Med 304:1210–1212, 1981

Thomson CD, Robinson MF: Selenium in human health and disease with emphasis on those aspects peculiar to New Zealand. Am J Clin Nutr 33:303–323, 1980

VanRij AM, Thomson CD, McKenzie JM, Robinson MF: Selenium deficiency in total parenteral nutrition. Am J Clin Nutr 32:2076–2085, 1979

5. Laboratory Values and Their Interpretation

Connie Stone Williams

Laboratory measurements yield useful material for evaluating nutrition status. Biochemical data obtained routinely in the clinical environment or in developmental research can often objectively estimate nutrition depletion or monitor nutrition support.

Generally, laboratory data employed in assessing nutrition status can be categorized into three main sections: (1) assessment of protein nutriture with laboratory data, (2) effect of stress and starvation on laboratory data, and (3) developmental research with laboratory data.

In the first section of this chapter, the assessment of protein nutriture includes serum albumin, serum transferrin, serum prealbumin or thyroxine-binding prealbumin, retinol-binding protein, creatinine–height index (CHI), and urine urea nitrogen (UUN).

The effect of stress and starvation on the various serum laboratory values of uric acid, cholesterol, creatinine, blood urea nitrogen (BUN), calcium and phosphorus, magnesium, zinc, white cell count, total lymphocyte count (TLC), and liver function tests is discussed in the second section.

The third section highlights the use of 3-methylhistidine excretion and indirect calorimetry as methods of developmental research with laboratory data.

ASSESSMENT OF PROTEIN NUTRITURE WITH LABORATORY DATA

Serum Albumin

Definition and Physiologic Function. Serum albumin is a protein of the blood that is synthesized by the hepatocyte, contributing a large body pool of 4 to 5 g/kg.[1] Albumin functions to maintain colloid oncotic pressure, which includes the movement of the extracellular fluid between the intravascular and interstitial compartments, and aids in carrying enzymes, hormones, drugs, metals, fatty acids, ions, and metabolites.[2]

Method of Testing and Normal Range. A measurement of serum albumin is obtained by a blood specimen and easily performed in many laboratories. In interpreting a serum albumin concentration, normal concentration levels are 3.5 to 5.5 g/dl.[3] In general, a serum albumin concentration from 2.8 to 3.5 g/dl represents moderate visceral protein depletion and less than 2.8 g/dl denotes severe depletion.[4] Due to its relatively long half-life of 17 to 20 days, albumin cannot indicate early protein malnutrition.[2] According to

Whitehead et al.,[5] a serum albumin of 3.0 g/dl is a marker for the appearance of early edema and kwashiorkor.

Nutritional Significance. Serum albumin is widely used as a biochemical method of determining visceral protein status.[4,6-8] A depressed serum albumin is utilized as the primary method of detecting inadequate intakes of protein and diagnosing protein–calorie malnutrition (PCM).[9,10] Bistrian et al.[4,7] investigated PCM in a municipal hospital. In these studies, serum albumin was correlated with other nutrition assessment parameters and substantiated a prevalence of malnutrition in approximately 50 percent of a surgical patient population and 44 percent of general medical patients. Similarly, Willcutts[6] found serum albumin, as part of the nutrition assessment, an aid in identifying moderate to severe malnutrition in 65 percent of the 1000 surgical patients in his study. Weinsier et al.[11] concluded a low serum albumin concentration is a common finding in PCM.

Serum albumin has some value in predicting the morbidity and mortality rates of surgical and nonsurgical patients. Since serum albumin or any other available laboratory technique is not totally specific for malnutrition, some investigators have proposed developing nutrition profiles or indexes combining several parameters to predict the morbidity and mortality rates of surgical patients.[12-14]

In 161 patients undergoing major elective surgery, Mullen et al.[14] found four of their nutrition assessment parameters measured preoperatively could assist in predicting major postoperative complications and survival. The equation that utilizes these parameters describes the possibility of complications for the surgical patient:

$$\text{Prognostic Nutrition Index (PNI) \%} =$$
$$158 - (16.6 \times \text{ALB}) - (0.78 \times \text{TSF}) -$$
$$(0.2 \times \text{TFN}) - (5.8 \times \text{DH})$$

where

ALB = serum albumin (g/dl)
TSF = triceps skinfold thickness (mm)
TFN = serum transferrin (mg/dl)
DH = delayed hypersensitivity (reaction to any of 3 recall antigens) 0 = nonreactive; 1 = less than 5 mm reactivity; 2 = greater than or equal to 5 mm reactivity.

This predictive model has been tested and validated by Mullen et al.[13] and Buzby [15] to identify the surgical patients who require preoperative nutrition support to reduce operative morbidity and mortality. In a study by Jones et al.,[16] however, the PNI was found inconclusive as a predictor of complications following trauma. Presently the PNI is used to predict the risk of morbidity and mortality for the surgical patient, while research continues to reconcile this discrepancy.

In the nonsurgical patient, Morath et al.[17] noted several nutrition deficits at postburn day 10, including a serum albumin of less than 3.0 g/dl, identifying those burn patients at risk for development of sepsis.

A study performed at the New England Deaconess Hospital[18] validated that albumin correlated with anergy, sepsis, and mortality. In this study's conclusion, a nutrition assessment with a serum albumin was found as a means to evaluate high-risk hospitalized patients and response to nutrition therapy.

Anderson and Wochos[19] found a low serum albumin was the most common nutrition-related laboratory measurement associated with infected patients and longer hospital stay.

With the inclusion of serum albumin, nutrition screening may serve as an indicator for the sophisticated or more complicated methods of nutrition assessment. For health · professionals without a nutrition support team in their institution, adequate time for a thorough nutrition assessment may be unavailable. Serum albumin can be utilized as a nutrition screening device since it is usually acquired by routine admission laboratory tests.[20]

After completion of nutrition screening on 500 consecutive admissions, Seltzer et al.[20] found an abnormal serum albumin presented a fourfold increase in complications and a sixfold increase in deaths. The use of an instant nutrition screening method appears to serve as a warning for future complications and deaths, although a simplified method of assessing nutrition status contains certain flaws. This immediate screening should not be expected to identify those patients with early signs of PCM that require more elaborate means of detection or patients developing malnutrition after admission to the institution. This would require additional laboratory data.

Factors That Affect Validity. There are various factors and incidents that interfere with the reliability of serum albumin. Hypoalbuminemia can occur in nephrotic syndrome, multiple myeloma, chronic constrictive pericarditis, leprosy, acute or chronic inflammation, hypervitaminosis A, rheumatoid arthritis, chronic renal insufficiency, hepatic failure, alcohol hepatitis, and protein-losing enteropathy.[3] In protein-losing enteropathy, hypoalbuminemia may be the result of excessive loss of plasma proteins in the intestinal lumen, which is usually secondary to a malabsorption syndrome.[21] Additionally, a decreased serum albumin occurs in individuals with trauma (i.e., burns), non-enteropathic diarrhea, fistulas, draining wounds, and infections.[22]

Albumin or blood may be given to a patient following an injury or surgery. After moderate hemorrhage, the body's blood volume should restore itself within 24 hours due to shifts of fluid and the aid of serum albumin. If the serum albumin is extremely deficient, albumin may be infused to maintain fluid within the vascular space. This may alter the serum albumin concentration.[21]

Fluid status influences plasma protein levels and can alter their interpretation.[2] In patients with dehydration, serum albumin is elevated as a result of diminished plasma volume rather than enhanced protein synthesis. This may result in a deceptively high serum albumin. When plasma volume is increased due to renal impairment or congestive heart failure, serum albumin appears deceptively low.

Serum albumin levels are affected by age. The hypoalbuminemia that occurs in the elderly is thought to be a part of a decreased rate of albumin synthesis which responds slowly to increases in protein intake.[23]

The tissue proteins, including serum albumin, contain approximately 25 percent of total body protein.[24] With a half-life of 80 days, total protein should normally range from 6.0 to 8.0 g/dl.[3] When minimal amounts of protein are ingested, total body protein and serum albumin decline proportionally.

Serum Transferrin

Definition and Physiologic Function. Serum transferrin, a beta globulin, serves to transport iron in the plasma.[25] It is synthesized by the liver and is bacteriostatic. The bacteriostatic quality of transferrin prevents growth of gram-negative bacteria by binding with free iron. Gram-negative bacteria also require iron for growth.[26]

Method of Testing and Normal Range. Levels of serum transferrin can be measured by radial immunodiffusion[27] or by an indirect measurement of total iron-binding capacity (TIBC). Use of the TIBC with one of several formulas can provide a close estimate of serum transferrin. Blackburn et al.[28] have suggested the most widely used formula for computing serum transferrin:

$$\text{Serum transferrin} = (0.8 \times \text{TIBC}) - 43$$

Another formula that converts TIBC to calculated transferrin is as follows:[29]

$$\text{Serum transferrin} = (0.68 \times \text{TIBC}) + 21$$

This controversy in calculating serum transferrin suggests that an infallible, universal conversion factor for serum transferrin from TIBC may not be possible.[29] Stromberg et al.[30] suggest variations in laboratory techniques may require each hospital or facility to develop its own predicting equation for indirect transferrin. Since serum transferrin can be directly measured, but is not immediately available at many facilities, there may be instances where this is not possible, and an indirect or calculated transferrin may be the only feasible alternative. Consequently, in current clinical practice, the most widely used and accepted calculation method for indirect transferrin is the formula from Blackburn et al.[28] as stated previously.

The standard value for serum transferrin is 170 to 250 mg/dl. TIBC should range from 250 to 410 μg/dl to be considered acceptable. The identification of variations from the norm has permitted detection of PCM.[31]

The degree of malnutrition can be interpreted with the parameter of serum transferrin. With a level of 150 to 170 mg/dl, a serum transferrin concentration can signal a mild visceral protein depletion. A moderate deficit can prevail with a serum transferrin of 100 to 150 mg/dl, and a severe deficit will be identified with a serum transferrin of less than 100 mg/dl.[2] Serum transferrin has a biologic half-life of 8 to 10 days that must be considered when evaluating nutrition deficits.[26]

Nutritional Significance. In the nutrition assessment of a patient, the serum transferrin assists in diagnosing visceral protein depletion.[32] A decrease in serum transferrin is associated with a limited supply of protein and a decrease in organ muscle mass.[33]

Serum transferrin levels of 170 mg/dl or less are early indicators that adequate nutrition support is necessary or an increase in mortality is possible.[34] In addition, patients with serum transferrin levels less than 220 mg/dl are identified as those at high risk for postoperative complications.[12] A serum transferrin level of less than 150 mg/dl is affirmed as useful in predicting patients at risk to develop future sepsis.[17]

The development of the prognostic nutritional index (PNI) as a method of identifying the high-risk surgical patient has validated serum transferrin as a useful tool.[14] This index has motivated others to use serum transferrin as a nutritional marker. Rainey-Macdonald and associates[35] combined serum albumin and serum transferrin to develop a practical method of evaluating clinical outcome. The combination of serum albumin and serum transferrin predicted clinical outcome and the weighted index

$$1.2 \ (SA) = + \ 0.013 \ (ST) - 6.43$$

where

SA = serum albumin
ST = serum transferrin

was most effective in identifying PCM that might necessitate further nutrition support.[35]

TIBC and serum transferrin share a linear relationship since most of the body's iron is carried by serum transferrin. Serum transferrin is ordinarily expressed in physiologic terms as TIBC. In iron deficiency anemia, TIBC is elevated and more serum transferrin is unbound. The amount of iron in the plasma is sufficient to saturate approximately one-third of the available transferrin. The remainder is the unsaturated iron-binding capacity. Plasma iron is decreased with iron deficiency anemia, so there is not enough iron to saturate the transferrin. Hemoglobin, the compound of red blood cells that requires iron for synthesis, is decreased out of proportion, which results in fewer red blood cells (RBCs).[3]

Factors That Affect Validity. Various factors can invalidate serum transferrin as an accurate method of assessing visceral protein status. Serum transferrin can be depressed in acute or chronic inflammation and chronic liver disease. As one of the plasma proteins that is synthesized in the liver, serum transferrin could be decreased with hepatic failure, thus destroying this criterion as a method of nutrition assessment.[3] Alterations of transferrin can be seen when transferrin is determined by TIBC since TIBC can be elevated by iron deficiency anemia.[1]

Serum transport protein concentrations, including levels of serum transferrin, can be altered by the degree of hydration. Fluid retention could falsely signify a low plasma protein concentration.[1]

Serum Prealbumin or Thyroxine-Binding Prealbumin

Definition and Physiologic Function. Serum prealbumin has a key role as a plasma transport protein; it carries thyroxine and assists in transport of retinol-binding protein.[1] Since the manufacturing of prealbumin requires the availability of amino acids and calories in the liver, it appears prealbumin could be used as an indication of endogenous protein synthesis.[36]

Method of Testing and Normal Range. Prealbumin is a direct measurement by radial immunodiffusion with a standard value of 15.7 to 29.6 mg/dl and a mean value of 22.4 mg/dl.[1] Mild visceral protein depletion can be identified with serum concentration levels between 10 and 15 mg/dl. Levels between 5 and 10 mg/dl can signify moderate visceral protein depletion, whereas less than 5 mg/dl represents a severe depletion.[27] Prealbumin has an estimated half-life of 2.5 to 3.0 days.[1]

Nutritional Significance. Research in the clinical importance of serum prealbumin as a measurement of visceral protein status continues. Ingelbleek and colleagues[37] concluded thyroxine-binding prealbumin responds rapidly to protein deprivation, and subsequently rises quickly with the reinstatement of adequate intake. Plasma prealbumin is documented as a more sensitive indicator of nutrition status and more responsive to dietary changes than serum albumin or serum transferrin.[38,39] Ogunshina and Hussain[40] discovered thyroxine-binding prealbumin measured the degree of malnutrition in children and detected mild malnutrition in some of the subjects, which could not be determined with other nutrition assessment parameters. These recent studies appear to signify the importance of prealbumin as a biochemical measurement for nutrition assessment.

Factors That Affect Validity. Since thyroxine-binding prealbumin is synthesized in the liver, an impaired hepatic function could create a decrease in prealbumin that is independent of any visceral protein deficiency.[36]

Retinol-Binding Protein

Definition and Physiologic Function. Another plasma protein that is synthesized in the liver and used as a signal for visceral protein depletion is retinol-binding protein.[1] Retinol, a form of vitamin A, is transported in the plasma with molecules of retinol-binding protein and serum prealbumin. Transport of retinol would be impossible without these two proteins. The reduction of retinol-binding protein can create a functional deficiency of vitamin A. Release of vitamin A from the liver is impaired without the availability of the plasma proteins for transport. With an adequate intake of protein and calories, the retinol-binding protein and prealbumin increase, and the vitamin A levels in the plasma are restored.[2]

Method of Testing and Normal Range. Providing acute changes in protein malnutrition, retinol-binding protein has a half-life of 12 hours[41] and is measured by radial immunodiffusion.[27] Normal serum concentrations range from 2.6 to 7.6 mg/dl with an average value of 5.1 mg/dl.[1]

Nutritional Significance. In examining the effectiveness of retinol-binding protein as a biochemical method of nutrition assessment, Shetty and co-workers[39] summarized that retinol-binding protein and thyroxine-binding prealbumin are more sensitive indexes of the adequacy of dietary protein and calories than are the concentrations of serum albumin and transferrin. Furthermore, their data substantiate the concept that serum retinol-binding protein responds more rapidly to increases in intake than serum prealbumin. Milano et al.[38] explored various plasma protein levels in response to nutrition stress. Retinol-binding protein was restored rapidly with increases in intake; however, it was difficult to analyze and not suggested for routine clinical use. Retinol-binding protein, as a biochemical measurement of visceral protein status, is used in research of nutrition status instead of in routine clinical practice.

Factors That Affect Validity. Since retinol-binding protein is metabolized by the kidneys, it can be elevated with renal disease.[42] Serum retinol-binding protein levels are depressed in chronic and acute liver disease.[43]

Creatinine–Height Index

Definition and Physiologic Function. The CHI serves as a laboratory method of assessing skeletal muscle.[28] Creatinine is the result of the breakdown of creatine. Significant in the energy transfer of skeletal muscle, creatine is synthesized by the liver and is deposited primarily within the body muscle mass.[1] A daily, remarkably constant rate of creatinine is obtained as creatine, either free or bound with phosphate, completes an irreversible breakdown to form creatinine. This constant rate of creatinine production is approximately 1.7 percent of the total creatine supply per day and is excreted unaltered in the urine.[43] A measurement of the urine creatinine excreted in 24 hours furnishes an estimate of the total body creatine or total body muscle mass.[1] One gram of creatinine excreted is equivalent to approximately 17 to 20 kg muscle.[44]

Method of Testing and Normal Range. An analysis of the 24-hour urinary creatinine excretion can be compared with a standard table of creatinine excretion based on sex and stature (Table 5–1). The actual creatinine excretion can be collated with what is expected and expressed as a percent using the CHI:[28]

$$CHI = \frac{\text{measured or actual 24-hour urine creatinine}}{\text{ideal 24-hour creatinine for stature}} \times 100$$

An alternate method of determining the CHI is the adult reference values of 23 mg/kg ideal body weight for males and 18 mg/kg ideal body weight for females.[32]

The comparison of actual creatinine excretion with a standard table of creatinine excretion based on sex, height, and weight is the preferred measurement for the CHI. Furthermore, if the body weight is the only measurement used in expressing the creatinine excretion, the CHI would be less reliable since fluid status can cause variations in body weight.[45]

Assuming an accurate creatinine measurement has been collected, a CHI of 60 to 80 percent of standard indicates a moderate deficit in body muscle mass. A value of less than 60 percent for CHI indicates a severe deficit of body muscle mass.[28]

Nutritional Significance. The CHI is used in assessing body muscle mass.[12,31,43,45] It is a more sensitive parameter than weight for height in measuring somatic muscle status.[25,46] Since there is no valid, ordinary, reasonably priced method of measuring muscle mass to evaluate CHI, however, the reliability of the CHI is difficult to assess in humans.[47,48]

Neutron activation analysis appears to provide better data for the assessment of an individual's total body nitrogen. This direct measurement of total body nitrogen replaces indirect measures of nitrogen input and output to determine body composition changes

TABLE 5–1. IDEAL URINARY CREATININE VALUES

Men			Women		
Height		Ideal Creatinine	Height		Ideal Creatinine
(cm)	(in)	(mg)	(cm)	(in)	(mg)
157.5	62	1288	147.3	58	830
160.0	63	1325	149.9	59	851
162.6	64	1359	152.4	60	875
165.1	65	1386	154.9	61	900
167.6	66	1426	157.5	62	925
170.2	67	1467	160.0	63	949
172.7	68	1513	162.6	64	977
175.3	69	1555	165.1	65	1006
177.8	70	1596	167.6	66	1044
180.3	71	1642	170.2	67	1076
182.9	72	1691	172.7	68	1109
185.4	73	1739	175.3	69	1141
188.0	74	1785	177.8	70	1174
190.5	75	1831	180.3	71	1206
193.0	76	1891	182.9	72	1240

Adapted from Blackburn GL, Bistrian BR, Maine BS, et al.: Nutritional and metabolic assessment of the hospitalized patient. JPEN 1:11, 1977.

with nutritional deprivation. The technique employs a noninvasive, fairly accurate method of testing with little discomfort to the patient.[47] The major disadvantage of neutron activation analysis is the small number of instruments in use.[48]

Factors That Affect Validity. The validity of the CHI is dependent upon the accuracy of the 24-hour urine sample. Failure of the nursing staff to obtain an accurate sample, the inability of the patient to remain continent, and laboratory and other technicians reluctantly unable to assist in obtaining the urine sample while the patient is in another department exemplify many of the problems that occur when collecting an accurate 24-hour urine sample. Three consecutive 24-hour samples serve as a more precise indicator of lean body mass (LBM) since there is a greater chance of obtaining one accurate 24-

hour urine sample[12,45] and daily variations may occur.[44]

Additional complications occur with the reliability of the CHI when the patient has abnormal renal function. Assuming the renal function is normal, the rate of creatinine production is equal to the rate of creatinine excretion in the urine.[49] With renal insufficiency, a false reading of the creatinine excreted is obtained or the collection of the 24-hour urine is impaired due to a minimal output of urine. As a result, the CHI appears significantly low.

Active physical exertion is necessary for an increase in lean body mass, as measured by the CHI. A bedfast patient without physical activity will display no increases in CHI, even though adequate nutrition is administered.[50]

Creatinine excretion reliability is altered when emotional stress is present. Although the reason for this is unclear, varying degrees of stressful conditions increase the diversity of an individual's creatinine excretion.[51]

Increased creatinine excretion can be produced with strenuous exercise. Srivastava et al.[52] demonstrated a 10 percent increase in urinary output of creatinine when normal individuals marched at different speeds for 3 hours. The cause of this phenomenon is not known.

Changes in excretion of creatinine are seen in the menstrual cycle. A 5 to 10 percent increase in creatinine excretion appears in the second half of the menstrual cycle followed by a decrease the days before and during menstruation.[53]

Sepsis, fever and trauma can create elevations in urinary creatinine removal.[54] Increases in creatinine excretion from 20 to 100 percent can manifest in some individuals following the initial posttraumatic phase.[54,55]

The components of an individual's diet influence the creatinine excretion. Consuming a protein-free diet will slightly reduce the amount of creatinine excreted since dietary protein is the main constitutent of the amino acid precursors of creatine. The amount of the creatine accumulated is dependent on the dietary intake of creatine. Consequently, the output of creatinine is greater as the intake of creatine increases. The only way to assure that the diet does not alter the creatinine excretion would be to place the individual on a constant creatine, meat-free diet with 60 to 80 g protein per day during the entire time of testing.[44] This should aid in eliminating most of the variations in creatinine excretion that are associated with the diet, but would not be suitable for many individuals in the clinical setting.

LBM declines with age, thereby reducing creatinine excretion in the elderly.[56] If the standards employed with younger adults are used for the elderly, many of the elderly would display a deficit of the CHI.

The aging process has a significant impact on height, which creates an additional problem with the use of the CHI in the elderly.[57] Height can decrease with age after maturity as the result of changes in the spine and a narrowing of the weight-bearing cartilages.[58] To accentuate this problem, it is often impossible to obtain an accurate height in bedfast patients, as well as ambulatory elderly patients, since many have kyphosis and vertebral compression and are unable to stand upright.[49] Consequently, if the patient is unable to stand upright, the clinician could obtain a height with a tape measure while the patient reclines. Although this measurement may not be completely precise, this current measurement is probably more accurate than the estimated height of the patient. Without an accurate determination of height, the CHI is useless.

To correct this lack of a suitable standard for body muscle mass in the elderly, Mitchell and Lipschitz[59] suggested arm length measurement as an alternative to height in the CHI. The changes in height attributed to senescence do not occur in the long bone length and thus total arm length remains constant.[60] Mitchell and Lipschitz[59] determined the creatinine excretion per cm total arm length would be a more reliable method of estimating body muscle mass and total arm length would be easily obtainable in the bedfast patient. Additional studies in this area may produce future biochemical methods for assessing body muscle mass. At the present time, the CHI is one clinically available method for measuring body muscle mass.

Urine Urea Nitrogen (UUN)

Definition and Physiologic Function. In humans, urea is the major byproduct of protein catabolism. Under normal conditions, approximately 80 to 90 percent of urinary nitrogen is comprised of urea.[61] The remainder must be estimated. Approximately 2 to 3 g of nitrogen is lost from normal stool and 0.5 to 1 g is excreted in hair, nails, sweat, and sloughed skin.[1] To obtain the UUN, a collection of a 24-hour urine sample is secured and analyzed.[28]

Method of Testing and Normal Range. The concept of nitrogen balance can serve as a useful indicator of the present adequacy of nutrition intake.[28] A nitrogen balance can express the difference between nitrogen intake and nitrogen output:[28,45]

$$\frac{\text{Nitrogen}}{\text{balance}} = \frac{\text{protein intake}}{6.25} - \frac{(\text{UUN} + 3}{\text{or } 4)}$$

The protein intake divided by 6.25 g protein/g N determines the nitrogen intake, and the nitrogen output is expressed by the UUN plus an addition of 3 *or* 4 g N for the insensible losses of feces, hair, nails, sloughed skin, and sweat.

Mullen et al.[1] suggested a substitute method of determining nitrogen balance:

$$\frac{\text{Nitrogen}}{\text{balance}} = \frac{\text{protein intake}}{6.25} - \frac{(\text{UUN} + 20\%}{\text{of total UUN}}$$
$$\text{loss } + 2 \text{ g})$$

Since only 80 to 90 percent of total urinary nitrogen is represented in the UUN, the addition of 20 percent of the UUN is included to complete the urinary nitrogen loss. The remaining 2 g is added to compensate for fecal and skin losses.

Since the insensible nitrogen losses cannot be objectively measured and are estimated in each of these formulas, the use of any of these formulas will compute the estimated nitrogen balance.

In normal healthy individuals, the rates of anabolism and catabolism are in a state of equilibrium or zero nitrogen balance.[25] With major trauma and stress, a hypermetabolic patient begins to experience a larger turnover in protein. Due to this increased loss of nitrogen, the patient must ingest enough protein to compensate for these tremendous losses.[21] A positive nitrogen balance suggests that the protein ingested is being conserved and utilized for rebuilding of protein deficits. A nitrogen intake, in the form of high quality protein, of approximately 4 to 6 g in excess of output is adequate to maintain and rebuild the patient with protein defi-

cits.[62] A negative nitrogen balance suggests protein catabolism and, if it persists, protein depletion can affect all organ systems adversely.[31]

Nutritional Significance. Measurement of the 24-hour UUN excretion can assist in estimating the rate of catabolism according to the degree of stress. In response to stress and increased protein demand, the body adapts by a rapid mobilization of its protein compartments. The increased utilization of amino acids as energy is reflected in increased production of urea and excretion of urea in the urine.[2] With infection, an estimated loss of 9 to 11 g/day of UUN can be expected. In major burns that are 30 percent or greater, 12 to 18 g/day of urea nitrogen may be expected in the urine.[28]

Factors That Affect Validity. The validity of the UUN is altered by difficulty in clinical collection of the 24-hour urine. Incontinence, spills, and inaccurate timing create an incomplete sample collection that estimates the nitrogen loss lower than the actual loss. This allows the patient's nitrogen balance to appear better than the actual balance.[32]

In patients with renal disease, the UUN decreases and the BUN increases. This makes it difficult to carefully estimate the urea excretion of these patients.[3]

In addition, fluid retention can alter the accuracy of the 24-hour urine sample by underestimating the nitrogen loss. Bacterial contamination of the specimen can alter the analysis.

The deficiency that exists in estimating the nitrogen balance is that this measurement does not effectively account for the protein turnover in the body.

EFFECT OF STRESS AND STARVATION ON OTHER SERUM LAB VALUES

Other serum lab values are affected by stress and starvation. These values are not specific for assessing malnutrition and, generally, are affected by many factors. For this reason, these other serum laboratory values are only briefly examined in this section. Several of the vitamins and minerals are more thoroughly discussed in Chapter 11 on vitamin and mineral requirements. A more extensive discussion on total lymphocyte count can be found in Chapter 7.

Uric Acid

A rise in serum uric acid occurs in starvation in response to a decreased urinary excretion of uric acid.[21] Purine bases aid in establishing the ribonucleotides of adenine, guanine, uracil, and cytosine. Uric acid is the metabolic end product of purines.[43] An increased serum uric acid level is the result of a higher destruction of purine bases. The normal range for serum uric acid is 3.0 to 7.5 mg/dl in females and 8.5 mg/dl or less in males.[3]

Cholesterol

Essential fatty acids (EFA) may be involved in the regulation of cholesterol metabolism since in the absence of fat intake, large amounts of cholesterol accumulate in the liver and lead to lowering of serum cholesterol levels. Hence, cholesterol absorption is enhanced by the presence of dietary fat and a decrease in serum cholesterol can be seen with fat malabsorption. In collecting the specimen for the serum cholesterol, it is necessary to fast overnight, or approximately 14 hours prior to the collection.[43]

Creatinine

Protein starvation causes a reduction of serum creatinine.[2] Normal levels for serum creatinine are 0.7 to 1.5 mg/dl. Impaired renal function causes an elevation of serum creatinine. Serum creatinine provides a more specific indicator of renal disease than BUN.[32]

Blood Urea Nitrogen (BUN)

The BUN is decreased in minimal protein intake and starvation.[3] With increased protein catabolism, the serum urea nitrogen increases.[26] The BUN may rise slightly in refeeding, especially in chronic renal insufficiency or secondary to dehydration.[32]

Calcium and Phosphorus

Serum calcium decreases gradually in the presence of starvation primarily due to a decrease in serum albumin and vitamin D.[21] In normal plasma, the protein-bound calcium accounts for about 46 percent of the total calcium; 81 percent of this protein-bound calcium is bound to albumin. This provides an explanation of the correlation between a low serum albmin and a low serum calcium. A decreased serum calcium is not a specific test of a calcium deficiency. Generally, as serum albumin status is restored, the serum calcium improves. Phosphorus affects bone resorption and collagen synthesis, assisting in calcium homeostasis. Hypophosphatemia can be evident in starvation or in patients on total parenteral solutions with low levels of additional phosphorus. A normal serum calcium concentration is 8.6 to 10.8 mg/dl.[32] Tetany can occur at serum calcium levels of 7 mg/dl or less.[2] A normal serum phosphorus concentration is 3.0 to 4.5 mg/dl.[3] (See Chapter 11, Vitamin and Mineral Requirements, for further discussion.)

Magnesium

Starvation, diarrhea, malabsorption, acute pancreatitis, intestinal fistulas, and the absence of magnesium in total parenteral nutrition (TPN) or total enteral nutrition can lead to a depressed serum magnesium. Symptoms of muscle spasms, tremors, personality changes, anorexia, and apathy can occur.[43] The metabolism of magnesium is similar to that of calcium and phosphorus; 1.5 to 2.5 mEq/liter or 1.8 or 3.0 mg/dl represents the normal range for serum magnesium.[3] Serum levels of less than 1.0 mEq/liter result in tetany.[2] (See Chapter 11 for further discussion.)

Zinc

A zinc deficiency can cause growth retardation, anorexia and impaired wound healing. A decrease in intake and a loss of taste acuity are signs of a zinc deficiency. Acute or chronic inflammatory stress can cause a depressed zinc level.[43] Serum zinc should range from 10.7 to 18.4 mmol/liter or 70 to 120 mg/dl.[21] Since the body stores of zinc are not readily available, regular dietary intakes are necessary to maintain serum zinc. Starvation presents with a depressed serum zinc level as circulating zinc levels are bound with plasma proteins. Thus, serum zinc does not always reflect the body stores of zinc, but the protein-bound zinc. It is necessary to obtain additional measurements to identify a zinc deficiency.[32] (See Chapter 11 for further discussion.)

White Blood Cell Count and Total Lymphocyte Count

Alterations of the white blood cell count (WBC) can exist in various hematologic, metabolic, infectious, inflammatory, and neoplastic disease processes. This leukocyte count with a blood smear is a common laboratory measurement to determine the severity of the disease process and can assist in the location of individuals with susceptibility to sepsis.[2]

There are five types of circulating leukocytes: neutrophils, lymphocytes, monocytes, eosinophils, and basophils. Neutrophils develop in the bone marrow and possess the ability to kill and digest microorganisms. Phagocytosis is a foremost responsibility of neutrophils. Lymphocytes serve to create immunoglobulins and regulate cellular immunity. The immunoglobulins attack and assist in removal of the foreign substances from the body. A total lymphocyte count and other types of leukocyte counts are obtained by multiplying the total leukocyte count by the percent of the type of white blood cell. From 1500 to 4000 cells per cubic millimeter represents a normal total lymphocyte count.[2]

A total lymphocyte count of less than 1000 per cubic millimeters can occur in patients with pneumonia, sepsis, administration of glucocorticosteroids, malignancies, uremia, congestive heart failure, myocardial infarction, lymphomas, aplastic anemia, lupus erythematosus, certain chemotherapeutic agents, and other diseases of the immune system.[2] This lymphopenia may suggest a decreased intake of protein secondary to PCM.[3]

An increase in the total or absolute lymphocyte count occurs in many infections such as infectious hepatitis, mumps, chronic tuberculosis, infectious mononucleosis, pertussis, adrenal insufficiency, lymphatic leukemia, German measles, or syphilis, and with fluctuating fever.[2,3]

Liver Function Tests

A fatty liver can be produced by a number of circumstances including (1) increased inflow of fatty acids, (2) increased amounts of fatty acids in the liver creating more triglyceride (TG) formation, (3) decreased synthesis of lipoproteins, and (4) decreased release of lipoproteins from the liver. Alcohol is one of the most frequent agents that cause a fatty liver, although the exact etiology is unclear. Other factors that can precipitate a fatty liver include PCM; obesity; poorly regulated, adult onset diabetes mellitus; prolonged TPN (accumulation of carbohydrates); and other chronic illnesses in which malabsorption of nutrients can occur (chronic pancreatitis, ulcerative colitis).[2]

Laboratory findings in fatty liver are usually the result of the underlying situations (i.e., malnutrition, frequently alcoholism). Liver function tests are generally normal in 50 percent of the cases, while some show minimal increases of alkaline phosphatase and the transaminases (SGOT, SGPT). The normal value for alkaline phosphatase is 1.5 to 4.5 units (the Bodansky method).[2] SGOT (glutamic–oxaloacetic) should range from 5 to 40 units/ml (Sigma–Frankel units) and SGPT (glutamic–pyruvic) should range from 5 to 35 units/ml (Sigma–Frankel units).

DEVELOPMENTAL RESEARCH WITH LABORATORY DATA

3-Methylhistidine Excretion

3-Methylhistidine excretion is an experimental laboratory test under investigation for possible usage in estimation of total somatic protein mass.[1] 3-Methylhistidine is an unusual amino acid that is present only in myofibrillar protein.[62] Formed by methylation of histidine residues after syntheses of actin and myosin, 3-methylhistidine excretion occurs when the myofibrillar protein is destroyed. All of the 3-methylhistidine is excreted unaltered in the urine. Therefore, a 24-hour urine collection, which can be obtained and measured for 3-methylhistidine, should represent somatic muscle turnover during the time of collection.[1]

Long et al.[62] employed a study on seven skeletal trauma patients and eight normal individuals to compare the usefulness of 3-methylhistidine excretion as a measurement of somatic protein status. It suggested that urinary excretion of 3-methylhistidine would be a poor indicator for muscle protein catabolism in the human.

There are several limitations to the use of 3-methylhistidine excretion. 3-methylhistidine excretion does not represent all muscle breakdown. In addition, age and sex, starvation, trauma, dietary intake of meat protein (which contains 3-methylhistidine), infection, and the accuracy of the urine sample influence the validity of this test. Furthermore, this technique of measuring 3-methylhistidine excretion requires an amino acid analyzer, which is not universally available.[1]

INDIRECT CALORIMETRY IN THE CLINICAL SETTING

Indirect calorimetry using a mobile metabolic cart is in use in larger facilities as a method of determining resting energy expenditure.[63] This equipment provides information concerning the volume of oxygen consumed, the volume of CO_2 produced, and the respiratory quotient. Indirect calorimetry computes actual, approximate needs of patients by estimating the types of fuel oxidized and their energy. One of the main advantages of indirect calorimetry as a measurement of resting energy expenditure is that it is not necessary to add calories for various degrees of stress.[63]

When comparing indirect calorimetry to direct calorimetry as a model, measurement of energy requirements is not always the same.[64–66] Carlson and Hsieh[67] displayed similarity in calculations for direct and indirect calorimetry only while the individual was not active. According to Webb et al.,[68] comparisons of these two measurements demonstrated an accuracy of ± 5 percent while the individual was resting and ± 20 percent while the individual was active during an experiment of 3 to 6 hours in length.

Further limitations to indirect calorimetry in the clinical setting include (1) the cost of equipment could be significant for many institutions and facilities; (2) experienced personnel would be necessary to operate and calibrate the analyzer, so training would be mandatory; (3) time to complete the measurement would be lengthy for the patient and tester (from 3 to 24 hours); (4) time for calibration and repair of the machine should be allowed; and (5) accuracy of the mobile cart could be questioned due to movement and continual calibration of the machine. Before indirect calorimetry is employed, the clinician should carefully weigh the advantage of actual versus calculated values for energy needs against the preceding disadvantages.

REFERENCES

1. Mullen JL, Crosby LO, Rombeau JL (eds): Symposium on surgical nutrition. Surg Clin North Am 61:3, 1981
2. Isselbacher KJ, Adams RD, Braunwald E, et al. (eds): Harrison's Principles of Internal Medicine, 9th ed. New York: McGraw-Hill, 1980
3. Wallach J: Interpretation of Diagnostic Tests, 3rd ed. Boston: Little, Brown, 1978
4. Bistrian BR, Blackburn GL, Vitale J, et al.: Prevalence of malnutrition in general medical patients. JAMA 235:1567, 1976
5. Whitehead RG, Coward WA, Lunn PG: Serum-albumin concentration and the onset of kwashiorkor. Lancet 1:63, 1973
6. Willcutts HD: Nutritional assessment of 1000 surgical patients in an affluent suburban community hospital. JPEN 1:25B, 1977
7. Bistrian BR, Blackburn GL, Hallowell E, Heddle R: Protein status of general surgical patients. JAMA 230:85B, 1974
8. Butterworth CE, Blackburn GL: Hospital malnutrition and how to assess the nutritional status of a patient. Nutr Today 18:March/April, 1976
9. Bollet AJ. Owens SO: Evaluation of nutritional status of selected hospitalized patients. Am J Clin Nutr 26:931, 1973
10. Prevost EA, Butterworth CE: Nutritional care of hospitalized patients (abstract). Clin Res 22:579, 1974
11. Weinsier RL, Hunker EM, Krumdieck CL, Butterworth CE: Hospital malnutrition. A prospective evaluation of general medical patients during the course of hospitalization. Am J Clin Nutr 32:418, 1979
12. Mullen JL, Gertner MH, Buzby GP, et al.: Implications of malnutrition in the surgical patient. Arch Surg 114:121, 1979
13. Mullen JL, Buzby GP, Matthews DC et al.: Reduction of operative morbidity and mortality by combined preoperative and postoperative nutritional support. Ann Surg 192:604, 1980
14. Mullen JL, Buzby GP, Waldman MT, et al.: Prediction of operative morbidity and mortality by preoperative nutritional assessment. Surg Forum 30:80, 1979
15. Buzby GP: Preoperative nutritional support—Nutritional indications for delaying surgery. Clin Consult Nutr Supp 2:April, 1982
16. Jones TN, Moore EE, Van Way CW: Factors influencing nutritional assessment in trauma patients. JPEN 5:559, 1981
17. Morath MA, Miller SF, Finley RK: Nutritional indicators of postburn sepsis. JPEN 5:488, 1981
18. Harvey KB, Ruggiero CS, Regan CS, et al.: Hospital morbidity-mortality risk factors using nutritional assessment. Clin Res 26:581A, 1978
19. Anderson CF, Wochos DN: The utility of serum albumin values in the nutritional assessment of hospitalized patients. Mayo Clin Proc 57:181, 1982
20. Seltzer MH, Bastidas JA, Cooper DM, et al.: Instant nutritional assessment. JPEN 3:157, 1979
21. Ballinger WF (ed): Manual of Surgical Nutrition. Philadelphia: W.B. Saunders, 1975
22. Golden MHN: Transport proteins as indices of protein status. Am J Clin Nutr 35:1159, 1982
23. Misra DP, Loudon JM, Staddon GE: Albumin metabolism in elderly patients. J Gerontol 30:304, 1975
24. Guthrie HA: Introductory Nutrition, 3rd ed. St. Louis: C.V. Mosby, 1975
25. Winborn AL, Banaszek NK, Freed BA, Kaminski MV: A protocol for nutritional assessment in a community hospital. J Am Diet Assoc 78:129, 1981
26. Guyton A: Basic Human Physiology: Normal Function and Mechanism of Disease. Philadelphia: W.B. Saunders, 1971
27. Mancini G. Carbonara AO, Heremans JF: Immunological quantitation of antigens by single radial immunodiffusion. Int J Immunochem 2:235, 1965
28. Blackburn GL, Bistrian BR, Maine BS, et al.: Nutritional and metabolic assessment of the hospitalized patient. JPEN 1:11, 1977
29. Miller SF, Morath MA, Finley RK: Comparison of derived and actual transferrin: A potential source of error in clinical nutritional assessment. J Trauma 21:548, 1981
30. Stromberg BV, Davis RJ, Danziger LH: Relationship of serum transferrin to total iron

binding capacity for nutritional assessment. JPEN 6:392, 1982

31. Weinsier RL, Butterworth CE: Handbook of Clinical Nutrition. St. Louis: C.V. Mosby, 1981

32. Labbe RF (ed): Laboratory assessment of nutritional status. Clin Lab Med December, 1981

33. Travill AS: The synthesis and degradation of liver-produced proteins. Gut 13:225, 1972

34. Kaminski MV, Fitzgerald MJ, Murphy RJ, et al.: Correlation of mortality with serum transferrin and anergy. JPEN 1:27, 1977

35. Rainey-Macdonald CG, Holliday RL, Wells GA, Donner AP: Validity of a two-variable nutritional index for use in selecting candidates for nutritional support. JPEN 7:15, 1983

36. Vanlandingham S, Spiekerman AM, Newmark SR: Prealbumin: A parameter of visceral protein levels during albumin infusion. JPEN 6:230, 1982

37. Ingelbleek Y, De Visscher M, De Nayer P: Measurement of prealbumin as index of protein–calorie malnutrition. Lancet 2:106, 1972

38. Milano G, Cooper EH, Coligher JC, et al.: Serum prealbumin, retinol-binding protein, transferrin, and albumin levels in patients with large bowel cancer. J Natl Cancer Inst 61:687, 1978

39. Shetty PS, Watrasiewicz KE, Jung RT, James WPT: Rapid turnover of transport proteins: An index of subclinical protein-energy malnutrition. Lancet 2:230, 1979

40. Ogunshina S, Hussain M: Plasma thyroxine-binding prealbumin as an index of mild protein energy malnutrition in Nigerian children. Am J Clin Nutr 33:794, 1980

41. Peterson PA: Demonstration in serum of two physiological forms of human retinol-binding protein. Eur J Clin Invest 1:437, 1971

42. Smith FR, Goodman DWS: The effects of diseases of the liver, thyroid and kidneys on the transport of vitamin A in human plasma. J Clin Invest 50:2426, 1971

43. Goodhart RS, Shils ME: Modern Nutrition in Health and Disease, 6th ed. New York: Lea & Febiger, 1980

44. Heymsfield B, Arteaga C, McManus C, et al.: Measurement of muscle mass in humans: Validity of the 24-hour urinary creatinine method. Am J Clin Nutr 37:478, 1983

45. Grant A: Nutritional Assessment Guidelines, 2nd ed. Berkeley, Calif: Cutter Laboratories, 1979

46. Bistrian BR, Blackburn GL, Sherman M, Scrimshaw NS: Therapeutic index of nutritional depletion in hospitalized patients. Surg Gynecol Obstet 141:512, 1975

47. Cohn SH, Vaswani AN, Vartsky D, et al.: In vivo quantification of body nitrogen for nutritional assessment. Am J Clin Nutr 35:1186, 1983

48. Heymsfield SB, McManus C, Stevens V, Smith, J: Muscle mass: Reliable indicator of protein–energy malnutrition severity and outcome. Am J Clin Nutr 35:1192, 1982

49. Lipschitz DA, Mitchell CO: Creatinine height index in the elderly. Third Ross Roundtable on Medical Issues. Columbus, Ohio: Ross Laboratories, 1982

50. Umapathy KP, Mack PB, Dozier EA: Effect of immobilization on urinary excretion of creatine and creatinine with certain possible ameliorating measures applied. Ind J Nutr Dietet 10:292, 1973

51. Scrimshaw NS, Habicht JP, Piche ML, et al.: Protein metabolism of young men during university examinations. Am J Clin Nutr 18:321, 1966

52. Srivastava SS, Mani KV, Soni CM, Bhati J: Effect of muscular exercises on urinary excretion of creatine and creatinine. Ind J Med Res 55:953, 1957

53. Smith OW: Creatinine excretion in women: Data collected in the course of urinalysis for female sex hormones. J Clin Endocrinol 2:1, 1942

54. Schiller WR, Long CL, Blakemore WS: Creatinine and nitrogen excretion in seriously ill and injured patients. Surg Gynecol Obstet 149:561, 1979

55. Threlfall CJ, Stoner HM, Galasko CSB: Patterns in the excretion of muscle markers after trauma and orthopedic surgery. J Trauma 21:140, 1981

56. Cockcroft DW, Gault MH: Prediction of creatinine clearance from serum creatinine. Nephron 16:31, 1976

57. Mitchell CO, Lipschitz DA: Detection of protein–calorie malnutrition in the elderly. Am J Clin Nutr 35:398, 1982

58. Trotter M, Gleser GC: The effect of aging on stature. Am J Phys Anthropol 9:311, 1951

59. Mitchell CO, Lipschitz DA: Arm length measurement as an alternative to height in nutritional assessment of the elderly. JPEN 6:266, 1982

60. Dequeker JV, Baeyens JP, Claessens J: The significance of stature as a clinical measurement of aging. J Am Geriatr Soc 17:169, 1969

61. Pittman JG, Cohen P: The pathogenesis of cardiac cachexia. N Engl J Med 271:403, 1964

62. Long CL, Birkhahn RH, Geiger JW, Blakemore WS: Contribution of skeletal muscle protein in elevated rates of whole body protein catabolism in trauma patients. Am J Clin Nutr 34:1087, 1981

63. McCamish MA, Dean RE, Ouellette TR: Assessing energy requirements of patients on respirators. JPEN 5:513, 1981

64. Burton AC: Human calorimetry: II. The average temperature of the tissues of the body. J Nutr 9:261, 1935

65. Pittet PH, Gygax PH, Jequier E: Thermic effect of glucose and amino acids in man studied by direct and indirect calorimetry. Brit J Nutr 31:343, 1974

66. Webb P, Annis JF: Cooling required to suppress sweating during work. J Appl Physiol 25:289, 1968

67. Carlson LD, Hsieh ACL: Control of Energy Exchange. New York: Macmillan, 1970

68. Webb P, Annis JF, Troutman SJ: Energy balance in man measured by direct and indirect calorimetry. Am J Clin Nutr 33:1287, 1980

6. Clinical Methods in Anthropometry

Rebecca L. Murray

Anthropometry is a science in which the body is described by a series of measurements of its external morphology. Its uses include evaluation of body circumferences for clothing design; evaluation of growth rates, body build analysis, and body composition analysis for determination of genetic, endocrine, nutritional, or disease-related problems as they affect both populations and individuals. According to Martorell,[1] nutrition anthropometry first gained acceptance in the early 1800s when the association between poverty and poor nutrition status on height and weight was established among French Army conscripts and among youngsters employed in English workhouses. It continues to hold wide acceptance among pediatricians and public health nutritionists in assessing nutrition status. In fact, the techniques, standards, and methods of interpreting anthropometry in assessing hospital malnutrition, as recommended by Bistrian and Blackburn,[2–4] were based on those of Dr. Derrick B. Jelliffe, a pediatrician and public health nutritionist. Dr. Jelliffe is widely known for his work with malnourished children in developing countries and as the author of WHO Monograph No. 53.[5]

Today, among hospitalized adults, anthropometric measures such as weight and triceps skinfolds are more commonly associated with the assessment of obesity and as a prognostic index in disorders related to overnutrition.[6–9] They have recently regained recognition, however, in assessing type and degree of hospital malnutrition.[10–12]

The major uses of anthropometrics in adult patients are:

1. To gain information on current body composition of fat, lean body mass (LBM), or skeletal muscle for the purpose of assessing nutrition status
2. As a prognostic index of morbidity and mortality related to malnutrition
3. To measure changes in body composition as a result of instituting nutrition therapy

ANTHROPOMETRIC EVALUATION OF BODY COMPOSITION

The nutrition assessment attempts to objectively classify type and degree of malnutrition on the basis of rate and extent of change in (1) body function and (2) body composition.

Body composition studies yield information on the amount and distribution of fat (and hence calorie reserves), protein in the muscle, viscera, and structural compartments and water. Examples of reliable methods used for analyzing body composition include radioisotope dilution studies, radiographic studies, e.g., computed tomography ("CT") scan, direct physical and chemical analysis at autopsy, and body density measurements. These are explained in Tables 6–1 and 6–2. It is sufficient here to state that these methods are costly, time consuming, and frequently neither available nor practical for the clinician or the patient. Therefore, Blackburn and colleagues[2–4] proposed the use of anthropometric studies in the clinical setting to estimate body composition and changes in the various body compartments because they are relatively simple and rapid to obtain, inexpensive, and noninvasive.

Generally, anthropometrics are the responsibility of the dietitian to carry out. This is a relatively new role and not all dietitians have formal training in it. This chapter will first address the validity and reproducibility of anthropometrics. The following areas will be covered:

1. Definition of body composition in terms of fat, protein, water, and minerals
2. Review and comparison of anthropometry with other methods of measuring body composition

3. Inter- and intraobserver reproducibility of anthropometric measurements
4. Limitations of anthropometry in the clinical setting:
   a. Availability of "normal" or preillness measurements
   b. Position of the subject (e.g., confined to bed versus able to stand)
   c. State of hydration

The second portion of this chapter addresses the anthropometric measurements themselves. There are five general types of anthropometric measurements:

1. Body mass (weight)
2. Diameters (e.g., height)
3. Circumferences
4. Skinfolds
5. Derived (e.g., arm muscle circumference)

The clinical significance of each type and site of measurement will be discussed as well as the proper technique for taking the measurement.

The third portion of this chapter discusses standards for comparison of anthropometric measurements and their interpretation.

VALIDITY AND REPRODUCIBILITY OF ANTHROPOMETRICS

DEFINITION OF BODY COMPOSITION

The cellular mass of the body is measured and defined in several different ways in the literature. With the exceptions noted, the following definitions of body composition are derived from Dr. Francis Moore's work.[13] The techniques in measuring body composition are derived from Garrow.[14]

Definitions and characteristics of:
1. Body cell mass (BCM) or lean body weight (LBW)
   a. All the cells in the body (protoplasm,

nucleus, cytoplasm, and cell membrane) by weight
   b. No fat except for 2 to 10 percent found in the cellular structure
   c. No extracellular supporting structures are included (skeleton, dermis, collagen, or extracellular proteins)
   d. No extracellular fluids (lymph, interstitial fluid, blood plasma)
   e. Accounts for 30 to 38 percent of total body weight—larger in males than females as well as in athletic individuals who have less fat stores
   f. Measured using one or a combination

of the following: dilution of 40 K isotope; neutron activation of nitrogen, sodium, calcium, or other elements; whole body conductivity

2. Lean body mass (LBM) (Table 6–3).
   a. The weight of the entire body minus *only* neutral fat
   b. Includes 2 to 10 percent "essential lipid" in cell membranes
   c. Includes all of the body cells (as above)
   d. Includes all of the structural proteins (skeleton, tendon, fascia, cartilage, dermis, hair)
   e. Includes all of the dissolved extracellular proteins (e.g., albumin, immunoglobulins, gastrointestinal enzymes)
   f. Accounts for 75 to 80 percent body weight, larger amounts in males than females, and in athletic or starved individuals who have less fat stores
   g. Measured by determining total body water (TBW) from deuterium or tritium dilution, and from total body nitrogen (TBN) by neutron activation

3. Fat-free mass (FFM)
   a. Same as LBM, except no fat at all is included, even that in the cellular membrane
   b. Accounts for 68 to 78 percent of body weight
   c. Measured by subtracting weight of total body fat (TBF), determined by underwater weighing to derive body density, from total weight
   d. Estimation of FFM can be derived from measurements of skinfold thickness[15,16]

4. Total body fat (TBF)
   a. All lipids in the body, including adipose tissue, cell membrane lipids, and lipid compounds circulating in plasma[13]
   b. Accounts for a mean of 15 to 39 percent of total body weight in normal adults[15] (less in males than females; increases with age)
   c. Measured by underwater weighing and plethysmography to derive body density, and from measurement of fat-soluble gases (experimental)[14]
   d. Is estimated by measurements of skinfold thickness[15]

5. Total muscle mass
   a. Includes striated (skeletal) and smooth (visceral organs) muscle,[17] although the literature varies greatly in definition of these
   b. Accounts for approximately 40 percent of body weight in males[13,18] and approximately 30 percent in females[13] (see Table 6–3)
   c. An independent, valid, noninvasive measure for measuring total muscle mass is not available[17,18]
   d. Indirect measurements of total muscle mass are made from 24-hour urinary excretion of creatinine, and 3-methylhistidine, from cross-sectional analysis using computer tomography, and from anthropometric measurements (midupper arm muscle circumference [MAMC] and midupper arm muscle area [MAMA])
   e. Measurement of TBN and total body potassium (TBK) by neutron activation and prediction of muscle and nonmuscle mass on the basis of nitrogen to potassium (N/K) ratio appears to be the most valid quantitative technique available at this time for determining muscle composition[19]

Fat, protein, water, and bone mineral provide the structural complex of the human body. In addition, fat, protein, and a small amount (approximately 225 g) of glycogen provide fuel during periods of fasting or increased metabolic need. The total supply of energy in the reference (70-kg man) is 166,000 kcal. Glycogen supplies only 900 of these kcal. Adipose tissue accounts for the majority of the fuel reserve—140,000 to 145,000 kcal in the 70-kg reference man compared to 20,000 to 25,000 kcal from protein. Fat stores are expendable. The body normally carries approximately 14 percent of its total weight as fat in males and approx-

TABLE 6–1. DESCRIPTION OF TECHNIQUES FOR MEASURING BODY COMPOSITION[a]

Method	Assumption
Total body water (TBW)	1. LBM has a constant water content. 2. Tracer dose of water will equilibrate with all body water in 3 to 4 hours. 3. Its volume of dilution equals total body water. 4. Total body weight − LBM = Total body fat.
Total body potassium (TBP)	1. BCM has a constant concentration of K^+. 2. 40 K is a naturally occurring radioisotope of K^+.
Neutron activation (NA)	1. LBM estimated from TBN concentration. 2. Muscle has lower N/K ratio than nonmuscle component of LBM. 3. Lipid or adipose tissue does not contain N or K^+.
Whole body conductivity (WBC)[b,c,d]	1. FFM conducts electricity better than fat.
Whole body density (WBD)	1. Density of fat is constant and different than density of FFM.
Fat-soluble gases (FSG)	1. Some anesthetic and rare gases are more soluble in fat than water. 2. TBF can be measured from absorption of these gases.
Radiographic analysis (RA)[e,f]	1. Measurement of area and volume of adipose tissue, muscle, and visceral organs can be obtained from a cross-sectional computed tomography image and a computer generated histogram of the image pixels.

Method	Procedures	Limitations
TBW	1. Tracer dose of water is isotopically labeled with ^3H, ^2H, or ^{18}O, injected, equilibrated, and the concentration measured.	1. Involves radiation to the subject to count isotope dilution. 2. The water content of fat-free tissue is increased during obesity, stress, and starvation leading to an underestimate of fat.
TBP	1. ^{40}K is a naturally occurring isotope. Concentration is measured by using a whole body counter.	1. Equipment for measuring is expensive. 2. Obese subjects have lower K^+ concentrations, leading to overestimates. 3. K^+ concentration of BCM is altered during stress and starvation, and during TPN.
NA	1. Isotopes of N, K^+, CA^{++} or other elements are radioactively labeled by irradiating the subject. 2. The radioactivity of the element is measured by whole body counter.	1. Expensive. 2. Ratio of N/K in nonmuscle lean tissue is not constant. 3. Not all elements are uniformly activated.

TABLE 6–1. (*Continued*)

Method	Procedures	Limitations
WBC	1. A solenoidal coil is driven by a 5 MHz oscillating radio frequency. 2. Difference in coil impedance measured when empty versus when the subject is inserted.	1. Edema, ascites, dehydration, and electrolyte imbalance will alter conductivity and interfere with reading. 2. Extent to which variation in body shape and size affect readings needs testing. 3. Variations in bone mass may affect reading.
WBD	1. Subject is submerged in tank with known volume of water. 2. Amount of water displaced measured. 3. Plethysmograph may be used in conjunction to record changes in air pressure around head, in lungs, and in gut.	1. Requires high degree of cooperation from subject. 2. Water is displaced by air trapped in lungs and gut, and will alter density measurements. (Plethysmography helps correct this.)
FSG	1. Rate of absorption and measured dilution of gas at stable state.	1. Inconvenient for subject due to length of time needed to reach equilibrium. 2. Depot fat is irregularly perfused and uptake curve is not smooth.
RA	1. Computer tomographic planimetry of the desired structure. 2. CT pixels give visual evidence of contrast in structure. 3. CT no. associated with the pixels, quantitate this contrast.	1. Low energy roentgen rays are preferentially absorbed as they pass through tissue leading to somewhat unpredictable changes in CT no. 2. The CT does not provide information on chemical composition of the structures, as do other methods. 3. Cost may be prohibitive. 4. Radiation dosage to the subject must be considered.

[a]From Garrow JS: New approaches to body composition. Am J Clin Nutr 35:1152–1158, 1982.[14]

[b]From Harrison GG, Van Itallie TB: Estimation of body composition: A new approach based on electromagnetic principles. Am J Clin Nutr 35:1176–1179, 1982.

[c]From Presta E, Wang J, Harrison GG, et al.: Measurement of total body electrical conductivity: A new method for estimation of body composition. Am J Clin Nutr 37:735–739, 1983.

[d]From Hoffer EC, Meador CK, Simpson DC: A relationship between whole body impedance and total body water volume. Proc of the First International Conference on Bioelectrical Impedance. NY Acad Sci 170:452–461, 1970.

[e]From Heymsfield SB, Olafson RP, Kutner MH, Nixon D: A radiographic method of quantifying protein–calorie undernutrition. Am J Clin Nutr 32:693–702, 1979.[37]

[f]From Heymsfield SB: Radiographic analysis of body composition: In Report of the Second Ross Conference on Medical Research, Nutritional Assessment—Present, Past and Future Status. Columbus, Ohio: Ross Laboratories, 1981, pp 91–94.

TABLE 6–2. GUIDE TO METHODS IN MEASURING BODY COMPOSITION

Method	Compartment	Inexpensive?	Easy?	Accurate?
Water ^{2}H or ^{18}O	LBM	**	**	***
^{3}H	LBM	***	**	**
Potassium (40 K)	BCM	**	***	***
N, Ca^{++} Neutron Activation	Muscle and non-muscle lean tissue	*	***	**
Conductivity	BCM, LBM	**	****	***?
Fat-soluble gas	TBF	?	?	?
Skinfold thickness	Subcutaneous fat	****	***	**
Muscle metabolic excretion (creatinine, 3 MH)	Muscle mass	****	***	?
Density				
By immersion	TBF	***	*	***
By plethysmograph	TBF	**	**	****

? denotes that there is not enough information for comparison

* to **** = least to most

Adapted from Garrow JS: New approaches to body composition. Am J Clin Nutr 35:1152–1158, 1982.[14]

imately 26 percent in females. While males function quite well with 5 percent of body weight as fat, approximately 10 percent body weight as fat appears to be necessary for females to maintain a normal menstrual cycle.[20]

Using protein as an energy substrate, however, endangers the body's functional and metabolic activities of which protein is the key component. Loss of body protein cannot occur indefinitely without impairing body function sufficiently so that death results. This occurs in a matter of days if fat stores have been used up and no other source of calories is made available. This is hastened by the fact that approximately 30 to 45 percent of total body protein is extracellular (e.g., collagen, keratin, elastin) and unavailable for metabolism[13]

The nutrition assessment attempts to quantify the amount of fat and protein available, the rate of its loss, and whether it is maintained or repleted during nutrition support. Obviously, it is not possible to do this by measuring the protein and fat directly (except with cadaver dissection) since they occur as constituents of the cellular mass, in combination with other substances. Estimates of change in body composition can be derived from changes in body weight, fluid balance, nitrogen balance, and calorie balance (see Table 6–4). Change in body weight by itself does not reflect the compositional change of any one compartment[21,22] but it has documented prognostic value in presurgery patients[23] and cancer patients.[24]

Anthropometry attempts to measure body protein and fat indirectly. Skinfold thickness measurements reflect the amount of subcutaneous fat. The triceps skinfold (TSF) is a relatively good index of body fat in females and children, while subscapular skinfold is better for young boys but not for adult males.[25,26] It has been shown, however, that TSF changes much more slowly, has a greater degree of variability than other indices of assessment, and correlates poorly with changes in composition measured by TBW and TBN in obesity,[27] aging,[26,28] starvation,[18,29,30] in cancer,[28] after surgery,[23] and during nutrition repletion with total parenteral nutrition (TPN)[31] and with diet alone.[32] In addition, deposition of fat differs with age, sex, and degree of adiposity.[33,34]

Change in muscle mass is an important index of the severity of protein–energy mal-

TABLE 6–3. COMPOSITION OF BODY MASS (STANDARD MAN, 20 TO 30 YEARS OF AGE, 70 KG)

Organ	Weight of Organ (kg)	% of Body Weight
Muscles	30.000	42.86
Skin and subcutaneous tissue	8.500	12.14
Skeleton (without bone marrow)	7.000	10.00
Bone marrow—"red and yellow"	3.000	4.28
Blood	5.400	7.71
Gastrointestinal tract	2.300	3.29
Liver	1.700	2.43
Brain	1.400	2.00
Lung (2)	0.950	1.36
Lymph Tissue	0.700	1.00
Heart	0.350	0.50
Kidney	0.300	0.43
Spleen	0.150	0.21
Urinary bladder	0.150	0.21
Pancreas	0.065	0.09
Eye (2)	0.030	0.04
Spinal Cord	0.030	0.04
Teeth	0.023	0.03
Miscellaneous (blood vessels, fat tissue, glands, cartilage, nerves, etc.)	7.952	11.36
Total	70.000	99.98

Data in this table proposed by Lisco of the Argonne National Laboratory on the basis of a careful evaluation of many sources, and adapted from Behnke AR, Wilmore JH: Application of the various field methods. In Evaluation and Regulation of Body Build and Composition. Englewood Cliffs, NJ. Prentice-Hall, 1974, p 58.

nutrition in both stress[35] and starvation.[36] Measurement of either MAMC or MAMA attempts to predict changes in total body muscle mass on the basis of changes either in the volume or in the cross-sectional area of one muscle group. The measurements, however, assume that the midupper arm is a perfect

cylinder, when, in fact, it is usually elliptic. The underlying muscle is in the shape of an off-centered "cloverleaf" and the subcutaneous fat is distributed unevenly around it.[37] Also assumed is accurate measurement of the triceps skinfold, which is difficult to obtain in the extremely obese, in the aged, or where dependent skin or edema alter compressibility of the skinfolds.[27,36,38] Furthermore, these measurements assume that muscle mass has a constant composition during starvation. In fact, Heymsfield et al.[18] have shown that change in muscle size in early semi-starvation is due to loss of glycogen stores, but that there is no significant change in dry protein or water. Glycogen accounts for 1.5 percent per gram wet weight of muscle tissue. They also showed that in chronic semi-starvation, there is a relative increase in water and collagen compared to the amount of total protein or noncollagenous protein lost from the wasted muscle. Therefore, the functional protein content of the muscle decreased more than the muscle size, or the energy and total protein content of the muscle tissue.

For these reasons, changes in MAMC and MAMA, which reflect changes in muscle size, do not correlate significantly with other measurements of muscle mass, such as creatinine height index (CHI)[17] or body protein, such as TBN measured by neutron activation analysis,[39] and thus are less reliable indices of nutrition status in starvation. Changes in MAMC do not correlate significantly with changes in albumin or serum transferrin in postsurgery patients either.[40] This is to be expected, as changes in "visceral" proteins are more marked in the initial stages of stress than are changes in somatic protein or fat stores. Changes in arm circumference related to height (QUAC stick),[41,42] however, correlate very highly with mortality rate in undernourished children. Therefore, it appears that stress, starvation, and growth and development each have different influences on changes in muscle volume and area that alter the usefulness of measured circumference or area as a nutrition indicator.

TABLE 6–4. ESTIMATING COMPOSITIONAL CHANGE OF WEIGHT LOSS[a]

Given the following:

1. Body weight = dry protein + mineral + water + fat **or**
   Body weight = FFM + fat.
2. FFM = 20% dry protein + 7% mineral + 72% water[b]
3. If weight of bone mineral is assumed to be constant, then:
   Δ Body weight = Δ dry protein + Δ water + Δ fat **or**
   Δ Body weight = Δ FFM (bone free) + Δ fat
4. Energy and Hydration Constants[c]
   a. 1 g body fat = 9.4 calories
   b. 1 g dry protein = 5.65 calories
   c. 1 g dry protein = 4.6 g FFM (bone free)

Calculate compositional change as follows:

1. Estimate energy expenditure in calories per day.
2. Calculate calorie balance.
3. Measure nitrogen losses in g N/day.
4. Calculate nitrogen balance.
5. Δ dry protein g/day = g N balance $\times$ 6.25 g dry protein/g N.
6. Δ fat g/day = $\dfrac{\text{calorie balance} - (\Delta \text{ dry protein} \times 5.6 \text{ cal/g protein})}{9.4 \text{ calories/g fat}}$
7. Δ water g/day = Δ body weight g/day − (Δ dry protein g/day − Δ fat g/day)
8. Δ FFM = Δ dry protein g/day $\times$ 4.6 g FFM/g dry protein.

[a]Murray RL, Schaffel NA, et al.: Body composition changes in the critically ill patient: Emphasis on water balance. JPEN 3:219, 1979.[22]

[b]Durnin JVGA, Womersley J: Body fat assessed from total body density and its estimation from skinfold thickness: Measurements on 481 men and women aged 16–72 years. Br J Nutr 32:77–97, 1974.[15]

[c]Heymsfield SB, Stevens V, Noel R, et al.: Biochemical composition of muscle in normal and semistarved human subjects: Relevance to anthropometric measurements. Am J Clin Nutr 36:131–142, 1982.[18]

Notwithstanding their difficulties and limitations, upper arm anthropometry is a quick, inexpensive, noninvasive means of evaluating body composition that is readily available to the clinician. Presently, there are no alternatives to it outside of the research setting.

Because of the limitations of anthropometric measurements as they are traditionally used, it would be desirable to find means of enhancing their predictive value. Durnin and Womersley's method for estimating TBF from the log of the sum of four skinfolds correlates very highly in normal subjects with measurements of TBF from densitometric studies[15] as well as with TBN and TBW by neutron activation.[28] It is also a valid means of estimating FFM, as the difference between body weight and TBF. In cancer patients[28] and in severely undernourished Colombian males,[29,30] however, this method underestimates TBF. The results appear to be influenced by age, sex, and the degree of adiposity.[26,27] Also, it is more difficult and time consuming to obtain skinfold measurements at multiple sites than at a single locus such as the TSF.

The body mass index, wt/ht^2, is another anthropometrically derived index that has a high degree of predictive value for TBF.[25] This index is easily obtained and calculated but has received little attention for clinical use in nutrition assessment. Clinical dietitians who are serious about developing the accuracy and usefulness of their nutrition assessment program would benefit by further investigating methods such as these.

Another limitation of anthropometry is

the difficulty in obtaining reproducible results. In the clinical setting, there are several factors that cause this:

1. *Inter- and intraobserver variation of measurement.* Wilmore and Behnke[43] found that when dealing with a group of highly trained anthropometrists, the reliability of the measurements is very good. In a study comparing two measurements taken by the same trained observer at 44 measurement sites on each of 133 males, 17 to 37 years of age, reliability coefficient ranged from $r = 0.917$ to $r = 0.977$. Six of the measurement sites, however, exhibited statistically significant differences of greater than 1 percent between the first and second trials. This indicates the importance of repeated measures being made if the discrepancy is greater than 1 percent within a set of measurements.

The individual performing the analysis has to be properly trained. This implies a thorough understanding of the anatomic landmarks, familiarity with the testing equipment, and sufficient practice under close supervision. Behnke and Wilmore[44] suggest that in order to determine whether the individual is properly trained, his/her analysis of a group of test subjects should be compared to those of a trained anthropometrist. Since this is not practical for many dietitians, it is suggested that one can at least test the reproducibility of one's own measurements on the same subjects, practicing until there is not greater than 1 percent discrepancy between the first and second set of measurements.

Standardization of technique among trained observers is also necessary. Variation in results between observers has been shown to mask true changes in anthropometric measurements.[45] It can be minimized with coordination of technique and repeated testing of observer performance using two-way analysis of variance.[46]

2. *Inability to compare patient's present anthropometric measurements with "normal" or preillness measurements.* Since the observer is frequently not familiar with the patient's normal or preillness anthropometrics, it is sometimes difficult to interpret whether the values obtained reflect nutritional deficit, fluid shifts, or are simply normal for that individual. However, with patients who are in the hospital for long-term stays, who return frequently to the hospital, or who are being followed on home enteral or parenteral therapy, interpretation of changes in anthropometric measurements taken serially will be easier.[39]

3. *Positioning the subject.* It is frequently impossible in the clinical situation to take measurements while the patient is in the upright position. Many patients are confined to bed or are unable to move. Jensen et al.[47] compared measurements on standing and recumbent patients and found no statistically significant differences between the measurements.

TABLE 6–5. VARIOUS MEMBERS OF THE BODY AS A PERCENTAGE OF TOTAL WEIGHT

Member	Percentage of Total Weight
Leg	
Below the knee	7.0
Above the knee	15.0
Whole leg	18.5
Arm	6.5
Trunk	43.0
Head	10.0
	100.0

From Brunnstrom S: *Clinical Kinesiology.* Philadelphia: F. A. Davis, 1962.[49]

In some cases, the site is not available for measurement (e.g., trauma, dressings, IV insertion). Other sites can be used instead. According to Garn et al.[48] the abdominal fat fold (2 cm to the right of the umbilicus) or the suprailiac crest fold appear to be as useful as the triceps or subscapular in assessing fat stores, although it is not possible to estimate LBM as with the MAMC. If an extremity has been amputated, an estimation of the weight of the member must be made to correct ideal body weight for comparison (Table 6–5).[49]

4. *State of hydration.* (See Chapter 12 on Fluid–Electrolyte Requirements.) Results of weight, circumference, and skinfold measurements will be affected by dehydration, edema, and ascites. If the site where the caliper pinched the skin remains pitted after the caliper is removed, edema is present. If the edema is localized, another site for measurement should be chosen. Error can be further minimized by obtaining weights and taking arm anthropometric measurements immediately after dialysis or periods of diuresis.

ANTHROPOMETRIC MEASUREMENTS

BODY MASS (WEIGHT)

Due to its wide use and general attainability, weight and weight changes remain the best general indicator of protein–calorie over- and undernutrition. Rate of weight change is a prognostic indicator of the body's ability to survive stress sustained from surgical or skeletal trauma,[23,51–53] from cancer and its treatments,[24,54] as well as from malnutrition alone. Degree of obesity is a prognostic indicator in diseases linked with overnutrition, such as adult onset diabetes mellitus and heart disease.[6–9] Serial measurements of weight are important in establishing whether the patient is responding to nutrition therapy. Dehydration, overhydration, edema, and ascites may account for sudden changes in weight. This can be established by comparing the patient's weight change with the balance of his fluid intake and output.[22] (See chapter 12 on Fluid–Electrolyte Balance.) This is of real importance in patients treated with TPN, as much of the initial weight gain may be from fluid.[31,55,56]

Equipment[57,58]

Scales should be sturdy, easy to move, and accurate to within ±0.1 kg. It is helpful if the scale can be read in both the English and metric equivalents; however, metric scales are preferable. Scales with digital displays are now available, but they are more expensive.

Scales featuring the beam or lever balance are recommended as spring scales become inaccurate more quickly as the spring stretches with use. Care should be taken to have the scales calibrated routinely at 6-month intervals according to the manufacturer's instructions, and serviced as needed by a qualified repairman. For adults, the scale should permit reading to the nearest tenth of a kilogram (or fourth of a pound if measuring in English units).

Some models of hospital platform scales can be adapted for the patient who is able to sit but not to stand by attaching a specially made chair. Bed scales for bedridden patients that can be wheeled from room to room are available in most hospitals. Also available are scales that can be placed permanently underneath the bed, taring the bed to allow weighing of the subject alone. This facilitates serial weighings for patients who cannot be lifted, such as those with spinal cord injuries.

Techniques

1. Weigh the patient upon admission and at stated intervals thereafter as condition requires and permits. Take weights at the same time each day, on the same scale with the subject clothed in the same general type of attire. Weighing should not be done after a full meal or if the patient has not voided.
2. Calibrate the scale to zero before the subject is weighed. If the beam pointer stabilizes above or below the center of the trigloop, then it needs to be adjusted according to the manufacturer's instructions before using it again.
3. Instruct the patient to stand on the platform or lie quietly in the middle of the bed, without touching anything else. Shoes should be removed and the minimum clothing worn (Fig. 6–1).
4. Note the measurement and record it immediately.
5. Compare present measurement with previous measurement(s) before the patient is removed from the scale, to determine if there are any incongruities or unusual changes.

Note should be made if any street clothing is worn. The average weight of street clothing without shoes is approximately 2 pounds. However, this varies greatly.

Other items may need to be tared or accounted for in weighing the patient, especially if he or she is weighed on a bedscale, e.g., bed linens, dressings, catheters, respiratory equipment. Standard hospital items such as these should be weighed, the average taken of three weights, then a record kept

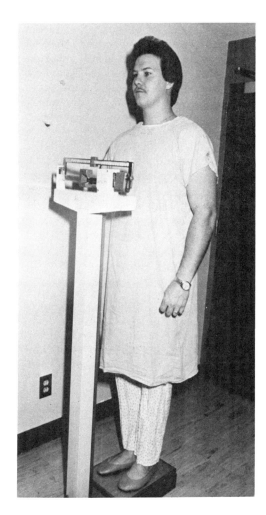

Figure 6–1. The patient stands in the middle of the platform scale without touching anything. Shoes should be removed; minimal clothing should be worn.

with the scales to assist in more accurate determinations of weight. Intravenous (IV) bags, chest tube collections, or Foley bags should be hung on a floor pole above the patient or held by an assistant, so that their weight does not add to that of the patient on the bedscale or floor scale.

Patients who are in traction or with casts present special problems as they frequently were not weighed before the cast or traction was placed. Although an accurate absolute weight is not attainable, it is still important to keep track of weight changes. Therefore, use the weight of the body plus hardware as a starting reference. Record on the nurse's graphic sheet the number of casts, pounds of traction, or other appliances present at the initial weight. Note changes from this during subsequent weighing. Also, account for alterations in weight due to amputation (see Table 6–5).

Patients' admission weight and height is best obtained during a nursing history. In hospitals where a preadmission work-up is obtained prior to the patient's hospitalization, height and weight can be measured then.

The height and weight should be measured by a trained observer rather than taking the patient's recall of his weight as self-reported weights are frequently over- or underestimated. Stunkard and Albaum,[59] in reviewing the research, found correlation coefficients of reported to measured weight ranging between 0.96 and 0.98 for groups of Americans. Their own research sampled 550 American men and women and yielded a correlation coefficient of 0.974. Pirie et al.[60] reported correlation coefficients of 0.92 for men and 0.94 for women, with men tending to overestimate their true weight except at higher weights, and women to underestimate their true weight. There was a time lapse of approximately 1 month between the time the subjects reported their weights and the time that they were weighed, however, which could account for the larger error. Pirie et al.[60] also reported correlation coefficients between reported and measured height of 0.93 for men and 0.94 for women. The men tended to underestimate and the women to overestimate their true height. Morgan et al.[61] asked 105 men and women at the Leeds General Infirmary what their usual weight or their weight before becoming ill was, and found that among 50 percent of these patients, the difference between their reported and measured weight exceeded 5 kg and ranged as

high as 15 kg discrepancy. There were no data regarding their length of stay in the hospital.

Calculating Rate of Change

To determine the rate of weight loss, compare the measured weight to preillness or usual weight, based on patient's recall, as well as to standard weights for a population of same age, sex, and height as the patient.

$$\frac{\%\ \text{ideal}}{\text{body weight}} = \frac{\text{actual weight}}{\text{standard weight}} \times 100$$

$$\%\ \text{usual weight} = \frac{\text{actual weight}}{\text{usual weight}} \times 100$$

$$\%\ \text{weight change} = \frac{\text{usual weight} - \text{actual weight}}{\text{usual weight}} \times 100$$

Interpretation of weight loss and weight that is below "standard" must take into account a consideration of what compartment of the body the weight loss occurred in—fat, protein, or water. Other anthropometric measurements are used to assess this as are certain biochemical indices.

Evaluating the rate of weight change is sometimes difficult as it is normal for weight to fluctuate from day to day by ±1.0 to 1.5 kg. Weight gain can be expected in postsurgery or posttrauma patients who have undergone fluid resuscitation with later weight loss attributed to diuresis. Patients with renal disease or ascites also may rapidly lose or gain large amounts of weight that is mostly water. Burn patients or patients with chronic diarrhea may exhibit sudden weight loss that is secondary to dehydration.[50] Moore[62] has noted that weight loss exceeding 500 g/day in postsurgery patients is most likely the result of dehydration or diuresis.

Interpretation of weight and weight change must also take into account age and growth determinants. Stroudt,[63] in a review of the U.S. Health and Nutrition Examination Survey (HANES I) data for height and weight in adults, noted an increase in weight through early adulthood, then a drop in weight in advanced old age. The average weight for males was the same at 65 to 74 years as it was at 18 to 24 years of age, then dropped 10 pounds from 75 to 79 years of age. Stroudt hypothesized that this trend to gain weight for height may be the construct of a gradual loss in stature due to changes in the vertebrae of the spine as a natural part of the aging process. Weight gain, however, may also be due to loss of LBM that occurs at reported rates that range from 0.13 to 0.42 kg/yr.[64] This loss of LBM leads to a decrease in basal energy expenditure (BEE) which, in the face of unchanged intake, promotes weight gain. Loss of weight in advanced old age is likely due to a combination of factors, including earlier mortality of the more obese, continued loss of LBM, and decrease in skeletal density.[63,64]

Blackburn et al.[4] gives guidelines in Table 6–6 for evaluating weight change.

To summarize, in evaluating weight loss, one should consider the following questions:

1. How reliable is the patient history concerning the rate and extent of weight loss? Can it be confirmed by comparing with prior measurements or by physical examination?
2. Has there been a recent change in food intake that accounts for this?
3. Has there been evidence of change in gastrointestinal (GI) function (malabsorption, maldigestion)?
4. Has there been any evidence of polyuria, diuresis, edema, or ascites?
5. What medical conditions or other stresses exist that could contribute to weight loss? (See Table 6–7.)

BONE AND GENERAL BODY DIAMETERS

Measurements are usually made from one bony prominence to another using a broad or narrow blade anthropometer or a small precision caliper. The fingers of both hands are

TABLE 6–6. EVALUATING RATE OF WEIGHT CHANGE[a]

Time	Significant Weight Loss (%)	Severe Weight Loss (%)
1 week	1–2	>2
1 month	5	>5
3 months	7.5	>7.5
6 months	10	>10

[a]Values charted are for % weight change.
From Blackburn GL, Bistrian BR, Maine BS, et al.: JPEN 1:11, 1977.[4]

placed over the bony prominence and the anthropometer is laid immediately over the identified landmark.

The most common measurement of a body diameter that is made in the hospital setting is stature. The next most common is measurement of the upper arm to determine the midpoint between the olecranon and acromion process. Various other body diameters have been tested as a means of predicting body frame size.

Height

Stature or standing height is the distance from the crown of the head to the soles of the feet. Accurate determination of height is important in nutrition assessment in order to calculate CHI, estimated BEE using the Harris–Benedict equation, and body surface area. Body weight is compared against height as a relative index of fatness.

The chief limitation in using height as a standard for comparison noted earlier in this text is that it decreases with age.[63,65] This shortening appears to occur chiefly in the trunk, but does not affect the extremities.[63,66] Mitchell and Lipschitz[66] compared total arm length (TAL) among a group of 100 young and elderly males and females (mean age 69.8 years). They found values of 0.68 and 0.63 respectively for the young and old populations between height and TAL. The

TABLE 6–7. VARIOUS ETIOLOGIES OF WEIGHT LOSS

Appetite Normal or Increased	Appetite Decreased

1. Increased caloric utilization
  a. Hyperthyroidism
  b. Anxiety
  c. Drugs—thyroid, amphetamines
  d. Trauma
  e. Fever
	1. Predominantly psychologic
	  a. Depression
	  b. Anorexia nervosa

2. Decreased intestinal adsorption
  a. Hypermotility
  b. Pancreatic deficiency
  c. Enteropathy
	2. Primarily gastrointestinal
	  a. Decreased adsorption: sprue, enteropathy, etc.
	  b. Obstruction: neoplasm, adhesions, etc.
	  c. Hepatobiliary disease

3. Abnormal loss
  a. Diabetes mellitus (glucosuria)
  b. Fistulas
  c. Intestinal parasites
  d. Surgical or traumatic wounds
	3. Systemic disturbances
	  a. Malignancy
	  b. Infection
	  c. Uremia
	  d. Cardiovascular disease
	  e. Pulmonary disease
	  f. Endocrine-metabolic
	    (1) Adrenal insufficiency
	    (2) Hypercalcemia
	    (3) Hypokalemia
	  g. Intoxications: lead, alcohol
	  h. Hematologic disorders:
	    (1) Myelofibrosis
	    (2) Leukemia

Adapted from Thorn GW, Adams, RD, Braunwald E, et al. (eds.): Harrison's Principles of Internal Medicine. 8th ed. New York: McGraw-Hill, 1977, p 227, Table 45-1.

regressions were parallel in both groups with slopes of 0.303 for the young and 0.337 for the elderly. The CHI also correlated significantly with mg creatinine/cm TAL (CTAL) in this group. In another study, Mitchell and Lipschitz[67] compared CHI with TAL between groups of well-nourished and malnourished young and elderly. They found that CTAL was a better discriminator of nutrition status in the young groups than CHI, and that it was similar to CHI in elderly males. There was no significant difference between well-nourished and mal-nourished elderly females in CTAL versus CHI.

TAL is easier to measure in bedridden patients than arm span, and not as readily affected by altered range of motion or clubbing deformities as in rheumatoid arthritis. It also avoids alterations in chest size due to kyphosis, osteoporosis, or lung disease.

TAL has potential use in other patient populations in whom accurate measurement of height is difficult, i.e., para- and quadraplegics, amputees, stroke, head injury, or whenever the patient is confined to bed or to a wheelchair.

Techniques. Jelliffe[57] and Behnke and Wilmore[44] advocate use of a movable block square attached to a scale that is fixed to a wall or other vertical flat surface for measuring stature. This equipment is rarely available in clinical settings. Jensen et al.[68] describes the proper use of the movable rod for measuring height on the platform scales. The examiner should be familiar with the available equipment before using it.

1. When possible, measure patients on admission. If the patient cannot be mea-

sured, note that the height is verbally reported or taken from past records.

2. Instruct the patient to remove shoes or other footwear having heels.
3. Have the patient step onto the platform of the scale with his or her back to the measuring rod.
4. Raise the measuring rod approximately 6 inches above the patient's head and extend the steel bar vertically over the head.
5. Instruct the patient to stand erect. The patient's line of sight should be horizontal and the heels and scapulas aligned with the measuring rod.
6. Lower the steel bar, crushing the hair if necessary, until it contacts the scalp (Fig. 6–2).
7. Allow the patient to step off the platform.
8. At the base of the adjustable portion of the measuring rod, read the height to the nearest one-fourth inch or half centimeter.
9. Immediately record the height on the appropriate form in the medical record.

Total Arm Length

TAL is measured as follows:[66]

1. The patient stands, sits, or lies with the arm outstretched to full length, palm up.
2. Mark the tip of the acromial process of the scapula and the end of the styloid process of the ulna with water-base felt pen or tape.
3. Keeping the patient's arm outstretched, measure the length between these two points with a steel measuring tape in centimeters.
4. Record the measurement immediately on the appropriate form.

The Midupper Arm

Reproducible location of the midpoint of the upper arm requires practice. Use a tape 7 to 12 mm wide for easy reading and made of

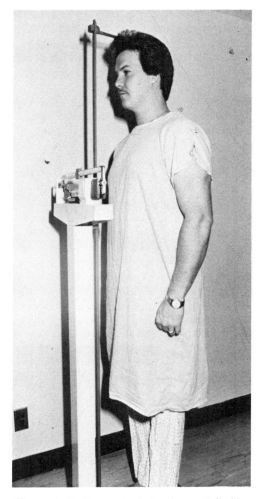

Figure 6–2. The patient stands erect, looking straight ahead while the steel bar is lowered until it contacts the scalp.

metal, fiberglass, or other nonstretchable material. (Cloth is not acceptable.) The tape should not be crimped during or between usage.

Use of the paper Inser-Tape (Ross Laboratories, Columbus, Ohio 43216) is acceptable. Steel tapes graded in millimeters are also available.

Epidemiologists commonly take measurements on the right arm whereas for purposes of assessment, measurements are usually made on the left or nondominant arm. Burgert and Anderson,[69] in comparing sites of measurement, found no significant difference in a heterogeneous population between right and left arm measurements, although in some individuals, significant differences did occur.

1. Instruct the patient to bend the arm at the elbow at a 90 degree angle, palm up (Fig. 6–3).
2. Stand behind the patient's arm.
3. Palpate the acromion process of the scapula (bony protrusion on the posterior of the upper shoulder at the end of the scapular ridge), and the olecranon process (the bony point of the elbow). Mark these spots after locating them with a water-base felt-tip pen or piece of tape to assist in accurate placement of the tape (Fig. 6–4).
4. If the Inser-Tape is used, the "Midpoint Measure" side should be visible and the

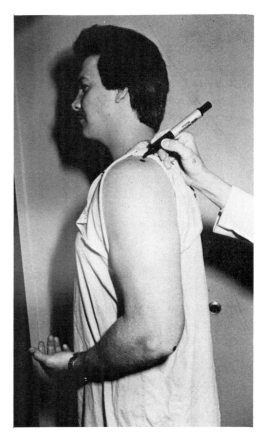

Figure 6–4. The acromion and olecranon processes are palpated and marked with a water-base felt-tip pen or a piece of tape.

tape adjusted vertically along the arm until the same measurement appears at the acromial process of the scapula and the olecranon process (Fig. 6–5).
5. If a measuring tape is used, measure the length between the two points and divide by two. Mark the midpoint with water-base felt-tip pen or tape (Fig. 6–6).
6. The midpoint of the arm is the point where the midpoint indicator of the Inser-Tape appears on the arm (half the distance between the two points as measured by the tape). Mark it accurately with felt-pen or tape (Fig. 6–6).

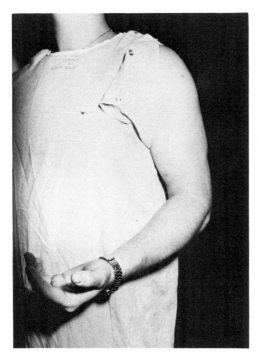

Figure 6–3. The patient bends the arm at a 90 degree angle, palm up.

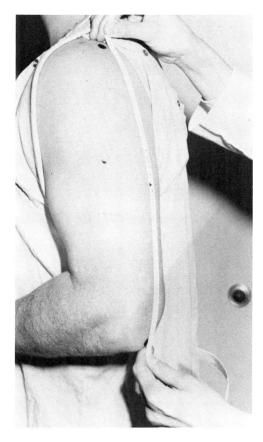

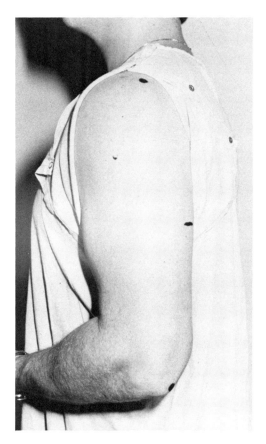

Figure 6–5. The insertion tape is adjusted vertically until the same measurement appears at the acromial process of the scapula and at the olecranon.

Figure 6–6. The midpoint of the upper arm is marked with a water-base felt-tip pen or tape.

7. Note on which arm the midpoint was marked. Take all subsequent arm measurements on the same side, if possible.

Frame Size

Besides the height and age, weight is also influenced by body width, bone thickness, muscularity, and trunk length relative to height. Body frame size reflects the sum effect of these four factors. The Metropolitan Life Insurance tables of "ideal" weight for height contained classifications of weight by frame size but failed to explain the criteria

for doing so.[7,8] Katch and Freedson[70] attempted to classify frame size based on measurements of height and biacromial and bitrochanteric diameters. Katch et al.[71] demonstrated that subjective appraisal was an invalid means of determining frame size. Their sample population, however, consisting of 295 caucasian university students, is too small and not representative. Also, their technique is too cumbersome to apply in a clinical setting. Frisancho and Flegel[72] have proposed measurement of elbow breadth as an index of frame size (Table 6–8). Their population is 16,494 persons 18 to 74 years of age from the U.S. Health and Nutrition Examination Survey (HANES I) of 1971 to

TABLE 6–8. FRAME SIZES BY ELBOW BREADTH OF U.S. BLACK AND WHITE ADULTS, HANES I, 1971–1974

Age (yr)	Frame Size (cm)		
	Small	Medium	Large
Caucasian Males			
18–24	≤6.7	>6.7, <7.5	≥7.5
25–34	≤6.7	>6.7, <7.5	≥7.5
35–44	≤6.9	>6.9, <7.6	≥7.6
45–54	≤6.9	>6.9, <7.7	≥7.7
55–64	≤6.9	>6.9, <7.7	≥7.7
65–74	≤6.9	>6.9, <7.7	≥7.7
Caucasian Females			
18–24	≤5.7	>5.7, <6.4	≥6.4
25–34	≤5.8	>5.8, <6.5	≥6.5
35–44	≤5.9	>5.9, <6.6	≥6.6
45–54	≤5.9	>5.9, <6.8	≥6.8
55–64	≤6.0	>6.0, <6.9	≥6.9
65–74	≤6.0	>6.0, <6.9	≥6.9
Black Males			
18–24	≤6.7	>6.7, <7.6	≥7.6
25–34	≤6.8	>6.8, <7.6	≥7.6
35–44	≤6.7	>6.7, <7.7	≥7.7
45–54	≤6.9	>6.9, <7.9	≥7.9
55–64	≤6.9	>6.9, <7.9	≥7.9
65–74	≤6.9	>6.9, <7.8	≥7.8
Black Females			
18–24	≤5.8	>5.8, <6.6	≥6.6
25–34	≤5.8	>5.8, <6.7	≥6.7
35–44	≤6.0	>6.0, <7.0	≥7.0
45–54	≤6.0	>6.0, <7.1	≥7.1
55–64	≤6.1	>6.1, <7.2	≥7.2
65–74	≤6.1	>6.1, <7.0	≥7.0

Adapted from Frisancho AR, Flegel PN: Am J Clin Nutr, 37:311–314, 1983, Table 2.[72]

1974. They compared elbow breadth, bitrochanteric breadth, and weight against age and against the log-transformed sum of the triceps and the subscapular skinfolds as a reflection of body fat. Elbow breadth was more independent of age than bitrochanteric breadth and of skinfolds than weight. It was a better discriminator of weight categorizations than stature. It is a readily obtained, highly replicable measurement that appears suitable for use in the clinical setting, but is not commonly employed there at this time. Further investigation of its application is needed.

Garn et al.[73] proposed measurement of bony chest breadth (BCB) as an index of body frame size, based on radiogrammetric data from 2201 males examined in the Western Scotland Health Survey. They established three frame size categories ("small," "medium," "large") that were characterized by differences of 10 to 12 kg body weight. Furthermore, they assert that the BCB is independent of TBF measured anthropometrically and radiogrammetrically. Their population, however, is not representative of the United States, does not include females, and further standardization of their technique is needed. Furthermore, radiography is more expensive and difficult to obtain than anthropometry. Studies relating the use of this technique in a U.S. population are needed before it can be recommended for use in the clinical setting.

Technique for Measuring Elbow Diameter

1. The examiner must be familiar with the use of a broad blade anthropometer.
2. The patient extends the arm forward perpendicular to the body and bends the elbow at a 90 degree angle with the palm of the hand toward the patient.
3. The examiner places the broad blade anthropometer at the condyles of the humerus, each blade of the anthropometer touching a condyle.
4. The examiner reads the distance between the condyles in centimeters.
5. The examiner records the measurement immediately on the appropriate form.

BODY CIRCUMFERENCE

In the nutrition assessment of adults, the midupper arm circumference (MAC) is the most common measurement of body circumference. It has little prognostic value in adults, but is usually measured in order to calculate MAMC or MAMA.

A steel or fiberglass tape measure is recommended as cloth tape measures tend to stretch. Zerfas[74] studied the design of conventional tape measures used in measuring MAC. He found it difficult to align them and keep them horizontal while trying to achieve orientation or the zero point. The thickness of the tape measure contributed to the measured circumference. Variations in placement and graduations of numerals also made accurate readings difficult. He found errors of 0.5 to 1.0 cm in reading MAC depending on the type of tape and technique used. Zerfas tested the insertion tape versus the conventional tape measure. He does not report the data, but he states that 1.8 percent of the trials had errors greater than 0.2 cm while only 0.1 percent exhibited an error greater than 1.0 cm.

Technique[44,74]

1. Instruct the patient to stand or sit with the patient's arm hanging fully extended and relaxed by the side of the body.
2. Loop the insertion tape or measuring tape around the arm at the previously marked midpoint level (Fig. 6–7).
3. Position the tape horizontally at the previously marked midpoint, then tighten it firmly around the contour of the arm, but not so tightly as to cause indentation or pinching of the contour (Fig. 6–8).
4. Note and record the measurement in centimeters on the appropriate form.
5. Compare the measurement with previous MAC measurements to check for discrepancies or changes.

SKINFOLDS

Measurement of skinfold thickness is a commonly used means of assessing subcutaneous

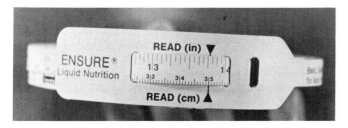

Figure 6–7. Loop the insertion tape through the slot so that the measurement can be read by centimeters through the window.

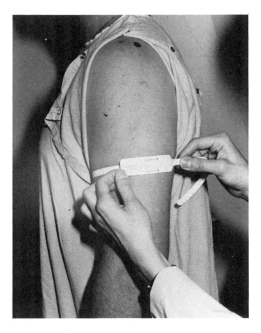

Figure 6–8. Position the looped insertion tape at the midpoint of the upper arm, tightening it firmly around the contour of the arm, without causing indentation of the contour.

fat. Specially designed calipers are needed to accomplish this. The calipers are calibrated to provide a constant tension (10 g/mm^2) over a range of 2 to 40 mm of caliper openings on a contact or "pinch" area of 20 to 40 mm^2 and should read to ±0.1 mm accuracy. They are used to measure a double thickness of skin with a layer of fat between. It is important to determine precisely the area where the calipers are to be applied and to maintain a constant distance between the caliper and the thumb and finger holding the skin, not letting go of the skin while taking the measurement. This minimizes differences due to variation in distribution of fat over different parts of the body. The calipers should be tested at least once a month, to assure their accuracy. A graduated metal calibration block can be ordered from the manufacturer of the caliper.

Lange skinfold calipers are the standard calipers used in the United States. They are manufactured by Cambridge Scientific Instruments, Cambridge, Maryland, according to the accepted standards (Fig. 6–9).

Although the plastic skinfold calipers are widely available, they do not give acceptably reproducible results. When compared to the Lange caliper, the measurements are significantly lower and therefore not accurate enough to predict body composition.[75] They tend to lose tension over time and to break easily. They are much cheaper than the standard calipers however, and are used frequently for this reason (Fig. 6–10).

Harpenden skinfold calipers are used primarily in Britain. They are available through Holtain Ltd., Bryberian Crymmych, Pembrokeshire, United Kingdom. Durnin and Womersley[15] found no significant difference between the results given by the Lange and those of the Harpenden caliper.

Skinfolds are limited in several ways as means of assessing an individual's fat stores:

1. Skinfold compressibility differs with each individual. Compressibility decreases with age[38] and with progressive dehydration.[76] Lee and Ng[33] measured thickness of skin and fat directly and compared them with skinfold measurements in 71 fresh male and female cadavers with ages varying from 1 month to 74 years of age. They found a mean correlation coefficient of 0.83 between skinfold and actual fat, with a range of 0.61 to 0.92 in the nine areas of the body that were measured. They suggested three reasons for discrepancies between actual fat layer and skinfold measurement: (1) differences in thickness of skin; (2) differences in compressibility of subcutaneous tissues, such as amount, density and fixation of fibrous tissue, content of blood vessels, hair follicles, glands, and total amount of fat; and (3) differences in skin tension over bone, muscle, and viscera.

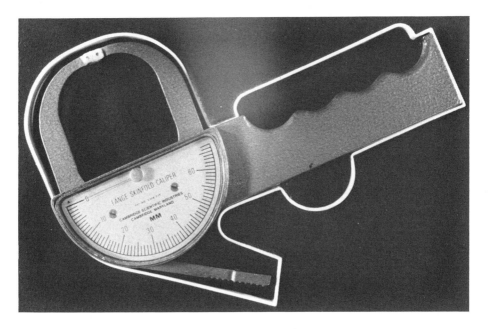

Figure 6–9. The Lange skinfold caliper. *(Courtesy of Cambridge Scientific Industries, P.O. Box 265, Moose Lodge Road, Cambridge, MD, 21613.)*

2. The skinfold measurements do not directly account for nonsubcutaneous fat that has been deposited between muscles or other places throughout the body.

Allen et al.[34] in a study of 87 Formosan men and women demonstrated that the ratio of subcutaneous to internal fat increased with increasing total body fat, as measured by underwater

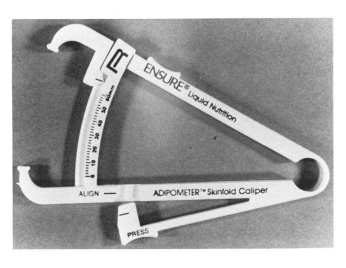

Figure 6–10. An example of a plastic skinfold caliper.

densitometry. Durnin and Womersley[15] also noted that changes in skinfold measurements at four sites were not linearly related to changes in adiposity measured densitometrically.

3. Subcutaneous fat is evenly distributed over the body. Individual differences occur due to sex, weight loss with aging, and in those who are athletic.[20,27,65,67] There is disagreement in the literature over which site is the most representative of TBF. It is generally agreed that skinfold measurements taken at more than one site correlate better with TBF than do single measurements.[15,16,26]

4. Although they are useful in assessing degree of body fatness,[6] skinfolds are difficult to obtain accurately in obese subjects and are not as good an index of weight loss as are changes in body circumferences in the obese.[27]

5. Skinfold measurements do not appear to be important predictors of outcome in stressed patients compared to other parameters of nutrition assessment.

Mullen et al.[77] found that 33 percent of 64 patients undergoing elective surgery in a Veterans Administration Hospital had triceps skinfolds (TSF) less than 90 percent of standard. In this group, according to the investigators, TSF did not predict morbidity or mortality but were important, along with weight changes, in detecting protein–calorie malnutrition (PCM).

Harvey et al.[21,23] studied 528 general medical–surgical patients referred to a nutrition support team. Patients who became septic had TSF that were 64 percent of standard compared to 209 nonseptic patients with TSF 79 percent of standard. Sixty-five patients died with a mean percent standard TSF 69 ± 5 percent compared to a mean of 81 ± 4 percent for those who survived. Harvey stated the difference was not significant.

Harvey et al.[54] also studied 161 cancer patients undergoing various forms of therapy; 111 survived with a mean percent standard TSF of 77 percent; 50 who died had a mean percent standard TSF of 69 percent.

Freeman et al.[78] evaluated the nutrition status of 65 patients with lung cancer undergoing chemotherapy both with and without total parenteral nutrition support. Patients with initial TSF greater than 74 percent standard, initial weight loss of less than 4 percent, and greater than the initial median for mean daily kilocalories had the lower mortality rate.

It is interesting that in the latter three studies, the TSF for those who survived were approximately 75 percent of standard. One wonders if perhaps Mullen set his standard of comparison too high or the results were indeterminate because the population studied was less stressed and had lower rates of morbidity and mortality than that of the other studies. One can also ask whether too much emphasis is being placed on changes in TSF during hospitalization, rather than on initial admission values and long-term follow-up. Finally one can conjecture about the possible influence of starvation apart from stress on TSF and on the sensitivity of TSF as a predictor of morbidity and mortality in a relatively energy depleted state, as in Freeman et al.'s population. Further investigation and definition of these factors is needed.

Techniques

Skinfolds that are frequently measured in clinical situations include:

- Triceps (Figs. 6–11, 6–12)
- Subscapular (Figs. 6–13, 6–14)
- Suprailiac crest (Fig. 6–15)
- Biceps (Fig. 6–16)

Choice of measurement site will be determined by the availability of the site on the individual, the purpose of the study, and the standards available for comparison.

A. Triceps Skinfold
  1. The Ambulatory Patient[44,57,79]
    a. Instruct the patient to stand with his arms hanging fully extended and relaxed, at his side, then stand behind the patient.

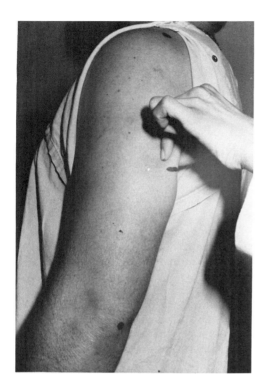

Figure 6–11. Gently grasp a double layer of skin and fat 1.0 cm above the midpoint of the upper arm, parallel to the long axis of the arm and in line with the olecranon process. Pull it away from the underlying muscle.

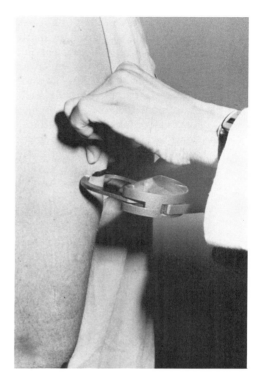

Figure 6–12. Still grasping the skinfold, align the jaws of the caliper horizontally at the midpoint mark. Release the arm of the caliper, wait 3 seconds, then take a reading. Repeat three times.

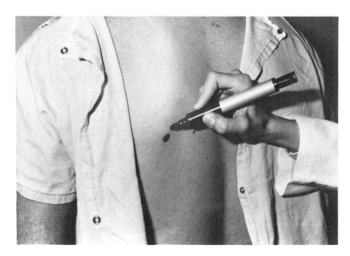

Figure 6–13. Palpate the tip of the scapula at its lower border. Mark with water-soluble felt-tip pen.

b. To ensure that only fat is grasped, not muscle, and that it is in the area of the triceps, have the patient press the hand, palm down, on the knee or other solid object. This will tighten the triceps so that it can be easily palpated. Have the subject relax before taking the reading.

c. Gently grasp a double layer of skin and fat about 1.0 cm above the previously marked midpoint, parallel to the long axis of the arm in a direct line with the olecranon process, and pull it away from the underlying muscle (Fig. 6–11).

d. Align the jaws of the caliper horizontally at the midpoint mark, while maintaining a gentle grip of the skinfold (Fig. 6–12).

e. Release the arm of the caliper, wait approximately 3 seconds, then take a reading.

f. Take three readings and average them.

g. Record measurements accurately in millimeters on the appropriate form, comparing them with previous measurements to determine possible change or errors in reading the caliper.

2. The Nonambulatory Patient[80]

For patients who are not able to stand for whatever reason, Jenson et al.[80] recommend measuring the triceps skinfold as follows:

a. The patient lies flat in bed, face up.

b. The patient's arm rests, fully extended, along the side with the hand on the thigh.

c. Take the measurements in the same way as with an ambulatory patient (see steps b through g, above).

The same general techniques applied in measurement of triceps skinfold apply in the measurement of other fatfolds.

B. Subscapular Skinfold[44]

1. Instruct the patient to stand, relaxed. Stand behind the subject.

2. Palpate the lower border of the scapula and mark it with water-soluble felt-pen or tape (Fig. 6–13).

3. Grasp the skinfold at the site with fingers on top, thumb below, and forefinger on the site at the lower tip of the scapula; the skinfold should angle 45 degrees from horizontal, medially upward, and laterally downward.

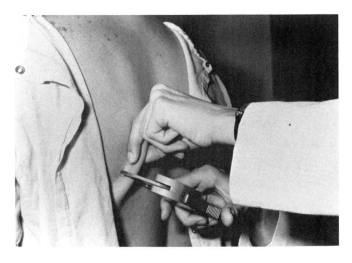

Figure 6–14. Grasp the skin and fat with fingers on top, thumb below and forefinger on the marked site of the scapula tip. With the fat fold at a 45 degree angle, medially upward and laterally downward, apply the caliper 1.0 cm below the site.

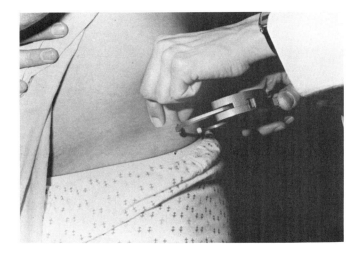

Figure 6–15. Palpate the crest of the ilium at the midaxillary line. Grasp a vertical fold of skin and fat, 1.0 cm above the mark. Align the jaws of the calipers horizontally at the mark, release the arm, wait 3 seconds, and take a reading.

4. Apply the caliper 1.0 cm below the site (Fig 6–14).
5. After approximately 3 seconds, take a reading.
6. Take three readings, average them, and record the average on the appropriate form.
C. Suprailiac Crest Skinfold[44]
   1. Grasp a vertical fold of skin and fat at the crest of the ilium at the midaxillary line (Fig. 6–15).
   2. Take three readings, average them, and record the average on the appropriate form.
D. Biceps Skinfold[44]
   1. Grasp a vertical fold of skin and fat at the previously marked midpoint on the upper arm over the biceps muscle (Fig. 6–16).
   2. Take three readings, average them, and record the average on the appropriate form.

DERIVED ANTHROPOMETRIC MEASUREMENTS

Midupper Arm Muscle Circumference

MAMC is an indirect indicator of muscle mass that is used extensively in many pro-

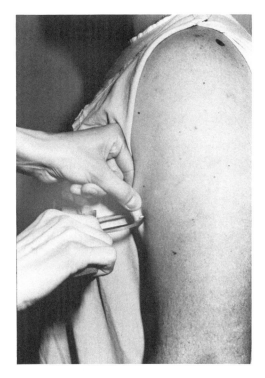

Figure 6–16. Grasp a vertical fold of skin and fat at the previously marked midpoint of the upper arm over the biceps muscle. Align the jaws of the caliper horizontally. Release the arm of the calipers. Wait 3 seconds and take a reading.

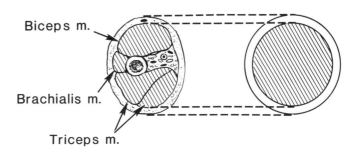

Figure 6–17. The relationship of actual to the theoretical midupper arm circumference, midupper arm muscle circumference, and midupper arm muscle area.

Biceps m.

Brachialis m.

Triceps m.

tocols for nutrition assessment.[57] The logic is that TSF is a measurement of the thickness or diameter of fat and skin overlaying the muscle. From this diameter, the area of fat surrounding the muscle can be calculated roughly, if the fat and muscle are both assumed to be circular. Then the fat is subtracted from the total arm circumference to yield the circumference of the muscle. The equation is as follows (Fig. 6–17):

$$\frac{MAMC}{(cm)} = \frac{MAC}{(cm)} - \frac{\pi \times TSF \ (mm)}{10}$$

where $\pi = 3.14$.

The potential uses and limitations of the MAMC were discussed earlier in the chapter.

Midarm Muscle Area and Bone-Free Midarm Muscle Area

MAMA quantitates the surface area of muscle, medial neurovascular sheath and bone at the cross-section of the midupper arm. When Heymsfield et al.[81] corrected MAMA for the area of bone, they found an average discrepancy of 7.7 percent between calculated values and values measured by CT. Bone-free MAMA (MAMA.BF) changes more rapidly than MAMC in response to PCM on a long-term basis. Like MAMC, however, short-term changes (daily or weekly) may be masked by shifts in hydration, and its exact relationship to body composition of functional protein, both muscle and nonmuscle, is difficult to establish.

MAMA.BF appears to be of some prog-

nostic value. Heymsfield et al.[36,81] found that nine patients with advanced PCM died within 1 to 2 weeks after their MAMA.BF dropped below 9 to 11 cm². They postulated that this was the minimal amount of muscle area compatible with survival, but also warned that the population sampled is small, the majority of the sample had cancer, and that further investigation is needed to validate this.

$$MAMA \ (cm^2) = MAC - \left[\frac{MAMC}{4\pi} \right]$$

$$MAMA.BF \ (cm^2) = \begin{array}{l} Males \quad MAMA - 10 \\ Females \ MAMA - 6.5 \end{array}$$

The Body Mass Index

The body mass index is an alternate means of describing degree of body fatness. The assumption is that weight, when corrected for height, is positively correlated to degree of adiposity. Therefore, the higher the body mass index, the greater the relative amount of fat it carries. It cannot, therefore, be considered a direct measurement of body composition, since weight gain or loss can occur because of changes in hydration or LBM. It is a useful descriptor, however, since measurement of skinfolds is not always possible.

There are several body mass indices, but the most frequently used is the Quetelet index (wt/ht²). Roche et al.[82] compared the TSF, biceps skinfold (BSF), subscapular skinfold (SSSF), wt/ht², wt/ht³, and wt/ht by percentiles with percentage body fat and

TBF derived from underwater measurement of body density in 539 adults and children. They found that wt/ht^2 was more highly correlated with TBF in children, adolescent girls, and adults and with percentage of body fat in men than the other measurements. Investigation of its application in the clinical setting is needed. Frisancho and Flegel[83] recommended that wt/ht^2 be used in addition to the other measurements of body fat, such as skinfolds, to assess body fatness or leanness rather than by itself.

$$\text{Quetelet index} = \text{wt/ht}^2 \times 100$$
$$\text{where wt} = \text{weight in kg}$$
$$\text{ht} = \text{height in cm}$$

Prediction of Percentage Body Fat From Summated Skinfolds

In patients who are able to stand, who do not exhibit signs of over- or underhydration and who are not extremely obese, the clinician can, if necessary, obtain a prediction of percentage body fat from the sum of four skinfolds according to the method of Durnin and Womersley.[15] This can be done either by calculating body density from the log of the sum of the four skinfolds (see Table 6–9), or by referring to a table (Table 6–10).

1. Measure the biceps, triceps, subscapular and suprailiac skinfolds in mm and weight in kg.
2. Calculate Σ by adding the four skinfolds.
3. Calculate the logarithm of Σ.

TABLE 6–9. ESTIMATION OF BODY DENSITY FROM THE LOGARITHM OF THE SUM OF FOUR SKINFOLD THICKNESSES

Age Range (yr)

Men:	17–19	D = 1.1620 − 0.0630 × (log Σ)
	20–29	D = 1.1631 − 0.0632 × (log Σ)
	30–39	D = 1.1422 − 0.0544 × (log Σ)
	40–49	D = 1.1620 − 0.0700 × (log Σ)
	50+	D = 1.1715 − 0.0779 × (log Σ)
Women:	16–19	D = 1.1549 − 0.0678 × (log Σ)
	20–29	D = 1.1599 − 0.0717 × (log Σ)
	30–39	D = 1.1423 − 0.0632 × (log Σ)
	40–49	D = 1.1333 − 0.0612 × (log Σ)
	50+	D = 1.1339 − 0.0645 × (log Σ)

Adapted from Durnin JVGA, Womersley J: Br J Nutr 32: 77–97, 1974, Table 5.[15]

4. Calculate body density (D, g/cc) using one of the equations in Table 6–9.
5. Calculate fat mass (FM):

$$\frac{\text{FM}}{\text{(kg)}} = \frac{\text{Body weight}}{\text{(kg)}} \times \left[\left(\frac{4.95}{\text{D}} \right) - 4.5 \right]$$

6. Calculate fat-free mass(FFM):

$$\text{FFM (kg)} = \text{Body weight (kg)} - \text{fat mass (kg)}$$

Table 6–10 incorporates the calculations in steps 3 through 5. Simply calculate Σ of the four skinfolds and obtain percentage FM from the table.

ANTHROPOMETRIC STANDARDS OF REFERENCE AND INTERPRETATION

Interpretation of anthropometric measurements is facilitated by comparing them to standards derived from a reference population. Jelliffe suggested standards of reference[5] that include the 1959 Metropolitan Life Insurance table of "desirable" weight for height, and tables of arm anthropometrics derived from a variety of sources (Tables 6–

TABLE 6–10. THE EQUIVALENT FAT CONTENT, AS A PERCENTAGE OF BODY WEIGHT, FOR THE SUM OF FOUR SKINFOLDS (BICEPS, TRICEPS, SUBSCAPULAR, AND SUPRAILIAC)

Skinfolds (mm)	Percentage Fat							
	Males				*Females*			
	17–29 (yr)	*30–39*	*40–49*	*50+*	*16–29*	*30–39*	*40–49*	*50+*
15	4.8				10.5			
20	8.1	12.2	12.2	12.6	14.1	17.0	19.8	21.4
25	10.5	14.2	15.0	15.6	16.8	19.4	22.2	24.0
30	12.9	16.2	17.7	18.6	19.5	21.8	24.5	26.6
35	14.7	17.7	19.6	20.8	21.5	23.7	26.4	28.5
40	16.4	19.2	21.4	22.9	23.4	25.5	28.2	30.3
45	17.7	20.4	23.0	24.7	25.0	26.9	29.6	31.9
50	19.0	21.5	24.6	26.5	26.5	28.2	31.0	33.4
55	20.1	22.5	25.9	27.9	27.8	29.4	32.1	34.6
60	21.2	23.5	27.1	29.2	29.1	30.6	33.2	35.7
65	22.2	24.3	28.2	30.4	30.2	31.6	34.1	36.7
70	23.1	25.1	29.3	31.6	31.2	32.5	35.0	37.7
75	24.0	25.9	30.3	32.7	32.2	33.4	35.9	38.7
80	24.8	26.6	31.2	33.8	33.1	34.3	36.7	39.6
85	25.5	27.2	32.1	34.8	34.0	35.1	37.5	40.4
90	26.2	27.8	33.0	35.8	34.8	35.8	38.3	41.2
95	26.9	28.4	33.7	36.6	35.6	36.5	39.0	41.9
100	27.6	29.0	34.4	37.4	36.4	37.2	39.7	42.6
105	28.2	29.6	35.1	38.2	37.1	37.9	40.4	43.3
110	28.8	30.1	35.8	39.0	37.8	38.6	41.0	43.9
115	29.4	30.6	36.4	39.7	38.4	39.1	41.5	44.5
120	30.0	31.1	37.0	40.4	39.0	39.6	42.0	45.1
125	30.5	31.5	37.6	41.1	39.6	40.1	42.5	45.7
130	31.0	31.9	38.2	41.8	40.2	40.6	43.0	46.2
135	31.5	32.3	38.7	42.4	40.8	41.1	43.5	46.7
140	32.0	32.7	39.2	43.0	41.3	41.6	44.0	47.2
145	32.5	33.1	39.7	43.6	41.8	42.1	44.5	47.7
150	32.9	33.5	40.2	44.1	42.3	42.6	45.0	48.2
155	33.3	33.9	40.7	44.6	42.8	43.1	45.4	48.7
160	33.7	34.3	41.2	45.1	43.3	43.6	45.8	49.2
165	34.1	34.6	41.6	45.6	43.7	44.0	46.2	49.6
170	34.5	34.8	42.0	46.1	44.1	44.4	46.6	50.0
175	34.9					44.8	47.0	50.4
180	35.3					45.2	47.4	50.8
185	35.6					45.6	47.8	51.2
190	35.9					45.9	48.2	51.6
195						46.2	48.5	52.0
200						46.5	48.8	52.4
205							49.1	52.7
210							49.4	53.0

From Durnin JVGA, Womersley J: Br J Nutr 32:77–97, 1974, Table 9.[15]

11 and 6–12). He also developed the method of interpreting anthropometric measurements as a percentage deviation from the reference level. Bistrian and Blackburn popularized the references and method. They are

TABLE 6–11. IDEAL WEIGHT FOR HEIGHT[a,b]

Females		Males	
Height (cm)	Weight (kg)	Height (cm)	Weight (kg)
140	44.9	157	58.6
141	45.4	158	59.3
142	45.9	159	59.9
143	46.4	160	60.5
144	47.0	161	61.1
145	47.5	162	61.7
146	48.0	163	62.3
147	48.6	164	62.9
148	49.2	165	63.5
149	49.8	166	64.0
150	50.4	167	64.6
151	51.0	168	65.2
152	51.5	169	65.9
153	52.0	170	66.6
154	52.5	171	67.3
155	53.1	172	68.0
156	53.7	173	68.7
157	54.3	174	69.4
158	54.9	175	70.1
159	55.5	176	70.8
160	56.2	177	71.6
161	56.9	178	72.4
162	57.6	179	73.3
163	58.3	180	74.2
164	58.9	181	75.0
165	59.5	182	75.8
166	60.1	183	76.5
167	60.7	184	77.3
168	61.4	185	78.1
169	62.1	186	78.9

[a]Society of Actuaries. Build and Blood Pressure Study, Chicago, 1959.
[b]This table represents the 1959 Metropolitan Life Insurance's data corrected to nude weight and height without shoes.

still commonly used in nutrition assessment today.

The purpose of this section is to broaden the clinician's knowledge of the background and use of acceptable methods for interpreting anthropometrics, to provide references available today, and to suggest standards and procedures for future practice.

In order to achieve a reliable comparison, anthropometric reference standards require the following characteristics:

1. Ideally, standards for all anthropometric measurements should be derived from the same or very similar sample populations.
2. The sample population from which the standards are derived must represent the population under clinical surveillance. Genetic and environmental factors that influence the body habitus include age, sex, race, ethnic and socioeconomic factors. Disease entities that influence body habitus should be controlled in the sample. The size of the total sample as well as the stratification of the sample with respect to these factors bears on its reliability as a standard of comparison and its potential application either to the general population, to minority groups, or to specific communities. The clinician applies these population standards to individuals, rather than to other populations. Therefore, standards should be used from populations to which the individual would logically belong. For example, Jelliffe's[5] standards for MAC and MAMC were not based on a large-scale population survey, but rather on several small surveys in Turkey, Greece, and Italy, and not all the measurements were derived from the same population. The source of the standards for TSF are from a reference by Jolliffe.[88] This allows a greater degree of error in the application and interpretation of the data and makes them less than acceptable as standards for comparison.

TABLE 6–12. REFERENCE VALUES FOR UPPER ARM ANTHROPOMETRY IN ADULTS[a,b]

Percent Deviation from Standard	Triceps Skinfold (mm)		Midarm Circumference (cm)		Midarm Muscle Circumference (cm)	
	(M)	**(F)**	**(M)**	**(F)**	**(M)**	**(F)**
Standard	12.5	16.5	29.3	28.5	25.3	23.2
90% Standard	11.3	14.9	26.3	25.7	22.8	20.9
90–60% Standard	11.3–7.5	14.9–9.9	26.3–17.6	25.7–17.1	22.8–15.2	20.9–13.9
<60% Standard	<7.5	<9.9	<17.6	<17.1	<15.2	<13.9

[a]Jelliffe DB: The Assessment of the Nutritional Status of the Community. WHO Monograph No. 53, WHO, Geneva, 1966.[5]
[b]Adapted from Blackburn GL, Bistrian BR, Maine BS, et al.: JPEN 1:11, 1977, Tables 3, 4 and 5.[4]

3. The methods for collecting raw data should be carefully standardized and reported. Seltzer and Mayer[6] cited the classic example of the 1959 Metropolitan Life Insurance Company tables that did not define the manner in which individuals were classified according to frame size. Although methods to objectively describe frame size have been proposed, these methods were not employed in the 1959 Build and Blood Pressure Study.[7] Measurements of weight were taken with clothes on and height was taken with shoes on. In

TABLE 6–13. 1979 METROPOLITAN LIFE INSURANCE COMPANY—HEIGHT AND WEIGHT TABLES

	Men[a]				**Women**[b]		
Height	**Small Frame**	**Med. Frame**	**Lg. Frame**	**Height**	**Small Frame**	**Med. Frame**	**Lg. Frame**
5'2"	128–134	131–141	138–150	4'10"	102–111	109–121	118–131
5'3"	130–136	133–143	140–153	4'11"	103–113	111–123	120–134
5'4"	132–138	135–145	142–156	5'0"	104–115	113–126	122–137
5'5"	134–140	137–148	144–160	5'1"	106–118	115–129	125–140
5'6"	136–142	139–151	146–164	5'2"	108–121	118–132	128–143
5'7"	138–145	142–154	149–168	5'3"	111–124	121–135	131–147
5'8"	140–148	145–157	152–172	5'4"	114–127	124–138	134–151
5'9"	142–151	148–160	155–176	5'5"	117–130	127–141	137–155
5'10"	144–154	151–163	158–180	5'6"	120–133	130–144	140–159
5'11"	146–157	154–166	161–184	5'7"	123–136	133–147	143–163
6'0"	149–160	157–170	164–188	5'8"	126–139	136–150	146–167
6'1"	152–164	160–174	168–192	5'9"	129–142	139–153	140–170
6'2"	155–168	164–178	172–197	5'10"	132–145	142–156	152–173
6'3"	158–172	167–182	176–202	5'11"	135–148	145–159	155–176
6'4"	162–176	171–187	181–207	6'0"	138–151	158–162	158–179

[a]Weight at ages 25 to 59 in shoes with 5 pounds of indoor clothing.
[b]Weight at ages 29 to 59 in shoes with 3 pounds of indoor clothing.
From Society of Actuaries. Build and Blood Pressure Study, 1979.

TABLE 6–14. AVERAGE WEIGHTS AND SELECTED PERCENTILES FOR EACH INCH/CM OF HEIGHT: WOMEN, AGED 18–74 YEARS, UNITED STATES 1971–74, HANES SURVEY

Height Inches	Cm	Percentiles	Age Group in Years — Weight in Pounds—Kilograms											
			18–24		25–34		35–44		45–54		55–64		64–74	
57"	144.8	95th	160	72.6	171	77.6	183	83.0	185	83.9	187	84.8	178	80.7
		90	150	68.0	159	72.1	170	77.1	172	78.0	175	79.4	167	75.7
		80	138	62.6	145	65.8	154	69.8	157	71.2	160	72.6	154	69.8
		50	114	51.7	118	53.5	125	56.7	129	58.5	132	59.9	130	59.0
		20	90	40.8	91	41.3	96	43.5	101	45.8	104	47.2	106	48.1
		10	78	35.4	77	34.9	80	36.3	86	39.0	89	40.4	93	42.2
		5	68	30.8	65	29.5	67	30.4	73	33.1	77	34.9	82	37.2
58"	147.3	95th	163	73.9	174	78.9	187	84.8	189	85.7	191	86.6	182	82.5
		90	153	69.4	162	73.5	174	78.9	176	79.8	179	81.2	171	77.6
		80	141	63.9	148	67.1	158	71.7	161	73.0	164	74.4	158	71.7
		50	117	53.1	121	54.9	129	58.5	133	60.3	136	61.7	134	60.8
		20	93	42.2	94	42.6	100	45.4	105	47.6	108	49.0	110	49.9
		10	81	36.7	80	36.3	84	38.1	90	40.8	93	42.2	97	44.0
		5	71	32.2	68	30.8	71	32.2	77	34.9	81	36.7	86	39.0
59"	149.9	95th	166	75.3	178	80.7	191	86.6	192	87.1	195	88.4	185	83.9
		90	156	70.7	166	75.3	178	80.7	179	81.2	183	83.0	174	78.9
		80	144	65.3	152	68.9	162	73.5	164	74.4	168	76.2	161	73.0
		50	120	54.4	125	56.7	133	60.3	136	61.7	140	63.5	137	62.1
		20	96	43.5	98	44.4	104	47.2	108	49.0	112	50.8	113	51.2
		10	84	38.1	84	38.1	88	39.9	93	42.2	97	44.0	100	45.4
		5	74	33.6	72	32.7	75	34.0	80	36.3	85	38.5	89	40.4
60"	152.4	95th	169	76.6	181	82.1	195	88.4	196	88.9	198	89.8	188	85.3
		90	159	72.1	169	76.6	182	82.5	183	83.0	186	84.4	177	80.3
		80	147	66.7	155	70.3	166	75.3	168	76.2	171	77.6	164	74.4
		50	123	55.8	128	58.0	137	62.1	140	63.5	143	64.9	140	63.5
		20	99	44.9	101	45.8	108	49.0	112	50.8	115	52.2	116	52.6
		10	87	39.5	87	39.5	92	41.7	97	44.0	100	45.4	103	46.7
		5	77	34.9	75	34.0	79	35.8	84	38.1	88	39.9	92	41.7

(continued)

TABLE 6–14. (Continued)

| Height | | Percentiles | 18–24 | | 25–34 | | 35–44 | | 45–54 | | 55–64 | | 64–74 | |
Inches	Cm													
						Weight in Pounds—Kilograms								
61″	154.9	95th	172	78.0	185	83.9	199	90.2	199	90.2	202	91.6	192	87.1
		90	162	73.5	175	79.4	186	84.4	186	84.4	190	86.2	181	82.1
		80	150	68.0	159	72.1	170	77.1	171	77.6	175	79.4	168	76.2
		50	126	57.1	132	59.9	141	63.9	143	64.9	147	66.7	144	65.3
		20	102	46.3	105	47.6	112	50.8	115	52.2	119	54.0	120	54.4
		10	90	40.8	91	41.3	96	43.5	100	45.4	104	47.2	107	43.5
		5	80	36.3	79	35.8	83	37.6	87	39.5	92	41.7	96	43.5
62″	157.5	95th	175	79.4	189	85.7	202	91.6	203	92.1	205	93.0	195	88.4
		90	165	74.8	177	80.3	189	85.7	190	86.2	193	87.5	184	83.4
		80	153	69.4	163	73.9	173	78.5	175	79.4	178	80.7	171	77.6
		50	129	58.5	136	61.7	144	65.3	147	66.7	150	68.0	147	66.7
		20	105	47.6	109	49.4	115	52.2	119	54.0	122	55.3	123	55.8
		10	93	42.2	95	43.1	99	44.9	104	47.2	107	48.5	110	49.9
		5	83	37.6	83	37.6	86	39.0	91	41.3	95	43.1	99	44.9
63″	160.0	95th	178	80.7	192	87.1	206	93.4	206	93.4	208	94.3	199	90.2
		90	168	76.2	180	81.6	193	87.5	193	87.5	196	88.9	188	85.3
		80	156	70.7	166	75.3	177	80.3	178	80.7	181	82.1	175	79.4
		50	132	59.9	139	63.0	148	67.1	150	68.0	153	69.4	151	68.5
		20	108	49.0	112	50.8	119	54.0	122	55.3	125	56.7	127	57.6
		10	96	43.5	98	44.4	103	46.7	107	48.5	110	49.9	114	51.7
		5	86	39.0	86	39.0	90	40.8	94	42.6	98	44.4	103	46.7
64″	162.6	95th	181	82.1	195	88.4	210	95.2	210	95.2	212	96.1	202	91.6
		90	171	77.6	183	83.0	197	89.3	197	89.3	200	90.7	191	86.6
		80	159	72.1	169	76.6	181	82.1	182	82.5	185	83.9	178	80.7
		50	135	61.2	142	64.4	152	68.9	154	69.8	157	71.2	154	69.8
		20	111	50.3	115	52.2	123	55.8	126	57.1	129	58.5	130	59.0
		10	90	40.8	101	45.8	107	48.5	110	49.9	114	51.7	117	53.1
		5	89	40.4	89	40.4	94	42.6	98	44.4	102	46.3	106	48.1

Age Group in Years

Height (in)	(cm)	%ile	lb	kg	lb	kg	lb	kg	lb	kg	lb	kg	lb	kg
65"	165.1	95th	184	83.4	199	90.2	214	97.1	214	97.1	215	97.5	206	93.4
		90	174	78.9	187	84.8	201	91.2	201	91.2	203	92.1	195	88.4
		80	162	73.5	173	78.5	185	83.9	186	84.4	188	85.3	182	82.5
		50	138	62.6	146	66.2	156	70.7	158	71.7	160	72.6	158	71.7
		20	114	51.7	119	54.0	127	57.6	130	59.0	132	59.9	134	60.8
		10	102	46.3	105	47.6	111	50.3	115	52.2	117	53.1	121	54.9
		5	92	41.7	93	42.2	98	44.4	102	46.3	105	47.6	110	49.9
66"	167.6	95th	187	84.8	203	92.1	217	98.4	217	98.4	219	99.3	209	94.8
		90	177	80.3	191	86.6	204	92.5	204	92.5	207	93.9	198	89.8
		80	165	74.8	177	80.3	188	85.3	189	85.7	192	87.1	185	83.9
		50	141	63.9	150	68.0	159	72.1	161	73.0	164	74.4	161	73.0
		20	117	53.1	123	55.8	130	59.0	133	60.3	136	61.7	137	62.1
		10	106	48.1	109	49.4	114	51.7	118	53.5	121	54.9	124	56.2
		5	95	43.1	97	44.0	101	45.8	105	47.6	109	49.4	113	51.2
67"	170.2	95th	190	86.2	206	93.4	221	100.2	221	100.2	222	100.7	213	96.6
		90	180	81.6	194	88.0	208	94.3	208	94.3	210	95.2	202	91.6
		80	168	76.2	180	81.6	192	87.1	193	87.5	195	88.4	189	85.7
		50	144	65.3	153	69.4	163	73.9	165	74.8	167	75.7	165	74.8
		20	120	54.4	126	57.1	134	60.8	137	62.1	139	63.0	141	63.9
		10	108	49.0	112	50.8	158	71.7	122	55.3	124	56.2	128	58.0
		5	98	44.4	100	45.4	105	47.6	109	49.4	112	50.8	117	53.1
68"	172.7	95th	193	87.5	210	95.2	225	102.0	224	102.0	226	102.5	217	98.4
		90	183	83.0	198	89.8	212	96.1	211	95.7	214	97.1	206	93.4
		80	171	77.6	184	83.4	196	88.9	196	88.9	199	90.2	193	87.5
		50	147	66.7	157	71.2	167	75.7	168	76.2	171	77.6	169	76.6
		20	123	55.8	130	59.0	138	62.6	140	63.5	143	64.9	145	65.8
		10	111	50.3	116	52.6	122	55.3	125	56.7	128	58.0	132	59.9
		5	101	45.8	104	47.2	109	49.4	112	50.8	116	52.6	121	54.9

Notes: Examined persons were measured without shoes; clothing ranged from 0.20 to 0.62 pound, which was not deducted from body weight. The weight values were computed from the regression equation of weight on height by age. The values above and below the expected mean value represent the $\pm.8416$, ±1.2816 and ±1.6449 standard error of the estimate covering within this range 60, 80, and 90 percent of the population around the expected mean respectively. The first range is expected thus to identify 20, 10, and 5 percent of the population of the specific height on either side of the range. Figures are the expected means.

Adapted from Table 5, Weight by Height and Age of Adults 18–74 years: United States, 1971–74; DHEW: Series 11, No. 208, 1979, Center for Disease Control, Atlanta, Ga. Tables copied with permission from Manual of Clinical Dietetics, 1982 Rev. Ed., Akron General Medical Center, Akron, Ohio, 44307.

TABLE 6-15. AVERAGE WEIGHTS AND SELECTED PERCENTILES FOR EACH INCH/CM OF HEIGHT: MEN, AGED 18-74 YEARS, UNITED STATES 1971-1974, HANES SURVEY

Height (Inches)	Height (Cm)	Percentiles	18-24	25-34	35-44	45-54	55-64	64-74
			Weight in Pounds—Kilograms					
62"	157.5	95th	175 / 79.4	191 / 86.6	188 / 85.3	194 / 88.0	190 / 86.2	186 / 84.4
		90	165 / 74.8	180 / 81.6	178 / 80.7	183 / 83.0	180 / 81.6	176 / 79.8
		80	153 / 69.4	167 / 75.7	166 / 75.3	171 / 77.6	167 / 75.7	165 / 74.8
		50	130 / 58.9	141 / 63.9	143 / 64.8	147 / 66.7	143 / 64.9	143 / 64.8
		20	107 / 48.5	115 / 52.2	120 / 54.4	123 / 55.8	119 / 54.0	121 / 54.9
		10	95 / 43.1	102 / 46.3	108 / 49.0	111 / 50.3	106 / 48.1	110 / 49.9
		5	85 / 38.5	91 / 41.3	98 / 44.4	100 / 45.4	96 / 43.5	100 / 45.3
63"	160.0	95th	180 / 81.6	195 / 88.4	193 / 87.5	199 / 90.2	194 / 88.0	190 / 86.2
		90	170 / 77.1	184 / 83.4	183 / 83.0	188 / 85.3	184 / 83.4	180 / 81.6
		80	158 / 71.6	171 / 77.5	171 / 77.5	176 / 79.8	171 / 77.6	169 / 76.6
		50	135 / 61.2	145 / 65.7	148 / 67.1	152 / 68.9	147 / 66.7	147 / 66.7
		20	112 / 50.8	119 / 54.0	125 / 56.7	128 / 58.0	123 / 55.8	125 / 56.7
		10	100 / 45.3	106 / 48.1	113 / 51.2	116 / 52.6	110 / 49.9	114 / 51.7
		5	90 / 40.8	95 / 43.1	103 / 46.7	105 / 47.6	100 / 45.4	104 / 47.2
64"	162.6	95th	185 / 83.9	200 / 90.7	198 / 89.8	203 / 92.1	200 / 90.7	194 / 88.0
		90	175 / 79.4	189 / 85.7	188 / 85.3	192 / 87.1	190 / 86.2	184 / 83.4
		80	163 / 73.9	176 / 79.8	176 / 79.8	180 / 81.6	177 / 80.3	173 / 78.5
		50	140 / 63.5	150 / 68.0	153 / 69.4	156 / 70.7	153 / 69.4	151 / 68.5
		20	117 / 53.1	124 / 56.2	130 / 58.9	132 / 59.9	129 / 58.5	129 / 58.5
		10	105 / 47.6	111 / 50.3	118 / 53.5	120 / 54.4	116 / 52.6	118 / 53.5
		5	95 / 43.1	100 / 45.4	108 / 49.0	109 / 49.4	106 / 48.1	108 / 49.0
65"	165.1	95th	190 / 86.2	206 / 93.4	203 / 92.1	207 / 93.9	205 / 93.0	199 / 90.2
		90	180 / 81.6	195 / 88.4	193 / 87.5	196 / 88.9	195 / 88.4	189 / 85.7
		80	168 / 76.2	182 / 82.5	181 / 82.1	184 / 83.4	182 / 82.5	178 / 80.7
		50	145 / 65.8	156 / 70.7	158 / 71.7	160 / 72.6	158 / 71.7	156 / 70.7
		20	122 / 55.3	130 / 59.0	135 / 61.2	136 / 61.7	134 / 60.8	134 / 60.8
		10	110 / 49.9	117 / 53.1	123 / 55.8	124 / 56.2	121 / 54.9	123 / 55.8
		5	100 / 45.4	106 / 48.1	113 / 51.2	113 / 51.2	111 / 50.3	113 / 51.2
66"	167.6	95th	195 / 88.4	210 / 95.2	208 / 94.3	211 / 95.7	210 / 95.2	203 / 92.1
		90	185 / 83.9	199 / 90.2	198 / 89.8	200 / 90.7	200 / 90.7	193 / 87.5
		80	173 / 78.5	186 / 84.4	186 / 84.4	188 / 85.3	187 / 84.8	182 / 82.5

(continued)

in	cm	%ile												
67"	170.2	50	150	68.0	160	72.6	163	73.9	164	74.4	163	73.9	160	72.6
		20	127	57.6	134	60.8	140	63.5	140	63.5	139	63.0	138	62.6
		10	115	52.2	121	54.9	128	58.0	128	58.0	126	57.1	127	57.6
		5	105	47.6	110	49.9	118	53.5	117	53.1	116	52.6	117	53.1
68"	172.7	95th	199	90.2	215	97.5	214	97.1	216	98.0	215	97.5	207	93.9
		90	189	85.7	204	92.5	204	92.5	205	93.0	205	93.0	197	89.3
		80	177	80.3	191	86.6	192	87.1	193	87.5	192	87.1	186	84.4
		50	154	69.8	165	74.8	169	76.6	169	76.6	168	76.2	164	74.4
		20	131	59.4	139	63.0	146	66.2	145	65.8	144	65.3	142	64.4
		10	119	54.0	126	57.1	134	60.8	133	60.3	131	59.4	131	59.4
		5	109	49.4	115	52.1	124	56.2	122	55.3	121	54.9	121	54.9
69"	175.3	95th	204	92.5	220	99.8	219	99.3	220	99.8	220	99.8	212	96.1
		90	194	88.0	209	94.8	209	94.8	209	94.8	210	95.2	202	91.6
		80	182	82.5	196	88.9	197	89.3	197	89.3	197	89.3	191	86.6
		50	159	72.1	170	77.1	174	78.9	173	78.5	173	78.5	169	76.6
		20	136	61.7	144	65.3	151	68.5	149	67.6	149	67.6	147	66.7
		10	124	56.2	131	59.4	139	63.0	137	62.1	136	61.7	136	61.7
		5	114	51.7	120	54.4	129	58.5	126	57.1	126	57.1	126	57.1
69"	175.3	95th	209	94.8	224	101.6	224	101.6	224	101.6	225	102.0	216	98.0
		90	199	90.2	213	96.6	214	97.1	213	96.6	215	97.5	206	93.4
		80	187	84.8	200	90.7	202	91.6	201	91.2	202	91.6	195	88.4
		50	164	74.4	174	78.9	179	81.2	177	80.3	178	80.7	173	78.5
		20	141	63.9	148	67.1	156	70.7	153	69.4	154	69.8	151	68.5
		10	129	58.5	135	61.2	144	65.3	141	63.9	141	63.9	140	63.5
		5	119	54.0	124	56.2	134	60.8	130	59.0	131	59.4	130	59.0
70"	177.8	95th	213	96.6	229	103.9	229	103.9	229	103.9	230	104.3	220	99.8
		90	203	92.1	218	98.9	212	96.1	218	98.9	220	99.8	210	95.2
		80	191	86.6	205	93.0	207	93.9	206	93.4	207	93.9	199	90.2
		50	168	76.2	179	81.2	184	83.4	182	82.5	183	83.0	177	80.3
		20	145	65.8	153	69.4	161	73.0	158	71.7	159	72.1	155	70.3
		10	133	60.3	140	63.5	149	67.6	146	66.2	144	66.2	140	65.3
		5	123	55.8	129	58.5	139	63.0	135	61.2	136	61.7	134	60.8
71"	180.3	95th	218	98.9	234	106.1	235	106.6	234	106.1	236	107.0	225	102.0
		90	208	94.3	223	101.1	225	102.0	223	101.1	226	102.5	215	97.5
		80	196	88.9	210	95.2	213	96.6	211	95.7	213	96.6	204	92.5
		50	173	78.5	184	83.4	190	86.2	187	84.8	189	85.7	182	82.5
		20	150	68.0	158	71.7	167	75.7	163	73.9	165	74.8	160	72.6
		10	138	62.6	145	65.8	155	70.3	151	68.5	152	68.9	149	67.6
		5	128	58.0	134	60.8	145	65.8	140	63.5	142	64.4	139	63.0

TABLE 6–15. (Continued)

Height		Percentiles	Age Group in Years											
Inches	Cm		18–24		25–34		35–44		45–54		55–64		64–74	
			Weight in Pounds—Kilograms											
72"	182.9	95th	223	101.1	239	108.4	239	108.4	238	107.9	240	108.8	229	103.0
		90	213	96.6	228	103.4	229	103.9	227	102.9	230	104.3	219	99.3
		80	201	91.2	215	97.5	217	98.4	215	97.5	217	98.4	208	94.3
		50	178	80.7	189	85.7	194	88.0	191	86.6	193	87.5	186	84.4
		20	155	70.3	163	73.9	171	77.6	167	75.7	169	76.6	164	74.4
		10	143	64.9	150	68.0	159	72.1	155	70.3	156	70.7	153	69.4
		5	133	60.3	139	63.0	149	67.6	144	65.3	146	66.2	143	64.9
73"	185.4	95th	228	103.4	244	110.7	245	111.1	243	110.2	244	110.7	233	105.7
		90	218	98.9	233	105.7	235	106.6	232	105.2	234	106.1	223	101.1
		80	206	93.4	220	99.8	223	101.1	220	99.8	221	100.2	212	96.1
		50	183	83.0	194	88.0	200	90.7	196	88.9	197	89.3	190	86.2
		20	160	72.6	168	76.2	177	80.3	172	78.6	173	78.5	168	76.2
		10	148	67.1	155	70.3	165	74.8	160	72.6	160	72.6	157	71.2
		5	138	62.6	144	65.3	155	70.3	149	67.6	150	68.0	147	66.7
74"	188.0	95th	233	105.7	249	112.9	250	113.4	247	112.0	250	113.4	237	107.5
		90	223	101.1	238	107.9	240	108.8	236	107.0	240	108.8	227	102.9
		80	211	95.7	225	102.0	228	103.4	224	101.6	227	102.9	216	98.0
		50	188	85.3	199	90.2	205	93.0	200	90.7	203	92.1	194	88.0
		20	165	74.8	173	78.5	182	82.5	176	79.8	179	81.2	172	78.0
		10	153	69.4	160	72.6	170	77.1	164	74.4	166	75.3	161	73.0
		5	143	64.9	149	67.6	160	72.6	153	69.4	156	70.7	151	68.5

Figures are the expected means.
See Table 6–14 for sources and notes.

134

TABLE 6-16. HEALTH AND NUTRITION EXAMINATION SURVEY I, 1971-1974: DATA ON TRICEPS SKINFOLDS OF WHITES IN UNITED STATES IN PERCENTILE FORM

Age Group (yr)	Males (mm)							Age Group (yr)	Females (mm)						
	5	10	25	50	75	90	95		5	10	25	50	75	90	95
1-1.9	6	7	8	10	12	14	16	1-1.9	6	7	8	10	12	14	16
2-2.9	6	7	8	10	12	14	15	2-2.9	6	8	9	10	12	15	16
3-3.9	6	7	8	10	11	14	15	3-3.9	7	8	9	11	12	14	15
4-4.9	6	6	8	9	11	12	14	4-4.9	7	8	8	10	12	14	16
5-5.9	6	6	8	9	11	14	15	5-5.9	6	7	8	10	12	15	18
6-6.9	5	6	7	8	10	13	16	6-6.9	6	6	8	10	12	14	16
7-7.9	5	6	7	9	12	15	17	7-7.9	6	7	9	11	13	16	18
8-8.9	5	6	7	8	10	13	16	8-8.9	6	8	9	12	15	18	24
9-9.9	6	6	7	10	13	17	18	9-9.9	8	8	10	13	16	20	22
10-10.9	6	6	8	10	14	18	21	10-10.9	7	8	10	12	17	23	27
11-11.9	6	6	8	11	16	20	24	11-11.9	7	8	10	13	18	24	28
12-12.9	6	6	8	11	14	22	28	12-12.9	8	9	11	14	18	23	27
13-13.9	5	5	7	10	14	22	26	13-13.9	8	8	12	15	21	26	30
14-14.9	4	5	7	9	14	21	24	14-14.9	9	10	13	16	21	26	28
15-15.9	4	5	6	8	11	18	24	15-15.9	8	10	12	17	21	25	32
16-16.9	4	5	6	8	12	16	22	16-16.9	10	12	15	18	22	26	31
17-17.9	5	5	6	8	12	16	19	17-17.9	10	12	13	19	24	30	37
18-18.9	4	5	6	9	13	20	24	18-18.9	10	12	15	18	22	26	30
19-24.9	4	5	7	10	15	20	22	19-24.9	10	11	14	18	24	30	34
25-34.9	5	6	8	12	16	20	24	25-34.9	10	12	16	21	27	34	37
35-44.9	5	6	8	12	16	20	23	35-44.9	12	14	18	23	29	35	38
45-54.9	6	6	8	12	15	20	25	45-54.9	12	16	20	25	30	36	40
55-64.9	5	6	8	11	14	19	22	55-64.9	12	16	20	25	31	36	38
65-74.9	4	6	8	11	15	19	22	65-74.9	12	14	18	24	29	34	36

Adapted from Frisancho R: New norms of upper limb fat and muscle areas for assessment of nutritional status. Am J Clin Nutr 34:2540-2545, 1980, Table 1.

some cases, height was reported rather than measured. In making the classifications for the mildly overweight, the data did not differentiate between overweight due to excess fat as opposed to excess musculature, as in athletes.

4. Data should be tabulated according to age and sex. Anthropometric data from upper age categories is limited at present. Tables are needed that report data for each decade over 50 years, rather than grouping it as "50+ years" or "65 and older."

5. Data should be reported in percentiles

rather than percentages or subjective criteria (e.g., "frame size"). General evaluation of obesity, emaciation, body fat content, and overall nutritional health is frequently determined solely by comparison of the individual's weight related to height to tables of average weight for height in a "normal" population, where:

$$\text{\% standard weight (or "ideal" weight)} = \frac{\text{measured weight}}{\text{standard weight}} \times 100$$

TABLE 6–17. HEALTH AND NUTRITION EXAMINATION SURVEY I, 1971–1974: DATA ON ARM CIRCUMFERENCE OF WHITES IN UNITED STATES IN PERCENTILE FORM

Age Group (yr)	Males (cm) 5	10	25	50	75	90	95	Age Group (yr)	Females (cm) 5	10	25	50	75	90	95
1–1.9	14.2	14.6	15.0	15.9	17.0	17.6	18.3	1–1.9	13.8	14.2	14.8	15.6	16.4	17.2	17.7
2–2.9	14.1	14.5	15.3	16.2	17.0	17.8	18.5	2–2.9	14.2	14.5	15.2	16.0	16.7	17.6	18.4
3–3.9	15.0	15.3	16.0	16.7	17.5	18.4	19.0	3–3.9	14.3	15.0	15.8	16.7	17.5	18.3	18.9
4–4.9	14.9	15.4	16.2	17.1	18.0	18.6	19.2	4–4.9	14.9	15.4	16.0	16.9	17.7	18.4	19.1
5–5.9	15.3	16.0	16.7	17.5	18.5	19.5	20.4	5–5.9	15.3	15.7	16.5	17.5	18.5	20.3	21.1
6–6.9	15.5	15.9	16.7	17.9	18.8	20.9	22.8	6–6.9	15.6	16.2	17.0	17.6	18.7	20.4	21.1
7–7.9	16.2	16.7	17.7	18.7	20.1	22.3	23.0	7–7.9	16.4	16.7	17.4	18.3	19.9	21.6	23.1
8–8.9	16.2	17.0	17.7	19.0	20.2	22.0	24.5	8–8.9	16.8	17.2	18.3	19.5	21.4	24.7	26.1
9–9.9	17.5	17.8	18.7	20.0	21.7	24.9	25.7	9–9.9	17.8	18.2	19.4	21.1	22.4	25.1	26.0
10–10.9	18.1	18.4	19.6	21.0	23.1	26.2	27.4	10–10.9	17.4	18.2	19.3	21.0	22.8	25.1	26.5
11–11.9	18.6	19.0	20.2	22.3	24.4	26.1	28.0	11–11.9	18.5	19.4	20.8	22.4	24.8	27.6	30.3
12–12.9	19.3	20.0	21.4	23.2	25.4	28.2	30.3	12–12.9	19.4	20.3	21.6	23.7	25.6	28.2	29.4
13–13.9	19.4	21.1	22.8	24.7	26.3	28.6	30.1	13–13.9	20.2	21.1	22.3	24.3	27.1	30.1	33.8
14–14.9	22.0	22.6	23.7	25.3	28.3	30.3	32.2	14–14.9	21.4	22.3	23.7	25.2	27.2	30.4	32.2
15–15.9	22.2	22.9	24.4	26.4	28.4	31.1	32.0	15–15.9	20.8	22.1	23.9	25.4	27.9	30.0	32.2
16–16.9	24.4	24.8	26.2	27.8	30.3	32.4	34.3	16–16.9	21.8	22.4	24.1	25.8	28.3	31.8	33.4
17–17.9	24.6	25.3	26.7	28.5	30.8	33.6	34.7	17–17.9	22.0	22.7	24.1	26.4	29.5	32.4	35.0
18–18.9	24.5	26.0	27.6	29.7	32.1	35.3	37.9	18–18.9	22.2	22.7	24.1	25.8	28.1	31.2	32.5
19–24.9	26.2	27.2	28.8	30.8	33.1	35.5	37.2	19–24.9	22.1	23.0	24.7	26.5	29.0	31.9	34.5
25–34.9	27.1	28.2	30.0	31.9	34.2	36.2	37.5	25–34.9	23.3	24.0	25.6	27.7	30.4	34.2	36.8
35–44.9	27.8	28.7	30.5	32.6	34.5	36.3	37.4	35–44.9	24.1	25.1	26.7	29.0	31.7	35.6	37.8
45–54.9	26.7	28.1	30.1	32.2	34.2	36.2	37.6	45–54.9	24.2	25.6	27.4	29.9	32.8	36.2	38.4
55–64.9	25.8	27.3	29.6	31.7	33.6	35.5	36.9	55–64.9	24.3	25.7	28.0	30.3	33.5	36.7	38.5
65–74.9	24.8	26.3	28.5	30.7	32.5	34.4	35.5	65–74.9	24.0	25.2	27.4	29.9	32.6	35.6	37.3

Adapted from Frisancho R: New norms of upper limb fat and muscle areas for assessment of nutritional status. Am J Clin Nutr 34:2540–2545, 1980, Table 2.

TABLE 6–18. HEALTH AND NUTRITION EXAMINATION SURVEY I, 1971–1974: DATA ON ARM MUSCLE CIRCUMFERENCE OF WHITES IN UNITED STATES IN PERCENTILE FORM

Age Group (yr)	Males (cm)							Age Group (yr)	Females (cm)						
	5	10	25	50	75	90	95		5	10	25	50	75	90	95
1–1.9	11.0	11.3	11.9	12.7	13.5	14.4	14.7	1–1.9	10.5	11.1	11.7	12.4	13.2	13.9	14.3
2–2.9	11.1	11.4	12.2	13.0	14.0	14.6	15.0	2–2.9	11.1	11.4	11.9	12.6	13.3	14.2	14.7
3–3.9	11.7	12.3	13.1	13.7	14.3	14.8	15.3	3–3.9	11.3	11.9	12.4	13.2	14.0	14.6	15.2
4–4.9	12.3	12.6	13.3	14.1	14.8	15.6	15.9	4–4.9	11.5	12.1	12.8	13.6	14.4	15.2	15.7
5–5.9	12.8	13.3	14.0	14.7	15.4	16.2	16.9	5–5.9	12.5	12.8	13.4	14.2	15.1	15.9	16.5
6–6.9	13.1	13.5	14.2	15.1	16.1	17.0	17.7	6–6.9	13.0	13.3	13.8	14.5	15.4	16.6	17.1
7–7.9	13.7	13.9	15.1	16.0	16.8	17.7	19.0	7–7.9	12.9	13.5	14.2	15.1	16.0	17.1	17.6
8–8.9	14.0	14.5	15.4	16.2	17.0	18.2	18.7	8–8.9	13.8	14.0	15.1	16.0	17.1	18.3	19.4
9–9.9	15.1	15.4	16.1	17.0	18.3	19.6	20.2	9–9.9	14.7	15.0	15.8	16.7	18.0	19.4	19.8
10–10.9	15.6	16.0	16.6	18.0	19.1	20.9	22.1	10–10.9	14.8	15.0	15.9	17.0	18.0	19.0	19.7
11–11.9	15.9	16.5	17.3	18.3	19.5	20.5	23.0	11–11.9	15.0	15.8	17.1	18.1	19.6	21.7	22.3
12–12.9	16.7	17.1	18.2	19.5	21.0	22.3	24.1	12–12.9	16.2	16.6	18.0	19.1	20.1	21.4	22.0
13–13.9	17.2	17.9	19.6	21.1	22.6	23.8	24.5	13–13.9	16.9	17.5	18.3	19.8	21.1	22.6	24.0
14–14.9	18.9	19.9	21.2	22.3	24.0	26.0	26.4	14–14.9	17.4	17.9	19.0	20.1	21.6	23.2	24.7
15–15.9	19.9	20.4	21.8	23.7	25.4	26.6	27.2	15–15.9	17.5	17.8	18.9	20.2	21.5	22.8	24.4
16–16.9	21.3	22.5	23.4	24.9	26.9	28.7	29.6	16–16.9	17.0	18.0	19.0	20.2	21.6	23.4	24.9
17–17.9	22.4	23.1	24.5	25.8	27.3	29.4	31.2	17–17.9	17.5	18.3	19.4	20.5	22.1	23.9	25.7
18–18.9	22.6	23.7	25.2	26.4	28.3	29.8	32.4	18–18.9	17.4	17.9	19.1	20.2	21.5	23.7	24.5
19–24.9	23.8	24.5	25.7	27.3	28.9	30.9	32.1	19–24.9	17.9	18.5	19.5	20.7	22.1	23.6	24.9
25–34.9	24.3	25.0	26.4	27.9	29.8	31.4	32.6	25–34.9	18.3	18.8	19.9	21.2	22.8	24.6	26.4
35–44.9	24.7	25.5	26.9	28.6	30.2	31.8	32.7	35–44.9	18.6	19.2	20.5	21.8	23.6	25.7	27.2
45–54.9	23.9	24.9	26.5	28.1	30.0	31.5	32.6	45–54.9	18.7	19.3	20.6	22.0	23.8	26.0	27.4
55–64.9	23.6	24.5	26.0	27.8	29.5	31.0	32.0	55–64.9	18.7	19.6	20.9	22.5	24.4	26.6	28.0
65–74.9	22.3	23.5	25.1	26.8	28.4	29.8	30.6	65–74.9	18.5	19.5	20.8	22.5	24.4	26.4	27.9

Adapted from Frisancho R: New norms of upper limb fat and muscle areas for assessment of nutritional status. Am J Clin Nutr 34:2540–2545, 1980, Table 2.

TABLE 6–19. HEALTH AND NUTRITION EXAMINATION SURVEY I, 1971–1974: DATA ON ARM MUSCLE AREA OF WHITES IN UNITED STATES IN PERCENTILE FORM

Age Group (yr)	Male (cm²)						
	5	10	25	50	75	90	95
1–1.9	95.6	101.4	113.3	127.8	144.7	164.4	172.0
2–2.9	97.3	104.0	119.0	134.5	155.7	169.0	178.7
3–3.9	109.5	120.1	135.7	148.4	161.8	175.0	185.3
4–4.9	120.7	126.4	140.8	157.9	174.7	192.6	200.8
5–5.9	129.8	141.1	155.0	172.0	188.4	208.9	228.5
6–6.9	136.0	144.7	160.5	181.5	205.6	229.7	249.3
7–7.9	149.7	154.8	180.8	202.7	224.6	249.4	288.6
8–8.9	155.0	166.4	189.5	208.9	229.6	262.8	278.8
9–9.9	181.1	188.4	206.7	228.8	265.7	305.3	325.7
10–10.9	193.0	202.7	218.2	257.5	290.3	348.6	388.2
11–11.9	201.6	215.6	238.2	267.0	302.2	335.9	422.6
12–12.9	221.6	233.9	264.9	302.2	349.6	396.8	464.0
13–13.9	236.3	254.6	304.4	355.3	408.1	450.2	479.4
14–14.9	283.0	314.7	358.6	396.3	457.5	536.8	553.0
15–15.9	313.8	331.7	378.8	448.1	513.4	563.1	590.0
16–16.9	362.5	404.4	435.2	495.1	575.3	657.6	698.0
17–17.9	399.8	425.2	477.7	528.6	595.0	688.6	772.6
18–18.9	407.0	448.1	506.6	555.2	637.4	706.7	835.5
19–24.9	450.8	477.7	527.4	591.3	666.0	760.6	820.0
25–34.9	469.4	496.3	554.1	621.4	706.7	784.7	843.6
35–44.9	484.4	518.1	574.0	649.0	726.5	803.4	848.8
45–54.9	454.6	494.6	558.9	629.7	714.2	791.8	845.8
55–64.9	442.2	478.3	538.1	614.4	691.9	767.0	814.9
65–74.9	397.3	441.1	503.1	571.6	643.2	707.4	745.3

Adapted from Frisancho R: New norms of upper limb fat and muscle areas for assessment of nutritional status. Am J Clin Nutr 34:2540–2545, 1980, Table 3.

The individual's weight is compared to average weight at the same height and same relative age, same sex, and occasionally also referenced to body build or frame size.

To consider a single data point as representative is to ignore the degree of variation that occurs normally. Percentiles, unlike percentages, describe the distribution of points along a bell-shaped curve.

6. The definition for normal limits as well as the limits considered diagnostic of malnutrition should reflect the body's ability to remain healthy and to withstand disease rather than simply be a value derived from an average of body measurements. For example, the Metropolitan Life Insurance Company's tables of "ideal" weights for heights, published in 1959,[7] indicate that there was a positive relationship between overweight and mortality related to heart disease. When the study was repeated

Age Group (yr)	Female (cm²)						
	5	10	25	50	75	90	95
1–1.9	88.5	97.3	108.4	122.1	137.8	153.5	162.1
2–2.9	97.3	102.9	111.9	126.9	140.5	159.5	172.7
3–3.9	101.4	113.3	122.7	139.6	156.3	169.0	184.6
4–4.9	105.8	117.1	131.3	147.5	164.4	183.2	195.8
5–5.9	123.8	130.1	142.3	159.8	182.5	201.2	215.9
6–6.9	135.4	141.4	151.3	168.3	187.7	218.2	232.3
7–7.9	133.0	144.1	160.2	181.5	204.5	233.2	246.9
8–8.9	151.3	156.6	180.8	203.4	232.7	265.7	299.6
9–9.9	172.3	178.8	197.6	222.7	257.1	298.7	311.2
10–10.9	174.0	178.4	201.9	229.6	258.3	287.3	309.3
11–11.9	178.4	198.7	231.6	261.2	307.1	373.9	395.3
12–12.9	209.2	218.2	257.9	290.4	322.5	365.5	384.7
13–13.9	226.9	242.6	265.7	313.0	352.9	408.1	456.8
14–14.9	241.8	256.2	287.4	322.0	370.4	429.4	485.0
15–15.9	242.6	251.8	284.7	324.8	368.9	412.3	475.6
16–16.9	230.8	256.7	286.5	324.8	371.8	435.3	494.6
17–17.9	244.2	267.4	299.6	333.6	388.3	455.2	525.1
18–18.9	239.8	253.8	291.7	324.3	369.4	446.1	476.7
19–24.9	253.8	272.8	302.6	340.6	387.7	443.9	494.0
25–34.9	266.1	282.6	314.8	357.3	413.8	480.6	554.1
35–44.9	275.0	294.8	335.9	378.3	442.8	524.0	587.7
45–54.9	278.4	295.6	337.8	385.8	452.0	537.5	596.4
55–64.9	278.4	306.3	347.7	404.5	475.0	563.2	624.7
65–74.9	273.7	301.8	344.4	401.9	473.9	556.6	621.4

in 1979,[8] however, although the average weights for each age category had increased by 1 to 17 pounds, the mortality rate had dropped (Table 6–13). Garn et al.[84] in a 16-year study on 2381 males from West Scotland, aged 45 to 75, showed that there were higher rates of mortality associated with lung cancer among lean males whereas in heavy males, there was a higher incidence of cardiovascular mortality. While much is yet to be learned about the relationship between body fatness and mortality, both of the above studies argue against the concept of a single "ideal" weight for height.

The use of the same percentages for all measurements to indicate depletion is misrepresentative since the normal variation for some measurements is greater than others. This would lead to misdiagnosis of malnutrition. Gray and Gray[89,90] cite the following example:

The amount of body fat and muscle is directly related to cross-sectional fat and muscle areas. . . . When the triceps skin-

TABLE 6–20. HEALTH AND NUTRITION EXAMINATION SURVEY I, 1971–1974: DATA ON ARM FAT AREA OF WHITES IN U.S. IN PERCENTILE FORM

Age Group (yr)	Male (cm²)						
	5	10	25	50	75	90	95
1–1.9	45.2	48.6	59.0	74.1	89.5	103.6	117.6
2–2.9	43.4	50.4	57.8	73.7	87.1	104.4	114.8
3–3.9	46.4	51.9	59.0	73.6	86.8	107.1	115.1
4–4.9	42.8	49.4	59.8	72.2	85.9	98.9	108.5
5–5.9	44.6	48.8	58.2	71.3	91.4	117.6	129.9
6–6.9	37.1	44.6	53.9	67.8	89.6	111.5	151.9
7–7.9	42.3	47.3	57.4	75.8	101.1	139.3	151.1
8–8.9	41.0	46.0	58.8	72.5	100.3	124.8	155.8
9–9.9	48.5	52.7	63.5	85.9	125.2	186.4	208.1
10–10.9	52.3	54.3	73.8	98.2	137.6	190.6	260.9
11–11.9	53.6	59.5	75.4	114.8	171.0	234.8	257.4
12–12.9	55.4	65.0	87.4	117.2	155.8	253.6	358.0
13–13.9	47.5	57.0	81.2	109.6	170.2	274.4	332.2
14–14.9	45.3	56.3	78.6	108.2	160.8	274.6	350.8
15–15.9	52.1	59.5	69.0	93.1	142.3	243.4	310.0
16–16.9	54.2	59.3	84.4	107.8	174.6	228.0	304.1
17–17.9	59.8	69.8	82.7	109.6	163.9	240.7	288.8
18–18.9	56.0	66.5	86.0	126.4	194.7	330.2	392.8
19–24.9	59.4	74.3	96.3	140.6	223.1	309.8	365.2
25–34.9	67.5	83.1	117.4	175.2	245.9	324.6	378.6
35–44.9	70.3	85.1	131.0	179.2	246.3	309.8	362.4
45–54.9	74.9	92.2	125.4	174.1	235.9	324.5	392.8
55–64.9	65.8	83.9	116.6	164.5	223.6	297.6	346.6
65–74.9	57.3	75.3	112.2	162.1	219.9	287.6	332.7

Adapted from Frisancho R: New norms of upper limb fat and muscle areas for assessment of nutritional status. Am J Clin Nutr 34:2540–2545, 1980, Table 3.

fold is 60 percent of standard, the cross-sectional fat area is also about 60 percent of standard. However, when the arm muscle circumference is 60 percent of standard, the cross-sectional muscle is 36 percent of standard. Thus, a decrease in the arm muscle circumference by a given percentage is more severe than a decrease in the triceps skinfold by the same percentage.[90]

In addition, Jelliffe does not represent the background data used to justify 60 to 90 per-

cent as "moderate depletion" or less than 60 percent as "severe depletion." (See Interpretation section below.)

In light of the above discussion, the question arises as to whether use of other references besides Jelliffe's for interpretation of anthropometry measurements would be more appropriate. Gray and Gray[89,90] compared Jelliffe's standards with weight data obtained from the Health and Nutrition Examination Survey (HANES) (Tables 6–14 through 6–20) and other anthropometric measurements reported from the Ten-State

Age Group (yr)	Female (cm²)						
	5	10	25	50	75	90	95
1–1.9	40.1	46.6	57.8	70.6	84.7	102.2	114.0
2–2.9	46.9	52.6	64.2	74.7	89.4	106.1	117.3
3–3.9	47.3	52.9	65.6	82.2	96.7	110.6	115.8
4–4.9	49.0	54.1	65.4	76.6	90.7	110.9	123.6
5–5.9	47.0	52.9	64.7	81.2	99.1	133.0	153.6
6–6.9	46.4	50.8	63.8	82.7	100.9	126.3	143.6
7–7.9	49.1	56.0	70.6	92.0	113.5	140.7	164.4
8–8.9	52.7	63.4	76.9	104.2	138.3	187.2	248.2
9–9.9	64.2	69.0	93.3	121.9	158.4	217.1	252.4
10–10.9	61.6	70.2	84.2	114.1	160.8	250.0	300.5
11–11.9	70.7	80.2	101.5	130.1	194.2	273.0	369.0
12–12.9	78.2	85.4	109.0	151.1	205.6	266.6	336.9
13–13.9	72.6	83.8	121.9	162.5	237.4	327.2	415.0
14–14.9	98.1	104.3	142.3	181.8	240.3	325.0	376.5
15–15.9	83.9	112.6	139.6	188.6	254.4	309.3	419.5
16–16.9	112.6	135.1	166.3	200.6	259.8	337.4	423.6
17–17.9	104.2	126.7	146.3	210.4	297.7	386.4	515.9
18–18.9	100.3	123.0	161.6	210.4	261.7	350.8	373.3
19–24.9	104.6	119.8	159.6	216.6	295.9	405.0	489.6
25–34.9	117.3	139.9	184.1	254.8	351.2	469.0	556.0
35–44.9	133.6	161.9	215.8	289.8	393.2	509.3	584.7
45–54.9	145.9	180.3	244.7	324.4	422.9	541.6	614.0
55–64.9	134.5	187.9	252.0	336.9	436.0	527.6	615.2
65–74.9	136.3	168.1	226.6	306.3	394.3	491.4	553.0

Nutrition Survey (TSNS). Their data indicated that American men sampled in the HANES and TSNS were heavier, more muscular, and less fat than Jelliffe's standards, while American women were heavier, less muscular, and fatter. They noted, however, that the TSNS was not representative of the total U.S. population but heavily weighted by members of low income and of minority groups. Burgert and Anderson[69] found this to be true also in comparing anthropometric measurements taken on 77 healthy volunteers with Jelliffe's standards.

The advantages of using the HANES stan-dards for weight and arm anthropometry are that all measurements are derived from the same population; the sample represents a fairly representative cross-section of the U.S. population with respect to age, sex, ethnicity, and socioeconomic background; methods of measurement are standardized and reproducible; and the data are represented in percentile form.

Bistrian[91] has suggested use of the 1959 Metropolitan Life Insurance Data for the reason that it is correlated with mortality rates, allowing the use of one standard for diagnosing both malnutrition and obesity.

The higher mortality rates, however, reported at below-average weights by both the 1979 Metropolitan statistics and Garn et al.[84,86] preclude the advisability of continuing to use one standard, specifically the 1959 Metropolitan Life Insurance tables.

Nonetheless, it is important to note that no other standards have been tested against hospital morbidity and mortality.

INTERPRETATION

Obesity is customarily defined in terms of weight. The criterion is 20 percent or more above the "standard" weight (meaning that derived from a table such as Metropolitan Life's). An abnormally low weight is considered to be 10 percent below the "standard" weight (or 10 percent below the usual weight, or a 10 percent weight loss, depending on which source is referenced). As previously noted, neither takes into account individual differences in body composition (see Table 6–5).

The methods of Jelliffe[5] and Bistrian and Blackburn[2–4] for interpreting leanness and obesity from upper arm measurements are similar. Their method is as follows:

$$\frac{\% \text{ deviation}}{\text{from standard}} = \frac{\text{actual measurement}}{\text{standard value} \times 100}$$

where:
normal = 90 to 110 percent of standard
moderate depletion = 60 to 90 percent of standard
severe depletion = < 60 percent of standard
obesity = > 120 percent of standard (for weight and TSF).

As stated earlier, these cutoff points have not been justified.

Gray and Gray,[89,90] Burgert and Anderson,[69] and Bishop and Ritchey[85] propose substituting percentiles for percentages as a method of comparison of all anthropometric measurements. Gray and Gray[89,90] suggest that values falling below the 5th percentile are more likely to correspond to severe depletion and values between the 5th and 15th to those at risk to become depleted. This is making the assumption, however, that the lowest 5 percent of the population is malnourished. This assumption still needs to be tested against morbidity and mortality rates in hospitalized patients.

Seltzer and Mayer[6] have suggested substituting the use of triceps skinfold for weight as a determinant of body fat and obesity. They have published figures indicating that the upper limits of triceps skinfold measurements for males 25 years of age is 20 mm and for females 25 years of age is 29 mm. Limitations on the use of TSF measurements in the clinical setting have been discussed elsewhere in this chapter.

In summary, the application of anthropometry to nutrition assessment of hospitalized patients requires careful attention to patient selection, technique, and the choice of standards used for interpretation. Presently, anthropometry has broader applications and more established validity in the nutrition assessment of populations than it does to the individual hospital patient. More research is needed on specific guidelines for the use of anthropometry in the differential diagnosis of chronic PCM versus acute protein malnutrition.

REFERENCES

1. Martorell R: Notes on the history of nutritional anthropometry. Fed Proc 40(11):2572–2576, 1981
2. Bistrian BR, Blackburn GL, Hallowell E, Hadelle R: Protein status of general surgical patients. JAMA 230:858, 1974
3. Bistrian BR, Blackburn GL, Vitale J, et al.: Prevalence of malnutrition in general medical patients. JAMA 235:1567, 1976
4. Blackburn GL, Bistrian BR, Maine BS, et al.: Nutritional and metabolic assessment of the hospitalized patient. JPEN 1:11, 1977
5. Jelliffe DB: The Assessment of Nutritional Status of the Community. WHO Monograph No. 53. Geneva, World Health Organization, 1966

6. Seltzer CC, Mayer J: A simple criterion of obesity. Post Grad Med 38:101–107, 1965

7. Build and Blood Pressure Study. Chicago, Society of Actuaries, 1959

8. Build and Blood Pressure Study. Chicago, Society of Actuaries, 1979

9. Keys A: Overweight, obesity, coronary heart disease and mortality. Nutr Rev 38(9):297–307, 1980

10. Butterworth CE: The skeleton in the hospital closet. Nutr Today March/April:4–8, 1974

11. Bollett AJ, Owens S: Evaluation of nutritional status of selected hospitalized patients. Am J Clin Nutr 26:931–938, 1973

12. Hill GL, Pickford I, Young GA, et al.: Malnutrition in surgical patients: An unrecognized problem. Lancet 1:689–692, 1977

13. Moore FD: Jonathan E. Rhoads Lecture: Energy and the maintenance of the body cell mass. JPEN 4:228–260, 1980

14. Garrow JS: New approach to body composition. Am J Clin Nutr 35:1152–1158, 1982

15. Durnin JVGA, Womersley J: Body fat assessed from total body density and its estimation from skinfold thickness: Measurements on 481 men and women aged from 16–72 years. Br J Nutr 32:77–97, 1974

16. Steinkamp RC, Cohen MPH, Siri WE, et al.: Measures of body fat and related factors in normal adults. (Parts I and II). J Chron Dis 18:1279–1289, 1291–1307, 1965

17. Heymsfield SB, Arteaga C. McManus C, et al.: Measurement of muscle mass in humans: Validity of the 24-hour urinary creatinine method. Am J Clin Nutr 37:478–494, 1983

18. Heymsfield SB, Stevens V, Noel R, et al.: Biochemical composition of muscle in normal and semistarved human subjects: Relevance to anthropometric measurements. Am J Clin Nutr 36:131–142, 1982

19. Cohn SH, Vaswani AN, Vartsky D, et al.: In vivo quantification of body nitrogen for nutritional assessment. Am J Clin Nutr 35:1186–1191, 1982

20. Behnke AF: Anthropometry. In Nutritional Assessment—Present Status, Future Directions and Prospects, Report of the 2nd Ross Conference on Medical Research. Columbus, Ohio: Ross Laboratories, pp 85–91, 1981

21. Yang MU, Van Itallie TB: Composition of weight loss during short term weight reduction: Metabolic responses of obese subjects to starvation and low calorie ketogenic and nonketogenic diets. J Clin Invest 58:722–730, 1976

22. Murray RL, Schaffel NA, Geiger JW, et al.: Body composition changes in the critically ill patient: Emphasis on water balance. JPEN 3:219–225, 1979

23. Harvey KB, Moldawer L, Bistrian B, Blackburn GL: Biological measures for the formulation of a hospital prognostic index. Am J Clin Nutr 34:2013–2022, 1981

24. Nixon D, Heymsfield SB, Ansley J, et al.: Protein-calorie undernutrition in hospitalized cancer patients. Am J Med 68:683–690, 1980

25. Roche AF, Siervogel RM, Chumlea WC, Webb P: Grading body fatness from limited anthropometric data. Am J Clin Nutr 34:2831–2838, 1981

26. Skinfold thickness and body fat. Nutr Rev 26:104–107, 1968

27. Bray G, Greenway F, Molitch ME, et al.: Use of anthropometric measures to assess weight loss. Am J Clin Nutr 31:769–773, 1978

28. Cohn SH, Ellis KJ, Vartsky D, et al.: Comparison of methods of estimating body fat in normal subjects and cancer patients. Am J Clin Nutr 34:2839–2847, 1981

29. Barac-Nietro M, Spurr GB, Lotero H, Maksud MG: Body composition in chronic undernutrition. Am J Clin Nutr 31:23–40, 1978

30. Spurr GB, Barac-Nieto M, Lotero H, Dahners HW: Comparisons of body fat estimated from total body water and skinfold thicknesses of undernourished men. Am J Clin Nutr 34:1944–1953, 1979

31. McNeill KG, Harrison JE, Mernagh JR, et al.: Changes in body protein, body potassium, and lean body mass during total parenteral nutrition. JPEN 6:106–108, 1982

32. Barac-Nieto M, Spurr GB, Lotero H, et al.: Body composition during nutritional repletion of severely undernourished men. Am J Clin Nutr 32:981–991, 1979

33. Lee M, Ng CK: Postmortem studies of skinfold caliper measurement and actual thickness of skin and subcutaneous tissue. Human Biol 37:91–103, 1965

34. Allen TH, Peng MT, Chen KP, et al.: Prediction of total adiposity from skinfolds and the curvilinear relationship between external and internal adiposity. Metabolism 34:346–352, 1956

35. Long CL, Birkhahn RH, Geiger JW, Blakemore WS: Contribution of skeletal muscle protein in elevated rates of whole body protein catabolism in trauma patients. Am J Clin Nutr 34:1087–1093, 1981

36. Heymsfield SB, McManus C, Stevens V, Smith

J: Muscle-mass: Reliable indicator of protein-energy malnutrition severity and outcome. Am J Clin Nutr 35:1192–1199, 1982

37. Heymsfield SB, Olafson RP, Kutner MH, Nixon DW: A radiographic method of quantifying protein-calorie undernutrition. Am J Clin Nutr 32:693–702, 1979

38. Brožek J, Kinzey W: Age changes in skinfold compressibility. Gerontology 15:45–51, 1960

39. Collins JP, McCarthy ID, Hill GL: Assessment of protein nutriture in surgical patients—the value of anthropometrics. Am J Clin Nutr 32:1527–1530, 1979

40. Young GA, Chem C, Hill GL: Assessment of protein-calorie malnutrition in surgical patients from plasma proteins and anthropometric measurements. Am J Clin Nutr 31:429–435, 1978

41. Loewenstein MS, Phillips JF: Evaluation of arm circumference measurement for determining nutritional status of children and its use in an acute epidemic of malnutrition: Owerri, Nigeria, following the Nigerian Civil War. Am J Clin Nutr 26:226–233, 1973

42. Sommer A, Loewenstein MS: Nutritional status and mortality: A prospective validation of the QUAC stick. Am J Clin Nutr 28:287–292, 1975

43. Wilmore J, Behnke AR: An anthropometric estimation of body density and lean body weight in young men. J Appl Physiol 25(4):25–31, 1969

44. Behnke AR, Wilmore JH: Field Methods. In Evaluation and Regulation of Body Build and Composition. Englewood Cliffs, NJ: Prentice-Hall, 1974, Chapter 2

45. Scholl DE, Hain WF, Mullen JL: Inter-observer reliability and usefulness of anthropometric measurements. Am J Clin Nutr 37:730(A), 1983

46. Hall JC, O'Quigley J, Giles GR, et al.: Upper limb anthropometry: The value of measurement variance studies. Am J Clin Nutr 33:1846–1851, 1980

47. Jensen T, Dudrick S, Johnston D: A comparison of triceps skinfold and arm circumference values measured in standard and supine positions (abstr). JPEN 3:513, 1979

48. Garn SM, Cole PE, Higgins IT: The abdominal and iliac fatfolds in nutritional assessment. Ecol Food Nutr 6:95–96, 1977

49. Brunnstrom S: Clinical Kinesiology. Philadelphia: F. A. Davis, 1962

50. Morath M, Miller SF, Finely RK: Nutritional

indicators of postburn bacteremic sepsis. JPEN 5:488–491, 1981

51. Studley HO: Percentage of weight loss: A basic indicator of surgical risk in patients with peptic ulcer. JAMA 106:458–460, 1936

52. Kinney JM, Duke JH, Long CL, Gump FE: Tissue fuel and weight loss after injury. J Clin Path 23(suppl):65–72, 1970

53. Seltzer M, Slocum BA, et al.: Instant nutritional assessment: Absolute weight loss and surgical mortality. JPEN 6:218–221, 1982

54. Harvey KB, Bothe A, Blackburn GL: Nutritional assessment and patient outcome during oncological therapy. Cancer 43:2065–2069, 1979

55. Yeung CK, Smith RC, Hill GL: Effect of an elemental diet on body composition. Gastroenterology 77:652–657, 1979

56. Dempsey DT, Crosby LO, Feurer ID, et al.: Interval weight change during nutritional support. Am J Clin Nutr 37:725, 1983A

57. Jelliffe DB: Direct nutritional assessment of human groups. In The Assessment of Nutritional Status of the Community. WHO monograph No. 53. Geneva, World Health Organization, 1966.

58. Jensen TG, Englert DM, Dudrick SJ: Procedure for measuring weight using a platform balance scale. In Nutritional Assessment. Norwalk, Conn: Appleton-Century-Crofts, 1983

59. Stunkard AJ, Albaum JM: Accuracy of self-reported weights. Am J Clin Nutr 34:1593–1599, 1981

60. Pirie P, Jacobs D, Jeffrey R, Hannan P: Distortion in self-reported weight and height data. J Am Diet Assoc 78:601–605, 1981

61. Morgan DB, Path MRC, Hill GL, et al.: The assessment of weight loss from a single measurement of body weight: The problems and limitations. Am J Clin Nutr 33:2101–2105, 1980

62. Moore FD: Metabolic Care of the Surgical Patient. Philadelphia: W. B. Saunders, 1959, pp 266–275

63. Stroudt HW: The anthropometry of the elderly. Hum Factors 23:29–37, 1981

64. Forbes GB: The adult decline in lean body mass. Hum Biol 48:161–173, 1976

65. Bowman B, Rosenberg I: Assessment of the nutritional status of the elderly. Am J Clin Nutr 35:1142–1151, 1982

66. Mitchell CO, Lipschitz D: Arm length measurement as an alternative to height in nutri-

tional assessment of the elderly. JPEN 6:226–229, 1982

67. Mitchell CO, Lipschitz D: The effect of age and sex on the routinely used measurements to assess the nutritional status of hospitalized patients. Am J Clin Nutr 36:340–349, 1982

68. Jensen TG, Englert DM, Dudrick SJ: Procedure for measuring stature using a balance scale. In Nutritional Assessment: A Manual for Practitioners. Norwalk, Conn: Appleton-Century-Crofts, 1983, pp 37–44

69. Burgert SL, Anderson CF: An evaluation of upper arm measurements used in nutritional assessments. Am J Clin Nutr 32:2136–2142, 1979

70. Katch VL, Freedson PS: Body size and shape: Derivation of the "HAT" frame size model. Am J Clin Nutr 36:669–675, 1982

71. Katch VL, Freedson PS, Katch FI, Smith L: Body frame size: Validity of self-appraisal. Am J Clin Nutr 36:676–679, 1982

72. Frisancho AR, Flegel PN: Elbow breadth as a measure of frame size for U.S. males and females. Am J Clin Nutr 37:311–314, 1983

73. Garn SM, Pesick SD, Hawthorne VM: The bony chest breadth as a frame size standard in nutritional assessment. Am J Clin Nutr 37:315–318, 1983

74. Zerfas AJ: The insertion tape: A new circumference tape for use in nutritional assessment. Am J Clin Nutr 28:782–787, 1975

75. Burgert SL, Andersen CF: A comparison of triceps skinfold values as measured by the plastic McGaw caliper and the Lange caliper. Am J Clin Nutr 32:1531, 1979

76. Laven GT: Skinfold compressibility—a measure of body composition and a source of error. Am J Clin Nutr 37:727, 1983A

77. Mullen JL, Gertner MH, Buzby GP, et al.: Implications of malnutrition in the surgical patient. Arch Surg 114:121–125, 1979

78. Freeman M, Frankmann C, Beck J, Valdiveiso M: Prognostic nutrition factors in lung cancer patients. JPEN 6:122–127, 1982

79. Jensen TG, Englert DM, Dudrick SJ: Procedure for measuring arm circumference in the standard position. In Nutritional Assessment: A Manual for Practitioners. Norwalk,

Conn: Appleton-Century-Crofts, 1983, pp 71–72

80. Jensen TG, Englert DM, Dudrick SJ: Procedure for measuring arm circumference and triceps skinfold in the supine position. In Nutritional Assessment: A Manual for Practitioners. Norwalk, Conn: Appleton-Century-Crofts, 1983, pp 79–80

81. Heymsfield SB, McManus C, Smith J, et al.: Anthropometric measurements of muscle mass: Revised equations for calculating bone-free arm muscle area. Am J Clin Nutr 36:680–690, 1982

82. Roche AF, Siervogel RM, Chumlea C, Webb P: Grading body fatness from limited anthropometric data. Am J Clin Nutr 34:2831–2838, 1981

83. Frisancho R, Flegel PN: Relative merits of old and new indices of body mass with reference to skinfold thickness. Am J Clin Nutr 36:697–699, 1982

84. Garn SM, Hawthorne VM, Pilkington JJ, Pesick SD: Fatness and mortality in the West of Scotland. Am J Clin Nutr 38:313–319, 1983

85. Bishop CW, Ritchey SJ: Evaluating upper arm anthropometric measurements. J Amer Diet Assoc 84:330–335, 1984

86. Garn SM, Hawthorne VM: The "New Metropolitan Weight Tables"(letter). Amer J Clin Nutr 39:490, 1984

87. Lew EA: Reply to letter by Garn and Hawthorne (letter). Am J Clin Nutr 39:491, 1984.

88. Jolliffe N: Clinical Nutrition, 2nd ed. New York: Harper, 1962

89. Gray GE, Gray LK: Validity of anthropometric norms used in the assessment of hospitalized patients. JPEN 3:366, 1979

90. Gray GE, Gray LK: Anthropometric measurements and their interpretation: Principles, practices and problems. J Am Diet Assoc 77:534–539, 1980

91. Bistrian B: Anthropometric norms used in assessment of hospitalized patients. (Letter to Editor.) Am J Clin Nutr 33(10):2211–2212, 1980

92. Frisancho AR: Triceps skinfold and upper arm muscle size forms for assessment of nutritional status. Am J Clin Nutr 27:1052–1058, 1974

7. Immune Function Tests
Nathaniel Clark

THE IMMUNE SYSTEM

The immune system of the human body is a very intricate and involved system. The overall goal of immune function is to protect the body from invading agents. This is accomplished by (1) destroying these agents directly by phagocytosis (the engulfing of microorganisms or other cells by phagocytes) or (2) forming specific antibodies and sensitized lymphocytes to them.[1] Lymphocytes and macrophages (two types of leukocytes) are the major cell types involved. Leukocytes (or white blood cells) can be distinguished and classified into several cell types each of which plays a role in the immune process. There are six classes of leukocytes, which are listed in Table 7–1. Most numerous are the polymorphonucleocytes (also called granulocytes or "polys"), which are 60 percent of the leukocyte population. They function mainly in a phagocytic role. These can be further divided into neutrophils, eosinophils, and basophils. The other major cell type is the lymphocytes, which compose typically 30 percent of the leukocyte population. Finally, there are the plasma cells and monocytes, immature cells that, in response to invading agents, enter target tissues and swell to become macrophages.

Two lymphocyte classes have been described: T-cells (thymus derived) and B-cells (bursal-equivalent derived). T-cells, which compose 70 to 80 percent of peripheral blood lymphocytes, are subdivided into supressors, helpers, and killers, each of which plays a role in the immune process. The relative proportion of each cell type is obviously critical. T-cells are the main effectors of "cell-mediated immunity" (CMI) (Fig. 7–1). B-cells, which are 12 to 15 percent of peripheral blood lymphocytes, function mainly to synthesize antibodies (IgM, -A, -D, -G, -E) in response to specific antigens (foreign proteins) forming the basis for "humoral immunity" (Fig. 7–1). These antibodies are carried as membrane-bound immunoglobulins. Upon contact with an antigen, clonal expansion occurs with differentiation to plasma cells. It is the plasma cells that synthesize the appropriate antibodies. In addition, as noted above, with inflammation macrophages are produced and these function to kill bacteria, fungi, and tumor cells. Macrophages are present in the thymus, liver, lung, peritoneum, spleen, and lymph nodes. They function sequentially in the induction of the immune

TABLE 7–1. TOTAL LEUKOCYTES (WHITE BLOOD CELLS) IN AVERAGE ADULT HUMAN: 7000 μL

Polymorphonuclear neutrophils	62.0%
Polymorphonuclear eosinophils	2.3%
Polymorphonuclear basophils	0.4%
Monocytes	5.3%
Lymphocytes	30.0%

From Guyton AC: Textbook of Medical Physiology. Philadelphia: W. B. Saunders, 1981, pp 74–83.[1]

response by processing and presenting immunogenic material to the lymphocytes.

Cell-mediated immunity (with T-cells) also is specific for a given antigen. Here T-cells are sensitized to foreign substances by a mechanism whereby an antigen is felt to interact with specially sensitized T-cells. These T-cells, upon activation, elaborate lymphokines. Lymphokines are lymphocyte mediators and amplify and regulate cell-mediated immunity by affecting macrophages, polys, as well as B- and T-cells. Three such lymphokines are chemotactic factor, migratory inhibitory factor, and macrophage-activating factor. As one might expect, if interested in

assessing the immune status of malnourished patients, one could examine each of the various portions of the immune system, whether cell-mediated or humoral.

RELATIONSHIP BETWEEN NUTRITION STATUS AND IMMUNE STATUS

Over the last 10 years, there have appeared increasing data regarding the relationship between nutrition status and immune status.[2] First in research based in developing countries (in mainly pediatric populations) and more recently in work done examining protein status and immune function, a relationship has been documented. What has emerged, in summary, is that protein depletion syndromes (particularly those involving visceral proteins) lead to decreased immune function.[3] This is not surprising as most immune cooperative activities are dependent on protein synthesis. When protein catabolism dominates anabolism, loss of immunocompetence often follows. Changes in cell-mediated immunity have been noted in malnutrition. Chandra[4] noted that patients with protein–calorie malnutrition (PCM) show (1) impaired cutaneous delayed hypersensitivity,

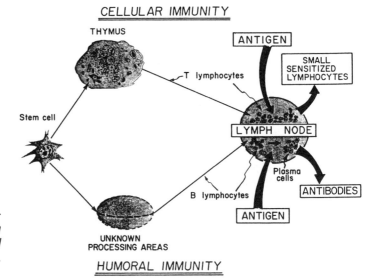

Figure 7–1. Cellular and humoral immunity. *(From Guyton AC: Textbook of Medical Physiology. Philadelphia: W. B. Saunders, 1981.)*

(2) decreased circulating T-cells, and (3) decreased lymphocyte stimulation response to mitogens. Humoral immunity appears to be less affected by nutrition status.[5] Secretory IgA levels and activity have been noted to be decreased, however.

TESTS OF IMMUNE FUNCTION[6]

Although immune function tests are often listed as one category of nutrition assessment tests, they are really quite different. While the bulk of the assessment tests assay nutrition status per se, immune function tests assess the result of altered nutrition status rather than simply its presence. The immune system confers to the patient the ability to meet the challenges of injury and infection.

Delayed Cutaneous Hypersensitivity (DCH)

Procedure. In this test 0.1 cc of a variety of antigens (usually 3 to 5) are injected intradermally in the forearm area and the response (redness and/or induration) is noted at 24 and 48 hours. A 5 mm or greater response is generally considered to be a positive response. Multiple antigens are used because a given patient will be immunoreactive only to those antigens that he or she has encountered previously. With multiple antigens, the chance that a patient will have been exposed to at least one antigen in the past increases. Commonly used antigens have been: Candida albicans, purified protein derivative (PPD), streptokinase–streptodornase (SK/SD), mumps, Tricophytin, and dinitrochlorobenzene (DNCB). The most commonly used antigens in current clinical use are Candida, PPD, mumps, and tetanus. Streptokinase–streptodornase (SK/SD or Varidase) is no longer available.

Complicating Factors. The major complicating factor in regard to the use of DCH testing in nutrition assessment is that many factors other than nutrition influence skin test response. Miller[7] reports that electrolyte imbalances, circulation problems, advanced age, uremia, liver disease, and concurrent infections all affect skin test reactivity. A more extensive list of interfering factors from Twomey et al.[8] appears in Table 7–2. A review of the literature on the effect of age on skin test reactivity specifically[9] indicates that while in some studies responses were altered in the elderly compared to the nonelderly, there is excellent evidence to indicate that this assessment test has both validity and prognostic significance in the elderly and forms an important part of the assessment process.

Bates et al.[10] have reviewed extensively the problems in DCH testing and make several important recommendations. They focus on what Twomey et al.[8] refer to as "technical" problems, specifically (1) the "booster effect," (2) reader variability, (3) dilution factors, and (4) the time course of interpretation. The "booster effect" refers to the finding that, with repeated testing, responses will be enhanced. This of course makes sense as an "acquired immunity" response to specific antigens is being tested and this improves with repeated exposure. This effect becomes most important in serial assessment protocols where repeat testing (preop versus postop, pretreatment versus posttreatment) is used.

Reader variability is a second area of concern. Bates et al.[10] quote Bearman et al.[11] as stating that "the variability from reader to reader is nearly as great as the biological variability from subject to subject." As one example, if a 5 mm response to a given antigen is necessary for a positive result to the test, one must be able to distinguish between a 4 mm and 6 mm response and this is difficult at best. Dilution factors are an obvious source of error. The correct antigen strength (and purity) must be known and used consistently. Finally, the time course of the interpretation is significant. While most assessment protocols use 24 and 48 hours as time points, some patients may not react fully until 72 hours.[12] Listed in Table 7–3

TABLE 7-2. NONNUTRITIONAL INFLUENCES ON SKIN TEST RESPONSE

Technical	Immune alterations
Antigen source and batch	Congenital
Preparation and storage	DiGeorge's syndrome
Method of administration	Thymic aplasia
Site of test	Acquired
Booster effect	SLE
Criteria of positivity	Rheumatoid arthritis
Reader variability	Trauma, burns, hemorrhage
Patient factors	Diseases—malignant
Age	Most solid tumors especially
Race	advancing stages
Geographic location	Lymphomas
Prior exposure to antigen	Leukemias
Circadian rhythm	Prior malignancy especially
Psychologic state	squamous cancer, lymphoma
Diseases—benign	Iatrogenic
Infections	Drugs
Viral	Immunosuppressants
Bacterial	Most antineoplastics
Fungal	Antiinflammatory
Metabolic	Anticoagulants
Uremia	H_2 blockers (cimetidine)
Liver diseases	? Aspirin
Inflammatory	X-ray therapy
Crohn's disease	General anesthesia
Ulcerative colitis	Surgery
Sarcoid	

From Twomey P, Ziegler D, Rombeau J: JPEN 6:50–58, 1982.[8]

TABLE 7-3. RECOMMENDATIONS FOR DELAYED HYPERSENSITIVITY TESTING

1. Use uniform dilutions.
2. Use uniform measurement techniques: Sokal[12] recommends placing a ball-point pen on the skin 1 to 2 cm away from the margin of the skin reaction and moving it slowly toward the center. When resistance at the edge of the induration is reached, the pen is lifted, and the procedure is repeated on the opposite side. The distance between the opposite lines is the diameter of induration.
3. Record the measurement of the erythema (redness) as well as induration. Both types of response have significance immunologically.
4. Use uniform interpretation techniques. A gradual scale including both the size of the erythema and induration is necessary (+1 to + 4 versus +).

From Bates SE, Suen JY, Tranum BL: Cancer 43:2306–2314, 1979.[10]

are the recommendations of Bates et al. regarding DCH testing.

Prognostic Significance. Christou et al.[13] prospectively studied surgical patients who were given skin tests for delayed cutaneous hypersensitivity. The rates of sepsis, mortality, and mortality due to sepsis were significantly higher in the anergic (immunoincompetent) versus immunocompetent group. The conclusion drawn here was that malnutrition led to a poorer prognosis. What next needed to be examined was whether nutrition support could (1) improve skin test response to intradermally placed antigens and (2) whether an improved skin test result would correlate with an improved prognosis. Meakins et al.[14] examined this and found that the mortality rate was decreased in those anergic patients who improved their response with nutrition support.

The most extensive analysis of the relationship between immune system status and prognosis has been done in research using multiple regression analysis. By this methodology, a patient's clinical course is analyzed by examining correlations between major events (sepsis, mortality) and various nutrition assessment data.

Buzby et al.[15] formulated a "Prognostic Nutrition Index" that estimates the risk of complications in surgical patients. It is computed using the formula:

Prognostic Nutrition Index (PNI in %) = 158 −16.6 (albumin concentration in g/dl) − 0.78 (triceps skinfold thickness in mm) − 0.20 (transferrin concentration in mg/dl) − 5.8 (delayed hypersensitivity response: 0 = anergy, 1 = <5mm response to any of three antigens, 2 = >5 mm response).

Patients were placed in four groups based on their risk status and their clinical course noted. Highly significant increases in the actual incidence of mortality, complications, sepsis, and major sepsis were noted as the predicted risk increased.

In similar work in another research center, Harvey et al.[16] formulated the "Hospital Prognostic Index." Here the probability of survival was predicted based on the following index:

Hospital Prognostic Index (HPI) = 0.91 (albumin concentration in g/dl) − 1.00 (delayed hypersensitivity response: 0 = anergy, 1 = a 5 mm or greater response to one or more antigens) − 1.44 (presence of sepsis: 1 = No, 2 = Yes) + 0.98 (diagnosis: 1 = cancer, 2 = noncancer) − 1.09.

From the result of this analysis, the probability of survival could be calculated. A value of −2 indicated a 10 percent probability of survival (nonseptic course, immune competence) and a +2 indicated a 90 percent probability of the above events. Further, an improvement in or maintenance of a positive response to delayed hypersensitivity testing was found to be the most accurate predictor of a favorable outcome.

New Technique. The Multitest CMI Delayed Hypersensitivity Skin Test kit is manufactured by Institute Merieux (Lyons, France). It is a sterile, disposable plastic, multipuncture applicator consisting of eight test heads preloaded with seven standardized antigens (tuberculin, tetanus toxoid, diptheria toxoid, Streptococcus, Candida, Trichophyton, and Proteus) in glycerin solution and a glycerin control. The placement of the antigens is similar to that with traditional antigen testing and the results are read at 24 and 48 hours as well. A positive response is noted if any of the antigens cause a reaction of 2 mm greater than the glycerin control.[17]

This new technique offers some theoretical advantages over traditional skin testing. It is felt to be more sensitive and specific because with seven antigens the number of false-negatives (due to lack of prior exposure to the antigens) should be decreased. Additionally, the doses are standardized, which eliminates a major complicating factor of the traditional technique as discussed above. Finally, it is felt to be more comfortable from the patient's point of view—which is a bonus. This system has been tested by Kniker et al.[18] and found to be very usable. With future studies comparing the predictive value of the results to those with traditional testing, we will see if this new technique offers better results.

Total Lymphocyte Count

Procedure. The total lymphocyte count is derived using the white blood count (WBC) and the differential:

Total lymphocyte count (TLC) = WBC × % lymphoctes in differential/100

For use as standards, Blackburn et al.[19] have recommended using 1500 to 1800 to represent mild depletion, 900 to 1500 to represent moderate depletion, and less than 900 to represent severe depletion.

Complicating Factors. Various co-existing conditions can affect the total lymphocyte count and need to be noted here. Surgical patients can have a decreased TLC and this is closely associated with the stress response as it is also correlated with serum albumin concentration. Additionally, a large wound can lead to a decrease in TLC due to migration of lymphocytes to the wound site. Finally, one might realize that a decreased TLC gives no real indication of which lymphocyte subpopulations have changed. A knowledge of the shifts in B-cell versus T-cell populations and of helper versus supressor ratios would be far more revealing.

Lymphocyte Blastogenesis and T-Cell Quantitation[7]

Methods. Lymphocytes are incubated in the presence of mitogens, which activate the carbohydrate receptors on the lymphocyte cell surfaces stimulating cell division. The commonly used mitogens are phytohemagglutinin (PHA), concanavalin A (Con A), pokeweed mitogen (PWM), and peanut agglutinin (PA). PHA, Con A, and PA are felt to stimulate T-lymphocytes (with macrophage involvement) and PWM stimulates B-cells (with T-cell and macrophage involvement). Quantification of lymphocyte multiplication is done by using 3H-thymidine uptake into DNA.

A more traditional technique used to quantitate thymus-dependent lymphocytes (T-cells) involves incubation of the lymphocytes with sheep red blood cells. T-cells will bind to the red blood cells (RBCs) forming rosettes which can be quantitated.

Comment. These are very useful methods that to date have had their major use in research rather than in the clinical setting. Chandra,[20] however, has listed lymphocyte-rosette assay as a "functional index" that should be employed in the clinical setting as well. As limitations, these tests do not identify the cause of the decreased stimulation or binding nor differentiate between decreased cell numbers, decreased cell surface receptors, or decreased levels of co-factors in the

reaction (particularly lymphokines). Additionally, with the stimulation assay, the mitogen preparations can differ markedly and alter the response seen.

Other Methods

Additional research methods used to examine the immune system are: (1) "Mixed leukocyte response," which is the ability of cells to divide in response to specific antigens. The level of blastogenic response is noted (using 3H-thymidine incorporation). (2) "Antibody production" in which one assays the levels of each of the five Ig classes, particularly IgA. Secretory IgA levels have been noted to be decreased with malnutrition. Ig synthesis levels cannot be determined from Ig levels alone. Ig synthesis requires T- and B-cell cooperation. Also, the increased levels of Igs accompanying the response to infection will often obscure any decreases in levels due to malnutrition. (3) "Complement levels" (particularly C3), can be assayed by radioimmunodiffusion. Complement levels are predicted to rise as part of the acute phase response to infection and to be decreased with malnutrition.

New Areas of Research

Leukocyte Endogenous Mediator (LEM or interleukin I) has been reported to stimulate lymphocyte proliferation in response to antigen. In addition, it may induce the fever and elicit the neutropenia and granulopoeisis that accompany the infective process.[21] Further, it may evoke the profound cellular, organic, and systemic alterations in trace minerals, nitrogen, hormone distribution, and metabolism that have been documented to accompany the metabolic response to injury. Due to the above, it has been postulated that LEM acts as a broad, but central, mediator or modulator of the development of and interactions among various aspects of non-specific and specific immunity.

This is a very exciting area of research due to the fact that while all the above phenomena accompany the infected state, and could therefore be seen as homeostatically positive, they also lead to the decline of the patient's nutrition status. Finally, the malnourished state is associated with decreased LEM levels. A vicious cycle is thus set up where the malnourished person becomes less and less able to immunologically meet the stresses of infection. The future promises to be exciting in this research area as we gain the ability to measure LEM levels in patients and decide whether LEM should be given to the patient with decreased levels.[22] In evaluating the value of a new assessment technique, one must consider the predictive value of this method and how it compares to current methods.[23] In this area, it is useful to consider the concepts of sensitivity, specificity, and predictive value. (See Chapter 8 for a more indepth discussion of these statistical methods.)

SUMMARY

In this chapter the current knowledge of immune function testing in nutrition assessment has been reviewed. The major components of the immune system (the cell-mediated and humoral systems) were described and their interactions discussed. The immune function tests presently in use both in the clinical and research setting were discussed as to how they are done, what the complicating factors are in terms of interpreting results from them, and what new tests are being developed. Emphasis was placed on delayed cutaneous hypersensitivity testing as this is the most widely used test to assess immune function in nutrition assessment protocols.

REFERENCES

1. Guyton AC: Resistance of the body to infection: The leukocytes, the tissue macrophage system, and inflammation. In Textbook of Medical Physiology. Philadelphia: W.B. Saunders, 1981, pp 74–83
2. Faulk WP, Demaeyer EM, Davies AJS: Some effects of malnutrition on immune response in man. Am J Clin Nutr 27:638–646, 1974
3. Bistrian BR: Assessment of protein energy malnutrition in surgical patients. In Hill G (ed.): Nutrition and the Surgical Patient. Edinburgh: Churchill Livingstone, 1981, pp 39–54
4. Chandra RK: Cell-mediated immunity in nutritional imbalance. Fed Proc 39:3088–3092, 1980
5. Stiehm ER: Humoral immunity in malnutrition. Fed Proc 39:3093–3097, 1980
6. Meakins JL, Nohr CW: Assessment of immunological responsiveness. In Kirkpatrick JR (ed.): Nutrition and Metabolism in the Surgical Patient. Mt. Kisco: Futura, 1983, pp 107–133
7. Miller CL: Immunological assays as measures of nutritional status: A review. JPEN 2:554–566, 1978
8. Twomey P, Ziegler D, Rombeau J: Utility of skin testing in nutritional assessment: A critical review. JPEN 6:50–58, 1982
9. Clark NG, Bistrian BR: Recognition of protein–calorie malnutrition in the hospitalized elderly. Geriatric Med Today (in press)
10. Bates SE, Suen JY, Tranum BL: Immunological skin testing and interpretation: A plea for uniformity. Cancer 43:2306–2314, 1979
11. Bearman JE, Kleinman H, Glyer VV, LaCroix OM: A study of variability in tuberculin test reading. Am Rev Respir Dis 90:913–919, 1964
12. Sokal JE: Measurement of delayed skin-test responses. N Engl J Med 293:501–502, 1975
13. Christou NV, Meakins JL, MacLean LD: The predictive role of delayed hypersensitivity in preoperative patients. Surg Gynecol Obstet 152:297–301, 1981
14. Meakins JL, Pietsch JB, Bubenick O, et al.: Delayed hypersensitivity: Indicator of acquired failure of host defenses in sepsis and trauma. Ann Surg 186:214–249, 1977
15. Buzby GP, Mullen JL, Mathews DC, et al.: Prognostic nutritional index in gastrointestinal surgery. Am J Surg 139:160–167, 1980
16. Harvey KB, Moldawer LL, Bistrian BR, Blackburn GL: Biological measures for the formation of a hospital prognostic index. Am J Clin Nutr 34:2013–2022, 1981

17. Package insert, "Skintest Antigens for Cellular Hypersensitivity Multitest CMI." Miami: Merieux Institute, Inc.

18. Kniker WT, Anderson CT, Roumiantzeff M: The Multi-test system: A standardized approach to evaluation of delayed hypersensitivity and cellular immunity. Ann Allergy 43:73–79, 1979

19. Blackburn GL, Bistrian BR, Maini BS, et al.: Nutritional and metabolic assessment of the hospitalized patient. JPEN 1:11–22, 1977

20. Chandra RK: Immunocompetence in nutritional assessment. Am J Clin Nutr 33:2694–2697, 1980

21. Keenan RA, Moldawer LL, Yang RD, et al.: An altered response by peripheral leukocytes to synthesize or release leukocyte endogenous mediator in critically ill, protein-malnourished patients. J Lab Clin Med 100:844–857, 1982

22. Moldawer LL, Sobrado J, Blackburn GL, Bistrian BR: A rationale for administering leukocyte endogenous mediator to protein malnourished, hospitalized patients. J Theor Biol 106:119–133, 1984

23. Dietz WH: Immune indices in the assessment of the nutritional status of hospitalized patients. Clin Nutr 2:11–15, 1983

8. Interpreting the Nutrition Assessment

Rebecca L. Murray

Interpreting the nutrition status assessment is a continuous process rather than a static event because the patient as a whole person is a dynamic entity. Evaluation of nutrition status is integral to the health care team's evaluation of all aspects of patients' present and changing medical, psychological, and socioeconomic status and their potential to recover and to resume their own care. The design of this manual as a systems approach to nutrition assessment and nutrition support reflects this philosophy.

The nutrition assessment process begins by gathering and synthesizing raw data to generate a nutrition care plan. The manner in which this is done depends on the political structure of the individual institution and the relationships between the members of its health care team. It is not the purpose of this chapter to define the role of the members of that team or to appoint any member as the sole arbitor and interpreter of the patient's nutrition status. It is the philosophy of this author that since the physician has the final responsibility for the patient, his or her decisions are also final. For that reason, the physician benefits from the professional input of other members of the health care team. The dietitian, in most clinical situations, is the team member with the most background in nutrition. Nutrition assessment is the responsibility of the generalist dietitian as well as the specialist. Both types of dietitians need to be conversant in the theory and practice of nutrition support. Both need to be available to the health care team on an ongoing basis.

The methods and standards used for assessing nutrition status should be agreed upon beforehand by all members of the health care team. This may be more easily carried out by appointing a nutrition committee or designating members of the nutrition support team to recommend policies and procedures. These people should then be charged with the responsibility of inservicing the other clinicians in the facility in the appropriate methods and procedures, auditing the implementation of the procedures and updating them periodically. Standardization of assessment protocols, when done properly, helps avoid duplication of services and prevents ordering of unnecessary tests. Readily available methods for assessing nutrition status facilitate early detection, prevention, and treatment of malnutrition.

Malnutrition indicates a state of dietary imbalance, characterized by the deficiency or excess of one or more nutrients. The focus of this chapter is the organization and analysis of the data base in order to determine the type and degree of malnutrition and its functional consequences. Development and application of the nutrition care plan will be touched on in this chapter and elaborated in subsequent chapters.

DATA ANALYSIS

Before interpreting the nutrition assessment, the clinician must first analyze the data, asking three key questions:

1. Is there reason to believe that the data contain significant errors that might render them unusable? For example, incomplete collection of sample, inappropriate timing of sample, inaccurate processing of laboratory samples, or incomplete data collection in the medical records may invalidate necessary information.
2. Are the parameters that are being measured valid indices of nutrition status, taking into account the patient's age, disease state, and clinical condition? For example, a low creatinine–height index (CHI) in an elderly patient may signify muscle wastage secondary to aging rather than muscle wasting secondary to protein malnutrition. An elevated serum transferrin may signify iron deficiency rather than simple protein malnutrition.
3. Are the data complete? Are additional data needed in order to confirm the assessment? For example, serum folate and B_{12} levels as well as a thorough review of the medication history may be necessary to confirm the etiology of megaloblastic anemia.

Table 8–1 summarizes the areas to consider in collecting data for a complete nutrition assessment. This is an outline of the thinking process used to justify the nutrition care plan. Standards of practice and clinical judgment dictate the amount of time and attention spent in investigating each area for the individual patient.

Guidelines for determining the accuracy and completeness of information necessary for the nutrition assessment have been given in Chapters 4 through 8. In addition, it is helpful if the data can be briefly scanned for completeness, and quickly charted. Forethought should be given to the personal records kept by the clinician on each patient assessed. Such records should include pertinent history, laboratory values, the final assessment, the nutrition care plan, and daily notes that monitor the patient's progress while undergoing nutrition therapy.

Flow sheets assist the clinician to monitor daily progress of the patient on nutrition support and make comparisons of subsequent assessments to the initial assessment. Thus, the clinician can see at a glance whether the patient is responding to therapy. Critical laboratory values, weights, vital signs, and a summary of fluid intake and output, caloric and protein intake, nitrogen and calorie balance should be included in the flow sheet. (Figure 8–1 is an example of such a flow sheet.)

THE PURPOSE OF THE NUTRITION ASSESSMENT

An individual or a team assesses a patient's nutrition status for basically four reasons:

1. To determine whether the patient is a candidate for short-term nutrition intervention
2. To determine whether the patient's present nutrition status will enable him to withstand acute stress or therapeutic intervention

TABLE 8–1. DATA BASE FOR ESTABLISHMENT OF THE NUTRITION CARE PLAN

I. Reason for the Nutrition Consultation
  A. To determine whether there is a need for short-term nutrition support (assessment of changes in body composition)
  B. To institute nutrition support for the appropriate candidate
  C. To evaluate the patient's potential for home nutrition support
  D. To determine the patient's ability to withstand surgery or other stress event (prognostic and statistical approach to nutrition assessment)
II. The Past Nutrition History
  A. Medical history
  B. Social history
  C. Medications and treatments
  D. Nutrient intake history
    1. Previous diet prescriptions
    2. Recent oral intake
    3. Previous nutrition support
    4. Dietary supplementation
    5. Weight history
    6. Changes in appetite, mechanical feeding problems, and GI function not covered above
III. Review of Systems—Examine each system for the following:
  Physical signs and symptoms of malnutrition (see Chapter 5)
  Presence of disease/dysfunction and its relationship to the following:
  Impact on organ failure
  Impact on delivery, absorption, and metabolism of nutrients
  Effect on GI function
  Effect on venous access
  A. Eyes   J. Nails
  B. Hair   K. Subcutaneous tissue
  C. Face   L. Muscular and skeletal systems
  D. Lips   M. Internal systems
  E. Tongue   1. Cardiovascular and pulmonary
  F. Teeth   2. Renal
  G. Gums   3. Gastrointestinal (including liver and pancreas)
  H. Glands   4. Nervous
  I. Skin
IV. Summarize Nutrition Assessment
  A. Deficiencies or excesses of nutrients—type and degree
    1. Initiating or exacerbating causes
    2. Factors that promote or prevent treatment
  B. Risk to patient of continued nutritional condition versus risk to patient of instituting nutrition support
  C. Nutrient requirements
    1. Basal
    2. Maintenance
    3. Repletion
V. Nutrition Care Plan
  A. Suggest mode of nutrition therapy to best optimize patient's overall condition
  B. Suggest monitoring procedures
  C. Suggest advancing/weaning patient on nutrition support
  D. Suggest home nutrition care

AKRON GENERAL MEDICAL CENTER

<u>NUTRITION SUPPORT FLOW SHEET</u>

	Mon.	Tues.	Wed.	Thurs.	Fri.	Sat.	Sun.
Date							
Weight							
Fluid Balance							
Temperature							
Blood Pressure							
Pulse							
Respiration							
Urine glu/Act							
Calories/Protein							
WBC							
Hgb							
Hct							
tot lymphs							
Pt. Pro time							
Cath tip cult.							
Urine cult.							
Blood cult.							
Urine vol/24°							
Creat. Clearance							
Urine creat. tot							
UUN							
N bal.							
Calorie bal.							
PPD							
Mumps							
Candida							

	Mon.	Tues.	Wed.	Thurs.	Fri.	Sat.	Sun.
Na mEq/L							
K mEq/L							
Cl mEq/L							
CO_2 mEq/6							
Glu mg%							
BUN mg%							
Creat. mg%							
Uric Acid mg%							
Ca mg%							
P mg%							
Alb g%							
Tot Pro g%							
SGOT U/L							
SGPT U/L							
LDH U/L							
Alk Phos U/L							
T. Bili mg%							
Fe mg%							
Chol mg%							
Trig mg%							
Amylase/Lipase							
Transferrin mg%							
Mg mg%							
Zn mg%							

Nutrition Therapy		Mon.	Tues.	Wed.	Thurs.	Fri.	Sat.	Sun.	Date	Clinical Course
A.A. ___ % cc/L										
Dex ___ % cc/L										
H$_2$O ___ cc/L										
NaCl ___ mEq/L										
NaAcetate ___ mEq/L										
KCl ___ mEq/L										
K Phos ___ mM/L										
Ca Glu ___ mEq/L										
MgSO$_4$ ___ mEq/L										
MVI-12 ___ amp/d										
tr. min. ___ cc/d										
ZnCl ___ mg/d										
hep										
ins										
Other										
HAF rate ___ cc hr.										
Other adds										
Fat ___ % cc hr.										
Fe										
Vit. K										
Other										
Non-pro cal/L										
gm N/L										
tot pro/L										
Tube fdg.										
conc.										
rate										
Diet										
Inter. Fdg.										

Date	Mon.	Tues.	Wed.	Thurs.	Fri.	Sat.	Sun.
P.O.							
Enteral							
HAF							
Lipid							
Dex							
Other							
Total In							
Urine							
Stool							
NG							
Other							
Total Out							

Figure 8–1. Sample flow sheet for monitoring nutrition assessment and support.

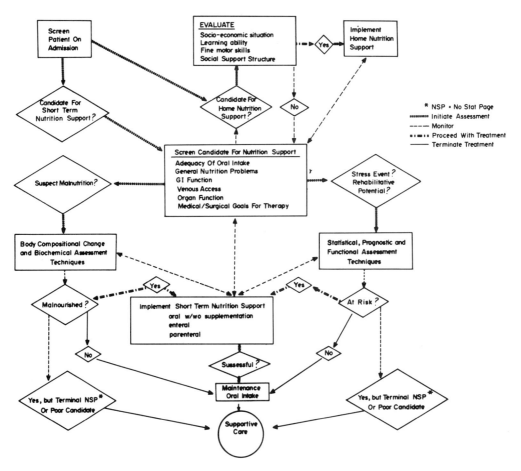

Figure 8–2. Decision matrix for establishing a nutrition care plan for nutrition support.

3. To determine whether the patient is a candidate for home nutrition support
4. To initiate and monitor nutrition support for the patient deemed to be an appropriate candidate

The choice of methodology used to assess the patient, recommend and institute therapy, and monitor the patient will depend on the reason for the initial assessment. The decision matrix in Figure 8–2 illustrates this. Before making any of the four above determinations in this matrix, the clinician does a limited assessment to get a general feel for

the patient's clinical picture and goals for therapy, as well as his or her nutrition problems. This limited assessment is a little broader in scope and usually occurs later during the patient's admission than does the admitting nutrition status screen.

The admission nutrition status screen includes just enough data to determine whether the patient is now or may become at nutrition risk. The data base is generally limited to a brief description of the patient's weight history, changes in gastrointestinal (GI) function, appetite, or ability to chew and swallow food, and a brief statement of previous nutrition therapy, pertinent medical history, and admission diagnosis. It may or may not include admission laboratory data (see Chapter 9). The admission screen should be so designed that a diet technician or other support personnel can collect the data and, under the supervision of the registered dietitian, decide whether or not the patient needs further nutrition intervention. On this basis, the registered dietitian implements limited and comprehensive assessments and communicates with the health care team.

The purposes of the limited assessment are:

1. To begin generating a nutrition problem list. The list will be very brief and very general at this point, and may not include anything more than the reason for the nutrition consult (e.g., persistent weight loss, inability to swallow, persistent diarrhea).
2. To determine the viability of the three major routes for nutrition support—oral, enteral, and parenteral—and preclude use of the oral route before investigating more expensive and invasive vehicles of nutrition support.
3. To integrate the goals of the nutrition care plan with the medical goals of treatment.
   a. To prevent institution of expensive and time-consuming testing and nutrition therapy in the patient who is terminally ill, or who has refused other life-sustaining treatment.
   b. To determine the anticipated length of time that the patient will be in the hospital, including a consideration of the patient's diagnoses and insurance coverage. This information will be necessary in deciding whether further nutrition assessment and short-term support will be feasible and whether home nutrition support will be feasible or necessary.
   c. To tailor the nutrition assessment and type of nutrition support to the patient's clinical condition.

The type and degree of organ malfunction may interfere with the results of standard parameters of nutrition assessment and indicate a need for additional or alternate tests. For example, synthesis of albumin and transferrin is impaired in end stage cirrhosis of the liver making them less sensitive as indices of protein nutriture. Serum levels of tryptophan, methionine, and branch chain amino acids (BCAA) may be indicated for patients in hepatic encephalopathy. In addition, the clinician must consider the relative risks of various methods for nutrition support to the patient exhibiting organ malfunction and the means needed to minimize the risk and potentiate the patient's response to nutrition support. (For example, the patient in hepatic encephalopathy will not tolerate protein in the standard amounts and with the standard distribution of amino acids. A patient with dysphagia secondary to a cardiovascular accident (CVA) may be a poor candidate for a nasogastric tube feeding because of the increased risk of aspiration but may respond well to nasoduodenal or jejunal tube feedings.)

This brief preliminary overview helps the clinician decide how to approach the patient and lessens the risk and the amount of time and money spent in assessing and treating the patient.

THE METHOD AND INTERPRETATION OF THE COMPREHENSIVE NUTRITION ASSESSMENT

As seen in Figure 8–2, there are basically two types of comprehensive nutrition assessment used in the clinical setting today:

1. The traditional categorization of nutrition status on the basis of biochemical and body compositional evidence of nutrient deficiency(ies)
2. The statistical prediction of prognosis and/or functional capabilities

Before going into a further explanation of these methods, let us pause for a minute to

TABLE 8–2. DETERMINING THE PREDICTIVE VALUE OF A TEST IN DISEASED AND HEALTHY SUBJECTS

	Number of Subjects with Positive Test Results	Number of Subjects with Negative Test Results	Total
Number of diseased subjects	TP	FN	TP + FN
Number of healthy subjects	FP	TN	FP + TN
Totals	TP + FP	FN + TN	TP + FP + TN + FN

1. Sensitivity (Se) $= \dfrac{TP}{TP + FN} \times 100$

2. Specificity (Sp) $= \dfrac{TN}{TN + FP} \times 100$

3. Predictive Value of a positive test result (V+) $= \dfrac{TP}{TP + FP} \times 100$

4. Predictive Value of a negative test result (V−) $= \dfrac{TN}{TN + FN}$

5. Prevalence of disease (actual P) $= \dfrac{TP + FN}{TP + FN + TN + FP}$

6. Prevalence of disease as diagnosed by this test:

(Dx P) $= \dfrac{TP + FP}{TP + FN + TN + FP}$ where

TP = The number of diseased patients correctly classified by the test (true-positive)
FP = The number of healthy patients falsely classified by the test (false-positive)
TN = The number of healthy patients correctly classified by the test (true-negative)
FN = The number of sick patients falsely classified by the test (false-negative)

explain some terms that will be used in discussing and critiquing these methods.

According to Galen and Gambino,[1] a test's "predictive value" (V + or −) is its ability to predict the presence or absence of disease. Determination of predictive value is based on the measurement of three variables:

1. Sensitivity (Se)—the number of times that the test is positive when disease is present (true-positive).
2. Specificity (Sp)—the number of times that the test is negative when there is no disease (true-negative).
3. Prevalence (actual P) of disease—the incidence (or frequency with which a disease occurs during a given time period) × the duration of the disease. For example, there may be an incidence of

folate deficiency among alcoholics of 10 percent per year and a prevalence of 25 percent; that is, 10 percent of the population is newly diagnosed with folate deficiency each year. But the prevalence, or number of existing cases of folate deficiency is higher.

Table 8–2 describes the method in which these three variables determine predictive value.

There are a few points to keep in mind:

1. No test can be both 100 percent sensitive and 100 percent specific.
2. V+ and V− can be changed by altering the levels at which the test is considered positive or negative.
3. An acceptable cut-off point for V+ or

V− is based on the number of false-negative (FN) and false-positive (FP) results that are considered tolerable, taking into account the prevalence of the disease, the severity of the disease, the cost of the test, and the availability and advantages of treatment.

4. The prevalence of the disease (actual P) alters the V+ of a test more than any other factor. Galen and Gambino[1] state that when the Se and Sp of a test both equal 95 percent and the actual P is 0.1 percent, the V+ is 1.9 percent. If the actual P increases to 5 percent, the V+ increases to 50 percent. And if the actual P increases to 50 percent, the V+ equals 95 percent.

5. According to Habicht,[2] the highest V+ is gained when Sp is high regardless of Se as long as Se is greater than zero.

Habicht[2] also makes the point that the best test and the best cut-off point for that test depend on whether it is used for screening, for determining actual P of the disease, or is used in surveillance. There is often an unrealistic burden placed on a single test, both as a reflection of past disease and as a predictor of future outcomes of the disease. In addition, the test results may not change in linear relationship with the degree of severity of the disease.

To conclude, in evaluating the usefulness of a test or group of tests in detecting malnutrition, that is, the test's Se and Sp, one must also determine the actual P of malnutrition, the purpose for using the test, and the stage or severity of malnutrition that the test is to detect. As will be seen, these calculations, though easy to make, have not been done in many cases. Practical experience or "eye-balling" the data is often substituted.

Let us take an example from the literature. Andersen and Wochos[3] assessed 47 patients admitted to a nephrology service, using weight for height less than 90 percent of ideal, triceps skinfold (TSF), mid-arm muscle circumference (MAMC), serum albumin < 3.4 g percent and total iron-binding capacity (TIBC) < 240 mg percent. Twenty-five of the 47 patients had serum albumin < 3.4 g percent. Of these 25 patients, 4 had proteinuria ≥ 3.5 g/day. Fifteen of the 47 patients had infections either on admission or subsequently. Eleven of the 15 had serum albumin < 3.4 g percent.

Based on this data, the V+ of serum albumin is calculated thusly:

	No. with Positive Test	No. with Negative Test	Totals
No. diseased subjects	21	4	25
No. "healthy" subjects	4	18	22
TOTALS	25	22	47

Se = 84%
Sp = 82%
V+ = 84%
V− = 82%
Actual P = 53%

Notice that in this example, proteinuria was considered the only reason for a false-positive result. If one were to consider infection as the etiology of decreased serum albumin rather than the result of malnutrition, as some do, then the actual P drops to 44.7 percent and the V+ drops to 58.3 percent. Note that the drop in actual P was only about 8 percent, but the drop in V+ was 40 percent!

In this study, the V+ was not enhanced by combining serum albumin with another test. Only 12 patients had a TIBC of < 240 mg percent and 9 of them also had a serum albumin < 3.4 g percent. Assuming that none of these patients are anemic and thus there are no FP or FN tests, then the actual P increases to 59.6 percent, and the V+ increases only to 85.7 percent. At this point, the clinician would have to decide whether the seriousness of malnutrition in a patient with renal disease warrants the additional cost of the TIBC to gain 1.7 percent advantage in detecting it. Additional study may be needed to decide this. This is a very small population and in a larger population of patients with renal disease or in a population having a different mixture of disorders that would affect the actual P of malnutrition, a higher V+ might be achieved by a combination of serum albumin plus TIBC.

Statistical analysis must be properly applied whenever nutrition assessment is investigated. The discerning and inquisitive dietitian can gain much by applying these principles in critiquing articles, in designing research, and in devising practical, cost-effective nutrition assessment protocols.

Compositional/Biochemical Methods in Comprehensive Nutrition Assessment

Generally, malnutrition is described on the basis of the deficient nutrient and severity of the depletion of bodily reserves of the nutrient. While malnutrition may refer to both over- and undernutrition and to macro- and micronutrient deficiencies, this chapter is principally concerned with the assessment of protein and calorie undernutrition. Undernutrition tends to occur in groups of two or more deficiencies. Protein and calorie deficiency are the most debilitating in the hospitalized patient, and are usually accompanied by other nutrient deficiencies.

Rudman and Bleier[4] note some principles common to deficiency syndromes:

1. Undernutrition can be either primary (due to inadequate food supply of essential nutrients) or secondary (due to a disease or its treatment).
2. Deficiencies develop in three stages:
   a. Stage 1—body reserves are drawn on to maintain normal blood values and normal function
   b. Stage 2—Blood levels of the nutrient or nutrient-dependent metabolite decline, but the patient remains asymptomatic
   c. Stage 3—Clinical signs and symptoms develop

   These stages are not exactly equivalent to the "mild, moderate, severe" categorization of malnutrition. The latter are usually applied to stages 2 and 3 only, because most deficiency syndromes lack techniques with which to assess stage 1. Stage 1 in protein malnutrition (PM) or in protein–calorie malnutrition (PCM), however, can be observed as an initial weight loss and negative nitrogen balance.
3. In assessing the patient for nutrient deficiencies associated with PM or PCM, consider first the deficiency syndromes typical to the patient's underlying disease and medical treatment. Then consider deficiencies related to the patient's individual patterns of eating and lifestyle.

   When losses of protein and energy exceed intake, the body draws on its own stores of fat and glycogen to meet energy need and from somatic and visceral mass to supply nitrogen and essential amino acids for protein synthesis. The techniques presently used to measure these stores in the clinical setting are described in Table 8–3. Previous chapters describe these methods, their limitations, and applications.

There are three types of protein and calorie malnutrition described by the use of these methods:[5] (1) Protein malnutrition (PM, or kwashiorkor*), or—the diet supplies calories chiefly in the form of carbohydrate (clear liquid diet, IV dextrose) with little or no protein intake. In addition, the body's ability to adapt to conserve protein sources in the hospitalized patient is usually confounded by a stress episode (surgery, leading

---

*Kwashiorkor means "the disease that occurs when a young child is displaced from his mother by another baby."

TABLE 8–3. NUTRITION ASSESSMENT TECHNIQUES COMMONLY AVAILABLE IN THE CLINICAL SETTING

I. Somatic (striated muscle) stores
  A. Physical assessment
    Physical appearance of muscle wastage
    Weakness, easy fatigability
  B. Anthropometric assessment
    Weight loss
    Midarm and midarm muscle circumference
    Midarm muscle area
    Fat free mass derived from anthropometric estimation of body density and fat mass
  C. Laboratory assessment
    Creatinine–height index
    3-methylhistidine excretion
    Nitrogen balance

II. Visceral (nonstriated muscle and circulatory proteins) stores
  A. Physical assessment
    Pallor
    Decubitus ulcers or wound dehiscence
    Edema, ascites
    Prone to infections
  B. Anthropometric assessment
    Radiologic or CT scan evidence of atrophy of heart, kidneys, etc.

  C. Laboratory assessment
    Nitrogen balance
    Serum albumin
    Serum transferrin or TIBC
    Retinol-binding protein
    Serum prealbumin
    Total lymphocyte count
    Delayed cutaneous hypersensitivity skin tests

III. Fat stores
  A. Physical assessment
    Loss of buccal fat pads, scaphoid abdomen, loss of fat pads in hips, thighs, upper arms
    Sunken eyes
    Dependent skin over extremities
  B. Anthropometric assessment
    Weight
    Triceps, biceps, suprailiac and subscapular skinfolds
  C. Laboratory assessment
    Energy expenditure measured via indirect calorimetry or estimated from Harris–Benedict equation and compared to energy intake

to infection, trauma), increased protein turnover, and loss. Hence, the onset is usually sudden (2 to 3 weeks). (2) Protein–calorie malnutrition (PCM, or marasmus†)—the diet is inadequate in both calories and protein. Typically, this is the result of simple starvation. Hence, the onset is slow, taking months to develop. (3) Combined malnutrition (mixed marasmus-kwashiorkor)—this is characterized by inadequate calories and protein intake with a sudden increase in demand for protein. Usually this results when a marasmic patient experiences a stress event. This upsets the adaptive mechanisms in starvation that are meant to spare lean body mass (LBM). The increased requirement for protein cannot be met by the body

from its own stores because LBM has previously been depleted through starvation. Without nutrition support, the clinical course deteriorates rapidly.

PM is, for the most part, a laboratory diagnosis based in the decline in the serum albumin, serum transferrin, and other circulatory protein. Edema is often present. Poor wound healing and development of decubitus ulcers are common, as are depressed cellular immune function and increased incidence of infection or sepsis. Clinical findings are usually absent at the outset. Fat reserves and LBM tend to be normal, or loss is masked by edema; thus the patient appears deceptively well nourished.

PCM is, on the other hand, chiefly a clinical diagnosis, characterized by obvious wastage of fat and muscle in the upper and lower extremities, scaphoid abdomen, and a

---

†Marasmus means "to waste away."

decrease in all anthropometric measurements. Radiologic examination may reveal atrophy of the heart and other visceral organs. However, the serum albumin usually remains above 2.8 g/dl and other circulatory proteins are unremarkable. The body's ability to maintain immune competence is generally well preserved, unless other factors intervene (e.g., chemotherapy, radiation therapy). Minor elective surgical procedures are usually tolerated fairly well and wound healing generally proceeds unimpaired. It is not until the stress level reaches grade 2 or 3 (see Table 8–8 on stress categorization) that the patient decompensates, developing mixed malnutrition with evidence of decreased circulatory proteins, delayed wound healing, infection, or sepsis.

Combined PCM is based on a combination of clinical and laboratory diagnoses. The laboratory values are similar to those found in PM. The history, however, is characterized by chronic debilitating disease with the onset of an acute event such as sepsis, hemorrhage, or a condition requiring surgical intervention that upsets the adaptive phase of starvation. The appearance is generally more wasted. There is often a history of gradual, unintentional weight loss. Measured deficits in somatic protein and fat stores are not unlikely. Clinical evidence of vitamin and of mineral deficiencies is more likely to develop.

Methods for detecting and assessing the severity of protein and calorie deficiencies are outlined in Tables 8–4 through 8–8.

A recent adjunct to the traditional method of assessing nutrition status just outlined is the method of categorizing stress developed by Cerra et al.[15] The expected risk of becoming malnourished and the type of nutrition therapy instituted to prevent it is dependent upon the patient's metabolic status. Chapter 10, "Protein and Energy Requirements," describes the alterations that occur in substrate metabolism during stress and starvation. In general the metabolic response to stress promotes proteolysis and lipolysis to support gluconeogenesis and ketogenesis. Peripheral muscle becomes insulin resistant

preferring BCAA, deaminated to form pyruvate, as an energy substrate. Thus, lactate production is increased. Serum glucose levels rise. There is an increased rate of ureagenesis, oxygen consumption, and energy expenditure. This response peaks at about 3 days then tapers until, without nutrition support, it resembles starvation.

The metabolic response to starvation is characterized by a decreased turnover of protein, with a marked decrease in ureagenesis, and conversion to fatty acids and ketone bodies as an energy substrate. This leads to a decreased demand for amino acids and for glucose. The peripheral muscle loses resistance to insulin. As insulin secretion drops, so do serum glucose levels. There is a drop in energy expenditure. These and other adaptive mechanisms occur to spare vital organ functions while meeting immediate requirements. If uninterrupted by a stress event, this adaptive process continues gradually until the body stores of fat and expendable protein can no longer provide adequate substrate, and vital functions are compromised.

Degree of stress response has long been clinically described as rate of increase of urine urea nitrogen (UUN) excretion.[18,19] Changes in plasma glucose, plasma lactate, ketone bodies, amino acid levels, oxygen consumption, resting energy expenditure, glucagon and insulin secretion, and excretion of 3-methylhistidine, however, reflect degree of stress as well. Cerra et al.[15] recognized this in their research and explained the clinical application of these factors in categorizing stress.[16] It is time consuming and expensive, however, to obtain all the laboratory values suggested in their previous method. More recently, Cerra[17] suggested a more streamlined approach that includes total urine nitrogen loss, plasma lactate, glucose, presence or absence of insulin resistance and, optionally, oxygen consumption (Table 8–8). These measurements are available in most clinical situations, and are less expensive to obtain.

Malnutrition is a potential reason for in-

TABLE 8–4. INTERPRETING THE RESULTS OF THE NUTRITION ASSESSMENT

Protein Malnutrition (Kwashiorkor)
Diet history
  Adequate calorie or high glucose intake
  Inadequate protein intake or stress state with increased losses of protein
Physical assessment and medical history
  Normal or obese appearance
  Moist skin
  Dull, sunken eyes
  Edema, ascites, or congestive heart failure
  Frequent decubitus ulcers and/or wound dehiscence
  Recent stress event (e.g., surgery, trauma, burns, infection, sepsis)
  Chronic protein loss (e.g., burns, decubiti, fistulas, dialysis)
  Secondary complications, including infection, sepsis, slow wound healing
  Increased LFTs, not associated with parenteral nutrition or primary liver disease
Assessment based on fat stores normal or greater than normal (e.g., weight, skinfolds); muscle mass normal or less than normal (e.g., CHI, MAMC); serum proteins lower than normal (e.g., serum albumin, transferrin, or TIBC); anergy

Protein–Calorie Malnutrition (Marasmus)
Diet history
  Inadequate intake of both calories and protein due to:
  1. Chronic losses (e.g., malabsorption, dialysis)
  2. Inability to ingest adequate calories and protein (e.g., obstruction of bowel, CVA with dysphagia)
  3. Unwilling to ingest adequate calories and protein (e.g., cancer cachexia, anorexia nervosa)
  4. Increased needs for growth not met (e.g., pregnancy, lactation, adolescence)

  5. Impaired metabolism of nutrients (e.g., diabetes mellitus, cirrhosis of liver)
Physical assessment and medical history
  Chronic disease (e.g., cancer, renal failure with dialysis, cirrhosis of the liver, rheumatoid arthritis, proteinuria, Crohn's disease, sprue, emphysema)
  Chronic losses (e.g., fistulas, decubiti, dialysis)
  Disease or surgery of the GI tract
  Frequent tests requiring NPO or clear liquid diet
  Drug–nutrient interactions (e.g., chemotherapy, corticosteroid therapy)
  Thin, wasted appearance of torso and extremities
  Skin wrinkled and dry, appears "aged"
  Sparse hair
  Bright eyes
Assessment based on fat stores less than normal (e.g., weight, skinfolds); muscle mass less than normal (e.g., CHI, MAMC); serum proteins normal or slightly decreased (e.g., serum albumin, transferrin or TIBC); anergy.

Combined Protein–Calorie Malnutrition
Diet history
  A stress event with episode of starvation immediately prior to or following it
Physical assessment and medical history
  Evidence of weight loss and muscle wastage, usually accompanied by edema or ascites
  Slow wound healing
  Usually accompanied by infection or sepsis
  Chronic losses due to malabsorption, fistula drainage, GI bleeding
  Frequently accompanied by respiratory, liver and/or other organ failure
Assessment based on fat stores less than normal (e.g., weight, skinfolds); muscle mass less than normal (e.g., CHI, MAMC); serum proteins less than normal (e.g., serum albumin, transferrin, TIBC); anergy.

creased morbidity and mortality among hospitalized patients. The standard approach to nutrition assessment is useful in detecting existing malnutrition, and categorization of metabolic stress is useful in determining the etiology of its development. Yet neither are designed to predict patient outcome. Recognizing this, Mullen et al.[20,21] designed a retrospective study to develop a linear predic-

tion model that related the risk of operative morbidity and mortality to baseline nutrition status. This model is called the Prognostic Nutrition Index (PNI). Buzby et al.[22] and Smale et al.[23] designed prospective studies to test the PNI on patients having abdominal surgery and cancer with surgical treatment, respectively.

Of 16 nutritional and immunologic factors

TABLE 8–5. GENERAL DIAGNOSTIC FEATURES OF MALNUTRITION

Maramus (Protein–Calorie Malnutrition)	Kwashiorkor (Protein Malnutrition)	Combined Marasmus–Kwashiorkor (Stress and Starvation)
Normal or ↓ serum albumin, serum transferrin, prealbumin, RBP, and TLC	↓↓ Serum albumin, serum transferrin, prealbumin, RBP, and TLC	↓↓ Serum albumin, serum transferrin, prealbumin, RBP, and TLC
May or may not be anergic	Anergic	Anergic
↓↓ MAMC and CHI	↓ or ↓↓ MAMC and CHI	↓ MAMC and CHI
↓↓ Weight and TSF	Normal or ↑ weight and TSF	↓ Weight and TSF
Emaciated appearance	Edema	Edema
Edema not usually present	Delayed wound healing	Delayed wound healing
Sparse, dry, easily plucked hair	↑ LFTs and fatty liver infiltration (not related to TPN)	
Delayed wound healing		

↓ = slightly decreased; ↓↓ = very decreased; ↑ = increased.

studied in developing the PNI, Mullen et al.[20] included 4 that they felt were sufficiently significant in predicting postoperative morbidity and mortality.

$$\text{Prognostic Nutritional Index (\%)} =$$
$$158 - 16.6\ (\text{ALB}) - 0.78\ (\text{TSF}) - 0.20\ (\text{TFN})$$
$$- 5.8(\text{DH})$$

where ALB = serum albumin (g/dl)
TSF = triceps skinfold (mm)
TFN = serum transferrin (mg/dl)
DH = delayed cutaneous hypersensitivity skin test (percent positive reaction)

Buzby et al.[22] found that of 100 patients undergoing gastrointestinal surgery, 28 patients experienced 44 different complications. There were 15 deaths. In 38 patients with a PNI less than 40 percent, 3 (8 percent) experienced complications and 1 (3 percent) died. In 23 patients with a PNI of 40 to 49 percent, 7 patients (30 percent) experienced complications and 1 (4.3 percent died). In 39 patients with a PNI greater than 50 percent, 18 patients (46 percent) experienced complications and 13 (33 percent) died. Thus, the PNI successfully predicted outcome in this group of patients.

Smale et al.[23] studied 159 cancer patients who underwent major surgery in treatment for the cancer. Fifty-four of the patients had preoperative total parenteral nutrition (TPN) and 105 did not. In 67 patients with a PNI less than 40 percent, 6 (21 percent) had complications and there were no deaths. Two of these patients received TPN and four did not. Of 92 patients with PNI greater than or equal to 40 percent, 47 (97 percent) had complications and 27 (55 percent) died. Twelve (31 percent) of the patients who had complications and 6 (15 percent) of these who died received TPN preoperatively and 35 (66 percent) not receiving TPN had complications and 21 (40 percent) died. Thus, in both of these studies, patients with a PNI greater than 40 percent appear at significantly greater risk for postoperative complication and death.

The PNI's usefulness, however, is limited to preoperative assessment. It is not useful in trauma patients[25] and it is not designed to predict survival in patients who do not undergo surgery. Harvey et al.[8] developed a discriminant function equation, called the Hospital Prognostic Index (HPI) from a retrospective study of 528 adult medical and surgical patients. They found that serum albumin was the single best predictor of mortality, and sepsis. Serum albumin below 2.2 g/dl was

TABLE 8-6. ALTERATIONS IN ORGAN FUNCTION SECONDARY TO PCM

General	Loss of LBM Loss of body fat Decreased protein turnover Edema (especially in kwash- iorkor) Muscle weakness Impaired cell-mediated immunity Impaired resistance to infection Delayed wound healing		Impaired ability to respond to antidiuretic hormone leading to increased retention of Na and of total and extracellular body water Decreased kidney mass Acidosis
Cardiovascular	Decreased RBC production Decreased blood volume Hemodilution Normochromic-normocytic anemia Decreased cardiac output Decrease in blood pressure Postural hypotension Diminished venous return Loss of heart muscle mass	Gastrointestinal tract and pancreas	Decreased enzyme production Decreased bile production Atrophy of intestinal villi Atrophy of pancreatic exocrine glands Diarrhea Malabsorption Steatorrhea Decreased absorption rate of glucose Bacterial overgrowth of intestine
Pulmonary	Decreased response to hypoxia Increased incidence of respira- tory infections Pulmonary edema (especially in kwashiorkor) Tissue anoxia	Liver	Decreased production of clotting factors Decreased production of trans- port proteins Atrophy Jaundice Fatty liver infiltration
Renal	Decreased plasma flow Decreased glomerular filtration rate Decreased tubular function Impaired ability to excrete acid load	Temperature regulation	Decreased resting energy expenditure (REE) Hypoglycemia Hypothermia
		Reproduction	Infertility Increased risk of fetal resorption or miscarriage Increased risk of low birth weight infant Impaired lactation

Condensed from Rudman D, Bleier JC: Protein and Energy Undernutrition. In Wintrobe MM, Thorn GW (eds.): Harrison's Principles of Internal Medicine, 10th ed. New York: McGraw-Hill, 1983, p 438;[4] Viteri F, Torún B: Protein–calorie malnutrition. In Goodhart RS, Shils ME (eds.): Modern Nutrition in Health and Disease, 6th ed. Philadelphia: Lea & Febiger, 1980, pp 697–720.[5]

associated with greater than a 75 percent probability of anergy, sepsis, and death during hospitalization. Harvey et al.[8] also developed discriminate function equations which were slightly better predictors than the single variables. The following equation, used to predict survival, has a 72 percent predictive value:

$$0.92 \ (ALB) - 1.00 \ (DH) - 1.44 \ (SEP) + 0.98 \ (DX) - 1.09$$

where

ALB = serum albumin (g/dl)
DH = delayed cutaneous hypersensitivity skin test interpreted as: positive response to one or more antigens = 1; negative response to all antigens = 2
SEP = sepsis, interpreted as: present = 1 not present = 2

TABLE 8–7. GENERAL ANTHROPOMETRIC AND LABORATORY ASSESSMENT VALUES[a]

Anthropometric/Laboratory Values	Degree of Impairment				Limitations
	Normal	Obese	Moderate Depletion	Severe Depletion	
Weight compared to height, age, sex (percentiles)[b,c]	15–50th	>80th	5–15th	<5th	• Weight change of 15 to 20 percentiles or more than 10 percent of usual body weight is significant, regardless of the patient's initial weight. • Fluid shifts often mask true change in LBM and fat. Check for signs of overhydration, edema, and ascites. Monitor I & O. Weight gain greater than 1/4 to 1/2 lb per day during TPN, after surgery, trauma, or prior to dialysis may reflect change in hydration. • Frequently, weight loss occurs initially in the starved patient started on nutrition therapy as edema is mobilized and serum oncotic pressure is normalized.
Triceps skinfold (percentiles)[b,c]	15–50th	>80th	5–15th	<5th	• As above, over- and underhydration affects results. • Difficult to obtain accuracy in the obese and the geriatric patient. • Not sensitive to short-term changes.
Midarm muscle circumference (percentiles)[b]	>15th	NA	5–15th	<5th	• As above, over and underhydration affects results. • Difficult to obtain accuracy in the obese and the geriatric patient. • Muscle atrophy, secondary to paralysis does not reflect nutrition status. • Not sensitive to short-term changes.
Creatinine-height index	>95%	75–95%	60–74%	<60%	• Falsely low secondary to altered renal function, to low urine output, and to incomplete urine collections. • Falsely high secondary to severe stress with rapid catabolism of muscle mass and to initiation of dietary meat after a period of meat-free diet or starvation.

170

					Interpretation/Comments
Albumin[d] (g/dl)	≥3.5	3.0–3.4	2.1–2.9	<2.2	• Falsely high with dehydration. • Altered synthesis occurs during hepatic disease and failure. • Conditions which affect albumin levels other than malnutrition include glomerulonephritis; hypervolemic states such as congestive heart failure; multiple organ hypersensitivity disease (e.g., SLE); allergic conditions, acute inflammatory response, acute burns, and protein-losing enteropathy.
Transferrin[e] (mg/dl)	>220	170–220	150–170	<150	• Falsely high in iron-deficiency anemia. • Falsely low in hypervolemic states such as congestive heart failure; in inflammatory reaction; and in chronic inflammation. • Altered synthesis occurs in hepatic disease and failure. • Increased loss occurs in hepatic disease and failure. • Increased loss occurs from chronically draining wounds and burn exudate. • Altered during pregnancy and estrogen therapy.
Total lymphocyte count (per mm³)[f]	>1800	1500–1800	800–1499	800	• Conditions other than malnutrition that cause lowered TLC levels include chemotherapy, sepsis, trauma, radiation therapy, thoracic duct fistula, thymectomy, steroid administration, immunologic deficiency states, agranulocytosis, SLE and other collagen disease, thymic aplasia, hypogammaglobulinemia, dysgammaglobulinemia, dyslymphocytoses.
Delayed cutaneous hypersensitivity skin test[g] (positive = ≥5 mm induration measured at 24 and 48 hours).	2 or more positive	NA	1 positive	0 positive	See Chapter 7 for discussion.

[a]For details regarding interpretation of data, see Chapters 5–7 on Laboratory Values and Their Interpretation, Anthropometric Evaluation and Tests of Immune Function.

[b]As suggested by Gray, Gray: J Am Diet Assoc 77:534, 1980, using percentiles derived from HANES I data.[7,10,13]

[c]Standards for obesity suggested by Seltzer and Mayer[12] fall above the 75th percentile for all age groups.

[d]From Harvey KB, Moldawer LL, et al.: Am J Clin Nutr 34:2013–2022, 1981.[8]

[e]From Mullen JL, Gertner M, et al.: Arch Surg 114:121–125, 1979;[20] Mullen JL, Buzby CP, Waldman TG, et al.: Surg Forum 30:80–82, 1979.[21]

[f]From Grant JP, Custer PB, Thurlow J: Surg Clin N Am 61(3):437–462, 1981;[11] Seltzer MH, Bastidas A, et al.: JPEN 3(3):157–159, 1979.[14]

[g]From Bates SE, Suen JY, Tranum BL: Cancer 43:2306–2314, 1979;[6] Twomey P, Zeigler D, Rombeau J: JPEN 6(1):50, 1982.[9]

TABLE 8–8. CLINICAL CATEGORIZATION OF METABOLIC STRESS[a]

Stress Level	Clinical Description	Glucose[b] (mg/dl)	Plasma Lactate[c] (m/L)	Insulin Resistance	Total Urinary Nitrogen Loss (g/day)	O₂ Consumption Index (ml/m²)[d]
0	Starvation	100 + 20	10 + 5	−	<5	90 ± 10
1	Elective surgery	150 ± 25	1200 ± 200	−	5–10	130 ± 6
2	Polytrauma	150 ± 25	1200 ± 200	±	10–15	150 ± 6
3	Sepsis	250 ± 50	2500 ± 500	+	>15	160 ± 10

[a]Adapted from Cerra FB: Pocket Manual of Surgical Nutrition. St. Louis. C.V. Mosby, 1984, Table 3-10.[17]
[b]In the absence of diabetes, pancreatitis, or steroid therapy.
[c]With normal lactate to pyruvate ratio between 1.5:1 to 20:1.
[d]Use is optional.

DX = diagnosis, interpreted as:
 cancer = 1
 noncancer = 2

The result of the equation must be compared to a discriminant function curve (Fig. 8–3) in order to obtain the probability of survival. According to Harvey et al.[8] a discriminate function (DF) of −2 represents a 10 percent probability of survival, which includes a nonseptic hospital course and maintenance of immune function. A DF of 0 represents a 50 percent probability of survival and a DF of +1 represents a 75 percent probability of survival.

Other attempts are being made to develop nutrition indices of prognosis.[25,26] The consensus among most of those who have developed such an index thus far appears to favor serum albumin, serum transferrin or TIBC, and delayed cutaneous hypersensitivity skin tests as most useful in predicting outcome.[8,21,26] It is interesting that these variables are more sensitive to the development of PM than to PCM. This may say something about the relative prevalence of this state in hospitalized patients.

There has been some debate in the literature as to the necessity of conducting objective nutrition assessment. A recent study by Detsky et al.[27] showed no significant difference between the number of patients judged to be malnourished by subjective assessment versus objective assessment. The results of a study by Pettigrew et al.[28] conflicted with this. Two surgeons, one with experience in nutrition assessment and one without, each conducted a history and physical examination on 98 patients who subsequently underwent an objective nutrition as-

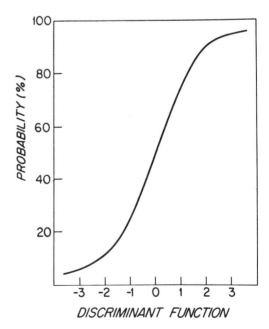

Figure 8–3. Probability of survival, nonseptic hospital course, or immune competence predicted from discriminant function value. *(Used with permission by Harvey KB, et al.: Am J Clin Nutr 34 (10):2018, 1981, Fig. 1.[8])*

sessment. They were able to correctly agree in classifying 83 percent of those patients whose weight was normal and 64 percent of those patients who were immune competent, but only 42 percent of those who were below the 10th percentile of wt/ht² and 31 percent of those who were immune incompetent. Jeejeebhoy[29] contested the significance of these results, stating that neither wt/ht² or delayed cutaneous hypersensitivity skin tests are reliable and both are questionable indices of function and outcome. Nevertheless, it is difficult to detect protein malnutrition without the aid of laboratory tests until it is advanced. And for those who are not trained to detect malnutrition, these results appear to indicate that an objective criterion is needed.

One of the major difficulties with objective assessment of nutrition status lies within the tests themselves. Anthropometric measurements are fairly specific but not sensitive in assessing marasmus. Serum albumin is neither sensitive nor specific because of its long half-life and the wide number of other conditions that influence it. It is nevertheless useful in screening.[14] Also, it continues to enjoy a reputation as the single best predictor of morbidity and mortality in a wide variety of conditions.[3,27,28]

Serum transferrin or TIBC is more responsive than serum albumin to changes in protein nutrition because of its shorter half-life, although not necessarily more specific. It is useful in the initial assessment and to determine presence and type of malnutrition as well as the efficacy of therapy.[8,22,23]

Prealbumin and thyroxine-bound retinol-binding protein are so extremely sensitive due to their short half-lives that they are of little utility in screening or as an initial assessment, since transient changes in dietary intake or minor stresses may alter them.[29] They may be useful, however, coupled with serum transferrin, in reassessment to evaluate short-term changes in caloric and protein intake.

Creatinine height index (CHI) is altered by renal function and by atrophy of muscle mass for reasons other than malnutrition.

Moreover, standards of normality are lacking for older populations. It is therefore sensitive but not specific. It is also the only noninvasive, readily obtained method of determining muscle mass in the clinical setting.[31]

Delayed cutaneous hypersensitivity (DCH) skin tests and total lymphocyte count (TLC) are also altered by a number of nonnutritional factors.[32] Both appear to lack sensitivity and specificity. In certain populations, however, DCH skin testing can be a useful tool in assessing the functional capability of the host to withstand surgery.[20–22]

Changes in muscle strength, measured with the handgrip dynamometer, correlate with changes in nutrition status during starvation in recent studies.[33,34] Its use, however, remains investigational.

MacLaren and Meguid[30] argue that more sophisticated techniques are needed in the clinical setting to objectively evaluate nutrition status. They urge a reconsideration of the experiences gained in diagnosing and treating PM and PCM in children. They also suggest classifying malnutrition by degree and type, rather than under one general category of malnutrition. This is an area which requires further study. Hopefully, the clinician will gain from this chapter an awareness of the potential use and application of present nutrition assessment techniques, rather than simply a knowledge of their limitations.

REFERENCES

1. Galen RS, Gambino SR: Beyond Normality: The Predictive Value and Efficiency of Medical Diagnosis. New York: Wiley, 1975
2. Habicht JP: Some characteristics of indicators of nutritional status for use in screening and surveillance. Am J Clin Nutr 33:531–535, 1980
3. Andersen CF, Wochos DN: The utility of serum albumin values in the nutritional assessment of hospitalized patients. Mayo Clin Proc 57:181–184, 1982
4. Rudman D, Bleier J: Assessment of Nutritional Status. In Petersdorf RG et al. (eds): Harrison's Principals of Internal Medicine,

10th ed. New York: McGraw-Hill, 1983, pp 433–436

5. Viteri FE, Torún B. Protein–calorie malnutrition. In Goodhart RS, Shils ME (eds): Modern Nutrition in Health and Disease, 6th ed. Philadelphia: Lea & Febiger, 1980, pp 697–720

6. Bates SE, Suen JY, Tranum BL: Immunological skin testing and interpretation: A plea for uniformity. Cancer 43:2306–2314, 1979

7. Frisancho AR: New norms of upper limb fat and muscle areas for assessment of nutritional status. Am J Clin Nutr 34:2540–2545, 1981

8. Harvey KB, Moldawer LL, Bistrian B, Blackburn G: Biological measures for the formulation of a hospital prognostic index. Am J Clin Nutr 34:2013–2022, 1981

9. Twomey P, Zeigler D, Rombeau J: Utility of skin testing in nutritional assessment: A critical review. JPEN 6:50–58, 1982

10. Vital and Health Statistics. Weight and height of adults 18–74 years of age. U.S. 1971–1974, DHEW Publication No. (PHS) 79–1656, Series 11, No. 212. Public Health Service, Washington, D.C.: Government Printing Office, 1979

11. Grant JP, Custer PB, Thurlow JT: Current techniques of nutritional assessment. Surg Clin N Amer 61(3):437–463, 1981

12. Seltzer CC, Mayer J. A simple criterion of obesity. Postgrad Med 38A:101–107, 1965

13. Gray GE, Gray LK: Anthropometric measurements and their interpretation: Principles, practices and problems. J Am Diet Assoc 77:534, 1980

14. Seltzer MH, Bastidas A, Cooper DM, et al.: Instant nutrition assessment. JPEN 3(3):157–159, 1979

15. Cerra FB, Upson D, Angelico R, et al.: Branch chains support postoperative protein synthesis. Surgery 92:192–198, 1982

16. Cerra FB: Profiles in Nutritional Management: The Trauma Patient. Chicago: Abbott Laboratories, Hospital Products Division, 1982

17. Cerra FB: Assessment of nutritional and metabolic status. In Pocket Manual of Surgical Nutrition. St. Louis: C.V. Mosby, 1984, pp 24–48

18. Rutten P, Blackburn GL, Flatt JP, et al.: Determination of optimal hyperalimentation infusion rate. J Surg Res 18:477, 1975

19. Blackburn GL, Bistrian B, Maini BS, et al.: Nutritional and metabolic assessment of the hospitalized patient. JPEN 1:11–22, 1977

20. Mullen JL, Gertner MH, Buzby GP, et al.: Implications of malnutrition in the surgical patient. Arch Surg 114:121–125, 1979

21. Mullen JL, Buzby GP, Waldman TG, et al.: Prediction of operative morbidity and mortality by preoperative nutritional assessment. Surg Forum 30:80–82, 1979

22. Buzby GP, Mullen JL, Matthews DC, et al.: Prognostic nutritional index in gastrointestinal surgery. Am J Surg 139:160–167, 1980

23. Smale BF, Mullen JL, Buzby GP, et al.: The efficacy of nutritional assessment and support in cancer surgery. Cancer 47:2375–2381, 1981

24. Blackburn GL, Harvey KB: Nutritional assessment as a routine in clinical medicine. Postgrad Med 71:46–63, 1982

25. Jones TN, Moore EE, Van Way CW: Factors influencing nutritional assessment in abdominal trauma patients. JPEN 7:115–116, 1983

26. Rainey-MacDonald CG, Holliday RC, Wells GA, Donner AP: Validity of a two-variable nutritional index for use in selecting candidates for nutrition support. JPEN 7:15–20, 1983

27. Detsky AS, Baker JP, Mendelsohn RA, et al.: Evaluating the accuracy of nutritional assessment techniques applied to hospitalized patients: Methodology and comparison. JPEN 8:153–159, 1984

28. Pettigrew RA, Charlesworth PM, Formilo RW, Hill GL: Assessment of nutritional depletion and immune competence: A comparison of clinical examination and objective measurements. JPEN 8:21–24, 1984

29. Jeejeebhoy K: Objective measurements of nutritional deficit (editorial). JPEN 8:1–2, 1984

30. McLaren DS, Meguid M: Nutritional assessment at the crossroads. JPEN 7:575–579, 1983

31. Heymsfield SB, McManus C, Stevens V, Smith J: Muscle mass: Reliable indicator of protein–energy malnutrition severity and outcome. Am J Clin Nutr 35:1192–1199, 1982

32. Englert DM, Dobbins D: Technical aspects in delayed hypersensitivity skin testing. Nutr Supp Serv 3:75–77, 1983

33. McRussell D, Leiter LA, Whitwell J, et al.: Skeletal muscle function during hypocaloric diets and fasting: A comparison with standard nutritional assessment parameters. Am J Clin Nutr 37:133–138, 1983

34. Lopes J, Russell DMcR, Whitwell J, Jeejeebhoy KN: Skeletal muscle function in malnutrition. Am J Clin Nutr 36:602–610, 1982

9. Screening Techniques

Terry Jensen

Malnutrition is often associated with general debility, weakness, apathy, indolent wound healing, and increased susceptibility to infections.[1-6] These and other complications have far-reaching medical and financial implications. Therefore, every effort must be made to recognize co-existing nutritional deficiencies in hospitalized patients and treat them along with the primary disease process. The development of clinically applicable, objective indicators of nutrition status has enabled clinicians to recognize and document a significant prevalence of malnutrition in hospitalized patient populations. Survey of patients of varying socioeconomic backgrounds and differing diagnoses admitted to a variety of institutions has detected a high incidence of previously undocumented malnutrition that once recognized may be corrected using a variety of nutrition support techniques.[7-13] Early recognition of nutrition aberrations, however, is essential if they are to be rectified prior to the onset of clinical complications.

The majority of clinicians recognize and acknowledge only the most extreme nutritional deficiencies. The history and physical examination may document massive weight loss, obesity, pitting edema, the presence of ascites, or a scaphoid abdomen and, therefore, provide only a rough assessment of more extreme nutrition aberrations. More subtle forms of depletion may escape attention as a result of limited use of more dependable and specific nutrition assessment techniques. Comprehensive profiles of anthropometric, biochemical and immunologic indicators have been implemented in numerous clinical situations and shown to identify patients with clinical and subclinical malnutrition.[14] These comprehensive nutrition assessment profiles indicate the need for appropriate nutrition therapy, provide guidelines for nutrition support, and evaluate patient response to nutrition intervention. The implementation of comprehensive nutrition assessment programs into traditional hospital settings, however, has presented a challenge for those involved with nutrition care. Additionally, comprehensive nutrition assessment may be inappropriate for all patients due to time, financial, and institutional limitations. A detailed assessment of every patient may be unnecessary and impractical and contribute unnecessarily to escalating medical costs. The development and utilization of standardized procedures for systematic screening assessment utilizing a limited but sufficient data base have evolved to assure that patients at risk for malnutrition are recognized and promptly receive further more comprehensive evaluation and treatment. Nutrition screening is the identification of high-risk patients who should be further evaluated by comprehensive nutrition assessment for specialized nutriton support. Streamlining nutrition assessment data collection in this manner allows prompt evaluation of more patients and allocation of available recourses to those most likely to benefit from intervention.

WHEN TO SCREEN

Screening assessment should begin as soon as possible after admission to the hospital. Because screening data must be collected, assimilated, and interpreted, 48 hours may be required to actually submit interpreted data to the medical record. Ideally, data collection for screening evaluation procedure should begin within 24 hours after admission unless comprehensive nutrition assessment is indicated. Patients with a diagnosis of cancer, burns, or multiple trauma, for example, need not be screened since these hypermetabolic states are associated with nutritional depletion as a result of injury and increased energy and nutrient requirements. Comprehensive nutrition assessment should automatically be instituted in these cases after the initial period of peak catabolism has subsided. Additionally, patients who are admitted for major emergency surgery cannot be screened until the metabolic response to injury or surgery has subsided. Initial hypermetabolism and blood loss will complicate immediate interpretation of laboratory data. In most cases, these patients are eventually candidates for initiation of comprehensive nutrition assessment.[15]

Large patient loads and limited professional staff time may make routine screening of all hospital admissions impractical or impossible in some clinical situations. Selective screening by diagnostic group has been sug-

TABLE 9–1. SELECTIVE SCREENING BY DISEASE CATEGORY

Medical
Cancer
Alcoholism
Gastrointestinal
Liver disease
Diabetes mellitus
Psychiatric
Cardiac
Pulmonary
Infections
Renal
Arthritis
Surgical
Abdominal
Cardiovascular
Head and neck
Burns
Urologic
Orthopedic
Neurosurgery
Medical and surgical
Pediatric
Geriatric

From Lundvick J, Phillips R: Nutritional screening of the oncology patient. Nutritional Support Services 3:21–24, 1983.[25]

gested as a more practical approach in these situations. Using this approach, a specific screening procedure is developed and implemented to identify high-risk patients with a specific diagnosis. Table 9–1 lists potential diagnostic categories for which this approach might be appropriate.[16]

Admission screening will of course fail to identify those patients who develop nutrition problems during hospitalization as a result of inadequate energy–nutrient intake, disease process, or medical–surgical treatment. Therefore, those patients who are NPO (nothing by mouth) for longer than 5 days and those with diagnosis or treatment plans that are associated with a high incidence of nutrition depletion should be reevaluated during hospitalization. A rescreening on an every 2-week or 10-day basis is recommended for these patients.

It is anticipated that with increased emphasis on decreasing the length of hospital stay and cost of hospitalization, many hospital services will move into the outpatient environment in the near future. A logical extension of screening assessment is into the outpatient clinic setting where patients can be assessed and receive appropriate nutrition intervention prior to actual admission to the hospital. In this manner, a further decrease in complications related to malnutrition and resulting length of hospital stay can be realized.

WHO SCREENS

While the need to screen patients for nutritional problems is unquestionable, the question of who actually performs the screening procedure and interprets the data is less well defined. Patients may be screened by dietitians, other dietetic personnel, nurses, or physicians depending upon the staff and capabilities in a particular setting. Physicians may devise methods to screen their own patient population. This can be done subjectively during the history and physical examination or objectively through the evaluation of routine admission laboratory data. Although this practice should be routinely encouraged to increase physician involvement in nutritional diagnosis and management, implementation of a routine screening procedure to complement physician screening is desirable. Implementation of a routine, automatic screening procedure assures prompt, systematic, and uniform evaluation of all patients regardless of physician interest or expertise in nutrition.

When a routine hospitalwide screening program is utilized, the dietitian may contribute significantly to the organization and operation of the program. The clinical dietitian is specifically trained and educated to interpret anthropometric, biochemical and other data relative to nutrition status. Therefore, a primary responsibility is to assist with cautious interpretation of data, considering interrelated clinical factors that may influence readings and results of tests used. Based upon this interpretation, the clinical dietitian may then recommend additional evaluation and assessment as well as appropriate nutrition intervention.[17] The dietitian is also qualified to define criteria and procedures for screening nutrition assessment, supervise all aspects of data collection and assimilation, and train appropriate personnel according to established procedures.

Dietetic technicians or nursing staff are frequently responsible for screening assessment data collection. Dietetic technicians have been employed effectively for both screening and comprehensive nutrition assessment data collection and assimilation.[18] Utilization of support personnel for some aspects of screening assessment data collection is usually essential to extend nutrition screening services to large numbers of hospitalized patients while freeing dietitians to assume other professional responsibilities. The dietitian, however, usually maintains responsibility for insuring that support personnel are adequately trained according to defined screening and referral procedures. By utilizing support personnel to actually collect and assimilate data, more productive use can be made of the specialized skills and limited time of the dietitian. The clinical dietitian can be most effectively utilized to interpret assimilated screening data, communicate this interpretation to the health care team, and recommend further assessment or therapy based upon the interpretation.[15] In this matter professional efforts are directed toward optimal utilization of assimilated data.

TECHNIQUES FOR SCREENING

Although screening techniques vary considerably in different practice settings, this assessment commonly utilizes demographic, subjective, and objective data that are collected routinely upon admission to the hospital.[19-26] Screening nutrition assessment techniques are often selected so that they can be completed by one person, interpreted soon after admission, are inexpensive, and require little or no additional laboratory testing. Additional laboratory testing is usually not required for screening nutrition assessment since the laboratory tests utilized are automatically ordered at admission for most patients. The selection of screening techniques is determined following consideration of available resources and resulting capabilities in a particular hospital or setting. Finally, the selection of screening nutrition assessment methods and criteria must be individualized for the specific patient population.

The primary resource that must be considered in the selection of techniques for screening nutrition assessment is, of course, personnel for staffing the program. Depending upon the complexity of the screening procedure and the availability of the patient and medical record, data collection usually requires from 5 to 15 minutes. Interpretation and communication of results may also require an additional 5 to 10 minutes of professional time. Dietetic technicians, dietitians, nurses, or other personnel may assume responsibility for screening nutrition assessment data collection depending upon the employment practices of the institution and other responsibilities of these practitioners. The dietitian is usually responsible for interpreting screening data and subsequently communicating them to the health care team. Selection of screening criteria will, therefore, depend partially upon the availability and priorities of these individuals.

Appropriate demographic, subjective, and objective data are selected and utilized for screening assessment. Selected data are usually organized on a computer or manual form for easier assimilation or interpretation.

DEMOGRAPHIC DATA

Demographic data frequently collected include patient name, room number, hospital identification number, attending physician and service, admission date, admitting diagnosis and/or chief complaint, age, and sex.

SUBJECTIVE DATA

Subjective data that may be utilized in the screening assessment are obtained primarily from two sources, the physician's history as recorded in the medical record and direct interview with the patient to elicit responses that are known to be associated with a high incidence of malnutrition. Review of the physician's history and physical examination may identify signs and symptoms of malnutrition or practices that are consistent with malnutrition. Subjective data that may be elicited directly from the patient include:

1. Usual weight, date usual weight was last recorded
2. Recent history of nausea, vomiting, diarrhea, dysphagia, or other gastrointestinal complaints
3. History of changes in appetite, food intake, body weight, elimination patterns
4. History of alcohol abuse

Although this information may be obtained by reviewing the medical record, less time may be required if the patient is asked directly.

OBJECTIVE DATA

Objective data utilized for screening assessment usually include weight/height, serum albumin, and white blood cell count. In some instances anthropometric measurement of arm circumference and triceps skinfold have also been used.

Weight/Height

Body weight is the most accessible and widely used index of nutrition status in hospitalized patients. As a simple measure of gross body composition, the body weight is a valuable screening indicator of nutrition risk when compared with usual weight, desirable weight, or both. Several surveys have verified that a significant proportion of hospitalized patients report recent weight loss or are below a desirable weight for their height.[8,11,12] Generally an unintentional weight loss of greater than 10 pounds within a 6-month period is considered significant.[27] A history of weight loss or a weight for height that is less than 85 percent of desirable weight has been related to functional consequences and complications of malnutrition.[27,28] Additionally, a significant increase in mortality has been positively correlated with a history of weight loss.[29] Seltzer et al.[30] have correlated an absolute weight loss of more than 10 pounds with a 19-fold increase in mortality in 4382 adult elective surgical patients at admission. Therefore, weight for height and history of weight change are usually included as screening assessment criteria. Weight and height may be ascertained from the medical record if these measurements are part of routine admission procedure. Measurements may have to be taken specifically for screening assessment, however, when they are not consistently measured and recorded for all patients. Desirable weight may be ascertained from the Health and Examination Survey.[31]

Laboratory Assessment

Because serum albumin concentration and data for calculation of total lymphocyte count (TLC) (from the complete blood count) are routinely obtained for many patients at admission, these tests have gained wide application as screening indicators of protein nutrition status and immune status.[14,21-25] Surveys done on selected patient populations in acute and chronic care facilities have documented a high incidence of hypoalbuminemia and total lymphocyte depression before and during hospitalization.[1,8-13] Additionally, these tests have been correlated repeatedly with increased morbidity and mortality rates. At one teaching hospital

in New Jersey, statistically significant correlations were reported between depressed albumin and lymphocyte levels and patient morbidity (a fourfold increase) and mortality (a sixfold increase) in 500 consecutive adult admissions.[21] The serum albumin concentration and TLC have also been identified as prognostic indicators for morbidity and mortality in surgical patient population[5,27] and in one study, surgical intensive care unit patients with depressed albumin levels and lymphocyte counts were reported to have twice the complication rate and 4.5 times the mortality rate of SICU patients with normal albumin levels and lymphocyte counts.[22] Lewis and Klein identified preoperative hypoalbuminemia and a depressed TLC as risk factors for postoperative sepsis in patients admitted for gastric and colonic operations.[4] Reinhardt et al.[13] reported a linear correlation between the level of hypoalbuminemia observed in a population of 2060 hospitalized veterans and the subsequent 30-day mortality rate in this group, while Bienia et al.[32] correlated low serum albumin concentration and TLC with an increased rate of infection and increased mortality rate in alcoholic and nonalcoholic hospitalized veterans. A low serum albumin concentration and TLC indicated imminent bacteremia sepsis in thermally injured patients who were evaluated on the 5th and 10th postburn days.[33,34] Therefore, the extensive documentation of high incidence of depression of these tests at admission and preoperatively coupled with the repeated significant correlation with increased morbidity and mortality justify the inclusion of these two tests as routine screening assessment indicators. A serum albumin concentration of less than 3.4 g/dl or TLC of less than 2000 cells/mm^3 warrants further nutrition evaluation.

Upper Arm Anthropometric Measurements

A low triceps skinfold measurement does indicate depletion of the primary caloric reserve of the body that may be critical to survival in those patients with increased energy–nutrient requirements and simultaneous low energy–nutrient intake. In these instances the triceps skinfold measurement may indicate the need for immediate and aggressive nutrition intervention. Although several surveys have documented that a significant proportion of hospitalized patients have depressed anthropometric measurements, a correlation of such measurements with morbidity and mortality in general medical and surgical patients has not been recorded.[8,11,12] The arm muscle circumference (AMC) has been reported as a significant predictor of morbidity in patients undergoing elective lower extremity orthopedic surgery.[35] Due to lack of correlation with morbidity and mortality data, however, inclusion of upper arm anthropometric measurements in screening assessment programs is rather uncommon unless the patient population is stressed or has high energy–nutrient requirements. Currently anthropometric assessment is the only method for clinical evaluation of subcutaneous fat and somatic protein energy stores.

SCREENING ASSESSMENT PROCEDURES

Several screening nutrition assessment procedures have been published. Seltzer et al.[21] use an Instant Nutritional Assessment that is comprised of only serum albumin concentration and TLC. Hooley[23] recommends evaluating history weight loss, serum albumin less than 3.5 g/dl, and presence of pathologic state with nutrition-related manifestation as indicators of nutrition risk. Jensen and Dudrick[14] recommend further evaluation based on a screening assessment comprised of weight/height, recent unintentional weight loss of more than 10 pounds, triceps skinfold or AMC less than 50th percentile, serum albumin concentration less than 3.5 g/dl, and/or TLC of less than 1800 cells/mm³. Additionally, a history of change in appetite or food intake, nausea, vomiting,

diarrhea, or recent surgery indicates potential nutrition risk, and a comprehensive profile is recommended. Lundvick and Phillips[25] consider weight history, serum albumin concentration, TLC, triceps skinfold, midarm circumference, and diet history for screening assessment of cancer patients. In various practice situations, selection of appropriate screening techniques is determined by philosophy of practitioners, institutional resources, and patient population.

SUMMARY

It is anticipated that with current cost-containment incentives and directives, the use of screening nutrition assessment will become common practice in both inpatient and outpatient medical care settings. Efforts to identify and treat malnutrition will decrease nutritionally related complications and therefore reduce the length of hospitalization in many cases. Screening nutrition assessment identifies the high-risk patient who will benefit most from nutrition intervention. The implementation of a procedure for routinely screening all admissions for nutrition status should, therefore, improve both the effectiveness and efficiency of nutritional care.

REFERENCES

1. Jensen JE, Jensen TG, Dudrick SJ, Smith TK: Nutrition and orthopaedic surgery. Nutr Supp Serv 4:27, 1984
2. Kaminski MV, Fitzgerald MJ, Murphy RJ, et al.: Correlation of mortality with serum transferrin and energy. JPEN 1:27, 1977
3. MacLean LD, Meakins JK, Taguchi K, et al.: Host resistance in sepsis and trauma. Ann Surg 182:207, 1975
4. Lewis TR, Klein H: Risk factors in postoperative sepsis: Significance of preoperative lymphocytopenia. J Surg Res 26:365, 1979
5. Mullen JL, Gertner MH, Buzby GP, et al.: Implications of malnutrition in the surgical patient. Arch Surg 114:121, 1979
6. Thompson WD: Effect of hypoproteinemia on wound disruption. Arch Surg 36:500, 1978

7. Jensen TG, Englert DM, Dudrick SJ, et al.: Delayed hypersensitivity skin testing: Response rates in a surgical population. J Am Diet Assoc 82:17, 1983

8. Hill GL, Blacket RL, Pickford I, et al.: Malnutrition in surgical patients: An unrecognized problem. Lancet 1:689, 1977

9. Weinsier RL, Hunker EM, Krumdieck CL, et al.: Hospital malnutrition: A prospective evaluation of general medicine patients during the course of hospitalization. Am J Clin Nutr 32:418, 1979

10. Willard MD: Protein–calorie malnutrition in a community hospital. JAMA 243:1720, 1980

11. Bistrian BR, Blackburn GL, Hallowell E, et al.: Protein status of general surgical patients. JAMA 230:858, 1974

12. Bistrian BR, Blackburn GL, Vitale J, et al.: Prevalence of malnutrition in general medical patients. JAMA 235:1567, 1976

13. Reinhardt GF, Myscofski JW, Wilkens DB, et al.: Incidence of hypoalbuminemia in a hospitalized veteran population (abstract). JPEN 4:81, 1980

14. Jensen TG, Dudrick SJ: Implementation of a multidisciplinary nutritional assessment program. J Am Diet Assoc 79(3):519–521, 1981

15. Jensen TG, Englert DM, Dudrick SJ: Nutritional Assessment: A Manual for Practioners. East Norwalk, Connecticut: Appleton-Century-Crofts, 1983

16. Lundvick J, Phillips R: Nutritional screening of the oncology patient. Nutritional Support Services 3:21–24, 1983

17. Role of the Dietitian in Nutritional Support. ASPEN Monograph, 1979

18. Jensen TG: Roles of the dietetic technician in nutritional assessment programs. ASPEN Monograph, 1980

19. Monteith M, Nakagawa A: A flow chart approach to nutritional screening and assessment in long-term care facilities. J Am Diet Assoc 75:684–686, 1975

20. Shapiro LR: Streamlining and implementing nutritional assessment: The dietary approach. J Am Diet Assoc 75:230–237, 1979

21. Seltzer MH, Bastidas JA, Cooper DM, et al.: Instant nutritional assessment. JPEN 3:157–159, 1979

22. Seltzer MH, Fletcher HS, Slocum BA, Engler PE: Instant nutritional assessment in an intensive care unit. JPEN 5:70–72, 1981

23. Hooley RA: Clinical nutritional assessment: A perspective. J Am Diet Assoc 77:682–686, 1980

24. McLaren DS: Assessment of nutritional status. Nutritional Support Services 3:15–19, 1983

25. Lundvick J, Phillips R: Nutritional screening of the oncology patient. Nutritional Support Services 3:21–24, 1983

26. Maillett JO: Evaluation of your assessment program. Nutritional Support Services 2:19–23, 1982

27. Harvey KB, Riggerio JA, Regan CS, et al.: Hospital morbidity-mortality risk factors using nutritional assessment (abstract). Clin Res 26:58A, 1978

28. Bistrian BR: Anthropometric norms used in assessment of hospitalized patients. Am J Clin Nutr 33:2211, 1980

29. Studley HO: Percentage of weight loss—A basic indication of surgical risk in patients with chronic peptic ulcer disease. JAMA 106:458, 1936

30. Seltzer MH, Slocum BA, Cataldi-Betcher EL: Instant nutritional assessment: Absolute weight loss and surgical mortality. JPEN 6:218, 1982

31. National Center for Health Statistics: Weight by Height and Age of Adults 18–74 Years: United States, 1971–1974. Rockville, MD: National Center for Health Statistics, 1979. Vital and Health Statistics, Series II: Data from National Health Survey, No. 208, DHEW pub. no. (PHS)79:1656

32. Bienia RM, Ratcliff S, Barbour GL: Malnutrition and hospital prognosis in the alcoholic patient. JPEN 6:301, 1982

33. Morath MA, Miller SF, Finley RK: Nutritional indicators of postburn bacteremic sepsis. JPEN 5:488, 1981

34. Jensen TG, Long JM, Dudrick SJ, et al.: Nutritional assessment indications of postburn complications. J Am Diet Assoc 85:68–72, 1985

35. Jensen JE, Jensen TG, Smith TK, et al.: Nutrition in orthopaedic surgery. J Bone Joint Sur 64A:1263, 1983

Part III. DETERMINING THE NUTRITION CARE PLAN

10. Protein and Energy Requirements

Rebecca L. Murray

Protein derives its name from a Greek word that means "of first importance." It is the fundamental structural compound of the body cell mass (BCM) as well as enzymes, hormones and antibodies synthesized by the BCM. Protein is the basic component of the nucleus without which synthesis of new cells and cellular constituents cannot take place.

Individual requirements for dietary protein and energy are determined by the number of cells in the body and the rate of protein synthesis and degradation. The goal of nutrition support is to preserve and, if necessary, replete body cell mass and function. Providing adequate protein, however, is not sufficient to do this. One must also provide adequate energy to support protein synthesis. Thus we shall consider these together.

It is important to understand normal body composition and factors that alter it in order to understand and be able to adapt protein and energy intake to meet individual requirements. Fat and protein plus a small amount of glycogen are the body's main sources of fuel during fasting. In the 70-kg reference man, the total stored energy supply is approximately 166,000 kcal. Glycogen stores are depleted initially during fasting, providing approximately 900 kcal in the reference man. Body fat is the main fuel reserve, providing approximately 140,000 to 145,000 kcal in the reference man. Only half of body protein is metabolically active, and this supplies 20,000 to 25,000 kcal in the reference man. Fat and glycogen stores are essentially expendable. Protein stores are not. Utilization of body protein as an energy substrate occurs at the sacrifice of lean body mass (LBM) and the functional and metabolic activities that it supports. This is the basic reason for the morbidity and mortality associated with protein–calorie malnutrition (PCM).

The purpose of the nutrition assessment is to objectively quantify body composition and functional capability. The reader is referred specifically to Chapter 6 for a more detailed description of body composition and methods used to measure its components.

After determining body composition, changes in body composition can be determined by metabolic balance techniques. By combining measurements of total energy expenditure and nitrogen (N) balance, it is possible to calculate the amount of fat lost during periods of starvation or food restriction. (See Table 6–4 in Chapter 6 entitled "Estimating Compositional Change of Weight Loss.")

If only N balance and weight change for a

given 24-hour period are known, however, then one can estimate the composition of weight loss as follows:

$$\Delta FFM = (\pm g \text{ N balance} \times 6.25 \text{ g dry protein/g N}) \times 4.6 \text{ g FFM/g dry protein}$$

$$FM = (\pm g \text{ body weight change}) - (\pm g \text{ FFM})$$

where $\pm$ means gain or loss of that compartment and where FM = fat mass and FFM = fat-free mass.

The rate of loss cumulated over a period of time and compared to estimated body stores of protein, fat, and water determines the extent of change in each compartment. It also serves as a guide for estimating protein, calorie, and fluid requirements in order to prevent further depletion of body stores and, when necessary, allow for repletion. Obviously, accurate determinations of nitrogen, calorie, and fluid balance influence the reliability of the methods. Furthermore, successful maintenance and repletion of body stores of protein, fat, and fluid requires provision of nutrients in a cost-effective form that allows digestion, absorption, and metabolism to occur without harm to the individual.

To assist the clinician in making these decisions, this chapter will attempt to cover practial theory and clinical guidelines in the following areas:

1. Techniques for determining N loss and energy expenditure
2. The effect of starvation and stress on energy and protein metabolism
3. Energy and protein requirements in specific disease states

NITROGEN EXCRETION AND NITROGEN BALANCE

In normal subjects the end products of N metabolism within the body are excreted in the urine, while unabsorbed protein coming from the diet or protein secreted into the lumen of the intestines is voided in the feces. In addition, some nitrogenous materials are lost from the skin as both soluble N (e.g., urea) and as shed epithelial cells. Finally minor routes of N loss are represented by nasal secretions, hair cuttings, menstrual fluid, and semen.

The major N compounds in the urine are urea, ammonia, uric acid, and creatinine. These respond differently to changes in protein intake. On a diet of normal protein content, urea accounts for more than 80 percent of urinary N. This proportion falls when a diet low in protein is consumed. During fasting, the absolute amount and percentage of ammonia N rise in response to acidosis. On the other hand, creatinine output tends to be independent of diet since it reflects the pool of creatine in muscle (Table 10–1).

The overall metabolism of protein in the body can be summarized by N balance. This represents the difference between N intake and N output.

$$\text{N balance} = \text{N intake} - \text{N loss}$$

$$\text{where N intake} = \frac{\dfrac{\text{g protein consumed}}{\text{per 24 hours}}}{\dfrac{6.25 \text{ g protein}}{\text{per g N}}}$$

and N loss = g urine urea N + g urine non-urea N + g fecal N + g dermal N

When N intake exceeds loss, the subject is considered to be in positive N balance. This indicates a state of anabolism, where synthesis of body tissue exceeds breakdown. Conversely, negative N balance indicates a catabolic state in which degradation of body tissue exceeds synthetic rate. When N intake equals N loss, the subject is considered to be in N equilibrium, a homeostatic state between tissue synthesis and degradation.

The determination of N balance requires a careful estimate of intake and of all routes of N loss, namely urine, feces, and dermal losses. The balance obtained is subject to the combined errors of measurement or estimation of the output and intake. N intake tends

TABLE 10–1. CONTRIBUTION TO URINE N LOSS IN ADULT HUMANS ON DIFFERENT NUTRITIONAL REGIMES

Urine N Component	Loss of N in g/day (Percentage of Whole)	
	High Protein Diet	Low Protein Diet
Total N	16.80 (100.0)	3.60 (100.0)
Urea N	14.70 (87.5)	2.20 (61.7)
Ammonia N	0.49 (3.0)	0.42 (11.3)
Uric Acid N	0.18 (1.1)	0.09 (2.5)
Creatinine N	0.58 (3.6)	0.60 (17.2)
Undetermined N	0.85 (4.9)	0.27 (7.3)

Adapted from Allison JB, Bird JWC: Elimination of nitrogen from the body. In Munro HN, Allison JB (eds): Mammalian Protein Metabolism, Vol. I. New York: Academic Press, 1964, p 488.

to be overestimated through unconsumed diet while output tends to be underestimated because of losses. There is thus a built-in bias toward a positive balance.

In addition, it is unusual to make direct measurements of obligatory N losses from the feces and skin. Generally, a correction factor is used or these sources of N loss are ignored. There is also a loss of N in the feces from dietary protein, enzymes, and desquamated intestinal cells that have not been fully digested and reabsorbed. This obligatory fecal N output of adults is about 12 mg N/kg body weight. Nitrogen is also lost from the skin in the form of desquamated cells, hair and nail clippings, and sweat. In studies of skin losses, the cutaneous N loss by adult men in a temperate environment with minimal sweat losses is about 5 mg/kg body weight when a protein-free diet is consumed.[40]

Minor sources of N loss, including ammonia in the breath, nasal secretions, menstrual flow in the female, and seminal fluid in the male average a total daily loss of approximately 2 mg N/kg body weight for men and 3 mg N/kg for women.[40]

Factors That Influence Nitrogen Balance

- Nitrogen balance is influenced by the biological value (BV) of the protein in the diet. The higher the BV, the more efficiently nitrogen is utilized.
- Nitrogen balance is positively influenced by needs for growth and development in children and pregnant women.
- There is a continuous relationship between energy intake and N balance from negative at low energy levels to positive at excessive intakes of energy. Conversely, when dietary protein is restricted, increased energy intake alone will not further improve N balance beyond a certain point. The conclusions are that N balance is the result of both protein intake and energy intake.
- Nitrogen balance in the normal subject is also influenced by changes in hormonal balance. Anabolic hormones (growth hormone, insulin, testosterone) influence N balance positively and catabolic hormones (corticosteroids, thyroxine) influence it negatively.
- Changes in renal function and hydration will alter the rate of N excretion. N balance should be corrected for daily change in serum blood urea nitrogen (BUN) levels.

Nitrogen Balance—Methods

Nitrogen balance is determined in the clinical setting by collecting a urine specimen over a 24-hour period and analyzing it for urea N only. Most hospitals do not have the equipment to do Kjeldahl nitrogen analysis to measure total urine N, nor is it necessary to do so since urea N accounts for most of the variation in N excretion.

Accurate N balance determinations are contingent on proper collection and handling of the specimen. Provide the patient with a clean bedpan or urinal in which to void. Instruct the patient to prevent feces from mixing with the urine sample during the collection period and to avoid dropping toilet paper in the sample.

The nurse measures the urine, then stores it in a clean (but not necessarily sterile) glass or plastic container supplied by the clinical laboratory in a refrigerator or in an ice bath. The container should contain an appropriate preservative such as toluene. The total volume of urine collected should be noted before any specimens are taken out for other tests.

Remind the nursing staff of the precautions that must be taken while a 24-hour urine is being collected. Signs at the patient's bed or on his door and in the dirty utility room may help staff remember that a collection is in process before the specimen is accidentally discarded.

Rutten et al.[41] estimate total N loss from urine urea N as follows:

Total N loss = urea N + 1.5 g N lost in feces and sloughed skin + (choose one of the following):

1.5 g N if urea N excretion is < 5 g/24 hr
2 g N if urea N excretion is 5 to 10 g/24 hr
2.5 g N if urea N excretion is > 10 g/24 hr

MacBurney and Wilmore[42] recommend factoring the urine urea N to obtain total urine N. Urine urea N (UUN) accounts for 80 to 90 percent of total urine N (TUN) in a normal subject on a regular mixed diet. In a stressed patient with an increased rate of protein catabolism or a patient on repletion total parenteral nutrition (TPN) or tube feeding formulas or a high protein diet, the urea N fraction will be higher than 90 percent. A starved patient may be expected to have a lower fraction of urea N to TUN. Thus TUN can be estimated by adjusting UUN.

On high protein intake or in stress:

$$\text{TUN (g/24 hr)} = \text{UUN (g/24 hr)} \times 1.1$$

On low protein intake or in starvation:

$$\text{TUN (g/24 hr)} = \text{UUN (g/24 hr)} \times 1.2$$

To estimate total N loss add 2 g N/day for normal fecal and dermal losses to TUN.

$$\text{Total N loss (g/24 hr)} = \text{TUN (g/24 hr)} + 2 \text{ g N/24 hr}$$

Questions about kidney function frequently arise when interpreting the results of the 24-hour UUN collection. It is possible to quickly predict creatinine clearance before ordering the urine collection by using the patient's serum creatinine value and body weight with the following method:[16]

$$\frac{\text{Creatinine clearance}}{\text{(ml/min)}} = \frac{(140 - \text{age})(\text{wt kg})}{72 \times \text{s. creatinine} \atop (\text{mg/100 ml})}$$

In order to derive N balance in the patient with compromised renal function, the clinician applies the principles of urea kinetic modeling as described by Sargent et al.[24] Their model is based on the fact that the patient's protein catabolic rate (PCR) in g/24 hr is directly related to the rate of urea nitrogen generation (GUN) in mg/min. This relationship is expressed as

$$\text{PCR (g/24 hr)} = [\text{GUN (mg/min)} + 1.2] \times 9.35$$

Hence, comparing PCR to total protein intake achieves the same information, expressed in terms of dry protein, that would be gained from N balance.

In order to calculate PCR, first calculate GUN. This is derived from changes in concentration of BUN in the total volume of body water (Vu), in residual clearance of urea nitrogen (KrUN) by the kidney, and in concentration of UUN over a known time interval (t).

GUN = amount of serum urea N × volume of serum cleared by kidney + urea N excreted in urine

Serum, in this case, is actually total body water (TBW). BUN is dissolved and distributed proportionately throughout the TBW. Sargent et al.[24] suggest use of the factors 0.58 for males and 0.55 for females multiplied by dry body weight in kilograms to estimate TBW. Percentage of TBW, however, decreases with age and with increasing adiposity. This author recommends use of Moore's nomogram for the prediction of percentage of TBW in normal adults (Fig. 10–1) using the patient's dry weight. The weight of accumulated fluid, edema, or ascites should then be added to TBW derived from the nomogram in order to estimate Vu.

The terms involved in calculating GUN are explained as follows:

KrUN = residual urea clearance by kidney (ml/min)
UUN = urine urea nitrogen concentration (mg/ml)
BUN = serum urea nitrogen (mg/ml)
Uv = volume of urine collection (ml)
t = time interval of urine collection (min)
Vu = estimated urea volume of body water (ml)
θ = time interval between blood samples (min)
BUN_1 = postdialysis BUN (mg/ml)
BUN_2 = predialysis BUN (mg/ml)
Vu_1 = urea volume of dry body weight (ml)
Vu_2 = Vu_1 + interdialytic weight gain (ml)
$\overline{BUN}$ = mean BUN
$-\dfrac{BUN_1 + BUN_2}{2}$ (mg/ml)

Note the differences in units of measurement.

There are four different clinical situations each with their own equation to which these terms apply (Fig. 10–2).

1. The nondialyzed, nutritionally stable patient: The following equation applies when progressive renal failure prevents clearance of excess urea from protein catabolism so that it accumulates in the

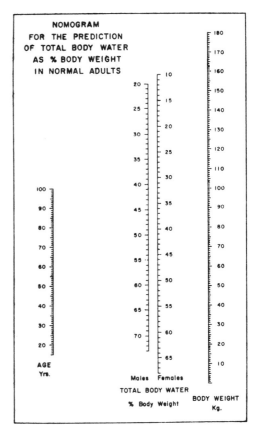

Figure 10–1. Nomogram for the prediction of total body water (as percent of body weight) in normal adults of both sexes. The nomogram is entered with observed age and body weight. A straightedge is laid across these points and the body water fraction read off from the appropriate column. *(From Moore FD, Olesen KH, McMurrey JD, et al.: The Body Cell Mass and Its Supporting Environment: Body Composition in Health and Disease. Philadelphia: W.B. Saunders, 1963, p 161, Fig. 85.[19])*

body. The BUN is higher than normal, but relatively constant. Therefore, it is necessary to determine KrUN and GUN only.

a. Calculate KrUN

$$KrUn = \frac{UUN}{BUN} \times \frac{Uv}{t}$$

Height _____ Age _____ Ideal Body Weight (kg) _____ Serum albumin (g/dl) _____ Prescribed Diet _____	Patient Stamp

CLINICAL

Vu_1 = Dry weight × % TBW

Vu_2 = Vu_1 + Wt. gain (mL)

Renal Function

$$KrUN = \frac{UUN}{\overline{BUN}} \times \frac{Uv}{t}$$

Protein Catabolic Rate

PCR = (GUN + 1.2) 9.35

KINETICS

1. Stable, no dialysis

   GUN = KrUN × BUN

2. Catabolic, no dialysis

   $$GUN = \left[\frac{(BUN_2 - BUN_1)(Vu)}{\theta}\right] + (KrUN \times \overline{BUN})$$

3. No urine urea, on dialysis

   $$GUN = \frac{(Vu_2 \times BUN_2) - (Vu_1 \times BUN_1)}{\theta}$$

4. With urine urea loss; on dialysis

   $$GUN = \left[\frac{(Vu_2 \times BUN_2) - (Vu_1 \times BUN_1)}{\theta}\right] + (KrUN \times \overline{BUN})$$

DATA   **DATES**

DATA					
Dry weight (post-dialysis; g)					
Interdialytic wt. gain (g)					
Urea volume$_1$ (Vu$_1$; mL)					
Urea volume$_2$ (Vu$_2$; mL)					
Collection time (t or θ, min)					
Urine volume (Uv; mL)					
Urine urea N (UUN; mg/mL)					
BUN$_1$ (mg/mL)					
BUN$_2$ (mg/mL)					
Mean BUN ($\overline{BUN}$, mg/mL)					
KrUN (mL/min)					
GUN (mg/min)					
Accumulated serum urea N (mg/min)					
Urine urea N excreted (mg/min)					
Protein Catabolic Rate (PCR; g/24 hrs)					

Figure 10–2. Urea kinetics worksheet for collection of clinical data and reporting results.

b. Calculate GUN

$$GUN = BUN \times KrUN$$

c. Calculate PCR

$$PCR = (GUN + 1.2) \times 9.35$$

2. The nondialyzed, nutritionally unstable (i.e., catabolic) patient: In this case, protein catabolism is occurring at a much faster rate than the rate at which the kidney can clear the urea. Therefore, the rapid rise in BUN must be accounted for in calculating the total amount of urea N produced.

a. Calculate KrUN

$$KrUn = \frac{UUN}{BUN} \times \frac{Uv}{t}$$

b. Calculate GUN

$$GUN = \frac{(BUN_2 - BUN_1)(Vu)}{\theta} + (KrUN \times \overline{BUN})$$

c. Calculate PCR

$$PCR = (GUN + 1.2) \times 9.35$$

3. The dialyzed patient without urea nitrogen loss in urine (e.g., anuria, polycystic disease): In conditions where there is no urea loss in urine, all urea generated from protein catabolism accumulates in the serum. Therefore, all that needs to be considered is GUN between two consecutive dialyses.

a. Calculate GUN

$$GUN = \frac{(Vu_2 \times BUN_2) - (Vu_1 \times BUN_1)}{\theta}$$

b. Calculate PCR

$$PCR = (GUN + 1.2) \times 9.35$$

4. The dialyzed patient with urea nitrogen loss in urine (e.g., oliguria): If there is sufficient renal function to allow some clearance of urea by the kidney, then urine urea must be considered along with changes in BUN between consecutive dialyses in order to calculate total GUN.

a. Calculate KrUN

$$KrUn = \frac{UUN}{BUN} \times \frac{Uv}{t}$$

b. Calculate GUN

$$GUN = \frac{(BUN_2 \times Vu_2) - (BUN_1 \times Vu_1)}{\theta} + (\overline{BUN} \times KrUN)$$

$$PCR = (GUN + 1.2) \times 9.35$$

The following is a case history in which urea kinetics proves helpful.

A 72-year-old man with a history of hypertension and atherosclerotic coronary artery disease is admitted to the hospital for a carotid endarterectomy.

During a routine admission nutrition status screen, the clinical dietitian notes that he is 170.2 cm tall, weighs 61.7 kg on admission, and has lost 7 kg unintentionally during the last 3 months. The laboratory data include serum albumin of 3 g/dl, BUN of 47 mg/dl, and serum creatinine of 2.7 mg/dl. The clinical dietitian calculates the creatinine clearance, according to the methods of Cockcroft and Gault[16] to be 21.6 ml/min.

$$\text{Creatinine clearance} = \frac{(140\text{-age})\ (\text{wt/kg})}{72 \times \text{s. creat.} (\text{mg/dl})}$$

$$= \frac{(140 - 72)(61.7 \text{ kg})}{72 \times 2.7 \text{ mg/dl}}$$

$$= 21.6 \text{ ml/min}$$

The clinical dietitian asks for a 24-hour urine for urea nitrogen to assess his protein requirements.

Data:
Uv = 1200 ml/24 hr
Urine urea N = 6 g/24 hr
UUN = 5 mg/ml
BUN_1 = 0.45 mg/ml
BUN_2 = 0.5 mg/ml
Total protein intake = 44.5 g/24 hr

Calculations:

In light of the patient's impaired renal function, rising BUN, and history of weight loss, the dietitian analyzes the data.

1. % TBW = 56%

2. $\text{KrUN (ml/min)} = \dfrac{\text{UUN}}{\text{BUN}} \times \dfrac{\text{UV}}{\text{t}}$

$$\times \frac{5.0}{0.47} \times \frac{1200}{1440}$$

$$= 8.86 \text{ ml/min}$$

3. $\text{GUN (mg/min)} = \dfrac{(\text{BUN}_2 - \text{BUN}_1)(\text{Vu})}{\theta}$

$$+ (\text{KrUN} \times \overline{\text{BUN}})$$

$$= \frac{(0.50 - 0.45)(34{,}552)}{1440}$$

$$+ (8.86 \times 0.47)$$

$$= 5.36 \text{ mg/min}$$

4. PCR (g/24 hr) = 5.36 + 1.2) × 9.35 = 61.3 g/24 hr.

Therefore, the patient's "balance" is negative by 16.8 g protein (equivalent to 2.7 g N) per day.

The patient then goes to surgery. Three days postop, he develops congestive failure, is placed on a ventilator, and is transferred to ICU. His renal function deteriorates and he is placed on hemodialysis. The dietitian in the ICU is asked to assess the patient's nutrition status prior to instituting nutrition support. The following data are obtained:

Physician's Orders:

Pre- and postdialysis BUN
Pre- and postdialysis weight
Timed urine collection for urea nitrogen to begin after dialysis and end just prior to the next dialysis

Laboratory Data:

Postdialysis weight = 67 kg
Predialysis weight = 70.5 kg

Postdialysis BUN (BUN$_1$) = 0.78 mg/ml
Predialysis BUN (BUN$_2$) = 0.89 mg/ml
θ = 1350 min
Uv = 275 ml
Urine urea nitrogen = 2.2 g/24 hr
UUN = 8 mg/ml
% TBW = 56%
Vu$_1$ = 39852 ml (assume dry weight = 61.7 kg and add 5300 ml of retained fluid)
Vu$_2$ = 43352 ml

Calculations:

1. $\text{KrUn (ml/min)} = \dfrac{\text{UUN}}{\text{BUN}} \times \dfrac{\text{Uv}}{\text{t}}$

$$= \frac{8.0}{0.84} \times \frac{275}{1350}$$

$$= 1.94 \text{ ml/min}$$

2. $\text{GUN} = \dfrac{(\text{BUN}_2 \times \text{Vu}_2) - (\text{BUN}_1 \times \text{Vu}_1)}{\theta}$

$$+ (\text{KrUN} \times \overline{\text{BUN}})$$

$$= \frac{(0.89 \times 43352) - (0.78 \times 39852)}{1350}$$

$$+ (1.94 \times 0.84) = 7.18 \text{ mg/ml}$$

3. PCR = (GUN + 1.2) × 9.35

$$= 78.4 \text{ g/24 hr}$$

On the basis of this information, the dietitian recommends a tube feeding formula to supply 80 g of protein.

24-HOUR FOOD INTAKE RECORDS

It is the responsibility of the dietitian to keep records of food intake over 24-hour intervals. These records are sometimes called "calorie counts," although intake of other nutrients may be estimated as well.

The purpose of the food intake record is to:

1. Gain an estimation of the patient's total intake of calories, protein, and other nutrients
2. Estimate protein and calorie intake in order to determine N and energy balance
3. Determine the adequacy of the patient's present intake as well as the value of initiating alternate feeding methods

Errors in 24-Hour Record of Food Intake

Discrepancies occur because of:

- Inaccurate or incomplete determination of the amount of food, beverages, or solutions consumed or infused
- Discrepancies between literature values of analyzed nutrient content
- Lack of communication between personnel responsible for initiating the calorie count, recording intake, calculating nutrient composition, and recording the results

Items to Include in a 24-Hour Record of Intake

Besides amounts of food consumed at meals, a system is needed that ensures recorded intake of between-meals snacks and food brought in from sources other than the hospital kitchen. An accurate description of food brought in from home, including brand names, ingredients used in the recipe, and method of preparation, assists the dietitian to estimate the food's nutrient composition.

In addition, the nutrient content of tube feedings, parenteral solutions, and commercially prepared vitamin, mineral, and calorie–protein supplements and their rate of infusion should be recorded separately on the intake sheet. The dietitian needs to know the formulation and the total volume of enteral and parenteral solutions delivered to the patient in order to calculate the nutrients infused.

Methods for determining intake include the following:[39]

1. Weigh back: The food and liquids are weighed on conventional kitchen scales before being trayed and sent to the patient. Unconsumed food is reweighed and that amount subtracted from the portion served to obtain the amount consumed.

   This is the most accurate and often least feasible method.

2. Portion control: The portion size of the food to be consumed by the patient is specified on the menu by the dietitian, and measured in the kitchen before the food is trayed and sent to the patient. The dietitian or other trained observer then examines the patient's tray and notes approximate amounts of unconsumed items.

   This is less complicated and time consuming than weigh backs and the controlled serving sizes gives the observer some idea of how much food was on the tray beforehand. Intake is, however, an estimate, rather than a measured quantity.

3. Observed estimation of food intake: The person who serves the tray to the patient notes the portion size of each food and beverage serving, then compares with unconsumed food to determine amount consumed. This is open to error as no attempt is made to measure food either prior to serving it or afterward. The observer should be trained, using food models and volumetric measurements of fluid to estimate quantities of food. The amount of foods and fluids consumed should be described as accurately as possible, by volume (i.e., ½ cup or 120 cc milk) or estimated portion (i.e., ½ hamburger with 2 tb of gravy). Knowing the capacity of various containers in which fluids are served facilitates this.

   In some cases, it is necessary to train the patient to record his or her own intake. This is often true for ambulatory patients. The patient should be provided with forms, instructions for filling them out, and taught to measure and estimate portion sizes of food consumed.

ENERGY EXPEDITURE

Definition of Terms

While the Recommended Dietary Allowances (RDA)[31] suggest mean energy requirements for normals, requirements vary greatly among individual subjects and are further altered by chronic disease infection and trauma. Therefore, in order to predict individual energy requirements, it is important to be familiar with the factors that contribute to total energy expenditure on a daily basis in the normal subject.

1. Basal metabolic rate (BMR) is the rate of free heat production of an individual measured by direct calorimetry in a neutral thermal environment, at least 12 hours postprandial. The subject is at ease mentally and physically, but not asleep and not doing external work. BMR is usually measured in the morning after the subject wakes up. BMR is the steady state at which the body is considered to be carrying out minimal cell respiration and function needed to maintain itself.[1] These conditions are difficult to achieve in the hospital setting.

 The central nervous system (CNS) accounts for approximately 18 percent of the BMR. The digestive and excretory systems account for approximately 27 percent and the circulatory and respiratory systems account for approximately 16 percent.[1,2] The remainder of the tissues utilize the final 39 percent of the BMR, with the LBM, especially skeletal muscle, accounting for the remainder of the metabolic demands.[2,3]

2. Resting energy expenditure (REE), sometimes called resting metabolic expenditure (RME) or basal energy expenditure (BEE), is a term that evolved in the last 30 years to describe the conditions under which energy expenditure is commonly measured in critically ill patients. The subject is at ease mentally and physically in a neutral thermal environment with a face mask or some other sort of headgear in place for measuring respiration via indirect calorimetry. REE ignores timing with respect to meals or sleep patterns.[7]

REE is generally considered to be greater than the predicted BMR by a factor of approximately 10 percent in order to account for variables such as the specific dynamic action of food.[7] At least one author has found no significant difference between REE measured by indirect calorimetry and predicted BMR.[8] This may be related to differences in the methods used for measuring these two entities.[5,6]

Methods for Measuring Energy Expenditure

Basal metabolic rate was first measured using direct calorimetry by Atwater, Benedict, Lusk, and DuBois, during the early 1900s. They demonstrated that man operates under the same thermodynamic laws that govern inanimate objects so convincingly that their work is seldom repeated today. They popularized the measurement of BMR by direct calorimetry as a test of thyroid function. However, this gave way to the faster, cheaper blood tests that were later developed.

Current research indicates that cellular heat production has three components:

1. Heat associated with the continuous process of anabolism–catabolism of tissue
2. Obligatory heat associated with various transport cycles (e.g., the Na^+ pump)
3. In warm-blooded animals, heat associated with regulation of body temperature

Direct calorimetry measures the total rate of heat loss from the body that is due to oxidation of energy substrates. A formula that demonstrates this concept is described by Jequier:[4]

$$M = S + (R+C+K+E) + W$$

where M = rate of free energy production

S = rate of storage of body heat
R = rate of radiant heat exchange
C = rate of convective heat transfer
K = rate of conductive heat transfer
E = rate of evaporative heat transfer
W = rate of work done against external forces.

In order to obtain BMR, the conditions would have to be such that there was no change in mean body temperature and no activity (S = O, W = O).

The calorimeter is an insulated chamber maintained at a constant temperature by water that circulates through channels in the wall of the chamber. Any change in the temperature of this water is accounted for by heat (R + C + K) given off by the subject inside the chamber. Evaporative heat losses (E) are determined by measuring changes in the temperature and amount of water vapor that is circulated through the chamber. For long-term studies, the weight and temperature of all foods consumed by the subject in the chamber and also of all excretions must be measured. The calorie content of food ingested and of excretion is measured in a bomb calorimeter.

The advantage of this system is that it gives an accuracy approaching 1 percent over time spans of up to 2 months on a normal patient in a closely supervised ward undergoing different levels of exercise. The disadvantages of direct calorimetry are that it is time consuming to conduct and expensive to set up the system. Measurement of habitual energy expenditure is precluded while the subject is confined to the chamber and cannot undertake the usual activities of daily living. This set-up is not useful for studying changes in energy metabolism in critically ill patients who need the facilities of an intensive care unit.[5,6]

A second method for measuring energy expenditure is called indirect calorimetry. In this method, O_2 consumption, CO_2 production, and N_2 excretion are measured to yield information on the rate of fuel oxidation. The concept is similar to direct calorimetry in that the formula M = S + (R + C + K + E) + W still holds.

In direct calorimetry, however, M is a measure of heat production, whereas indirect calorimetry measures the rate of oxidation of fuel, or as Webb[6] calls it, the rate of "metabolic free energy conversion."

Weir[10] developed the technique in 1949. It began to find application as a practical means of studying energy expenditure in the critically ill patient as investigations in the use of mechanical ventilators and total parenteral nutrition uncovered information on requirements for gas exchange and nutrients needed to support the stressed patient.[7,8,11]

A typical situation for measuring gas exchange for indirect calorimetry is as follows: The patient's head is placed in a sealed plastic canopy or he breathes into a face mask with hoses attached to a continuous gas analyzer. A mixture of air with a known concentration of CO_2, O_2 and N_2 is pumped to the patient, then back to the gas analyzer at a constant rate. As the patient breathes, the concentrations of O_2 and CO_2 in the canopy change. The gas analyzer measures this change in concentration and traces the measurements on a spirometer. Measurements are taken for a period of 30 to 45 minutes from three to five times per day. From these measurements, the REE can be calculated from a series of equations.

The advantage of indirect calorimetry is its greater flexibility. The equipment can be easily designed for use in a critical care area where the patient can receive appropriate professional care with a minimal degree of isolation needed during the study period. Thus it has the advantage of being able to determine energy expenditure in the patient's habitual environment. Although the equipment is, in most instances, still too cumbersome to be able to measure the patient's energy expenditure for many types of activity, measurements can be taken while the patient is sitting, walking, or lying down. It is less time consuming for the patient than direct calorimetry. This method is still fairly precise, having an internal error of 3 to 5 percent for subjects at rest.[7,8]

In addition, Webb[5,6] measured metabolic free-energy conservation via indirect calorimetry and sum of energy losses via direct calorimetry for 24 hours in each of six males, consuming a usual diet and at rest. He found that the measurements agreed within ± 3 percent. In subsequent measurements taken while the subjects were exercising or fasting, however, the energy expenditure measured as heat loss via direct calorimetry was less than the expenditure measured as oxidized energy via indirect calorimetry by factors of from 8 to 23 percent, indicating that perhaps not all of the oxidative energy is being accounted for as changes in heat production. For the time being, let it be said that caution should be exercised in comparing the results of indirect calorimetric measurements to methods for estimating energy expenditure that have been derived from direct calorimetry.

The disadvantage in using indirect calorimetry is that it does not take into account small exchanges of CO_2, O_2, and N_2 that are known to occur in the bowel or through the skin, but that may be a significant contribution in some patients, especially burn patients and patients with malabsorptive disorders. Errors can occur in the collection and storage of gases for later analysis as it is difficult to design a collection system that is completely free of leaks. Dysfunctions in respiration in the critically ill patient lead to abnormal exchanges of CO_2, O_2, and N_2 (e.g., hypoxia and hypercapnea). Many types of respiratory support systems do not allow for accurate collection of respired gases for analysis, therefore the effects of respiratory disturbances on oxidative exchange have not been fully studied in the critically ill patient. Increases in REE may occur due to anxiety on the part of the patient at having the face mask placed on or because of having his head sealed inside the plastic canopy.[6–8,12]

The problem associated with extrapolating energy expenditure from REE instead of BMR is that measurement of REE does not

control for the increased heat production due to the specific dynamic action of foods. There is some question, however, as to the significance of this.[8]

Attempts made to relate heart rate to energy expenditure as reflected by oxygen consumption have proven unsuccessful in both normals[20,21] and critically ill patients.[22]

Factors That Affect the Resting Rate of Energy Expediture in Control Subjects

The amount of LBM rather than total body weight is the most important variable in the control of the individual's BMR. This is because of the large amount of oxygen LBM consumes in order to synthesize protein, maintain the sodium pump, and carry out the other metabolic activities peculiar to maintenance of its cellular structure.[3,43]

Age and sex influence BMR. This is very likely due to the changes in LBM that occur during growth and with aging, however, as well as to the smaller proportion of LBM found in females as compared to males.[3,13,15,43] BMR decreases by 1 to 2 percent per decade in adults between 20 and 75 years of age.[28] This is taken into account in equations used to estimate BMR.

Body surface area (BSA), body weight, and amount of body fat have also been implicated as factors that are positively correlated with BMR. This may be due to the increased work of respiration and transportation of nutrients to and from all parts of the cell mass as body size increases. It more likely reflects the increase in LBM that accompanies increased body mass. Several investigators[13–15] have noted that smaller individuals expend more energy per square meter of BSA, reflecting the relatively larger amount of LBM versus fat.

Since BMR, by definition, is measured in a thermoneutral environment, studies dealing with changes in energy expenditure in nonthermoneutral environments deal with measurements of REE. REE is essentially independent of environmental influences if the temperature is maintained between 22 and 35°C for clothed or unclothed men. Shivering increases REE by approximately 36 percent.[1] Small, usually insignificant, decreases in REE occur in environments where the temperature is greater than 35°C[17] If the subject is not acclimatized, however, there may be an increase in REE due to sweating and discomfort.[1]

Methods for Estimating BMR and REE

Because most hospitals do not have the means to measure continuous energy expenditure, factorial methods have been developed and compared to actual measurements to determine their validity.

1. Harris–Benedict Equation.

BMR for males = 66.4730 + (13.7516 W) + (5.0033 H) − (6.7550 A)

BMR for females = 655.095 + (9.563 W) + (1.8496 H) − (4.6756 A)
where
    W = weight in kilograms
    H = standing height in centimeters
    A = age in years

Harris and Benedict[18] derived these equations from the BMRs measured via direct calorimetry on normal adults. Long et al.[8] compared predicted BMR, using the above equations, against measured REE via indirect calorimetry. They found a percent variation of −3.9 ± 2.6 in 9 normal males and −1.8 ± 1.3 in 11 normal females.

Wilmore[23] states that the standards achieved using this formula are high, representing the results of studies done on untrained subjects. As the subject gained experience, the metabolic rate dropped 8 to 9 percent over a period of days.

2. Klieber.

Because the relationship of energy expenditure to body weight is not linear, Kleiber[25] analyzed Harris and Benedict's[18]

data and related them to "metabolic body size."

He proposed that REE could be calculated as follows:

REE (kcal/day) = 70 × weight$^{3/4}$
or REE (kcal/hr) = 3 × weight$^{3/4}$
where weight = kg body weight

He retains age and sex differences in considering the data. He does not, however, take into account differences in LBM or BSA between individuals.

3. Dubois and Dubois, Boothby et al., and Fleisch.

Energy expenditure is frequently estimated using body surface because it reflects both height and weight. Dubois and Dubois[26] developed the following formula for determining body surface area (BSA).

BSA = wt$^{0.425}$ × ht$^{0.725}$ × 0.007184
where BSA = body surface area in sq m
    wt = body weight in kg
    ht = height in cm

While many clinicians have used the standards of Boothby et al[27] for calculating BMR, more recently Wilmore[23] popularized Fleisch's[28] standards as they were the composite of 24 sets of published standards and were felt to be the more complete and accurate. Wilmore does point out that they give results that are approximately 8 percent lower than Boothby's (Tables 10–2, 10–3).

4. Miscellaneous.

Cunningham[3] estimated that LBM accounted for approximately 70 percent of the variability in Harris and Benedict's studies on BMR. Both Cunningham[3] and Roza and Shizgal[43] reanalyzed Harris and Benedict's original data. Using methods developed by Moore et al.[19] to estimate LBM and BCM respectively, they devised formulas that estimate REE based on LBM and BCM. Their equations were independent of age and sex and had 95 percent confidence limits for the slope of the regression equation. Cunningham[3] found a prediction error of 10 per-

TABLE 10–2. MEAN BASAL ENERGY PRODUCTION BASED ON BODY AREA, AGE, AND SEX

Age Last Birthday (yr)	Males		Females	
	$kcal/m^2/hr$	$kcal/m^2/24\ hr$	$kcal/m^2/hr$	$kcal/m^2/24\ hr$
6	53.3	1279	50.7	1217
7	52.5	1260	50.1	1202
8	51.9	1245	45.9	1102
9	51.0	1224	46.4	1114
10	48.3	1159	45.9	1102
11	47.7	1145	46.1	1106
12	46.9	1126	43.4	1042
13	45.5	1092	43.6	1046
14	46.6	1118	42.0	1008
15	46.2	1109	40.0	960
16	46.1	1106	39.6	950
17	44.8	1075	37.4	898
18	45.0	1080	37.0	888
19	41.8	1003	35.7	857
20	42.5	1020	36.7	881
22	42.3	1015	35.7	857
24	41.3	991	35.8	859
26	39.2	941	36.6	878
28	41.0	984	36.4	874
30	40.0	960	35.3	847
35	39.2	941	35.8	859
40	38.0	912	35.4	850
45	37.7	905	35.0	840
50	36.9	886	33.9	814
55	35.5	852	33.2	797
60	35.2	845	34.7	833

Adapted from Boothby WM, Berkson J, Dunn HL: Am J Physiol 116:468, 1936, Table 1.[27]

cent for the equation on normal subjects while Roza and Shizgal[43] found a prediction error of 14 percent. Roza and Shizgal[43] also tested their equation on a group of 74 nonseptic, afebrile general surgery patients before starting parenteral nutrition (PN) therapy. Thirty-three of the subjects were normally nourished and 41 were malnourished. Body composition was determined by multiple isotope dilution in all patients. Lacking the equipment with which to measure REE, the authors substituted O_2 consumption in the equation. While their formula accurately predicted O_2 consumption in normally nourished patients, it significantly underestimated oxygen consumption in the malnourished group. They recommended direct measurement of REE in malnourished patients rather than use of the Harris–Benedict equation for estimating it. They had no apparent explanation for the high O_2 consumption in their malnourished patients, a

TABLE 10-3. METABOLIC RATES IN MALES AND FEMALES BASED ON BODY SURFACE AREA

Age (yr)	kcal/m²/24 hr	
	Males	*Females*
1	1272	1272
2	1258	1258
3	1231	1229
4	1207	1195
5	1183	1162
6	1159	1128
7	1135	1090
8	1111	1051
9	1085	1027
10	1056	1020
11	1032	1008
12	1020	991
13	1015	967
14	1010	941
15	1003	910
16	994	886
17	979	871
18	960	862
19	941	852
20	926	847
25	900	845
30	883	842
35	876	840
40	871	838
45	869	828
50	859	814
55	850	799
60	838	785
65	826	773
70	811	761
75 and over	797	751

From Fleisch A: Le metabolisme basal standard et sa determination au moyen du "Metabocalculator." Helv Med Acta 18:23–44, 1951.[28]

phenomenon that contrasts with the general view that O_2 consumption decreases during starvation. The relationship between estimated energy expenditure and LBM or BCM needs further study.

None of these methods of predicting energy expenditure are entirely accurate over the long term. Mahalko and Johnson[37] studied actual energy intake in 22 normal male subjects who maintained their weight on a constant energy intake over a 99- to 213-day period in a metabolic ward. These measured intakes were compared with estimated energy needs derived from:

1. 24-hour recall diet history
2. Food frequency questionnaire
3. Physical activity history
4. Harris–Bennedict formula calculating BMR with
   a. Factor of 50 percent of BMR added to estimate activity demands
   b. Factors of 30, 50, and 70 percent of BMR added to individualize activity demands for light, medium, and heavy activity, respectively
5. Mayo Foundation nomogram, with additional energy for activity added as described above
6. Kleiber formula for estimating BMR with additional energy for activity as described above
7. The American Diabetes Association and American Dietetics Association, "A Guide for Professionals," which estimates energy needs at 13, 15, and 20 calories per pound ideal body weight for light, medium, and heavy activity, respectively
8. The Recommended Dietary Allowance[31] for energy for an average size man

They found that the Harris–Bennedict, Kleiber, and Mayo methods estimated energy needs at approximately 10 percent less than the actual needs. The Harris–Bennedict formula, with individualized activity factors, was most accurate of the three but there was no significant difference between them.

TABLE 10–4. DAILY ENERGY EXPENDITURES OF ADULT NORMAL SUBJECTS

	Man (70 kg)		Woman (55 kg)	
Activity Category	*Rate (kcal/min)*	*% Increase Above RME*	*Rate (kcal/min)*	*% Increase Above RME*
Sleeping, reclining	1.0–1.2	0–20	0.9–1.1	0–10
Very light Seated and standing activities, laboratory work, driving autos and trucks, ironing, sewing	up to 2.5	up to 150	up to 2.0	up to 100
Light Walking on level: 2.5 to 3.0 mph, tailoring, pressing, garage work, restaurant trades, washing clothes, shopping with a light load, golf, sailing, table tennis, volleyball	2.5–4.9	150–400	2.0–3.9	100–300
Moderate Walking 3.5–4.0 mph, plastering, weeding, scrubbing floors, stacking and loading bales, cycling, skiing, tennis, dancing	5.0–7.4	400–650	4.0–5.9	300–500
Heavy Walking with a load uphill, tree felling, work with pick and shovel, basketball, swimming, climbing, football	7.5–12.0	650–1100	6.0–10.0	500–1000

Adapted from The National Research Council, Recommended Dietary Allowances, 9th ed. Washington, D.C.: National Academy of Sciences, 1980, Table 4.[31]

The food frequency and activity history was in error by approximately 30 percent, the diet history by approximately 20 percent, and the ADA Guide and RDA gave errors that ranged between 10 and 15 percent.

Thus, the Harris–Benedict formula comes the closest to estimating the energy requirements in normal males under controlled conditions. In the hospital setting, the Harris–Benedict formula with factors added to account for activity and stress is recommended as a starting point. Individual needs can be tailored from this estimate, using serial weights and N balance to reflect adequacy of energy intake.

Effect of Activity on Energy Expenditure

In the normal subject, the rate and duration of activity is the major variable in determining the individual's energy needs. For the critically ill patient, activity does not increase energy expenditure greatly until the patient becomes ambulatory. Long et al.[8,30] measured the activities of ten normal subjects under hospital ward conditions. They found mean expenditures that were 8 percent above resting for normals who were sitting up, 17 percent above resting when standing, and 137 percent above resting when walking in the hall at approximately 1.5 mph. These values for activity are comparable to literature values used in determining the 1980 RDA[31] for energy (Table 10–4.) These figures can be used to calculate energy expenditure by keeping records of the time spent in doing each type of activity during the day, and cumulating the results. Mahalko and Johnson[37] found that, in normal subjects carrying out normal activities of daily living, this was no more accurate than increasing the estimated BMR derived from the Harris–Benedict or Kleiber formula by 50 percent.

ESTIMATING CALORIE AND PROTEIN REQUIREMENTS IN STRESS AND STARVATION—GENERAL PRINCIPLES[13,44-46]

1. The objective is to provide adequate calories and protein to spare breakdown and loss of BCM.
2. Calories without N will spare protein breakdown somewhat, and protein without calories will spare the BCM somewhat. No significant benefit is derived, however, unless both calories and protein are supplied.
3. On a fixed, adequate protein intake, the level of energy intake decides the degree to which protein is spared. On a fixed and adequate calorie intake, the level of protein intake determines the degree to which protein will be spared and whether rate of protein synthesis will exceed catabolism.
4. The substrate from which the energy is derived may also be a factor in preventing protein breakdown. For example, at low levels of intake, approximately 125 g/day, glucose is more effective than fat in sparing protein. This is because the CNS has an absolute requirement for glucose that, during starvation, can be met via gluconeogenesis from endogenous protein stores. Gluconeogenesis requires about 250 g of endogenous protein, however, to make this same amount of glucose.
5. Both glucose and lipid need to be included in the patient's regimen to prevent increased production of CO_2 with high concentrations of glucose that stresses pulmonary reserve. This also allows better control of serum glucose and triglyceride (TG) levels.
6. There is an absolute requirement for fat in the diet to prevent essential fatty acid (EFA) deficiency. At least 4 percent of total calorie intake should be provided as linoleic and linolenic acids.
7. Individual requirements for calories

and protein vary greatly and change constantly due to a variety of factors that are discussed in this chapter. Daily body weights, N balance, and, when available, measured REE should be monitored routinely in order to individualize requirements.

EFFECT OF STARVATION ON BODY COMPOSITION[9,13,19,36]

The body can tolerate loss of large amounts of fat stores in starvation. There is an obligatory loss of BCM, however, that accompanies loss of fat in starvation. In the normal adult, the available stored energy amounts to about 250 g of glycogen, 6000 g of protein, and 15,000 g of fat. When a person starves, glycogenolysis takes place to maintain blood glucose levels. Glycogen stores, which supply about 900 kcal, are usually exhausted within 15 to 20 hours. Next, protein is mobilized from skeletal muscles, deaminated, converted to glucose in the liver, and released into the bloodstream to maintain the blood glucose level. Initially, the body may use as much as 75 g of protein per day to maintain blood glucose concentration. The nitrogen that is deaminated is excreted in the urine. Consequently, urinary N excretion is increased, which reflects a negative N balance of about −12 g N per day.

This use of body protein for energy is very costly. The body adapts by using a more dispensable body energy store—fat. This process of adaptation takes 3 to 4 days, but soon the body is mobilizing fatty acids for energy and using only about 25 g of protein per day for energy, and N balance decreases to about −4 g N (Table 10-5).

The liver also converts some fatty acids to ketone bodies, which all tissues of the body, including the brain, can metabolize for energy. In this stage, the urinary N loss will become even less, and the negative N balance will improve further, from −4 to −2 g N per day. In the final phase of starvation, fat

TABLE 10–5. STAGES OF ADAPTATION DURING STARVATION

Stage I—(Days 2–4)
 Depletion of endogenous glycogen stores
 Increase in urinary N loss due to catabolism of
   LBM to support gluconeogenesis
 Negative N Balance = −12 to −15 g/day

Stage II—(Days 5–40)
 Gradual decrease in urinary N loss and reduction
   in BMR as LBM decreases and protein is con-
   served
 Negative N Balance: − 4 g/day
 Body fat primary source of energy
 Serum fatty acids ↑
 Serum Ketones ↑
 Serum insulin ↓

Stage III—(Ketoadaptation)
 Decrease in urinary N loss as glucose-burning
   tissue adapts to ketones as an energy source
 Negative N balance: −2 to −4 g/day
 In absence of CHO intake, urinary N losses reflect
   rate of gluconeogenesis

Stage IV
 Depletion of endogenous fat stores
 ↑ utilization of body proteins to supply energy de-
   mands
 Loss of more than one-third total body protein
 Edema
 Death

Adapted from Krause MV, Mahan LK: Food, Nutrition and
Diet Therapy, 6th ed. Philadelphia: W. B. Saunders, 1979, p
695, Table 35–1.[38]

stores are used up, and the entire energy requirement must be met by visceral organ and
plasma proteins. Depletion of these proteins
is signaled by edema and finally results in
death.

Healthy humans of normal weight will not
tolerate the loss of more than 35 to 40 percent of their body weight. Losses of this size
(about 300 g of N in the male and 200 g of N
in the female) represent a loss of 1200 to
1800 g of body protein, or about one-third of
the total body protein. This is fatal.

The process of conversion to the economic
utilization of stored fat for energy depends on
a progressive decrease in circulating insulin,
which falls from a basal level of 16 to 20

U/ml to less than 12 U/ml. When this hap-
pens, fatty acid mobilization and ketone body
production are promoted. Severe ketonemia
will stimulate insulin secretion, however,
and since insulin strongly inhibits ketogenesis, a feedback control exists that prevents ketosis from reaching pathologic levels. This is not the situation with diabetics,
who have no insulin to control the ketogenesis when it becomes excessive. Table
10–5 summarizes the phases of starvation
and the changes that take place in a person
who is fasting completely but is otherwise
healthy.

EFFECT OF STARVATION ON REE[9,13,19,36]

During a period of starvation, the body appears to convert from glucose oxidation as
the main energy substrate to oxidation of endogenous calorie sources, principally fat.
During this transition, amino acids are mobilized to support gluconeogenesis in the liver
and kidney, thus decreasing the subject's
BCM. Since BCM is most active in the metabolic oxidation of foodstuffs, the REE drops
as it is depleted. At the same time, the CNS,
which normally requires 100 to 150 g of
glucose a day, shifts to ketones as a major
energy source, since free fatty acids (FFA) do
not readily cross the blood brain barrier. The
red muscle fibers also adapt to long chain
fatty acids as an energy substrate, thus sparing the branch chain amino acids (BCAA) as
an energy substrate. Tissues such as liver,
heart, lungs, and kidney can oxidize fats or
glucose interchangeably depending on the
availability of the substrate. Because ketones are more similar to glucose than fats,
they are oxidized by any tissue with a tricar-
boxylic acid cycle except the liver. This adaptive response and the decreased REE put less
burden on the host to catabolize nitrogenous
stores for energy production.

In contrast, the subject who is both
stressed and starved is unable to produce ketones, to stem gluconeogenesis, and therefore

to adapt to conserve protein and energy until the stressor is abated. For this reason, malnutrition occurs much more quickly in the stressed and starved subject.[13,36]

The liver and brain are the most highly oxidative organs, accounting for approximately 40 percent of the total REE. The skeletal muscles contribute approximately 25 percent of the REE, although they account for a much larger portion of body mass. REE does not drop in direct relationship with loss of BCM, since most of the loss at first is derived from skeletal muscle.

Total metabolic expenditure (TME) is an estimate of the total number of kilocalories expended by the body over a 24-hour period. It is derived by adjusting an estimate of normal REE with appropriate factors to account for changes in energy expenditure related to activity and to metabolic processes (i.e., starvation and stress). (See Table 10–6 and Fig. 10–3.)

During starvation, approximately 75 g of protein and 160 g of adipose tissue are metabolized each day for every 1800 calories utilized, although as starvation progresses, the contribution of protein decreases to 20 g per day and that of fat increases. All endogenous proteins are utilized including plasma and liver enzymes, skeletal muscle, and digestive enzymes. Serum albumin is lost at the rate of 1 g albumin per 30 g tissue protein loss. As the rate of gluconeogenesis de-

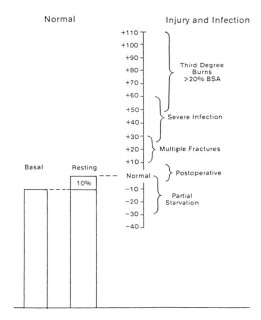

Figure 10–3. Resting energy expenditure. *(From Elwyn DH: Nutritional requirements of adult surgical patients. Crit Care Med 8:9–20, 1980.[46])*

creases, protein catabolism provides as little as 5 percent of TME, adipose tissue provides approximately 60 percent of the TME, 10 percent is derived from the conversion of FFA to ketones, and 25 percent is derived from the metabolism of ketones by peripheral tissues.

In stress superimposed on starvation, the rate of increase in energy expenditure and loss of N in the urine is reduced due to the prior depletion of body stores. The stress response, however, upsets the finely tuned adaptation of the host to the starvation, and the slight increase in protein catabolism and energy expenditure is less well tolerated by the host, so that malnutrition and "nitrogen death" occur more rapidly.

An individual starved for many weeks or months is extremely receptive to diet. Rates of N anabolism easily achieve up to 10 g/kg/day, far in excess of normal recovery anabolic rates (3 to 5 g/kg/day). This can be

TABLE 10–6. FORMULA FOR ESTIMATION OF TOTAL METABOLIC EXPENDITURE (TME)

TME = REE + IF + AF

where TME = Total metabolic expenditure in kcal/ 24 hr

REE = Resting energy expenditure in kcal/ 24 hr

IF = Injury factor, the percentage increase in REE due to injury, stress or the decrease due to starvation

AF = Activity factor, the percentage increase in REE related to work, exercise accomplished at low intakes and at low calorie/N ratios so long as the diet can be digested and absorbed by the patient. With a stress event imposed on starvation, less N is mobilized and the period of obligate N loss or net catabolism is of shorter duration than in a normally nourished patient.

Clinically, the starvation situation is sometimes erroneously considered an emergency that requires immediate institution of high dose central vein TPN or a high density enteral feeding in order to correct quickly. The situation is not the same, however, as with blood loss or dehydration. The chronically starved person is so avid for N and induction of protein synthesis occurs at such low calorie/N ratios that peripheral vein TPN or a more dilute enteral feeding is acceptable. Refeeding a long-starved individual by central vein using hyperosmotic TPN solutions should be initiated slowly. Enzyme induction in the liver may take a few days to adapt to large carbohydrate and amino acid (AA) loads. Also, the increase in REE that occurs after refeeding may exceed the heart's ability to meet oxygen transport needs.[9]

According to Moore,[13] in starvation alone N loss stabilizes at about 6 g N/m^2/day during the first week in the fasting adult male. Giving AA alone (100 to 120 g/day or 13 to 20 g N) reduces this net loss to about 4 g N/m^2/day, but at the cost of a large urinary urea N excretion (about 19 to 21 g N/day). By contrast, glucose (750 g/day) infused without AA reduces N loss to the "nitrogen floor" of about 1.8 g N/m^2/day. The individual, however, cannot attain positive N balance unless AA are infused along with the glucose.

In starvation, in the fasting normal subject, in trauma, stress, or sepsis, simultaneous presentation of glucose with AA makes it possible for the cell mass to utilize infused AA much more efficiently for protein synthesis. According to Moore, [13] the normal individual uses protein more efficiently at a kcal/N ratio of around 200 nonprotein kcal/g N. An unstressed individual who has been starved for several days passes into positive

N balance at a nonprotein kcal/N ratio as low as 50. In acute trauma and febrile illness, establishment of net protein synthesis requires a kcal/N ratio as high as 300 to 350 nonprotein kcal/g N. (Giving that high amount of kcal/N ratio, however, is not recommended during stress, as will be discussed later.)

In the fasting normal subject given no N base for protein synthesis and no other carbohydrate, glycerol accounts for most of the metabolic effects of IV fat emulsion for sparing protein rather than the fatty acids. Glycerol yields, on a weight basis, the same caloric value as glucose (about 3.79 cal/g). Glycerol alone or whole fat, provided intravenously without other substances, reduces N loss in starvation, but this occurs only to a minor extent and with a marked increase in ketosis.

When AA are provided intravenously with a fat emulsion, the long chain fatty acids support protein synthesis more efficiently than a solution of AA with glycerol alone. Calorie for calorie, fat does not appear to be quite as efficient as carbohydrate in starved subjects in sparing protein, although the difference is of little significance.[45,57]

Glucose and AA promote net protein synthesis more efficiently than either fat emulsion and AA or combination of fat, glucose, and AA during TPN in both starved, normal, and stressed patients.[45,57] The difference appears to occur primarily during the first few days of infusion and is of little significance clinically. Neither does there appear to be a reason for routinely giving only glucose or only lipid as an energy substrate in TPN.[13,45,46,57] Intravenous fat emulsions provide EFA to patients who cannot obtain them orally and fat lowers respiratory quotient (RQ).

There is, however, much controversy over the optimal proportion of fat to glucose in different conditions. In stressed patients, who remain hypercatabolic, higher concentrations of glucose appear beneficial in preventing hypertriglyceridemia and fatty liver. For most patients, there does not appear to be a reason to deviate from the ratio of fat to carbohydrate energy that exists in the normal diet except in cases of altered digestion or metabolism.[46]

EFFECT OF STRESS AND SEPSIS ON BODY COMPOSITION[19,23,33—35,58—60]

Stress is the result of force exerted on a biologic organism or system. If the quantity of the stress is sufficient to upset homeostasis of the biologic system, then pathologic changes occur. In the human being, these pathologic changes have certain characteristics in common regardless of the nature of the stressor or the degree of stress. This collection of changes is called "the catabolic response to stress." These systemic alterations occur as a result of injury and are the net effect of damage to individual cells, the number of cells involved, and extent of damage. This net effect characterizes the degree of stress.

Stress secondary to trauma exhibits first an "ebb phase," then a "flow phase" (Table 10–7). The "ebb phase" is characterized by contraction of circulatory volume. The main therapeutic goal is replacement of blood loss,

TABLE 10–7. METABOLIC RESPONSE TO STRESS

Initial "Flow Phase" of Stress	
Neural and Hormonal Changes ⟶	*Physiologic Changes*
↑ Sympathetic activity	—Hyperglycemia
↑ Ventromedial hypothalamic (VMH) activity	—Peripheral insulin resistance
↑ Epinephrine release	↑ Rate of gluconeogenesis
↑ Glucagon secretion	↓ Uptake of glucose by skeletal muscle
↑ Glucocorticoid release	↑ Protein catabolism
↑ Mineralocorticoid release	↑ Urine urea nitrogen
↓ Serum insulin release	↑ REE and O_2 consumption
↑ Growth hormone release	Fluid and sodium retention
	↑ Potassium excretion
	—Ileus
	—Anorexia
	↑ Clearance of fatty acids by peripheral muscle with ↓ plasma fatty acids

Adaptive "Flow Phase" of Stress	
Neural and Hormonal Changes ⟶	*Physiologic Changes*
↓ VMH activity	↑ Rate of gluconeogenesis, but not as high as initial phase
↑ Parasympathetic activity	↓ Serum glucose levels, but still higher than normal
↓ Sympathetic activity	↓ Protein catabolism, but still higher than normal
↑ Glucagon secretion	↓ Urine urea nitrogen
↓ Serum insulin release	↓ REE and O_2 consumption
Glucocorticoids normal	—Diuresis
Mineralocorticoids normal	↑ Plasma fatty acids
	—Ketonemia and ketonuria
	—Return of appetite

rehydration, and hemodynamic stabilization. It generally lasts no more than 24 to 48 hours. If the patient survives, the flow phase follows. This is characterized by increase in circulatory volume and a number of metabolic alterations, commonly referred to collectively as "hypercatabolism," which affect the patient's nutrition status, as will be discussed later. The stress response reaches its peak 3 to 6 days after the initial injury, then gradually abates over a 2- to 3-week period until the patient's metabolic profile either returns to normal (in the presence of nutrition support) or begins to resemble that of starvation (in the absence of nutrition support). Subsequent stress events will lengthen the course of stress response (e.g., surgical repair of blunt trauma to the viscera, delayed open reduction and internal fixation of a long bone fracture, repeated plastic surgeries to repair facial lacerations). The onset of infection and sepsis generally heightens the stress response.[60]

With the onset of the "flow phase" of traumatic stress, oxygen consumption and energy expenditure increase as the body temperature rises with fever or as temperature increases at the site of the wound. This heat production favors protein synthesis, helps fight infection, and supports cell proliferation and wound healing. The cell, however, relies on glucose to support inflammation and wound repair. The body has limited stores of glucose that are depleted during starvation within 24 hours. Therefore, a complex sympathetic nervous reaction occurs, leading to increased proteolysis of skeletal muscle and of gluconeogenesis. In turn, these processes supply more AA and energy to the wound as substrate for repair.

This sympathetic activity also causes release of glucagon by the pancreas and of glucocorticoids and epinephrine by the adrenals. These hormones inhibit the release of insulin and antagonize its actions. The net effect of this response is a reduced concentration of serum insulin, hyperglycemia, and a resistance to insulin by the peripheral tissues. The lack of insulin in response to

glucose and the tissue resistance to insulin action prevent muscle tissue from utilizing glucose, and a local fuel deficit develops.

Protein catabolism during stress assists in meeting energy requirements. The skeletal muscle uses BCAA for energy and the liver uses the remaining AA mobilized from the skeletal muscles to synthesize the proteins needed during stress: immunoglobulins, leukocytes, and lymphocytes to fight infection; hemoglobin or albumin to replace blood loss; collagen to begin tissue healing; and the enzymes necessary to make all of these proteins.

In trauma and sepsis, REE increases in proportion to the degree of stress from the injury or infection (Table 10–8; see Fig. 10–3 above). This is accompanied by an obligatory increase in gluconeogenesis. Apparently glucose is oxidized in preference to free fatty acids in the acute phase. Although lipolysis does occur and body fat stores are an impor-

TABLE 10–8. GUIDELINES FOR PREDICTING INCREASE IN RESTING ENERGY EXPENDITURE (REE) DUE TO INJURY[a]

Injury	Injury Factor (% Increase Above BEE)
Elective surgery	20
Skeletal trauma	30
Blunt trauma	35
Trauma with steroids	60
Sepsis	80
Burns	>100
Increase in body temperature per 1°C	13

[a]These figures represent energy expenditures that occur at the peak of the stress response, generally about 3 days after injury. As the stress abates, energy expenditure gradually decreases over a 2- to 3-week period until it returns to baseline. Estimates of energy expenditure should be tailored accordingly.
From Long CL, Schaffel N, Geiger JW, et al: Metabolic response to injury and illness: Estimation of energy and protein needs from indirect calorimetry and nitrogen balance. JPEN 3(6):452–456, 1979.

tant source of energy in trauma and septic patients, ketone production is depressed. Protein, chiefly from catabolized skeletal muscle, is mobilized at an increased rate to supply AA precursors for gluconeogenesis. The skeletal muscles appear to favor BCAA (leucine, isoleucine, and valine) as energy substrates. As protein is mobilized, the excess NH_3 that results aminates pyruvate to form alanine. The alanine is shunted to the liver where it is used in gluconeogenesis.

An increased number of AA deaminate to supply carbon fragments for gluconeogenesis. The resulting N is excreted as urea N in the urine.

Sympathetic nervous activity also stimulates the release of mineralocorticoids from the adrenal gland. These cause fluid and sodium retention and potassium excretion.

The increased rate of blood flow, characteristic of the catabolic response to stress, supports needs for substrate at the site of the injury for growth and repair. It is also necessary to maintain adequate organ perfusion and defense against microbial invasion. Therefore, in severe injury, cardiac output may rise 2 to 3 times above normal after plasma volume is restored.

If stress continues, the body's sympathetic activity should also continue. If the sympathetic response stops when the body is still under stress, then the stress overpowers the body. Assuming that the stress continues and that the body can maintain its sympathetic response and overcome the stress, the body begins to adjust somewhat to prolonged stress and enters an adaptive catabolic phase (see Table 10–7). In this phase, less skeletal protein is used to meet energy needs and more fatty acids and ketone bodies are used for energy, so that the N balance is not quite as negative. Lower blood glucose levels and lower rates of UUN excretion are the clinical signs that the body has entered the adaptive phase. During the adaptive phase, nutritional intake is used more efficiently because the levels of epinephrine and glucocorticoids decrease and so does their interference with the action of insulin.

Reoccurence of hyperglycemia means that the stress level has increased stimulating sympathetic activity and insulin resistance.

As the stress is relieved through treatment or by its own natural course, the sympathetic response decreases, the parasympathetic activity increases and the patient begins to feel hungry. Nutritional care should be aimed at putting the patient into anabolism and restoring the tissue protein lost during stress.

In addition to the wastage of nutrients caused by the stress response, there are gastrointestinal losses of nutrients from vomiting and diarrhea. Demands on the host's defense system to synthesize phagocytes, leukocytes, immunoglobulins, and nonspecific proteins further increase nutrient requirements. Additional losses occur due to blood loss from wounds or during surgery and from drainage sights. The amount of protein administered, either parenterally or enterally during the acute injury phase, must be much greater than that which is lost in the urine in order to replace these losses. While the starved patient is "avid" for N and protein synthesis, the posttraumatic patient is "refractory" to N administration and attempts to promote protein synthesis. Abatement of the stressors is essential to reversal of this sequence. This is the main objective of clinical management and surgical care. Once the stressors are controlled the metabolic-caloric-endocrine disorder subsides, and the patient, if given appropriate nutrition, will pass into a prolonged period of convalescent anabolism, first of protein resynthesis and then of fat.

The stress response to infection and sepsis in the early stages is very similar to that of stress due to trauma. There is an increase in energy expenditure and UUN loss. Gluconeogenic rate increases. Ketogenesis is inhibited. Lipolytic rate is increased due to the increased glucagon:insulin ratio. Free fatty acids (FFA) continue to serve as an energy substrate in peripheral tissue but at a reduced rate. Hepatic lipogenesis is stimulated due to the increased FFA cleared from plasma, the increased glucagon: insulin ratio, the increased availability of glucose, and the suppression of ketogenesis.

In late sepsis, lipid metabolism alters markedly. Serum triglycerides become elevated, and fatty liver infiltrations are apparent on biopsy. This reflects decreased peripheral lipid clearance and increased hepatic lipogenesis. Respiratory quotient increases, reflecting the decreased utilization of fat for energy in the face of increased production.[59,60] Gluconeogenesis cannot be suppressed by 5 percent IV dextrose solutions.[29] Unchecked sepsis in its terminal stages is characterized by multisystem organ failure, failed wound healing, anemia, decreased plasma protein levels, and death.[58,59]

The net effect of the catabolic stress response is a hormonal environment that protects and defends the body at the expense of skeletal muscle. It is a beneficial response to stress that includes negative N balance as a necessary side effect. During this catabolic response, which peaks at 3 to 6 days after injury, then declines gradually over a period of 2 to 3 weeks, there is increased rate of nitrogen, sulfur, phosphorus, potassium, magnesium, zinc, and creatinine lost in the urine.

The rate of urea N excretion and therefore skeletal muscle wastage appears to be a function of the amount of muscle mass at the time of injury. Young males who have larger muscle masses excrete N at higher rates than do females, older people, or people who were starved prior to the injury. A decrease in size of visceral organs also occurs, as does loss of body fat. The rate of loss is determined by the extent of the injury, the degree of fever, the extent of the infection, the length of time that the patient received inadequate nutrition to offset these losses, and the length of time that it takes to correct the underlying medical problems.

The body can tolerate loss of fat stores. Loss of more than 40 percent of the body cell mass, however, is fatal. If the stress of the surgery, trauma, or infection is mild and oral intake is resumed soon thereafter, the body tolerates the small loss of nitrogenous substances well. In severe and prolonged stress, however, such as a major burn complicated with sepsis and starvation, the patient may die a "nitrogen death."

GUIDELINES FOR IMPLEMENTING NUTRITION THERAPY

Trauma and Sepsis

After elective surgery, uncomplicated trauma, and low grade infections, patients do not generally sustain high nutrient losses secondary to catabolism. If well nourished prior to the stress event, these patients tolerate postop IV 5 percent dextrose alone until oral intake resumes. If the patient cannot resume oral intake within 5 to 7 days, postop nutrition support should be instituted.[8,46]

With sepsis and polytrauma, on the other hand, the stress is more severe and the nutrient losses secondary to catabolism are higher. Total parenteral or enteral nutrition support should be considered within 3 days of the stress event, regardless of prior nutrition status, in order to replace losses and, hopefully, maintain LBM.[8,46,60] (Refer to Table 10–9 for maintenance calorie and protein guidelines.)

Parenteral infusions containing 35 to 50 percent of crystalline AA as BCAA have been shown to promote positive N balance earlier in severe stress than standard crystalline AA solutions.[61,62] There is inadequate evidence on patient outcome, however, to warrant the additional expense of using high BCAA infusions. The use of BCAA is not indicated in minor stress or in starvation (level 0 and 1 stress) but may be in polytrauma and sepsis (level 2 and 3 stress). (Refer to Table 8–8 in Chapter 8 on Categorization of Stress.) Furthermore, infusion of BCAA alone, as in so-called "protein-sparing" therapy, is not warranted. Adequate calories should be provided to spare protein and promote protein synthesis.

TABLE 10–9. CONSIDERATIONS IN THE PROVISION OF MAINTENANCE LEVEL MACRONUTRIENTS DURING NUTRITION SUPPORT

Stress Level	Clinical Description	% Increase in Resting Energy Expenditure (REE)	Nonprotein Calorie to Nitrogen Ratio (kcal/g N)	Total Calories (kcal/kg/day)	Protein (g/kg/day)	Recommended Distribution of Calories			Consider Use of High BCAA Solution
						% CHO	% Fat	% Protein	
0	Starved[a]	−10 to −40	150/1	28	1.0	60	25	15	—
1	Elective general surgery	+10	150–200/1	25	0.8–1.0	50–55	30–35	15–20	—
2	Polytrauma	+20–30	100/1	32	1.5	50	30	20	+
3	Sepsis, early	+25–60[b]	100/1	40	2.0	40	35	25	+
3	Sepsis, late	+25–60	100/1	50	2.0–2.5	70	—[c]	30	+

[a]This level of calorie and protein intake will promote anabolism while preventing organic failure commonly seen in depleted patients secondary to substrate overload.
[b]13 percent increase in REE for each 1°C increase in body temperature.
[c]Hypertriglyceridemia present.
Adapted from Long CL, Schaffel N, Geiger JW, et al: JPEN 3(6):452–456, 1979;[8] Elwyn D: Crit Care Med 8:9–20, 1980;[46] Sheldon G, Peterson SR: JPEN 4:376–383, 1980;[50] Cerra FB: Pocket Manual of Surgical Nutrition. St. Louis: C. V. Mosby, 1984, Table 5–2.[60]

Cancer[48,49,55,56]

Calorie expenditure and N losses vary considerably, probably due more to the combined effects of prior BCM depletion, sex, age, presence of infections, and the effects of cancer therapy than to the metabolic demands of the tumor itself. REE does appear to be increased in many patients having Hodgkin's disease or leukemia.[48] More significantly, inefficient use of dietary energy necessitates greater energy intakes to meet cellular demands for energy. Tumors appear to have high rates of anaerobic glycolysis, metabolizing the resulting lactate to glucose via the Cori cycle. The Cori cycle produces less adenosine triphosphate (ATP) than the Krebs cycle. Also it has been shown that fatty acid oxidation is not suppressed by infusions of glucose. Hypothetically, the cancer patient may convert glucose to fat before oxidizing it. This is also less efficient in terms of the amount of energy derived.

Protein synthetic rate appears to be impaired and rate of protein breakdown increased in muscle cells from patients with cancer. Evidence regarding the effect of chemotherapy and radiation therapy on metabolic rate, energy expenditure, and protein turnover is conflicting.

There are no specific calorie and protein requirements established for cancer patients. Current recommendations are to estimate REE from the Harris–Benedict equation and apply the factors most appropriate to the patient's clinical condition and activity level to obtain estimated total calorie expenditure for maintenance of body weight and LBM (see Tables 10–4, 10–8, 10–9). Provide a standard distribution of calories unless an underlying disease process or clinical complication warrants differently. Provide protein at 0.8 to 1.2 g/kg and 150 nonprotein kcal/g N for daily maintenance intake. Adjust this prescription according to the patient's clinical condition and stress level. If the patient is underweight, give an additional 500 to 1000 nonprotein kcal per day to allow for weight gain. Then monitor weight, N balance, and other standard parameters of nutrition status, adjusting calorie and protein intake according to the patient's changing needs.

Thermal Injury[8,54]

The metabolic response to thermal injury bears many similarities to that of trauma or sepsis. It is exacerbated by loss of integument, leading to increased evaporative heat loss and increased loss of protein as albumin through burn wound exudate. Calorie expenditure often exceeds 100 percent of REE in patients with burns covering more than 30 percent of their BSA.

To maintain weight and promote wound healing, the minimal levels of protein and calories provided in the nutrition support regimen are calculated according to Curreri's formula:[54]

$$
\begin{aligned}
\text{Calories} &= (25 \text{ kcal} \times \text{body wt in kg}) + \\
&\quad (40 \text{ kcal} \times \% \text{ BSA burned}) \\
\text{Protein (g)} &= (1 \text{ g protein/kg body weight}) \\
&\quad + (3 \text{ g protein/}\% \text{ BSA burned})
\end{aligned}
$$

Provide a normal distribution of nonprotein calories. In 18 burn patients receiving TPN without lipid, glucose infusions exceeding 5 to 7 mg/kg/day were associated with increased CO_2 production and RQ exceeding 1 but not with increased protein metabolism.[63] In nine autopsied burn patients who had received TPN without lipid infusions, fatty liver infiltrates were found.[63]

Nonprotein calorie to N ratios less than 135:1 appear beneficial in promoting protein synthesis for burn patients who require more than 3000 kcal/day to maintain weight.[64]

Hormonal Influences[8,53]

Hypersecretion or chronic administration of thyroid hormone and the corticosteroids increase metabolic rate and protein catabolism. Catecholamines, corticosteroids, and thyroid hormone induce protein mobilization from peripheral tissues, increase urinary N excretion, and enhance uptake of AA by the liver and other viscera. Catecholamines stimulate glycogenolysis in muscle and inhibit glycogen synthesis. Both catecholamines and corticosteroids stimulate gluconeogenesis in the liver and inhibit insulin secretion, thus impairing peripheral uptake of glucose. Thyroid hormone acts primarily on the liver to increase the supply of glucose for oxidation by stimulating liver glycogenolysis and gluconeogenesis. Catecholamines and corticosteroids stimulate lipolysis and inhibit lipogenesis. Thyroid hormone enhances FFA mobilization from adipose tissue and increases FFA oxidation.

The overall effect in all cases is weight loss, loss of fat stores, muscle wasting, and glucose intolerance. Dubois[52] measured BMRs in hyperthyroid patients of 15 to 80 percent above normal.

In Cushing's syndrome, provision of 1 g protein/kg body weight with adequate calories will usually maintain the subject in positive N balance. Adjust carbohydrate intake if the patient exhibits glucose intolerance.

In head trauma patients who are given Decadron to decrease cerebral edema, the maximal increase in REE was measured at 60 percent above normal, over twice that measured in uncomplicated skeletal trauma, while N excretion was measured at 0.338 ± 0.106 g/kg/d.[8] Nutrition support should be tailored to cover these higher rates of loss.

Myocardial Injury, Vascular and Pulmonary Disease[50,51]

Energy expenditure and N losses in patients with cardiac or pulmonary disease are not well documented. Other factors in the patient's clinical condition probably influence them more than the disease itself. For example, the patient may develop increased requirements secondary to infection or sepsis. In chronic vascular disease with subsequent "cardiac cachexia," or after a stroke, requirements usually decrease secondary to starva-

tion. In obstructive pulmonary disease, the work needed to breathe may increase energy expenditure, while at the same time the patient's appetite is depressed and ability to eat hampered due to mucous secretion from the lungs.

Treatment depends on the patient's previous state of nutrition. If the patient is cachectic, then the treatment regimen should be as outlined under the section on starvation. Enteral alimentation is preferred. The heart burns FFA preferentially and in ischemic heart disease FFA may be more beneficial than glucose. On the other hand, excessively high levels of FFA tend to suppress heart function. If fluid retention and congestion is a problem, the TPN or enteral solution should be concentrated in the same manner as solutions used in renal failure.

Glucose as the sole or major source of nonprotein calories in TPN has been shown to increase CO_2 production, RQ, and minute ventilation in both depleted and hypermetabolic patients.[51] This poses a risk of increased CO_2 retention in patients with pulmonary disease or malfunction, which may necessitate ventilatory support. Supplying 33 to 50 percent of nonprotein calories as IV lipid emulsion has been shown to decrease CO_2 production, RQ, and minute ventilation.[65] Fat emulsions, however, may impair pulmonary diffusing capacity in some individuals when given in high concentrations.[66]

Semistarvation (5 percent IV dextrose infusions for 7 days or more) leads to depression of ventilatory drive (the pulmonary response to hypercapnea or hypoxia). Addition of 3.5 percent AA to the 5 percent IV dextrose improves ventilatory drive in normals.[68] In semistarved patients on ventilators, ventilatory drive and ventilatory sensitivity to CO_2 is positively correlated with increasing concentration of amino acids in isocaloric TPN solutions.[67]

Provide the patient with compromised pulmonary function calories sufficient to meet increased needs for stress or for weight gain according to the guidelines in Table 10–9.

Optimal distribution of calories has not been determined. Askanazi et al.[69] recommended supplying nonprotein calories in the form of both carbohydrate and fat, avoiding extreme concentrations (either 100 percent of fat or 100 percent of glucose as nonprotein calories). Generally, 50 percent of nonprotein calories as glucose and 50 percent as fat are provided when attempting to lower RQ and minute ventilation. Askanazi et al.[69] suggest Elwyn's[46] recommendations for protein intake in surgical patients as guidelines for initiating nutrition therapy in patients with pulmonary malfunction. These are 1.25 to 1.9 g protein/kg/day to maintain LBM and 1.5 to 2.5 g protein/kg/day to promote restoration of LBM.

Liver Disease

Liver disease and failure pose special nutrition problems because of the liver's key role in metabolism. Liver degeneration, fibrosis, and cirrhosis interfere with normal nutrient absorption and metabolism. Fat malabsorption is common in liver disease for a variety of reasons, including reduced conjugated bile salt secretion, pancreatic insufficiency, and neomycin administration.[70] Either hyper- or hypoglycemia may occur due to decreased rates of glucose uptake and impaired glycogenolysis and gluconeogenesis, which delay release of glucose from the diseased liver.[70,71]

Protein metabolism is impaired, although the reasons have not been fully explained. Decreased rate of plasma protein synthesis, increased serum ammonia levels, and decreased metabolism of phenylalanine and tryptophan lead to increased serum levels of these AA. There are also decreased serum levels of the BCAA isoleucine, leucine, and valine. Tryptophan levels remain unchanged.[72] The decreased competition between the aromatic amino acids (AAA) phenylalanine, tyrosine, and tryptophan and the BCAA at the blood brain barrier allows greater uptake of the AAA into the brain. This in turn may stimulate synthesis of the

neurotransmitter serotonin, and decrease synthesis of the neurotransmitters dopamine and norepinephrine,[73] accounting for development of hepatic encephalopathy.[72,73] Inadequate dietary intake of choline, leading to decreased production of the neurotransmitter acetylcholine, has also been implicated in the etiology of hepatic encephalopathy.[73] Elevated serum ammonia levels and increased levels of false neurotransmitters, however, may account for some of the aberrations characteristics of hepatic encephalopathy.[74] Enteral and parenteral nutrition solutions that are high in BCAA, but low in AAA have been developed and used clinically in an attempt to offset the altered serum AA patterns. They have been successful in improving symptoms of hepatic encephalopathy and N balance in some, but not all cases.[75,76] Horst[77] recommends reserving use of high BCAA nutrition therapy for protein-intolerant patients with liver failure and hepatic encephalopathy when conventional therapy (e.g., lactulose, neomycin) proves unsuccessful.

In acute liver disease, such as viral or alcoholic hepatitis, adequate nutrition is important in the recovery process. Fat need not be restricted unless it causes nausea and vomiting.[71] Calorie intake should be adequate to maintain and, if necessary, gain weight and spare protein for synthesis. Calorie requirements vary depending on the degree of stress, presence or absence of fever, and previous nutrition status (see Table 10–9 for guidelines). Recommendations for protein intake during acute liver disease vary, but generally recognize at least 1 g protein/kg body wt/day as necessary to meet needs for synthesis and repair.[70,71]

In chronic cirrhosis, the diet should remain high in calories to prevent weight loss and spare protein. Providing 0.8 to 1 g protein/kg/day promotes protein anabolism usually without precipitating encephalopathy.[71] A moderate restriction of dietary fat (40 to 50 g per day) is usually sufficient to prevent symptoms of steatorrhea and cramping abdominal pain. If jaundice develops or pancreatitis recurs, however, the dietary fat should be further restricted[71,73] Often this is accomplished by instituting PN or a defined formula diet that provides less than 10 percent of total calories as fat.

In acute encephalopathy or coma, withhold protein initially until neurologic symptoms begin to subside.[77] Provide calories in the form of IV dextrose or lipid emulsions, polycose tube feedings, or clear liquids, such as ginger ale. Cautiously increase protein intake in 10 to 15 g/day increments until neurologic symptoms worsen or serum ammonia levels rise or until an intake of 0.8 to 1 g/kg/day is achieved.[71,77] In chronic hepatic encephalopathy, 40 to 60 g of protein per day is usually sufficient to promote N balance and prevent exacerbation of symptoms. Provision of less than 40 g protein as a daily routine, however, is not recommended. [71,77]

Renal Failure

Nutrient requirements differ greatly in renal failure depending on the etiology of the kidney failure, the underlying disease process, the degree of kidney function remaining, and the type of treatment instituted. Following are some general guidelines:

1. Acute Renal Failure (ARF): The etiology of ARF is diverse and so is the nutrition care it necessitates. In ARF secondary to trauma, there is apparently both a decrease in rate of protein synthesis[78] and an increase in rate of protein catabolism.[79] The general approach is to provide calories in an amount consistent with the patient's stress state and nutrition status and enough protein in the form of essential amino acids (EAA) and nonessential amino acids (NEAA) to cover PCR. (Refer to the section on urea kinetics.) Prophylactic dialysis is generally necessary in order to provide the high amounts of protein needed during the catabolic state for these patients.
2. Chronic Renal Failure (CRF): Initially, the patient with CRF should be provided

about 30 to 35 kcal/kg/day in order to spare protein and maintain weight.[80] Hyperglycemia and impaired glucose tolerance are common side effects of uremia, but their causes are not well understood. Presence of insulin antagonists with uremia, inhibition of glycogen synthesis, or a combination of these have all been suggested.[81] Hypertriglyceridemia accompanied by increased secretion of very low density lipoproteins is also a common side effect of uremia.[82] Reaven et al.[82] found that decreasing the caloric distribution of carbohydrate in the diet from 50 to 35 percent lowered serum glucose, postprandial insulin response, and serum triglycerides in 27 patients with CRF.[82] Provision and distribution of calories needs to be tailored to the individual's needs.

a. Chronic renal failure—predialysis: In order to control uremia and postpone the need to institute dialysis, protein intake must be controlled. Generally, 0.6 g protein/kg/day maintains nutrition status without wastage of LBM.[83] Sixty-five to 75 percent of the protein provided should be of high biologic value.[80] Ketoanalogs have not been demonstrated as significantly more useful in controlling uremia than EAA or mixed proteins in patients on diets.[84,85]

b. Chronic renal failure—hemodialysis: For patients on hemodialysis, 1.0 to 1.2 g protein/kg/day is recommended for maintenance of LBM.[80] Use of ketoanalogs and EAA preparation are not indicated for the patient on hemodialysis.

c. Chronic renal failure—continuous ambulatory peritoneal dialysis (CAPD): In CAPD, about 2 liters of dialysate are pumped through the patient's peritoneum several times a day. The dialysate contains dextrose in concentrations ranging from 1.5 to 4.25 percent per liter. Since approximately 80 percent of this glucose is absorbed, calorie requirements to maintain body weight are lower, approximately 25 to 30 kcal/kg/day[86] On the other hand, protein loss in the dialysate is greater with CAPD than with hemodialysis. Therefore, protein requirements to maintain LBM are higher. Intakes of 1.2 to 1.5 g/kg/day are recommended to maintain LBM.[86]

REFERENCES

1. Goldman RF: Effect of environment and metabolism. In Report of the First Ross Conference on Medical Research: Assessment of Energy Metabolism in Health and Disease. Columbus, Ohio: Ross Laboratories, 1980, p 117

2. Grande F: Energy expenditure of organs and tissues. In Report of the First Ross Conference on Medical Research: Assessment of Energy Metabolism in Health and Disease. Columbus, Ohio: Ross Laboratories, 1980, pp 88–92

3. Cunningham JJ: A reanalysis of the factors influencing basal metabolic rate in normal adults. Am J Clin Nutr 33:2372–2374, 1980

4. Jequier E: Studies with direct calorimetry in humans: Thermal body insulation and thermoregulatory responses during exercise. In Report of the First Ross Conference on Medical Research: Assessment of Energy Metabolism in Health and Disease. Columbus, Ohio: Ross Laboratories, 1980, pp 15–20

5. Webb P, Annis JF, Troutman SJ: Energy balance in man measured by direct and indirect calorimetry. Am J Clin Nutr 33:1287–1298, 1980

6. Webb P: The measurement of energy exchange in man: An analysis. Am J Clin Nutr 33:1299–1310, 1980

7. Kinney JM, Duke JH, Long CL, Gump FE: Tissue fuel and weight loss after injury. J Clin Path 23 (suppl 4):65–72, 1970

8. Long CL, Schaffel N, Geiger JW, et al.: Metabolic response to injury and illness: Estimation of energy and protein needs from indirect calorimetry and nitrogen balance. JPEN 3(6):452–456, 1979

9. Viteri FE, Torún B: Protein–calorie malnutrition. In Goodhart RS, Shils M (eds): Modern Nutrition in Health and Disease, 6th ed. Phil-

adephia: Lea & Febiger, 1980, pp 697–720

10. Weir JB deV: New methods for calculating metabolic rate with special reference to protein metabolism. J Physiol 109:1, 1949

11. Gazzaniga AB, Polachek JR, Wilson AF, Day AT: Indirect calorimetry as a guide to caloric replacement during total parenteral nutrition. Am J Surg 136:128–133, 1978

12. Johnson RE: Techniques for measuring gas exchange. In Report of the First Ross Conference on Medical Research: Assessment of Energy Metabolism in Health and Disease. Columbus, Ohio: Ross Laboratories, 1980, pp 32–36

13. Moore FD: Energy and the maintenance of body cell mass. JPEN 4:228, 1980

14. Flatt JP: Energetics of intermediary metabolism. In Report of the First Ross Conference on Medical Research: Assessment of Energy Metabolism in Health and Disease. Columbus, Ohio: Ross Laboratories, 1980, pp 77–87

15. Danforth E: Nutritionally induced alterations in metabolism. In Report of the First Ross Conference on Medical Research: Assessment of Energy Metabolism in Health and Disease. Columbus, Ohio: Ross Laboratories, 1980, pp 139–141

16. Cockcroft DW, Gault MH: Prediction of creatinine clearance from serum creatinine. Nephron 16:31–41, 1976

17. Wyndham CH, Strydom NB, von Rensburg AJ, et al.: Relation between VO_2 max and body temperature in hot-humid air conditions. J Appl Physiol 29:45, 1970

18. Harris JA, Benedict FG: A biometric study of basal metabolism in man. Washington, D.C.: Carnegie Institute of Washington, Pub. No. 279, 1919

19. Moore FD, Olesen KH, McMurrey JD, et al.: The Body Cell Mass And Its Supporting Environment: Body Composition in Health and Disease. Philadelphia: W. B. Saunders, 1963

20. Bergren G, Christensen EH: Heart rate and body temperature as indices of metabolic rate during work. Arbeits Physiologie 14:255, 1950

21. Acheson KJ, Campbell JT, Edholm OG. et al.: The measurement of daily energy expenditure: An evaluation of some techniques. Am J Clin Nutr 33:1155–1164, 1980

22. Dennis RS, Long CL, Hall T, Blakemore WS: The clinical use of pulse rates to determine daily energy expenditure in trauma and surgical patients. JPEN 4:597A, 1980

23. Wilmore DW: The Metabolic Care of the Critically Ill. New York: Plenum, 1977, pp 18–27

24. Sargent J, Gotch F, Borah M, et al.: Urea kinetics: A guide to nurtitional management of renal failure. Am J Clin Nutr 31:1696–1702, 1978
25. Kleiber M: The Fire of Life—An Introduction to Animal Energetics. New York: John Wiley, 1961
26. Dubois D, Dubois EF: Clinical calorimetry: A formula to estimate the approximate surface area if weight and height be known. Arch Intern Med 17:683, 1916
27. Boothby WM, Berkson J, Dunn HL: Studies of the energy metabolism of normal individuals. Am J Physiol 116:468, 1936
28. Fleisch A: Le metabolisme basal standard et sa determination au moyen du "metabocalculator." Helv Med Acta 18:23–44, 1951
29. Long CL, Kinney JM, Geiger JW: Nonsuppressability of gluconeogenesis by glucose in septic patients. Metabolism 25(2):193–200, 1976
30. Long CL, Kopp K, Kinney JM: Energy demands during ambulation in surgical convalescence. Surg Forum 20:93–94, 1969
31. The National Research Council: Recommended Dietary Allowances, 9th ed. Washington, D.C.: The National Academy of Sciences, 1980
32. Moore FD: Endocrine-metabolic response to surgery and injury: Summary of remarks. JPEN 4:173–174, 1980
33. Birkhahn R: Alternate or supplemental energy sources. JPEN 5:24–31, 1981
34. Cuthbertson D: Metabolic response to injury and its nutritional implications: Retrospect and prospect. JPEN 3:108–136, 1979
35. Flear CTG, Bhattacharya SS, Singh CM: Solute and water exchanges between cells and extracellular fluids in health and disturbances after trauma. JPEN 4:98–120, 1980
36. Grande F, Keys A: Body weight, body composition and calorie status. In Goodhart RS, Shils ME (eds): Modern Nutrition in Health and Disease, 6th ed. Philadelphia: Lea & Febiger, 1980, pp 27–31
37. Mahalko JR, Johnson LK: Accuracy of predictions of long term energy needs. J Am Diet Assoc 77:557–561, 1980
38. Krause MV, Mahan LK: Food, Nutrition and Diet Therapy, 6th ed. Philadelphia: W. B. Saunders, 1979
39. White EC, McNamara DJ, Ahrens EH Jr: Validation of a dietary record system for the estimation of daily cholesterol intake in individual outpatients. Am J Clin Nutr 34:199, 1981
40. Munro HN, Crim MC: The proteins and amino acids. In Goodhart RS, Shils ME, (eds): Modern Nutrition in Health and Disease, 6th ed. Philadelphia: Lea & Febiger, 1980, pp 51–98
41. Rutten P, Blackburn GL, Flatt JP, et al.: Determination of optimal hyperalimentation infusion rate. J Surg Res 18:477, 1975
42. MacBurney M, Wilmore D: Rational decision making in nutrition care. Surg Clin North Am 61(3):571–582, 1981
43. Roza AM, Shizgal HM: The Harris-Benedict equation reevaluated: Resting energy requirements and the body cell mass. Am J Clin Nutr 40(1):168–182, 1984
44. Calloway DH, Spector H: Nitrogen balance as related to calorie and protein intake in active young men. Am J Clin Nutr 2:405, 1955
45. Wolfe BM, Culebras JM, Tweedle DE, et al.: Effect of glucose on the nitrogen-sparing effects of carbohydrate and fat on amino acid utilization in fasting man. Ann Surg 186:518–540, 1977
46. Elwyn D: Nutritional requirements of adult surgical patients. Crit Care Med 8:9–20, 1980
47. Spanier AH, Shizgal HM: Calorie requirements of the critically ill patient receiving intravenous hyperalimentation. Am J Surg 133:99, 1977
48. Young V: Energy metabolism and requirements of the cancer patient. Cancer Res 37:2336–2347, 1977
49. Maghissi K, Teasdale PR: Parenteral feeding in patients with carcinoma of the esophagus treated by surgery: Energy and nitrogen requirements JPEN 4:371, 1980
50. Sheldon G, Petersen SR: Malnutrition and cardiopulmonary function: Relation to oxygen transport. JPEN 4:376–383, 1980
51. Askanazi J, Rosenbaum SH, Hayman AI, et al.: Respiratory changes induced by the large glucose loads of total parenteral nutrition. JAMA 243(14):1444–1447, 1980
52. Dubois E: Basal Metabolism in Health and Disease. New York: Lea & Febiger, 1924
53. Eisenstein A, Singh SP: Hormonal control of nutrient metabolism. In Goodhart RS, Shils ME (eds): Modern Nutrition in Health and Disease, 6th ed. Philadelphia: Lea & Febiger, 1980, pp 537–559
54. Curreri P: Nutritional replacement modalities. J Trauma 19:906–908, 1979
55. Lipschitz DA, Mitchell CO: Enteral hyperali-

mentation and hemopoietic toxicity caused by chemotherapy of small cell lung cancer. JPEN 4:593, 1980

56. Young CR, Smith RC, Hill GL: Effect of an elemental diet on body composition: A comparison with intravenous nutrition. Gastroenterology 77:652–657, 1979

57. Wretlind A: Development of fat emulsions JPEN 5:230–235, 1981

58. Beisel WR, Wannemacher RW: Gluconeogenesis, ureagenesis and ketogenesis during sepsis. JPEN 4:277–285, 1980

59. Cerra FB, Seigel JH, Border JR, et al: The hepatic failure of sepsis: Cellular versus substrate. Surgery 86:409–422, 1979

60. Cerra FB: Pocket Manual of Surgical Nutrition. St. Louis: C. V. Mosby, 1984

61. Cerra FB, Upson D, Angelico R, et al.: Branched chain amino acids support postoperative protein synthesis. Surgery 92:192–199, 1982

62. Freund H, Hoover HC, Atamian S, Fischer J: Infusion of the branched chain amino acids in postoperative patients. Ann Surg 190:18–23, 1979

63. Burke JF, Wolfe RR, Mullany CJ, et al.: Glucose requirements following burn injury. Ann Surg 190(3):274–285, 1979

64. Hiebert JM, Anderson RG, Edlich RF, Rodeheaver GT: Fueling the burned patient: When does enteric nitrogen to calorie ratio influence nitrogen balance? (abstr) Am Burn Assoc Meeting, April, 1981

65. Askanazi J, Rosenbaum SH, Nordenstrom J, et al.: Nutrition for the patient with respiratory failure (abstr) Anesthesiology 51(3):S192, 1979

66. Greene HL, Hazlett D, Demaree R: Relationship between intralipid-induced hyperlipemia and pulmonary function. Am J Clin Nutr 29:127, 1976

67. Askanazi J, Rosenbaum SH, Hayman AI, et al.: Effects of parenteral nutrition on ventilatory drive (abstr). Anesthesiology 53(3):S185, 1980

68. Weissman C, Askanazi J, Rosenbaum SH, et al.: Amino acids and respiration. Ann Intern Med 98(1):41–44, 1983

69. Askanazi J, Weissman C, Rosenbaum SH, et al.: Nutrition and the respiratory system. Crit Care Med 10(3):163–172, 1983

70. Floch MH: Nutritional and Diet Therapy in Gastrointestinal Disease. New York: Plenum, 1981

71. Zeman FS: Clinical Nutrition and Dietetics. Lexington, Mass: D. C. Heath, 1983

72. Munro HN, Fernstrom JD, Wurtman RJ, et al.: Insulin, plasma amino acid imbalance, and hepatic coma. Lancet 1:722, 1975

73. Zeisel SH, Sheard NF: Nutrition and neurotransmitters: Clinical implications. Outline of presentation at the conference on Advances in Hyperalimentation: A Practical Approach, Harvard Medical School, September 12–14, 1984

74. Bernardini P, Fischer JE: Amino acid imbalance and hepatic encephalopathy. Annu Rev Nutr 2:419, 1982

75. Rossi-Fannelli F, Riggio O, Cangiano C, et al.: Branched-chain amino acids vs. lactulose in the treatment of hepatic coma—a controlled study. Dig Dis Sci 27:929, 1982

76. McGhee A, Henderson M, Warren WD, et al.: Comparison of the effects of Hepatic-Aid and a casein modular diet on encephalopathy, plasma amino acids and nitrogen balance in cirrhotic patients. Ann Surg 197:288, 1983

77. Horst D: Nutritional support in liver disease. Outline of talk given at conference on Advances in Hyperalimentation: A Practical Approach, Harvard Medical School, September 12–14, 1984

78. O'Keefe SJD, Sender PM, James WPT: "Catabolic" loss of body nitrogen in response to surgery. Lancet 2:1035, 1974

79. Hörl WA, Heidland A: Enhanced proteolytic activity—cause of protein catabolism in acute renal failure. Am J Clin Nutr 33:1423–1427, 1980

80. Roppler JD: Nutritional management of chronic renal failure. Postgrad Med 64:135–144, 1978

81. Quintanilla A, Shambaugh GE, Gibson TP, Craig R: Glucose metabolism in uremia. Am J Clin Nutr 33(7):1446–1450, 1980

82. Reaven GM, Swenson RS, Sanfelippo ML: An inquiry into the mechanism of hypertriglyceridemia in patients with chronic renal failure. Am J Clin Nutr 33:1476–1484, 1980

83. Fullerson RL: The renal nutrition field in review: The increasing emphasis on protein and calories. Contemp Dialysis, December 1982, pp 58–61

84. Giordano C: Amino acids and ketoacids—advantages and pitfalls. Am J Clin Nutr 33:1649–1653, 1980

85. Kampf D, Fischer HC, Kessel M: Efficacy of an unselected protein diet (24 g) with minor oral

supply of essential amino acids and ketoana-logues compared with a selective protein diet (40 g) in chronic renal failure. Am J Clin Nutr 33:1673–1677, 1980

86. Baig F, Brubaker KA, Ali AS: Nutritional im-plications in CAPD. Contemp Dialysis, March 1982, pp 37–41

11. Vitamin and Mineral Requirements
Charlette Gallagher-Allred

The essentiality of vitamins and minerals to health has been known for centuries. In the 2nd century BC, Cato the Elder identified that cabbage could cure an illness that today is believed to have been scurvy. In the 13th century, scurvy was described. During the 17th century, other deficiency symptoms, such as beriberi were recognized. At this time certain factors, later called vitamins, were recognized by their absence, not by their presence. It was not until several centuries later that certain foods were recommended as protective against deficiency diseases. In 1911 these protective factors were named vitamins, called then vitamine from vital amine, by Funk.

During the present century much has been learned concerning the metabolism and function, sources, and deficiency/toxicity states of vitamins and minerals. Use of total parenteral nutrition (TPN) within the last 20 years, often as the sole source of nutrients for nourishing individuals, has added a new dimension for studying vitamins and minerals. There are still wide gaps in our understanding of vitamin and mineral metabolism, however. Although we are able today to recognize specific vitamin and mineral deficiencies and to cure them with appropriate nutrients, we have yet to determine much about their actual biochemical functioning in metabolic processes. It is the purpose of this chapter to summarize current knowledge about vitamins and minerals, including functions, absorption, utilization, and deficiency/toxicity states. In addition, recommendations for oral and intravenous intakes are summarized. Dietary nutrient sources along with selected commercial enteral and parenteral preparations are also reviewed.

GENERAL FUNCTIONS OF VITAMINS AND MINERALS

Vitamins

Although vitamins and minerals constitute only a small part of human tissue, they are essential in many vital processes. Vitamins are potent organic compounds that cannot be synthesized by the organism but must be obtained from the diet, and their absence or improper absorption results in specific deficiency diseases. Fat-soluble vitamins, especially vitamins A and D, may function as hormones. Others, including the vitamin B complex, function as biologic catalysts or coenzymes in the many varied enzyme systems of the body. Vitamins, minerals (particularly calcium, zinc, and magnesium), or both make up the prosthetic portion of complete enzymes (holoenzyme). The prosthetic portion of the enzyme serves to activate the protein portion (apoenzyme) of the enzyme, which is composed of specific amino acids determined by the genetic code.

Minerals

In general, the vitamin portion of the enzyme is called the co-enzyme, and the mineral portion is called the activator. Minerals serve four major roles in the human organism: (1) as enzyme activators, (2) as structural components, (3) as integral components of organic compounds, and (4) as major factors in regulation of acid–base and fluid–electrolyte balance. Minerals may be classified as macro- or microelements depending on the amount of each that is required in the diet. Macroelements include calcium, phosphorus, magnesium, sodium, potassium, chloride, and sulfur. Microelements, or trace elements, include iron, zinc, copper, chromium, cobalt, manganese, selenium, fluorine, iodine, molybdenum, vanadium, tin, silicon, and nickel.

Current knowledge of the physiology, functions, and food sources of fat-soluble and water-soluble vitamins (Table 11–1) and the macro- and microelements (Table 11–2) has been summarized. A schematic summary of the gastrointestinal (GI) sites of absorption of these nutrients is depicted in Figure 11–1.

VITAMIN AND MINERAL REQUIREMENTS IN TOTAL PARENTERAL NUTRITION

Vitamin and mineral requirements for patients receiving enteral feedings are not thought to be significantly different than when oral feedings are administered. Vitamin and mineral requirements for patients receiving TPN, however, have not been determined with certainty and are constantly under study. Determination of nutrient requirements is difficult and is plagued with problems in controlling the variables which

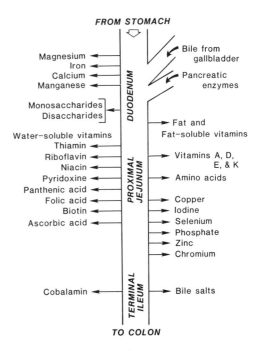

Figure 11–1. Summary of nutrient absorption sites.

are essential to control when guidelines are to be developed for general use. Laboratory tests appropriate for measuring efficacy of vitamin and mineral supplementation via TPN solutions are shown in Table 11–3. The appropriateness of these tests will be confirmed with future TPN research.

Vitamins

General. The Nutrition Advisory Group of the American Medical Association (AMA) Department of Foods and Nutrition has recommended specific amounts of essential parenteral vitamins for infants and children up to 11 years of age and for those age 11 or older. These recommendations, published in 1979, are shown in Table 11–1 under the heading "Needs and Allowances." When published, these recommendations were stated to be based largely on the oral Recommended Dietary Allowances (RDA) and were to be used as tentative guidelines, requiring research and revision as warranted. Many researchers have stressed that the AMA's 1979 recommendations are probably an underestimation of actual needs, citing that the figures are based on needs of nonstressed individuals with normometabolic states. Patients receiving TPN are often stressed and/or hypermetabolic. The content and quantity of TPN administered will depend in part upon the following needs of patients:

1. Need for reversal of nutrient depletion
2. Need associated with fever, infection, or other stresses
3. Need for anabolic processes
4. Need for compensation of excessive urinary losses when administered by a venous catheter

The fact that most patients who receive TPN are highly stressed and catabolic, and therefore need additional kilocalories and protein, may well indicate that they also need additional vitamins and minerals for anabolism and metabolism.[1] For example, thiamin, niacin, and riboflavin needs appear to be positively related to energy intake and body mass, and pyridoxine appears to be positively associated with protein intake. Increased needs of these vitamins can be expected when increased energy and nitrogen are administered to the catabolic patient.[2]

A recent report indicates that large amounts of fat-soluble vitamins given via TPN adhere to bags and tubing and may therefore never reach the patient.[3] Gills et al.[3] found that the average amount of the administered dose theoretically received by the TPN patient was only 31 percent for vitamin A, 68 percent for vitamin D, and 64 percent for vitamin E. It is imperative that measures be found for improving delivery, such as solubilizing the vitamins in an aqueous medium and reducing the lipophilic properties of the inner surfaces of the TPN bags and tubing. Proper covering of TPN bags and tubing is also essential to inhibit the effect of light on losses of nutrients such as riboflavin and lysine.

With the increasing use of self-administered TPN at home, the importance of ease and sanitation in solution mixing and delivery has become paramount. In a recent study, researchers demonstrated that giving ascorbic acid, thiamin, niacin, pyridoxine, and folacin twice weekly, rather than daily, can be safe and adequate to maintain vitamin status.[4] This may make home delivery of TPN solutions easier and safer.

Folacin. Patients receiving TPN may require vitamins and minerals in amounts greater than general guidelines if the patient had marginal stores or frank deficiency states prior to a period of stress or TPN administration. For example, Stromberg et al.[2] found that 200 μg/day of folacin was adequate for maintenance in 15 patients receiving TPN for postsurgical complications, but this amount could not reliably correct a deficiency state. In this study, researchers reported no low serum levels of riboflavin, pyridoxine, or vitamin B_{12} on intakes of approximately 50 percent of the AMA's guidelines. Stromberg,[2] however, stressed that in patients with subclinical vitamin B_{12} deficiency, subacute combined degeneration of the spinal cord could be precipitated by folacin therapy. Several studies of folate deficiency in patients receiving TPN have been recently summarized.[5]

Biotin. TPN vitamin solutions have traditionally included major water-soluble and fat-soluble vitamins, but have often been lacking in some vitamins whose requirements are small. One such vitamin is biotin. It is generally thought that biotin deficiency is rare, occurring only in one of two situations: (1) if patients consume a biotin-free diet and take oral antibiotics to destroy synthesis of biotin by gut flora, or (2) if one consumes large amounts of raw egg whites which contain avidin that binds biotin and thereby renders it unavailable for absorption. Biotin deficiency can be produced in patients on prolonged solutions of TPN devoid of biotin.[6–8] Such patients may develop al-

TABLE 11–1. SUMMARY OF VITAMINS IN HUMAN NUTRITION[1–8,26–29]

Vitamin	Function	Metabolism	Needs and Allowances
Thiamin Vitamin B_1	As cofactor thiamin pyrophosphate (TPP) or co-carboxylase in decarboxylation of pyruvate to acetyl CoA and alpha-ketoglutarate to succinyl CoA in tricarboxylic acid cycle (TCA), and in decarboxylation of alpha-keto analogs of branch chain amino acids. As TPP in transketolase reaction in pentose-phosphate shunt, an alternate pathway for glucose oxidation, production of ribose-5-phosphate for nucleic acid synthesis and production of NADPH for fatty acid synthesis.	Absorption: Small intestine by diffusion and active transport requiring sodium and ATP. Transport: Blood Storage: Limited Excretion: Urine and perspiration	RDA: Men = 1.2–1.5 mg Women = 1.0–1.1 mg Pregnancy = 1.4–1.5 mg Lactation = 1.5–1.6 mg Infants = 0.3–0.5 mg Children = 0.7–1.4 mg RDA based on 0.5 mg per 1000 kcal intake. Protein and fat intake may spare thiamin requirement. Alcohol and carbohydrate intake may increase requirement. Requirement increased with fever, exercise, surgery, hyperthyroidism, alcoholism. Parenteral Needs: Adults = 3 mg/day Children = 1.2 mg/day
Riboflavin Vitamin B_2	As coenzyme FAD or FMN to catalyze oxidation-phosophorylation reactions in mitochondria of cells to produce ATP (amino acid oxidase, xanthine oxidase, glutathione reductase). As FAD in dehydrogenase reactions in TCA cycle to convert succinate to fumarate, and in fatty acid betaoxidation. Essential in pyridoxine activation. Essential for growth, synthesis of corticosteroids, RBC, and thyroid enzymes.	Absorption: Small intestine. May require phosphorylation in intestinal mucosa prior to absorption. Increased gut absorption with presence of food. Transport: Blood Storage: Limited Excretion: Urinary metabolites	RDA: Men = 1.4–1.6 mg Women = 1.2–1.3 mg Pregnancy = 1.5–1.6 mg Lactation = 1.7–1.8 mg Infancy = 0.4–0.6 mg Children = 0.8–1.4 mg RDA based on 0.6 mg per 1000 kcal intake Requirements probably relate more to body mass than calorie intake. Requirements increase with growth, wound healing. Parenteral Needs: Adults = 3.6 mg/day Children = 1.4 mg/day

Deficiency	Toxicity	Enteral and Parenteral Sources	Chemistry
Beriberi. Fatigue, emotional instability, depression, irritability, retarded growth, bradycardia, weakened heart muscle, cardiac failure, ascites, peripheral edema, lowered body temperature. Slowed CNS function due to low blood glucose and destruction of brain cells, nerve fibers, peripheral nerves. Deep muscle pain in calf of leg; may progress to paralysis and muscle atrophy. GI symptoms of indigestion, constipation, anorexia, weight loss, gastric atony, HCl deficiency. Alcoholic polyneuropathy (Wernicke-Korsakoff's syndrome). Reduced erythrocyte transketolase activity.	None known except in amounts thousands of times larger than needs resulting in death by depression of respiratory center. Anaphylactic shock in man is rare but can occur when given in large amounts IV.	Foods: Pork, liver, organ meats, lean meat, poultry, egg yolk, fish, dried beans and peas, wheat germ, soybeans, peanuts, whole grains, enriched grain products Enteral Sources: Thiamin chloride Thiamin hydrochloride Parenteral Sources: Thiamin hydrochloride	Crystalline yellow-white powder, salty, nutty taste. Heat stable in acid. Heat unstable in alkali. Loss with alkali, long cooking time, high temperature, large amount of water.
Ariboflavinosis. Head disorders include cheilosis, angular stomatitis, glossitis, bleeding gums, dermatitis around nose, occular disorders (cornea vascularization). Other symptoms include growth retardation, scrotum dermatitis, reproductive abnormalities, fatty liver, hypoglycemia.	None known	Foods: Milk, cheese, organ meats, lean meats, eggs, green leafy vegetables, enriched cereals and breads. Enteral Sources: Riboflavin Parenteral Sources: Riboflavin phosphate	Yellow-green fluorescent pigment Slightly water soluble. Destroyed by alkali, visible or UV light, stable to heat, acid, oxygen. Little loss with cooking

(continued)

TABLE 11–1. (*Continued*)

Vitamin	Function	Metabolism	Needs and Allowances
Niacin Nicotinic acid	In nicotinamide form as NAD/NADH or NADP/NADPH in dehydrogenase reactions, serving as hydrogen acceptors and donors. Functions in glycolysis, alcohol metabolism, fatty acid synthesis, TCA cycle oxidative phosphorylation.	Absorption: Small intestine, passive diffusion Transport: Blood Storage: Limited Excretion: Urine as N-methylnicotinamide and 2-pyridone	RDA: Men = 18–19 mg NE (Niacin Equivalents) Women = 13–15 mg NE Pregnancy = 15–17 mg NE Lactation = 18–20 mg NE Infants = 6–8 mg NE Children = 9–16 mg NE RDA for adults based on 6.6 mg NE per 1000 kcal intake Tryptophan can contribute to NE (60 mg tryptophan = 1 mg niacin and on average protein is 1 percent tryptophan). Parenteral Needs: Adults = 40 mg/day Children = 17 mg/day
Pyridoxine Vitamin B_6	In pyridoxal-phosphate coenzyme form involved in nonoxidative degradation of amino acids including transamination (GOT, GPT), deamination, desulfuration, and dehydration. Decarboxylation reactions including synthesis of epinephrine and norepinephrine from tyrosine, histamine from histidine, serotonin from tryptophan. Synthesis of niacin from tryptophan. Synthesis of sphingolipids and myelin sheath. Maintenance of cellular immunity. Synthesis of porphyrins. As part of phosphorylase (storage form of B_6), facilitates release of glycogen from liver and muscle.	Absorption: Small intestine, passive diffusion. Some bacterial synthesis in gut. Transport: Blood Storage: Limited Excretion: Urine as 4-pyridoxic acid, pyridoxal, pyridoxamine, pyridoxine.	RDA: Men = 1.8–2.2 mg Women = 1.8–2 mg Pregnancy = 2.4–2.6 mg Lactation = 2.3–2.5 mg Infants = 0.3–0.6 mg Children = 0.9–1.3 mg Requirement increases as protein intake increases, with oral contraceptive use, and with penicillamine, isoniazid, cycloserine, and semicarbaside administration. Parenteral Needs: Adults = 4 mg/day Children = 1 mg/day

Deficiency	Toxicity	Enteral and Parenteral Sources	Chemistry
Pellagra, characterized by dermatitis (bilateral), dementia, diarrhea, death. GI symptoms include anorexia, indigestion, sore tongue, inflamed gut and mouth membranes. CNS and mental changes include tremors, neuritis, confusion, lassitude. Also seen are skin eruptions and muscle weakness.	Skin flushing, vasodilating effects, headaches, increased metabolic activity, tingling of extremities, GI tract irritation, possible liver damage.	Foods: Tryptophan-Niacin equivalents: Milk, eggs, lean meat, organ meats, poultry, fish, Brewer's yeast, peanuts, peanut butter, enriched or whole grain products. Enteral Source: Niacinamide Parenteral Source: Niacinamide	White crystal. Water soluble. Stable when dry. Stable in heat, light, air, acid, alkali. Little loss with cooking.
GI symptoms include nausea, vomiting, mucous membrane lesions, cheilosis, glossitis, stomatitis. Kidney problems include increased urinary oxalate and urea excretion and renal stone formation. Also see anemia, seborrheic dermatitis, peripheral neuritis, depression. Biochemical findings include increased xanthurenic acid excretion, decreased SGOT and SGPT activities, decreased DNA and mRNA synthesis, and impaired immune response.	Sleepiness Liver damage	Foods: Yeast, wheat germ, pork, liver, whole grains, meat, legumes, potatoes, bananas, oatmeal, soybeans, nuts Enteral Source: Pyridoxine hydrochloride Parenteral Source: Pyridoxine hydrochloride	White, crystal, odorless. Soluble in water and alcohol. Stable in heat with acid. Unstable in alkali and light.

(continued)

TABLE 11–1. (*Continued*)

Vitamin	Function	Metabolism	Needs and Allowances
Pantothenic acid	As part of coenzyme A in TCA cycle in transfer of acyl groups and in transfer of acetyl groups. Synthesis of cholesterol, steroid hormones. Synthesis of phospholipids, ketones, fatty acids. Beta oxidation of fatty acid. Degradation of alcohol. Synthesis of porphyrin for hemoglobin and cytochromes. Metabolism of some amino acids.	Absorption: Upper small intestine, probable gut synthesis by bacteria Transport: Blood Storage: Limited Excretion: Urine and feces	RDA: Not established; safe and adequate daily intakes as follows: Adults = 4–7 mg Children = 3–5 mg Infants = 2–3 mg Normal diet = 10–15 mg/day Decreased serum or tissue content found in patients with Korsakoff's psychoses, chronic ulcerative colitis, and granulomatous colitis. Parenteral Needs: Adults = 15 mg/day Children = 5 mg/day
Biotin	Activator for many enzyme systems including CO_2 fixation from compounds in fat synthesis, acetyl CoA carboxylase, propionyl CoA carboxylase, beta methylcrotonyl carboxylase, pyruvate carboxylase, methylmalonyl CoA transcarboxylase. Essential in cholesterol synthesis and gluconeogenesis and in deamination of amino acids.	Absorption: Proximal small intestine and colon. Probably active transport. Gut synthesis by bacteria. Decreased absorption in achlorhydria. Transport: Blood Storage: Limited, liver Excretion: Urine, feces	RDA: Not established; safe and adequate daily intakes as follows: Adults = 100–200 µg Children = 65–120 µg Infants = 35–50 µg Average daily intake = 100–300 µg/day Parenteral Needs: Adults = 60 µg/day Treat deficiency with 100–300 µg/day. Children = 20 µg/day
Folacin Pteroylglutamic acid	As tetrahydrofolate in transfer of single carbon units in synthesis of DNA, RNA, methionine, serine. Synthesis of purines (guanine, adenine) and pyrimidine (thymine) to form DNA, RNA. Oxidation of histidine to glutamic acid. Formation of heme, RBC, WBC.	Absorption: Entire small bowel, especially in proximal third of small intestine following deconjugation; mainly by active transport with some passive diffusion. Gut bacterial synthesis. Transport: Plasma bound to many plasma proteins and glycoproteins.	RDA: Men = 400 µg Women = 400 µg Pregnancy = 800 µg Lactation = 500 µg Infants = 30–45 µg Children = 100–300 µg Alcohol increases requirement. Parenteral Needs: Adults = 400 µg/day Children = 140 µg/day

Deficiency	Toxicity	Enteral and Parenteral Sources	Chemistry
Rare. When antagonists are given, may cause "burning feet syndrome" with spastic gait. GI symptoms include anorexia, nausea, cramps, ulcer. Other problems include loss of cellular immunity, adrenal gland malfunction, fatigue, insomnia, growth retardation, dermatitis, anemia, leukopenia, hypoglycemia.	None known Possible diarrhea	Foods: "Widespread" Egg, liver, organ meats, salmon, yeast, cereals, all animal and plant sources. Enteral Source: Calcium pantothenate Parenteral Source: Dexpanthanol Calcium pantothenate	White, crystal. Stable in neutral solution. Readily lost with acid, alkali, dry heat.
Rare. Can occur by eating raw egg whites, biotin deficient diet and decreased gut flora. GI symptoms of anorexia, nausea, facial rash. Blood changes include hypercholesterolemia, decreased protein synthesis, anemia, hypoglycemia. Also find dermatitis, paresthesia. EKG changes, conjunctivitis, lethargy.	None known	Foods: Liver, milk, meat, organ meats, egg yolk, yeast, soybeans, nuts, mushrooms, fruits Enteral Source: Biotin Parenteral Source: Biotin	An acid, soluble in water and alcohol, heat stable. Unstable in oxygen, alkali and strong acid.
Poor growth, megaloblastic anemia, glossitis, GI disturbances, irritability, forgetfulness. Deficiency may occur in alcoholism, blind loop syndrome, gluten-induced enteropathy, sprue, alcoholism, and with Dilantin administration	None known Large doses will antagonize anticonvulsants contributing to epileptic seizures	Foods: All foods, liver, kidney and lima beans, fruits, dark green leafy vegetables, beef, potatoes, whole grain products Enteral Source: Folic acid Parenteral Source: Folic acid	Yellow crystal. Water soluble. Unstable to heat in acid. Stable to light when in solution. Lost with high temperature processing such as dried milk.

(continued)

TABLE 11–1. (*Continued*)

Vitamin	Function	Metabolism	Needs and Allowances
Folacin Pteroylglutamic acid (cont.)	Control macrocytic anemia of pregnancy, sprue, and infancy. Correct pernicious anemia but not neurologic lesions.	Storage: Liver, normal stores will last 3–6 mo after cessation of folate ingestion. Excretion: Urine and bile. Enterohepatic circulation important in normal serum folate.	
Cobalamine Vitamin B_{12}	The extrinsic factor of food essential in treatment/prevention of pernicious anemia. Synthesis of single carbon units in synthesis of DNA, RNA, RBC, myelin, purine and pyrimidines. Essential in carbohydrate, fat, and protein metabolism. Essential in converting homocysteine to methionine, and methylmalonate to succinate. Essential in synthesis of folate. Component of mutase enzyme in malonyl CoA degradation.	Absorption: Ileum, requiring intrinsic factor and HCl from stomach, into portal vein. Transport: Bound to plasma B_{12}-binding proteins (Transcobalamin I, II, III) Storage: Liver, kidney Normal stores last 3–6 years after cessation of B_{12} absorption Excretion: Bile, urine, saliva	RDA: Men = 3 μg Women = 3 μg Pregnancy = 4 μg Lactation = 4 μg Infants = 0.5–1.5 μg Children = 2–3 μg Needs increase with bacterial overgrowth, Zollinger-Ellison's syndrome, tropical sprue, diverticulitis, cancer, administration of neomycin, colchicine, PAS. Parenteral Needs: (daily) Adults = 5 μg Children = 1 μg IV treatment for deficiency may be 0.5–1 mg
Ascorbic acid Vitamin C	Hydrogen acceptor or donor. Water-soluble antioxidant which becomes oxidized to protect other antioxidants such as vitamins E and A and the essential fatty acids. Essential in integrity of cell structure, cartilage, dentine, bone, capillaries. Essential in synthesis of collagen, conversion of proline to hydroxyproline. Promotes wound healing, resistance to infection.	Absorption: Upper small intestine probably by passive diffusion. Transport: Blood Storage: Adrenal cortex, kidney, liver, spleen Excretion: Urine	RDA: Men = 60 mg Women = 50–60 mg Pregnancy = 70–80 mg Lactation = 90–100 mg Infants = 35 mg Children = 45 mg Needs increase with fever, infection, stress, acidosis, alkalosis, exercise, injury, smoking. Parenteral Needs: Adults = 100 mg Children = 80 mg

Deficiency	Toxicity	Enteral and Parenteral Sources	Chemistry
Pernicious (megalo-blastic) anemia. Glossitis, neurologic (peripheral nerve, spinal cord or cerebral damage) and mental disorders (psychoses, hallucinations). Deficiency may result from inadequate absorption, vegan diet, alcoholism, poverty, abnormal intrinsic factor secretion, gastric atrophy or gastrectomy, ilectomy, gluten-induced enteropathy, ileitis.	None known	Foods: Liver, kidney, poultry, milk, eggs, meat, fish, cheese. Not found in foods of plant origin. Enteral Source: Cyanocobalamine Parenteral Source: Cyanocobalamine	Contains cobalt chelated in ring structure. Water soluble. Destroyed by acid, alkali, light, oxygen, high vitamin C amounts.
GI problems including anorexia, swollen and inflamed gums, loose teeth. Muscle and cartilage problems including weakness, weight loss, slow growth, stiff limbs, spread legs, swollen ankles and wrist joints, rib juncture enlargement. Also hemorrhage, infection, anemia, neuroses.	Rebound scurvy. Urate, cystine and oxalate stone development; gout. False tests for urine sugar. False tests for fecal occult blood. GI distress, nausea, diarrhea. Electrolyte disturbances. Headaches. Hemolysis. Interference with anticoagulant therapy. Possible mutagenic effects.	Foods: Citrus foods, liver, broccoli, raw leafy vegetables, spinach, turnip/mustard/collard greens, kale, parsley, sweet peppers, guava, cabbage, potatoes, strawberries, papaya, cauliflower, black currants Enteral Source: Ascorbic acid Parenteral Source: Ascorbic acid	White crystal. Water soluble. Stable when dry or in acid solutions. Destroyed by heat, air, alkali. Not lost with freezing.

(continued)

TABLE 11–1. (*Continued*)

Vitamin	Function	Metabolism	Needs and Allowances
Ascorbic acid Vitamin C (cont.)	Essential in oxidation of phenylalanine to tyrosine, and in norepinephrine synthesis. Essential in steroid hormone synthesis. Reduces ferric to ferrous iron to aid in iron absorption.		
Vitamin A Retinol	Combines with opsin to form rhodopsin of retina necessary for normal dim light vision. Growth and development of skeletal and soft tissues, protein synthesis and bone cell differentiation. Enamel formation of teeth. Maintenance of normal epithelial structure and differentiation of basal cells into mucous secreting epithelial cells. Reproduction and lactation.	Absorption: As retinol esters formed in intestinal mucosa cells via chylomicron with other fat-soluble compound absorption into lymph. Provitamin A conversion to vitamin A occurs in intestine wall. Requires bile. Transport: Through lymphatics via chylomicrons en route to storage or through blood attached to retinol-binding protein and prealbumin en route to tissues with metabolic requirement for vitamin A. Storage: Liver, body fat depots Excretion: Feces via biliary excretion	RDA: Men = 1000 μg RE (Retinol Equivalents) Women = 800 μg RE Pregnancy = 1000 μg RE Lactation = 1200 μg RE Infants = 400–420 μg RE Children = 400–700 μg RE Requirement increases with refeeding protein malnourished patients. Parenteral Needs: Adults = 660 μg RE Children = 460 μg RE Treat night blindness with 30,000 IU/day for several days via cod or halibut liver oil. Treat corneal damage with 500,000 IU daily. Provide orally unless fat malabsorption, then give parenterally.
Vitamin D Calciferol	Normal mineralization and formation of bones, teeth. Absorption of calcium and phosphorus from gut and kidney, and maintenance of normal serum calcium and phosphorus.	Absorption: Via chylomicron with other fat-soluble compound absorption into lymph from jejunum and/or ileum. Requires bile. Can be synthesized in skin by UV light on provitamin D_3.	RDA: Men = 5–10 μg Women = 5–10 μg Pregnancy = 10–15 μg Lactation = 10–15 μg Infants = 10 μg Children = 10 μg 10 μg cholecalciferol = 400 IU vitamin D

Deficiency	Toxicity	Enteral and Parenteral Sources	Chemistry
Xeropthalmia. Night blindness. Keratomalacia. Goose flesh. Reproductive failure. Deficiency may occur secondary to protein–calorie malnutrition, celiac disease, obstructive jaundice, infective hepatitis, cystic fibrosis, bile acid deficiency.	Hydrocephalus. Pseudotumor cerebri. Major symptoms include enlarged liver, spleen, cirrhosis (yellow skin except sclera of eyes with hypercarotenemia). Also GI symptoms of vomiting, nausea. Stunted growth, changes in leg length, fragile bones, bone pain, coarse and lost hair, scaly and dry skin, nose bleeds, anemia, headaches, insomnia, blurred vision, fatigue, malaise.	Foods: Fish liver oils, liver, kidney, butter, fortified margarine, egg yolk, whole or fortified skim or 2% milk, cream, cheese. Provitamin A found in dark green leafy vegetables, yellow vegetables and fruits, greens, carrots, sweet potato, squash, apricot, peach, cantaloupe. Enteral Source: Vitamin A palmitate Parenteral Source: Vitamin A	Beta carotene produces 2 molecules of vitamin A. Pale, yellow crystalline alcohol. Fat-soluble. Heat and light stable. Destroyed by oxidation, UV light, acid, high temperature, dehydration. Vitamin E prevents oxidation.
Rickets, osteomalacia, bone fragility, noncalcified broad epiphyseal plate. Cardiac arrhythmias. Deficiency may occur secondary to fat malabsorption, chronic pan-	Hypervitaminosis D. Characterized by excess bone calcification and stiffness, soft tissue calcification, kidney stone development and kidney insufficiency, hypercalcemia.	Foods: Fish liver oils, butter, cream, whole and fortified milk, egg yolk, liver. Enteral Source: Vitamin D_3 Parenteral Source: Vitamin D_3	Fat-soluble. Highly stable to heat, oxidation, acid, and base.

(continued)

TABLE 11–1. (*Continued*)

Vitamin	Function	Metabolism	Needs and Allowances
Vitamin D Calciferol (cont.)		Transport: Through lymphatics via chylomicron, through blood via globulin. Activated by liver and kidney to 1,25-dihydroxychole-calciferol. Storage: Liver Excretion: Via bile	Treat vitamin D resistant rickets in children with 50,000–100,000 IU daily Parenteral Needs: Adults = 5 μg Children = 10 μg
Vitamin E Tocopherol	Intracellular antioxidant to prevent formation of peroxides from polyunsaturated fatty acids; prevent oxidation of vitamins A and C, prevent cellular membrane deterioration by lipid peroxidation.	Absorption: Via chylomicron with other fat-soluble compound absorption into lymph. Transport: Blood Storage: Liver Excretion: As urinary metabolites	RDA: Men = 8–10 mg TE (Tocopherol Equivalents) Women = 8 mg TE Pregnancy = 10 mg TE Lactation = 11 mg TE Infants = 3–4 mg TE Children = 5–7 mg TE Parenteral Needs: Adults = 10 mg TE Children = 7 mg TE
Vitamin K	Prothrombin (factor II) synthesis and synthesis of several related proteins involved in blood clotting (factors VII, IX, X). May participate in tissue respiration.	Absorption: Upper small intestine with absorption of other fat-soluble compounds via chylomicron into lymph. Vitamin K produced by GI flora has limited ileal/colon absorption. Transport: Via chylomicron through lymphatics Storage: Liver, skin, muscle Excretion: As urinary metabolites	RDA: Not established; safe and adequate daily intakes as follows: Adults = 70–140 μg Children = 15–60 μg Infants = 10–20 μg Parenteral Needs: Adults = 0.7–2 mg Children = 0.2 mg as phylloquinone

From references 1–8, 26–29.

Deficiency	Toxicity	Enteral and Parenteral Sources	Chemistry
creatitis, celiac disease, biliary obstruction, liver or kidney disease, hypoparathyroidism.	Also see headaches, anorexia, nausea, vomiting, constipation, hypertension, cardiac arrhythmia, polyuria, polydypsia.		
Hemolysis and megaloblastic anemia in infants fed cow's milk. Some pediatricians supplement vitamin E from 10th day onward in premature infants who are artificially fed. Edema, skin lesions, elevated platelets in premature infants receiving formulas high in PUFA. Creatinuria, muscle weakness, hemolysis in patients with severe fat malabsorption.	Interference with vitamin K and blood clotting causing delayed clot time (especially in patients on anticoagulant therapy), headaches, nausea, fatigue, dizziness, GI pain, muscle weakness, hypoglycemia, blurred vision by antagonizing vitamin A.	Foods: Wheat germ, cereal germ, vegetable and seed oils, nuts, legumes, eggs, green plants, milk, fat, meat, liver, fish. Enteral Source: Vitamin E acetate Parenteral Source: Vitamin E acetate	Oily yellow liquid, fat soluble. Heat and acid stable. Oxidized in alkali, oxygen, rancid fat, iron, lead, UV light.
Hemorrhage, prolonged prothrombin time, blood loss. May occur secondary to obstructive jaundice, bile fistula, sprue, pellegra, regional ileitis, ulcerative colitis, chronic liver disease, premature newborn infants, antibiotic therapy.	Hemolytic anemia with RBC destruction.	Foods: Leafy green vegetables, broccoli, lettuce, spinach, greens, cauliflower, tomatoes, liver, wheat bran, soybean oil, cheese, egg yolk, green tea, fish oil. Enteral Source: Phylloquinone Parenteral Source: Phylloquinone hydrochloride Phylloquinone acetate	Fat soluble. Heat stable. Destroyed by sunlight and alkali.

TABLE 11–2. SUMMARY OF MINERALS IN HUMAN NUTRITION[9,11,13 – 15,18,20,23,26 – 28,30 – 47]

Mineral	Function	Metabolism
Calcium	Major component of bone hydroxyapatite and teeth. Essential in muscle contraction and nerve irritability. Activator for several enzymes. Essential in blood coagulation.	Absorption: Acid media of small intestine according to need. Facilitated by vitamin D, vitamin C, lactose, lysine, arginine, and parathyroid hormone (indirectly via 1,25-dihydroxycholecalciferol). Inhibited by oxalate, phytate, fat malabsorption, alkali. Transport: Plasma as free or complexed to albumin or globulin, calcium binding protein. Storage: Skeleton, teeth Excretion: Feces, urine, sweat
Phosphorus	Major component of bone hydroxyapatite and teeth. Essential component of phosphorylation reactions in metabolism of carbohydrate, protein, and fat, and in energy production. Component of nucleic acids, phospholipids, phosphocreatine, nucleoproteins, lecithin. Part of acid–base buffer system. Major intracellular anion.	Absorption: Upper small intestine as free phosphate. Facilitated by parathyroid hormone. Inhibited by phytates, oxalates, malabsorption. Transport: Plasma as unfilterable phosphate (e.g. $CaPO_4$), ultrafilterable phosphate (e.g. HPO_4^- or H_2PO_4). Storage: Bone and teeth with some in tissues, membranes, skeletal muscle, nervous tissue Excretion: Urine, feces

Needs and Allowances	Deficiency	Toxicity	Enteral and Parenteral Sources
RDA: Men = 800–1200 mg Women = 800–1200 mg Infants = 360–540 mg Children = 800 mg Pregnancy = 1200–1600 mg Lactation = 1200–1600 mg Parenteral Needs: Adults = 600 mg per day Children = 20–40 mg per kg body wt Very low birthweight infants = 60–100 mg/kg Hypercalcemia can be induced by high levels of amino acid infusion and may result in bone loss of calcium and metabolic bone disease. Urinary calcium losses increase with cyclic TPN (versus continuous drip) administration.	Hypocalcemic tetany (Chvostek and Trousseau signs), rickets, osteomalacia, osteoporosis, bleeding tendencies. Defiency may be caused by malabsorption, vitamin D deficiency, diuresis, magnesium toxicity, prolonged inadequate intake. Hypocalcemia may be due to hypoalbuminemia.	Excessive bone and soft tissue calcification, stiffness. Kidney problems including renal insufficiency, kidney stone development, suppression of parathyroid hormone secretion and subsequent hypophosphatemia and hypochloremic alkalosis. GI problems, including pancreatitis, nausea, vomiting. Also cardiac arrhythmia, weakness. Hypercalcemia may be caused by rapid bone destruction.	Food: Milk, cheese, dark green vegetables, clams, salmon, oysters, shrimp, meat. Enteral Sources: Calcium caseinate Calcium phosphate Calcium carbonate Parenteral Sources: Calcium gluconate
RDA: Men = 800–1200 mg Women = 800–1200 mg Infants = 240–360 mg Children = 800 mg Pregnancy = 1200–1600 mg Lactation = 1200–1600 mg Parenteral Needs: Adults = 600 mg per day Children = 20–40 mg per kg body weight Very low birthweight infants = 60–100 mg/kg Cyclic TPN results in increased urinary phosphorus compared to continuous drip TPN.	Rare. Anorexia, weakness, paresthesias, malaise, bone pain, cardiac failure, glucose intolerance. Deficiency caused by malabsorption, vitamin D deficiency, magnesium and aluminum hydroxide antacid administration, diuretic use, renal disease, diabetic ketosis treatment, alcoholism, respiratory alkalosis.	Rare. Neuroexcitability, tetany, convulsions. Hyperphosphatemia may be due to renal disease, hypoparathyroid secretion.	Food: Milk, cheese, meat, poultry, fish, cola beverages with phosphoric acid, nuts, legumes, breads, cereals Enteral Sources: Calcium phosphate Parenteral Sources: Sodium phosphate Potassium phosphate

(continued)

TABLE 11–2. (*Continued*)

Mineral	Function	Metabolism
Magnesium	Component of bone, teeth, and other tissues. Affects nerve and muscle irritability. Activator of enzyme reactions in glycolysis, e.g., glucokinase, all kinase reactions involving ATP. Center of chlorophyll molecule. Essential in protein synthesis. Essential in potassium and calcium balances.	Absorption: Upper small intestine, inhibited by diarrhea, fat malabsorption, sprue Transport: Plasma as free, complexed or protein-bound (serum is 30% albumin bound) Storage: Bone, teeth muscle, other organs, blood Excretion: Feces, urine increased by alcohol abuse, loop diuretics, osmotic diuresis, gentamicin and amphotericin B administration, *cisplatin* treatment
Iron	Constituent of hemoglobin, myoglobin, oxidative-phosphorylation, cytochromes, cytochrome oxidase. Essential in heme molecule in oxygen and electron transport.	Absorption: Duodenum in acid media according to need. Facilitated by vitamin C, HCl, meat, poultry, fish. Used iron reabsorbed via enterohepatic system. Inhibited by oxalate, phytate, tannic acid, alkali, fiber, cobalt, diarrhea, zinc, EDTA, manganese, copper. Transport: Blood bound to transferrin, RBC, free plasma iron. Storage: As ferritin and hemosiderin in liver, spleen, bone marrow, reticuloendothelial tissues. Excretion: Urine, bile, feces, sweat, hemorrhage, menstrual loss.

Needs and Allowances	Deficiency	Toxicity	Enteral and Parenteral Sources
RDA: Men = 350–400 mg Women = 300 mg Infants = 50–70 mg Children = 150–250 mg Pregnancy = 450 mg Lactation = 450 mg Parenteral Needs: Adults = 10–20 mEq/day Renal failure = 0–10 mEq/day Diuretic therapy, ethanol abuse, anabolism, osmotic diuresis, *cisplatin*, aminoglycoside, amphotericin therapy = 20–40 mEq Symptomatic deficiency syndrome = 40–50 mEq Magnesium urinary loss is greater with cyclic TPN administration than continuous drip administration.	Neuromuscular irritability including tremor, hyperreflexia, Chvostek sign, seizure, hallucinations, anxiety. Cardiac irritability including ventricular and supraventricular irritability, sudden death. Refractory hypokalemia and hypocalcemia, failure to thrive, decreased immunoglobulin concentration, paralysis, dysphagia. A fall in serum may be secondary to elevated free fatty acids and may cause cardiac irritability. Deficiency may be caused by alcoholism, prolonged losses via GI secretions, burns, renal disease with tubular dysfunction, diabetic ketoacidosis, long-term diuretic use, cirrhosis.	Cathartic effect, transient hypotension, respiratory depression, coma, paralysis and loss of deep tendon reflex. Toxicity may be caused by hyperparathyroidism, aldosterone deficiency and renal failure with antacid ingestion.	Food: Vegetables, whole grains, cereals, nuts, legumes, meat, seafood, milk, seeds, Mg-containing antacids Enteral Sources: Magnesium chloride Magnesium sulfate Parenteral Sources: Magnesium chloride Magnesium sulfate
RDA: Men = 10–18 mg Women = 10–18 mg Infants = 10–15 mg Children = 10–15 mg Pregnancy and lactation require enteral iron supplementation of 30–60 mg Parenteral Needs: Adults = 1–7 mg Children = 1–7 mg	Hypochromic, microcytic anemia. Due to anemia, see shortness of breath, paleness, nail clubbing and brittleness, malaise and lassitude, irritability, decline in work capacity, decreased resistance to infection, stomatitis, dysphagia, postcricoid esophageal stricture	RBC hemolysis, skin discoloration, diarrhea, GI distress, nausea, vomiting, muscle-joint pain. Iron overload may be due to idiopathic hemochromatosis, excess intake via supplements or TPN, chronic alcoholism or chronic liver disease, portal cirrhosis, pancreatic insufficiency, transfusional hemosiderosis.	Food: Liver, meat, egg yolk, legumes, dried fruits, enriched breads and cereals, dark green vegetables, broccoli, greens Enteral Sources: Ferrous sulfate Ferrous chloride Parenteral Sources: Iron dextran

(continued)

TABLE 11–2. (*Continued*)

Mineral	Function	Metabolism
Manganese	Can substitute for magnesium in some enzyme reactions. Essential in oxidative phosphorylation reactions. Essential in cholesterol synthesis. Activates transferases, hydrolases, lyases, isomerases, ligases, cholinesterase, arginase. Component of pyruvate decarboxylase. Essential in mucopolysaccharide synthesis for bone growth. Maintains structure and function of pancreatic beta cells.	Absorption: Active transport similar to iron in duodenum. Facilitated with iron deficiency. Inhibited by calcium, phosphorus, diarrhea. Transport: Plasma on transmanganin (possibly same as transferrin). Storage: Mitochondria, liver, kidney, bone, GI mucosa, pancreas, pituitary gland, pineal gland, lactating mammary glands. Excretion: feces, bile
Copper	Essential for hemoglobin synthesis, iron mobilization, bone mineralization, synthesis of aortic elastin, connective tissue metabolism, melanin formation, myelin sheath and phospholipid integrity. Activator in enzymes including tyrosinase, uricase, ascorbic acid oxidase, monoamine oxidase, dopamine-hydroxylase, cytochrome oxidase. Essential in electron transport system. Component of erythrocuprin.	Absorption: Duodenum. Facilitated by acid media. Inhibited by calcium, zinc, iron, diarrhea. Transport: Plasma on ceruloplasmin or albumin Storage: Liver, brain, kidney, heart, hair, eye, bone marrow Excretion: Feces, bile
Chromium	Cofactor with insulin at cellular level. Constituent of proteolytic enzymes. Essential in glucose utilization for lipogenesis, glycogen synthesis, cholesterol synthesis, incorporation of amino acids into protein, growth.	Absorption: Poor. Inhibited by acid media, diarrhea. Transport: Serum on siderophilin (transferrin) in competition for iron. Storage: Skin, fat, adrenal gland, brain, muscle. Excretion: Urine, some bile, feces, skin

Needs and Allowances	Deficiency	Toxicity	Enteral and Parenteral Sources
RDA: Not established; safe and adequate daily intakes as follows: Adults = 2.5–5 mg Children and adolescents = 1–2.5 mg Infants = 1–2 mg Parenteral Needs: Adults = 0.15–0.8 mg Children = 2–10 μg/kg body weight	Impaired growth, decreased mucopolysaccharide synthesis of cartilage, neonatal ataxia, nervous instability, abnormal glucose tolerance, testicular degeneration, sterility, hair color change, dermatitis	Least toxic trace mineral. Psychological disorder resembling schizophrenia, crippling neurologic disorder. Pulmonary changes, asthenia, anorexia, apathy, headache, impotence, leg cramps, speech disturbances.	Food: Whole grains, nuts, legumes, tea, cloves, leafy green vegetables, blueberries Enteral Sources: Manganese sulfate Parenteral Sources: Manganese chloride Manganese sulfate
RDA: Not established; safe and adequate daily intakes as follows: Adults = 2–3 mg Children and adolescents = 1–2.5 mg Infants = 0.5–1 mg Parenteral Needs: Adults = 0.5–1.5 mg Children = 20 μg/kg body weight For adults add 0.4–0.5 mg for intestinal loss	Hypochromic, normocytic anemia. Skeletal problems including poor bone mineralization, neonatal ataxia, decreased collagen synthesis, osteoporosis. Also infertility, cardiovascular disease, poor growth, neutropenia, abnormal pigmentation of hair (Menke's kinky hair syndrome)	Anemia, hemochromatosis, cirrhosis, Wilson's disease, hypercupremia, bronze skin color, bronze ring around iris, nausea, vomiting, metallic taste, epigastric pain, diarrhea, headache, dizziness, weakness.	Foods: Liver, kidney, drinking water, shellfish, oysters, legumes, nuts, cocoa, whole grains, raisins Enteral Sources: Cupric sulfate Parenteral Sources: Copper sulfate Copper chloride
RDA: Not established; safe and adequate daily intakes as follows: Adults = 0.05–0.2 mg Children and adolescents = 0.02–0.2 mg Infants = 0.01–0.06 mg Parenteral Needs: Adults = 10–15 μg Children = 0.14–0.2 μg/kg body weight For adults add 20 μg for intestinal loss	Decreased glucose tolerance, insulin resistance, decreased growth, disturbance in protein metabolism, increased blood lipids, peripheral neuropathy, ataxia.	Low incidence.	Foods: Brown sugar, bran, Brewer's yeast, Torula yeast, whole grain, meat, clams, natural cheeses Enteral Sources: Chromic chloride Parenteral Sources: Chromic chloride

(continued)

TABLE 11–2. (*Continued*)

Mineral	Function	Metabolism
Zinc	Component of metalloenzymes, alcohol dehydrogenase, carbonic anhydrase, carboxypeptidase, alkaline phosphatase. Component of metalloproteins, metallothionein. Component of insulin. Enhances protein synthesis, nucleic acid metabolism, cellular immune response. Component of an enzyme essential for vitamin A function.	Absorption: Small intestine, distal. Inhibited by fiber, phosphate, phytate, alcohol, oxalate, clay, copper, diarrhea, iron, calcium. Transport: Plasma on albumin and globulins. Storage: Liver, pancreas, muscle, bone, eye, prostate. Excretion: Feces, pancreatic and GI secretions, urine
Selenium	Replaces sulfur in sulfur-containing compounds in tissues occurring as selenocysteine and selenomethionine in protein-bound and nonprotein-bound forms. Component of myoglobin, cytochrome C, myosin, aldolase, nucleoproteins. Acts synergestically with vitamin E as nonspecific antioxidant to protect membranes and tissues against peroxidation. Component of glutathione peroxidase. May be important in synthesis of coenzyme Q in respiratory chain. Required for incorporation of pyrimidines into nucleic acid structure.	Absorption: Duodenum. Depends on solubility of selenium compound ingested and on ratio of dietary selenium to sulfur. Transport: Plasma, bound to protein. Storage: Liver, kidney, pancreas, pituitary gland, heart, spleen, fatty tissues. Excretion: Urine, feces, lungs
Iodine	Constituent of thyroid hormones that influence basal metabolism, growth, differentiation, maturation, neuromuscular functioning, CNS functioning.	Absorption: Complete and rapid as iodide via small intestine Transport: Blood, free or on protein as iodide Storage: As thyroglobulin in thyroid gland, as thyroid hormones, saliva, gastric mucosa, liver Excretion: Urine

Needs and Allowances	Deficiency	Toxicity	Enteral and Parenteral Sources
RDA: Men = 15 mg Women = 15 mg Infants = 3–5 mg Children = 10 mg Pregnancy = 20 mg Lactation = 25 mg Needs are increased with trauma, burns, tissue repair, anabolism. Parenteral Needs: Adults = 2.5–4 mg Children = 100–300 μg/ kg body weight For adults add 12–24 mg for GI loss with diarrhea	Acrodermatitis enteropathica. Characterized by growth retardation, sexual immaturity, rough/dry skin, alopecia, decreased wound healing and decreased cellular immunity and granulocyte function. Also see glucose intolerance, decreased taste and smell, diarrhea, anorexia, hepatosplenomegaly, iron deficiency anemia, mental depression, lethargy, apathy, impaired dark adaption.	Low incidence. GI problems including pancreatitis, hyperamylasemia, acute GI irritation, vomiting. Blood dyscrasias including copper and iron deficiency, anemia, thrombocytopenia. Also transient flushing and sweating, blurred vision, hypotension, pulmonary edema, renal failure.	Food: Shellfish, seafood, liver, meat, nuts, wheat germ, yeast, oysters, milk Enteral Sources: Zinc sulfate Parenteral Sources: Zinc chloride Zinc sulfate
RDA: Not established; safe and adequate daily intakes as follows: Adults = 0.05–0.2 mg Children and adolescents = 0.02–0.2 mg Infants = 0.01–0.06 mg Parenteral Needs: Adults = 40–120 μg	Pancreatic fibrosis, malabsorption, growth retardation, muscle pain. Compromised immune status due to deficiency is reversed with selenium supplementation. Also cardiomyopathy, cataract formation.	GI problems including dental caries, anorexia, emaciation. Also impaired vision, lethargy, paralysis, anemia, respiratory and cardiac failure, liver damage.	Food: Brewer's yeast, cereal grains, onions, organ meats, meats, eggs, seafood. Depends on selenium content of soil. Enteral Sources: Sodium selenite Parenteral Sources: Sodium selenite Selenomethionine
RDA: Men = 150 μg Women = 150 μg Infants = 40–50 μg Children = 70–120 μg Pregnancy = 175 μg Lactation = 200 μg Parenteral Needs: Adults = 70–140 μg	Goiter, myxedema. Characterized by sluggishness, apathy, slowed breathing, decreased reproduction, sterility, pale/ gray/doughy skin. See decreased thyroid function, BMR, free thyroxine in blood. Antithyroid drugs include propylthiouracil, methimazole, PAS, sulfonamide, thiocyanate, perchlorate, lithium.	Thyrotoxicosis, Graves' disease, hyperthyroidism. Characterized by nervousness, irritability, emotional instability, muscle tremors, hyperactive sweat glands.	Food: Seafood, fish, iodized salt and bread Enteral Sources: Sodium iodide Potassium iodide Parenteral Sources: Sodium iodide Potassium iodide

(continued)

TABLE 11–2. (*Continued*)

Mineral	Function	Metabolism
Iodine (cont.)		
Molybdenum	An unequivocal requirement for human growth and maintenance has not been determined.	Absorption: Readily absorbed from GI tract
		Transport:
	Constituent of xanthine oxidase, which is involved in purine degradation to uric acid.	In blood attached to protein for storage in tissues as part of enzymes
	Constituent of sulfite oxidase to convert sulfite to sulfate.	Storage: All animal tissues contain small amounts.
	Constituent of aldehyde oxidase.	Liver, kidney, bone, skin contain largest quantities
	Interrelationship with copper and sulfate.	Excretion: Urine, bile

From references 9, 11, 13–15, 18, 20, 23, 26, 27, 30–47.

opecia, conjunctivitis, irritability, lethargy, depression, muscle pain, hypotonia, paresthesias, and a rash around the eyes, nose, and mouth. Adding 60 µg of biotin daily to TPN solutions as recommended by the AMA has been found to reverse these symptoms.[9] It is therefore important to consider biotin deficiency as a possible nutritional diagnosis involving skin lesions in addition to zinc or essential fatty acid (EFA) deficiencies or vitamin A toxicity. As TPN research continues, deficiencies of other vitamins may be revealed.

Minerals

General. Determinations of mineral requirements for patients on TPN are as difficult as determinations for vitamins. It is almost impossible to predict mineral requirements in situations of abnormal losses that often occur in patients on TPN such as loss of body fluids (exudates, fistulas, enteropathies) or excess breakdown of body tissues as in hyper-

catabolic states (burns, ulcers). As in the case of vitamins, formulations have been used that allow for growth in infants and maintenance or weight gain in adults. A tentative range of mineral doses for infants, children, and adults is given in Table 11–2 and may be used as a guide for patients in whom there are no serious gastrointestinal or renal losses.

Calcium, Phosphorus, Magnesium, and Vitamin D. Interactions between calcium, phosphorus, and magnesium are an important consideration in determining content of these minerals in TPN solutions. For example, a low serum calcium level in malnourished patients can be caused by magnesium deficiency; magnesium deficiency tends to increase urinary calcium loss, which may indicate a need for more magnesium in the TPN solution if the cause is renal in origin.[10,11] The importance of administering approximately equal amounts of calcium and phosphorus can be seen through maintenance of adequate bone mineralization without induc-

Needs and Allowances	Deficiency	Toxicity	Enteral and Parenteral Sources
	Dietary goitrins include cabbage family vegetables, rutabagas, turnips.		
RDA: Not established; safe and adequate daily intakes as follows: Adults = 0.15–0.5 mg Children and adolescents = 0.05–0.15 mg Infants = 0.03–0.08 mg Parenteral Needs: Adults = 20–30 µg/day Many physicians do not recommend adding to TPN solutions until research indicates needs.	Headaches, night blindness, tachycardia, irritability, nausea, lethargy, coma, abnormal purine degradation, abnormal metabolism of sulfur-containing amino acids, decreased intestinal and liver xanthine oxidase activity.	Gout-like syndrome with elevated blood molybdenum, uric acid and xanthine oxidase, elevated urinary copper.	Food: Meat, grains, legumes. Concentration in foods vary according to soil content. Enteral Sources: Molbydenum Parenteral Sources: Ammonium molybdenate

ing soft tissue calcification. In order to avoid forming a calcium–phosphate precipitate when added to crystalline amino acid IV solutions, the phosphate ion should be first mixed with the amino acid (AA) solution and then the calcium ion should be mixed with the dextrose solution before being added to the amino acids.[12]

Systematic evaluation of calcium and vitamin D requirements during TPN is needed. Low serum calcium levels are rare even with calcium depletion. Normal serum levels can be found in TPN patients with clinical symptoms of rickets and metabolic bone disease.[13] In these patients, an elevated serum alkaline phosphatase level was a more rapid and consistent indicator of deficiency than was the serum level of calcium. A low serum calcium level clinically occurs more frequently as a consequence of hypoalbuminemia than it does secondary to calcium deficiency. Shils[11] suggests that, after low serum albumin, the most likely cause of hypocalcemia is magnesium deficiency. Measurements of skeletal mineralization provide the most definitive means of assessing calcium status, although these measurements do not indicate deficiency until it is severe.

Hypercalciuria frequently occurs with TPN administration probably as a reflection of the vitamin D, protein, or carbohydrate content of the TPN solution, and not as a reflection of excess calcium intake. Bone calcium loss, hypercalcemia, hypercalciuria, and kidney stones may result if TPN patients are immobilized.

Metabolic bone disease and negative calcium balance have recently received attention as a result of long-term TPN administration in adults.[14,15] Studies by Shike et al.[14] and Klein et al.[15] report that the striking consequence of TPN was the elevation of urinary calcium excretion. Shike's group[14] found that when vitamin D was removed from the TPN solution, reduction of urinary calcium occurred as well as a decrease in bone pain. Further research is needed to determine if the metabolism of vitamin D is

TABLE 11–3. LABORATORY TESTS FOR NUTRIENT MONITORING WITH TPN ADMINISTRATION

Nutrient	Appropriate Tests
Vitamins	
Thiamin	Urine thiamin
	Erythrocyte transketolase
Riboflavin	Erythrocyte glutathione reductase activity
	Urine riboflavin/g creatinine
Niacin	N-methylnicotinamide test
	2-Pyridone test
Pyridoxine	Tryptophan load test
	Serum transaminase tests
	Urinary pyridoxine
	Serum pyridoxine
Pantothenic acid	Urinary pantothenic acid
Biotin	Urinary biotin
	Whole blood biotin
Folacin	Serum and RBC folacin
	FIGLU test if facilities available
Cobalamine	Serum B_{12}
	Schilling test
Ascorbic acid	Serum ascorbic acid
	WBC ascorbic acid
Vitamin A	Serum vitamin A
Vitamin D	Serum alkaline phosphatase
Vitamin E	Plasma tocopherol
	Erythrocyte hemolysis test
Vitamin K	Clotting time tests
	Plasma vitamin K
Minerals	
Calcium	Serum calcium
Phosphorus	Plasma or serum phosphorus
Magnesium	Serum magnesium
Iron	Serum iron
	Hemoglobin and hematocrit
	RBC indices
	Transferrin
Manganese	Serum manganese
	Urine manganese
Copper	Plasma copper
	Serum ceruloplasmin
Chromium	Urine chromium
Zinc	Serum or plasma zinc
	Urine zinc
Selenium	Urine selenium
Iodide	Thyroid function tests
Molybdenum	Urine molybdenum

altered with TPN and what the vitamin and mineral interrelationships are that affect bone mineralization in TPN-nourished patients.

According to Shils,[11] factors that must be taken into account when deciding the amount of calcium to be included in a TPN solution should include parathyroid status, age, state of bone mineralization, heparin usage, magnesium repletion, and degree of calcium mobilization. An additional factor may include the sulfate and sulfur-containing amino acid content of the diet.[16] The postmenopausal woman who is essentially bedfast is a prime candidate for bone loss of calcium due to age, decreased estrogen level, and degree of immobility. Immobilization can increase serum calcium levels secondary to bone demineralization, and reversing demineralization can occur with physical stress (e.g., physical therapy, ambulation) and calcium supplementation via TPN.

According to Allen,[13] calcium is routinely added to TPN regimens for infants and children, but frequently overlooked for adults. Allen[13] notes that calcium is often added to TPN solutions for adults only when hypocalcemia (corrected for serum protein level) occurs. Because serum calcium concentration is of limited help in detecting negative calcium balance, bone demineralization and common sense should dictate that calcium supplements should be given to adults routinely if metabolic bone disease is to be prevented.

Slone et al.[17] have recently recommended that calcium intake from TPN solutions be 15 mEq/day which is higher than that recommended by the AMA, 1979.[9] Often, calcium is added to protein hydrolysates, (but not crystalline amino acid solutions), a factor that must be considered when deciding upon the amount of calcium to be added to the final TPN solution. Allen[13] has reviews of calcium and vitamin D studies in TPN and recommends a minimum of 600 mg/day of calcium be included in TPN formulas, with higher intakes recommended for patients with increased urinary calcium secondary to immobilization and for those with depleted bone calcium levels.

Shils[11] has demonstrated hypophosphatemia in patients on prolonged TPN feedings when phosphate was not included either with casein hydrolysate or as an additive to the basic solution. As with calcium, avoidance of soft tissue calcification is important, but too little phosphorus in TPN solutions has been found to induce symptoms of hypophosphatemia, which include reduced red blood cell glycolysis, reduced 2,3-diphosphoglycerate and adenosine triphosphate (ATP) concentrations, and increased hemoglobin–oxygen affinity, paresthesias, obtundation, and hyperventilation.

The magnesium level in serum will depend on the balance resulting from the amount administered, its release from tissue breakdown, renal excretion, and gastrointestinal losses. While elevated serum levels may indicate excess intake and/or renal impairment, a low serum level is not often observed until significant depletion of exhangeable stores has occurred and therapeutic intervention has been initiated.[18] Deficiency symptoms can occur when TPN administration is given in maintenance quantities, but resulting lean tissue catabolism is stopped and a fall in serum level occurs quickly. This is an indication for increasing the TPN solution content of magnesium. Urinary magnesium excretion is helpful in evaluating an individual's magnesium status, but like the serum level, it does not directly correlate with body stores under all conditions. Red blood cell (RBC) magnesium is not a valuable diagnostic parameter due to the long half-life of the RBC.

Symptoms of magnesium deficiency include hyperneuromuscular activity, convulsive seizures, and cardiac arrhythmia or cardiac arrest, symptoms similar to the tetany seen when blood levels of calcium are low. Phinney[18] has identified guidelines for magnesium therapy in parenteral nutrition, which are summarized in Table 11–2.

In patients receiving TPN who have renal insufficiency, plasma content of fluid, magnesium, potassium, sodium, phosphorus, and calcium should be carefully monitored. Cardiovascular, hepatic, and endocrine dysfunction will also markedly influence the need for water, sodium, and potassium, and periodic determinations of urine and serum ion levels will afford a rational basis for adjusting dosages.

Trace Elements in General. Trace elements must also be integral components of TPN solutions. Not always is TPN "total" in providing adequate amounts of trace minerals. In 1977 a Nutrition Advisory Group of the Department of Foods and Nutrition, AMA, convened to discuss trace element requirements and develop guidelines for parenteral intake. At that time, iron, iodine, cobalt (as vitamin B_{12}), zinc, and copper were recognized as essential for humans. Chromium and manganese were cited as candidates for essentiality in TPN solutions as well. Recently published reports indicate that copper, chromium, selenium, and zinc are often omitted or included in inadequate amounts in TPN solutions, and deficiencies of these minerals can be produced through prolonged administration of TPN formulas.[19]

Iron. The iron requirement in adults receiving TPN is small unless the patient has prolonged blood loss without adequate replacement. Iron needs of adults can be met by monthly administration via intramuscular or intravenous routes. Iron is needed in TPN solutions given to infants or children by weekly or biweekly administration. In patients of all ages, serum iron measurements and/or periodic estimates of hemoglobin, hematocrit, and erythrocyte indices are useful indicators of iron stores.

Copper. Copper deficiency can occur with prolonged TPN administration of solutions low in copper. A low plasma copper level may not, however, necessarily reflect body stores. Copper can be present in TPN solutions as a contaminant,[20] and although this is an unreliable source, it may prevent or slow the development of symptoms of copper deficiency.

A copper deficiency manifests itself as anemia, leukopenia, and neutropenia. In addition, children often develop osteoporosis. Blood dyscrasias and skeletal manifestations respond readily to copper supplements, and use of supplemental copper is indicated in all TPN solutions except in patients with cholestatic liver disease. Because the chief route for copper excretion is via bile, there is minimal copper loss in patients with cholestatic liver disease or conditions when bile excretion is decreased; therefore TPN solutions do not need to include copper for patients with these disorders.

Urinary copper losses of patients on TPN are higher than the amount lost in patients fed enterally. When copper is given intravenously, most of it arrives at the kidney. Shike et al.[21] report that the amount of copper in TPN solutions does not affect the amount lost in either stool or urine; they report that excessive copper given via TPN appears to be retained and caution that in prolonged home TPN copper toxicity can occur.

Lowry et al.[22] have recently recommended 60 to 65 µg/kg body weight of copper in TPN solutions, finding this level produced normal blood copper levels and positive urinary balance in tumor-bearing patients. Shike et al.[21] report the adult daily copper requirement in TPN is 0.3 mg/day. Requirements are increased to 0.5 mg/day in patients with increased gastrointestinal losses or secretions secondary to disease and decreased to 0.2 mg/day in the presence of liver excretory function abnormalities.

Zinc. As a component of many enzyme systems including DNA and RNA synthesis, zinc is an essential nutrient that must be included in TPN solutions. Circulating levels of alkaline phosphatase, a zinc enzyme, reflect zinc status during TPN. Lowry et al.[22] have produced positive urinary balance and normal blood levels of zinc in tumor-bearing patients when supplemented with 70 to 80 µg/kg body weight. More recently, Solomons[23] has suggested daily intravenous (IV) zinc intake for premature infants, in-

fants, children, adults, and catabolic adults.

The RDA for zinc has been modified based on its relatively poor gastrointestinal absorption (20 to 40 percent) to provide a recommended minimum intake of 3 mg daily in TPN solutions.[11] Generally, protein hydrolysates have higher zinc concentrations than do the synthetic mixtures of crystalline AA in present-day use. Without supplementation, crystalline amino acids do not provide adequate zinc intake. Zinc can leach into solution when TPN fluids are in prolonged contact with rubber tubing or stoppers. Inadequate intake of zinc has been demonstrated by poor wound healing, growth retardation, depressed cellular immunity, and acrodermatitic skin lesions. TPN patients who develop acrodermatitis have been found to have mental disturbances (apathy, depression, confusion, irritability) and depressed levels of albumin, transferrin, and prealbumin, all of which return to normal when zinc administration is adequate.

Serum or plasma zinc is the most accessible parameter of zinc status. An appropriate method to follow zinc nutriture with TPN would be to obtain a baseline determination at the onset of TPN and measure circulating zinc levels serially, remembering infections and low albumin concentrations can depress zinc levels even when stores are adequate. A normal zinc level does not provide assurance of zinc adequacy, especially in premature infants who are not born with full body reserves. Infants deposit 60 percent of their total body reserves during the last trimester of pregnancy and therefore need extra zinc, which represents an important concern if they require TPN.

Chromium. Although less common than copper or zinc deficiencies, chromium deficiency can occur with prolonged TPN use. Chromium deficiency manifests itself as glucose intolerance, weight loss, and sometimes peripheral neuropathy.

Selenium. Serum selenium levels appear useful in monitoring selenium status and efficacy of selenium supplementation. If patients have low selenium stores due to poor intake, perhaps because of living in areas with low selenium-containing soil, they may become depleted quickly if TPN solutions are void of selenium. Supplementation with 100 μg daily should correct the deficiency and allow serum levels to return to normal.

Iodide. Shils and Jacobs[24] reported plasma iodide levels in home TPN patients who had not received iodide in their daily TPN regimens. Serial plasma levels declined in most patients but none demonstrated low thyroid function. It was postulated that cutaneously applied povidone–iodine (as a topical antimicrobial agent) together with some dietary iodide serve as adequate sources of iodide for the patients studied. It was further recommended that plasma iodide and thyroid function studies be periodically monitored in TPN patients not given iodide on a regular basis.

SUMMARY

Parenteral solutions of vitamins and minerals have been available for several years. Single entity parenteral solutions of essential trace minerals such as manganese, copper, chromium, and zinc are recently available. As TPN-induced deficiencies of nutrients become recognized, such as rare molybdenum deficiency,[25] solutions of these nutrients will necessarily become available for use in TPN solutions. The availability of single entity trace elements should permit the TPN team to adjust dosages to meet specific needs without risking an overdose. Fixed multiple trace element solutions are not recommended because such solutions present a risk of overdosage. The AMA Nutrition Advisory Group has recommended several guidelines for use of trace minerals in TPN solutions.[9] Chapter 18 includes a discussion of the formulation of parenteral solutions.

REFERENCES

1. Robinson LA, Mabry CD, Wright BT: Vitamin regimens in parenteral nutrition: A dilemma. JPEN 6:76–77, 1982
2. Stromberg P, Shenkin A, Campbell RA, et al.: Vitamin status during total parenteral nutrition. JPEN 5:295–299, 1981
3. Gillis J, Jones G, Pencharz P: Delivery of vitamins A, D, and E in total parenteral nutrition solutions. JPEN 7:11–14, 1983
4. Howard L, Bigaouette J, Chu R, et al.: Water soluble vitamin requirements in home parenteral nutrition patients. Am J Clin Nutr 37:421–428, 1983
5. Anonymous: Further studies of acute folate deficiency developing during total parenteral nutrition. Nutr Rev 41:51–53, 1983
6. McClain CJ, Baker H, Onstad GR: Biotin deficiency in an adult during home parenteral nutrition. JAMA 247:3116–3117, 1982
7. Innis SM, Allardyce DB: Possible biotin deficiency in adults receiving long-term total parenteral nutrition. Am J Clin Nutr 37:185–187, 1983
8. Mock DM, Delorimer AA, Liebman WM, et al.: Biotin deficiency: An unusual complication of parenteral alimentation. N Engl J Med 304:820–823, 1981
9. American Medical Association Department of Foods and Nutrition: Guidelines for essential trace element preparations for parenteral use. JAMA 241:2051–2054, 1979
10. Guyton AC: Textbook of Medical Physiology, 6th ed. Philadelphia: W. B. Saunders, 1981
11. Shils ME: Guidelines for total parenteral nutrition. JAMA 220:1721–1729, 1972
12. Kaminski MW, Harris DF, Collin CF, Sommers GA: Electrolyte compatability in a synthetic amino acid hyperalimentation solution. Am J Hosp Pharm 31:244–246, 1974
13. Allen L: Calcium nutriture in total parenteral nutrition. Clin Nutr 2:18–22, 1983
14. Shike M, Harrison JE, Sturtridge WC, et al.: Metabolic bone disease in patients receiving long-term total parenteral nutrition. Ann Int Med 92:343–350, 1980
15. Klein GL, Ament ME, Bluestone R, et al.: Bone disease associated with total parenteral nutrition. Lancet 2:1041–1044, 1980
16. Cole DEC, Zlotkin SH: Increased sulfate as an etiological factor in the hypercalciuria associated with total parenteral nutrition. Am J Clin Nutr 37:108–113, 1983

17. Slone GM, White DE, Brennan MF: Calcium and phosphorus metabolism during total parenteral nutrition. Ann Surg 197:1–6, 1983
18. Phinney S: Magnesium nutriture in total parenteral nutrition. Clin Nutr 2:14–17, 1983
19. Phillips GD, Garnys VP: Trace element balance in adults receiving parenteral nutrition: Preliminary data. JPEN 5:11–14, 1981
20. Shike M: Copper nutriture in total parenteral nutrition. Clin Nutr 2:5–7, 1983
21. Shike M, Roulet M, Kurian R, et al.: Copper metabolism and requirements in total parenteral nutrition. Gastroenterology 81:290–297, 1981
22. Lowry SF, Smith JC, Brennan MF: Zinc and copper replacement during total parenteral nutrition. Am J Clin Nutr 34:1853–1860, 1981
23. Solomons N: Zinc nutriture in total parenteral nutrition. Clin Nutr 2:8–13, 1983
24. Shils ME, Jacobs DH: Plasma iodide levels and thyroid function studies in long-term home TPN patients (abstr). Am J Clin Nutr 37:731, 1983
25. Abumrad NN, Schneider AJ, Steel D, Rogers LS: Amino acid intolerance during prolonged total parenteral nutrition reversed by molybdate therapy. Am J Clin Nutr 34:2551–2559, 1981
26. Goodhart RS, Shils ME: Modern Nutrition in Health and Disease, 6th ed. Philadelphia: Lea & Febiger, 1980
27. Grant JP: Handbook of Total Parenteral Nutrition. Philadelphia: W. B. Saunders, 1980
28. Food and Nutrition Board, National Research Council: Recommended Dietary Allowances, 9th ed. Washington, D.C.: National Academy of Sciences, 1980
29. Anonymous: Multivitamin preparations for parenteral use: A statement by the nutrition advisory group. JPEN 3:258–262, 1979
30. Underwood EJ: Trace Elements in Human and Animal Nutrition, 4th ed. New York: Academic Press, 1971
31. Solomons NE, Layden TJ, Rosenberg IH: Plasma trace metals during total parenteral alimentation. Gastroenterology 70:1022–1025, 1976
32. Fleming CR, Hodges RE, Hurley LS: A prospective study of serum copper and zinc levels in patients receiving total parenteral nutrition. Am J Clin Nutr 29:70–77, 1976
33. Arakawa T, Tamura T, Igarashi Y, et al.: Zinc deficiency in two infants during total parenteral alimentation for diarrhea. Am J Clin Nutr 29:197–204, 1976
34. Gordon W, White PJ: Zinc deficiency in total parenteral nutrition. S Afr Med J 54:823–824, 1978
35. Kasarskis EJ, Schuma A: Serum alkaline phosphatase after treatment of zinc deficiency in humans. Am J Clin Nutr 33:2609–2612, 1980
36. Pekarek R, Sandstead HH, Jacob RH, Barcome DF: Abnormal cellular immune responses during acquired zinc deficiency. Am J Clin Nutr 32:1466–1471, 1979
37. Rude RK, Singer FR: Magnesium deficiency and excess. Ann Rev Med 32:245–259, 1981
38. Jeejeebhoy KN, Chu RC, Marliss EB, et al.: Chromium deficiency, glucose intolerance, and neuropathy reversed by chromium supplementation in a patient receiving long-term parenteral nutrition. Am J Clin Nutr 30:531–538, 1977
39. Freund H, Atamian S, Fischer JE: Chromium deficiency during total parenteral nutrition. JAMA 241:496–498, 1979
40. Thomson CD, Robinson MF: Selenium in human health and disease with emphasis on those aspects peculiar to New Zealand. Am J Clin Nutr 33:303–323, 1980
41. Van Rij AM, McKenzie JM, Robinson MF, Thomson CD: Selenium and total parenteral nutrition. JPEN 3:235–239, 1979
42. Van Rij AM, Thomson CD, McKenzie JW, Robinson MF: Selenium deficiency in total parenteral nutrition. Am J Clin Nutr 32:2076–2085, 1979
43. Bengoa JM, Sitrin MD, Wood RJ, Rosenberg IH: Amino acid induced hypercalciuria during total parenteral nutrition (TPN). Am J Clin Nutr 37:717–722, 1983
44. Shils ME, Jacobs DH, Cunningham-Rundles S: Selenium deficiency and immune functions in home TPN patients. Am J Clin Nutr 37:716–719, 1983
45. Wood RJ, Bengoa JM, Sitrin MD, Rosenberg IH: Increased urinary losses of calcium, phosphorus and magnesium in patients receiving cyclic versus continuous total parenteral nutrition. Am J Clin Nutr 37:721–723, 1983
46. Mertz W: The significance of trace elements for health. Nutr Today 18:26–31, 1983
47. Leape L, Valaes T: Rickets in low birthweight infants receiving TPN. J Ped Surg 2:665–674, 1976

12. Fluid and Electrolyte Requirements

Charlette Gallagher-Allred

The environment of any living organism profoundly affects its well-being. Although many external influences contribute to the environment of the human organism as a whole, the environment of the living cell is regulated solely by the internal environment. Regulation of body processes is essential if the body is to operate as an integrated whole and to maintain a stable internal environment for cells to live and function. Major nutrients essential in this regulation of cellular homeostasis are water and several electrolytes.

Small changes in fluid, electrolyte, and pH conditions of tissue fluid bathing each cell can cause profound physiologic damage incompatible with life. Such imbalances may occur as a major or minor feature of illness, trauma, or surgical procedures. Under such circumstances, it is important to anticipate and necessary to correct deficits and imbalances by replacing fluids and electrolytes.

Although the physician is the major health care team member who treats fluid–electrolyte and acid–base imbalances in patients, the nutrition support dietitian is expected to develop realistic goals for providing fluid and electrolytes and should be able to recognize signs of hydration and electrolyte imbalance and bring this to the attention of the physician and health care team. It is therefore the purpose of this chapter to (1) describe ways in which nutrients are involved in maintenance of normal fluid–electrolyte balance and acid–base balance, and to (2) enhance the nutrition support dietitian's clinical understanding of fluid–electrolyte therapy in correcting imbalances.

FLUID AND ELECTROLYTE BALANCE

Maintaining fluid and electrolyte balance is essential in providing a proper internal environment for cellular function. Specifically, maintaining fluid and electrolyte balance involves regulating compartmental nutrients of water, sodium, potassium, magnesium, calcium, phosphate (as HPO_4^- and $H_2PO_3^-$), and sulfate (SO_4^-). Approximately 60 percent of an adult male's weight is water whereas 50 percent of an adult female's weight is water; the leaner the individual the greater the proportion of water to total body weight. Fluid is distributed into compartments of the body separated by semipermeable membranes. Water within the cells, intracellular water, accounts for two-thirds of the total body water and 30 to 40 percent of body weight. Water within the spaces between cells, extracellular water, accounts for one-third of the total body water, approximately 20 percent of body weight, and consists of blood plasma, interstitial fluid, and lymph.

HORMONAL CONTROL OF FLUID–ELECTROLYTE BALANCE

Antidiuretic Hormone

Antidiuretic hormone (vasopressin) and thirst are the major controls affecting water balance, which is regulated to maintain the osmolality of extracellular fluid (ECF). Secretion of antidiuretic hormone (ADH) from the posterior pituitary gland is normally stimulated by (1) decreased vascular or ECF volume, as with acute hemorrhagic hypovolemia, (2) increased osmolality of ECF, and (3) drugs such as morphine. Excessive or inappropriate secretion may be caused by ectopic hormone production via oat cell carcinoma of the lung, acute and chronic lung diseases, encephalitis, head trauma, meningitis, myxedema, and with administration of drugs such as chlorpropamide, cyclophosphamide, and Vincristine. Antidiuretic hormone exerts its water retention properties by decreasing the permeability of the renal tubules to water, thus decreasing urine volume and increasing urine osmolality. The clinical picture is characterized by increased intracellular fluid (ICF) and ECF volume and therefore dilutional hyponatremia and hypotonicity.

On the other hand, ADH secretion is decreased under conditions such as (1) increased vascular or extracellular volume (ECV), (2) decreased osmolality of ECF, and (3) drug administration such as alcohol, lithium carbonate, and narcotic antagonists. Diabetes insipidus is characterized by a deficiency of ADH, usually resulting from a pituitary or hypothalamic lesion, head injury, or renal tubular resistance to hormone action. In the absence of ADH or its effects, urine volume is high with low urine osmolality. The clinical picture presents as decreased ICF and ECF, hypernatremia, and hyperosmolality.

Aldosterone

Aldosterone is secreted from the adrenal cortex, and exerts a major effect on fluid–electrolyte balance by controlling sodium absorption from the kidneys. The hormonal effect of aldosterone is to increase sodium reabsorption at the site of the renal tubules. Aldosterone also affects other ions involved in electrolyte balance; aldosterone increases renal excretion of potassium and hydrogen and enhances chloride reabsorption. Loss of potassium and hydrogen with excess aldosterone may lead to alkalosis.

Aldosterone secretion, thus sodium reabsorption, may be enhanced by salt deprivation, potassium loading, decreased cardiac output, hypovolemia, trauma, burns, or surgery. Primary hyperaldosteronism can result due to an adrenal tumor, whereas secondary hyperaldosteronism may occur with congestive heart failure, cirrhosis, and nephrotic syndrome. Clinically, a primary sodium excess, as with hyperaldosteronism, presents as thirst, increased ICF and ECF, hypernatremia, and hypertonicity.

Diminished aldosterone secretion, on the other hand, may result from salt loading, potassium depletion, hypervolemia, and recumbent posture. Clinically, patients present with a primary sodium deficit characterized by increased ICF, decreased ECV, hypovolemia, hyponatremia, and hypertonicity.

MAINTENANCE OF FLUID HOMEOSTASIS

Fluid balance involves the maintenance of the appropriate fluid contents of plasma and interstitial fluid. The nutrition support clinician should be knowledgeable regarding the etiology, clinical picture, and treatment when the following two major imbalances occur: (1) plasma-to-interstitial fluid shift, and (2) interstitial-to-plasma fluid shift.

Plasma-to-Interstitial Fluid Shift

The maintenance of balance between plasma and interstitial fluid is complex, involves many factors, and is governed by the fact that capillary membrane pores are permeable to water and electrolytes but are not readily permeable to plasma proteins and compounds except those of small molecular size. At the capillary membrane level, the pressures favoring transfer of fluid from the plasma space into the interstitial fluid space normally are (1) capillary hydrostatic pressure (17 mm Hg), (2) negative interstitial fluid pressure (7 mm Hg), and (3) interstitial fluid colloid osmotic pressure (4.5 mm Hg). These three factors are opposed by the plasma colloid osmotic pressure (28 mm Hg), which favors transfer of fluid from the interstitial fluid space to the plasma. The net effect of these factors is a slight force favoring the transfer of fluid from plasma to interstitial space.

An abnormally high plasma-to-interstitial fluid shift can be caused by a variety of factors and is often listed as the condition of edema, ascites, and anasarca. Conditions that may produce a plasma-to-interstitial fluid shift include increased capillary permeability, burns, severe trauma, crushing injury, surgery, infections, peritonitis, GI obstruction or bleeding, and blood vessel occlusion. The clinical picture may present as hypovolemia, shock, pallor, weakness, tachycardia, hypertension, oliguria, and apprehension, while laboratory findings suggest hemoconcentration with elevated hemoglobin, hematocrit, and red blood cell count.

The primary goals of therapy for plasma-to-interstitial fluid shift imbalance include (1) the restoration and maintenance of effective intravascular volume for prevention of shock, and (2) the treatment of the underlying condition. Intravenous (IV) therapy is generally required to restore plasma deficit. Solutions chosen are generally those whose composition and tonicity resemble the ECF in electrolytes and which may also contain albumin, plasma proteins, and dextran (a synthetic plasma volume expander). The patient's weight, blood pressure, heart rate, hemoglobin, hematocrit, plasma protein level, central venous pressure, and urine output are useful parameters to be continuously monitored in assessing the efficacy of treatment.

In correcting the plasma-to-interstitial fluid imbalance, the clinician must be careful to avoid a large rebound interstitial-to-plasma fluid shift whereby sequestered ECF is mobilized and reenters the vascular space. Mobilization of ECF occurs normally if the amount is not large and kidney function is normal.

Interstitial-to-Plasma Fluid Shift

The typical interstitial-to-plasma fluid shift is characterized by hypervolemia and may occur during the recovery phase of an underlying event when sequestered fluid is mobilized and returned to the intravascular compartment (e.g., day 2 or 3 in postburn patients, postoperative period, and recovery from crushing injury). Congestion may result especially if cardiac or renal function is impaired. Administration of large amounts of plasma proteins or dextran may also cause interstitial-to-plasma fluid shift.

The clinical findings of interstitial-to-plasma fluid shift are hypervolemia and engorgement of peripheral veins, air hunger, moist lung rales, cardiac dilation, and bounding pulse. Laboratory findings include hemodilution with decreased hemoglobin, hematocrit, and red blood cell count. Treatment should begin preventively, avoiding excess intravenous therapy. Use of diuretics is appropriate and, in life-threatening conditions, phlebotomy and plasmapheresis may be employed.

Normally, water intake and output balance each other on a daily basis to maintain proper compartmental distribution. The simplest way to monitor water balance is to determine daily body weight. Body weight of a normal adult may vary as much as 2 kilograms in 48 hours, due to changes in the amount of fluid and salt. A weight change of 1 kilogram (2.2 pounds) represents a fluid loss or gain of approximately 1 liter.

Table 12–1 provides a summary of functions of water, factors that increase requirements, and causes and manifestations of deficiency and excess.

MAINTENANCE OF ELECTROLYTE HOMEOSTASIS

Maintenance of a proper osmotic equilibrium between blood plasma and interstitial fluids and between interstitial fluid and ICF is dependent upon osmotic pressure. Most of the membranes of the body are semi-permeable, meaning they allow free exchange of water and many uncharged molecules between fluid compartments but partially or completely inhibit passage of large molecules, charged ions, and other dissolved particles such as glucose. Osmotic pressure is dependent upon the number of ions present on each side of a semi-permeable membrane irrespective of any charge they may carry. It is defined as the pressure exerted by dissolved particles on either side of a semi-permeable membrane, which results in water movement from an area of lower concentration to an area of higher concentration. Water movement will continue until the concentration of dissolved particles is equal on both sides. The unit of measurement of osmotic activity is the milliosmole (mOsm). Electrolytes (ionizable or nonionizable) and other substances such as glucose, urea, and protein, exert an osmotic effect. Sodium and chloride, because they are highest in extracellular concentration, exert the greatest effect on extracellular osmotic pressure, whereas potassium and bicarbonate, due to their high concentrations within cells, exert the major effect on intracellular osmotic pressure. As can be expected, if there is a significant gain or loss of any of these major electrolytes or other dissolved substances in

any fluid compartment, a change in osmotic pressure will result in an increase in water content of the compartment with the larger number of particles. The contribution of various constituents of normal human serum to the total serum osmotic pressure is shown in Table 12–2.

Measuring serum osmolality can be done directly but requires a few hours' time. Sometimes a quick estimate of serum osmolality is necessary. The serum sodium level can be used as a rough estimation of serum osmolality. Serum sodium comprises approximately 50 percent of the osmotically active components in serum. Therefore serum osmolality can be approximated by multiplying serum sodium concentration by two. If a patient has significant hyperglycemia, which increases serum osmolality, multiplying serum sodium by a factor of two would underestimate serum osmolality by not accounting for the osmolality of glucose. Of course, measuring serum osmolality directly provides greater accuracy than estimation.

Table 12–1 provides a summary of the major minerals involved in fluid and electrolyte balance. Functions, requirements, factors that increase requirements, and causes and manifestations of deficiency and excess of sodium, potassium, chloride, and sulfate are summarized in addition to water. (See Chapter 11, Vitamin and Mineral Requirements, Table 11–2 for similar information on phosphate, calcium and magnesium.)

FLUID AND ELECTROLYTE CHANGES IN DEHYDRATION

Pure water depletion or water deficit occurs when the water content of the body becomes depleted due either to excessive loss or inadequate intake. In water deficit, total body solute content remains essentially unchanged, thus the intracellular and extracellular compartments become hypertonic. Pure water depletion representing a loss of approximately 10 percent of total body water is a

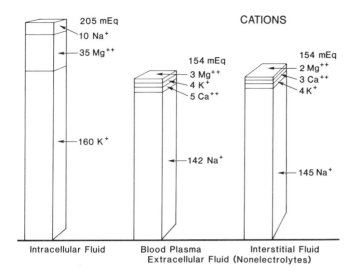

Figure 12–1. Cation content of various fluids.

medically serious condition whereas a loss from 20 to 22 percent is usually fatal.

Dehydration involves not only a change in water balance but also a change in charge differential of electrolytes. Electrolytes are chemical compounds that dissociate in water to form ions, such as salts, acids, and bases, and they carry either a positive or negative electrical charge. A charge differential must be constantly maintained or a cell will quickly die, as can happen in severe dehydration.

The measurement of the total combining power of electrolytes in the major body compartments, represented by milliequivalents (mEq) is an indication of the number of electrical charges within that compartment. As can be seen in Figures 12–1 and 12–2, positive cations and negative anions are balanced within cells; plasma and interstitial fluid (as measures of ECF) contain the same total electrolyte concentration, both of which are significantly less than the electrolyte

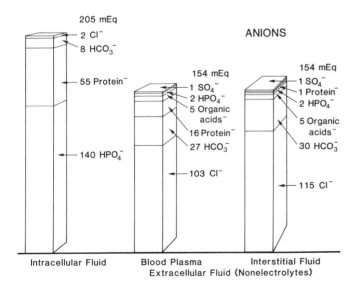

Figure 12–2. Anion content of various fluids.

TABLE 12–1. CHARACTERISTICS OF MAJOR BODY FLUIDS AND ELECTROLYTES

Nutrient	Functions	Factors That Increase Requirements	Deficiency and Clinical Manifestations
Water	Regulate body temperature. Aid in digestion, absorption, circulation and excretion of nutrients and blood solutes. Elimination of wastes. Major component of blood, cells, lymph, extracellular fluid, mucus, digestive juices, (saliva, gastric secretions, bile, pancreatic juice, intestinal secretions). Structural component of cells. Lubrication of joints. Milieu for chemical reactions.	Increased loss via kidney: Decreased ADH, aldosterone Uncontrolled diabetes mellitus Large renal solute load Diuretic therapy Chronic renal failure Increased loss via skin and lungs: Increased respiration Fever Hot, dry environment Skin trauma, e.g., burns, hemorrhage Prolonged heavy exercise with sweating Increased loss via GI tract: Diarrhea, decreased absorption Vomiting GI suction Fistula drainage	Dehydration-hypovolemia manifestations: Dry skin, dry mucous membranes, decreased saliva, wrinkly tongue, husky voice Decreased urine output (UO) with increased specific gravity Rapid pulse, respiration, postural hypotension, tachycardia Body weight loss, fatigue Elevated hematocrit, Na, K, hyperosmolality, hemoconcentration Kidney damage due to inadequate perfusion Thirst Elevated body temperature Mental changes, giddiness, convulsions, coma, death Plasma and extracellular fluid volume depletion Dehydration—hypovolemia caused by inadequate fluid intake, factors that increase requirements greater than intake, renal failure, diabetes insipidus.
Sodium	Maintenance of osmotic pressure in extracellular fluid. Maintenance of acid–base balance. Component of chemical reactions inside cells. Regulates body water and electrolytes by influencing kidney reabsorption. Maintains cellular permeability via Na–K–ATPase pump. Transmission of nerve impulses.	Increased loss via kidney: Salt-losing nephrosis, SIADH, hypoaldosteronism Diuretic therapy (thiazide, furosemide) Increased thyroxine and BMR Osmotic diuresis Addison's disease Ascites Increased loss via skin and lungs: Prolonged sweating Fever Burns	Hyponatremia caused by: Extracellular fluid volume depletion (see above) Extracellular fluid excess and edema Acute and chronic renal failure SIADH, hypoaldosteronism and adrenal failure Severe polydypsia Sickle-cell syndrome Osmotic diuresis Potent and prolonged diuretic therapy Defective urinary dilution

Excess and Clinical Manifestations	Requirement	Sources	Other Comments
Hypervolemia-fluid overload: Puffy eyelids Edema, ascites, pleural effusion or edema Weight gain Hemodilution, low hgb/hct, low blood solutes, hyponatremia Apathy, staring, confusion, convulsions Hypervolemia may be due to: Excessive ADH Oral or parenteral fluid overload Excess Na$^+$ retention Portal hypertension Chronic renal failure Malnutrition Congestive heart failure Cirrhosis Cushing's syndrome Myxedema Toxemia of pregnancy Absorption of excess water with TURP or enemas	Losses usually balance with intake Urine = 1500 ml/day Perspiration = 450 ml/day Respiration = 350 ml/day Feces = 200–250 ml/day ———————— 2500 ml/day Minimal UO with maximal urinary solute concentration (1400 mOsm/L for healthy adult and 700 mOsm/L for healthy young infant) is ≅ 1700 ml for adult and 600 ml for infant. Reasonable allowance is 1 ml/kcal for adults and 1.5 ml/kcal for infants. When greater than 3 L water/day are required to replace sweat losses, 2–7 g NaCl/L is needed.	Ingested beverages, liquids, and foods. Water of oxidation.	Simplest way to monitor water balance is via body weight.
Hypernatremia caused by: Extrarenal loss of water Diabetes insipidus Osmotic diuresis Excess salt administration without water Cushing's disease Primary hyperaldosteronism High protein tube feeding without adequate fluid Manifestations: Thirst Elevated blood osmolality, Na$^+$, Cl$^-$ Confusion, obtundation,	Minimum requirement = 12–15 mEq/day Maximum daily tolerance = 400 mEq Urine excretion usually balances intake/24 hours. Kidney can excrete sodium-free urine if necessary. Recommended safe and adequate daily dietary intake for adults = 1100–5300 mg (48–143 mEq)	Usual diet is 3–6 g/day. Sources include regular table salt, processed foods, cured meats, milk, dairy products, breads, cereals, canned vegetables, shellfish.	Major body location is in extracellular fluid. Total body exchangeable Na$^+$ is 2700–3800 mEq Serum sodium concentration does not always accurately reflect sodium balance or total body content of sodium.

(continued)

TABLE 12–1. (*Continued*)

Nutrient	Functions	Factors That Increase Requirements	Deficiency and Clinical Manifestations
Sodium (cont.)	Normal muscle irritability and contractility. GI absorption of monosaccharides and amino acids.	Increased loss via GI tract: Diarrhea, vomiting Sodium exchange resins increasing fecal Na+ Fistula drainage Cholera, flu GI suction High fluid intake	Manifestations: anorexia, nausea, vomiting Extracellular volume contraction Decreased plasma Na+ and Cl− Edema, CHF, decreased GFR, circulatory failure, shock Lethargy, giddiness, stupor, coma Muscle twitches Hypotension, tachycardia Abdominal cramps Diarrhea Low urine specific gravity
Potassium	Catalyst in chemical reaction for energy synthesis. Synthesis and deposition of glycogen and protein. Maintain osmotic pressure. Maintain fluid–electrolyte with acid–base balance. Transmission of nerve impulses. Maintain muscle activity. Component of Na–K–ATP-ase pump. Component of sweat, saliva, gastric juice. Major intracellular cation. Cofactor in enzymatic metabolic processes. Determines resting membrane potential for neuromuscular and cardiac function.	Elevated adrenal steroids increase urinary K+. Stress, increased epinephrine, norepinephrine. Tissue, injury, burn. Diuretic abuse. Pre- and postoperative stress. Testosterone. Anabolic conditions. Vomiting. Diarrhea, fistulas. Heat stress. Low Na+ diet. Colostomy, ileostomy, intestine resection, ulcerative colitis, Zollinger-Ellison's syndrome.	Hypokalemia caused by: Diuretic therapy Surgery GI suction, diarrhea, villous adenoma, nausea, vomiting Wound healing Sweat, fever, hot environment Exercise, anabolism K+-free IV fluid administration Cushing's syndrome, glucocorticoid excess K+-losing nephritis, pyelonephritis, renal tubular acidosis, respiratory metabolic alkalosis, leukemia Hyperaldosteronism, Na+ loading Glycogen and lean body mass synthesis and storage TPN and insulin, fluid overhydration Pancreatic drainage, GI or biliary fistulas, ureterosigmoidostomy Osmotic diuresis Excessive enemas K+ exchange resins

Excess and Clinical Manifestations	Requirement	Sources	Other Comments
coma Increased neuromuscular activity Urine is hypertonic to plasma Hypertension Dry, sticky mucous membranes			

Hyperkalemia caused by:
  K$^+$ leakage from cells by burns, crushing injury, fever, thyrotoxicosis, glycogenolysis, catabolism
  Decreased urine output with kidney disease, acute renal failure, chronic renal failure, uremia
  Addison's disease, hypoaldosteronism
  Spironolactone, triamterene therapy
  Shock, dehydration, decreased blood volume, decreased renal blood flow, decreased UO
  Acidosis
  Uncontrolled diabetes mellitus
  Excessive intake
  Blood transfusions
  Excess K$^+$ causes digitoxin to be toxic
Manifestations:
  Cardiac arrest in diastole with tall T-wave, prolonged PR interval, depressed ST segment, lengthened QRS complex
  Anuria, oliguria
	Daily turnover = 50–150 mEq/day
	Minimum daily needs = 30 mEq/day
	Maximum tolerance = 400 mEq/day
	Major storage of K$^+$ is intracellular
	Usual intake = 50–180 mEq/day
	Recommended safe and adequate daily dietary intake for adults = 1875–5625 mg (48–144 mEq)
		Meat, milk, fresh and dried fruits and juices, vegetables, nuts, salt substitute, cereals.	Kidney does not conserve K$^+$ well. Can see K$^+$ depletion in 1 week if adult receives no K$^+$ but does receive Na$^+$.
			Total body exchangeable K$^+$ = 3200 mEq for males and 2300 mEq for women.
			In the breakdown of body tissues, potassium and protein are excreted in a fixed ratio of 1 mEq K$^+$ to 2 g protein.
			Serum K$^+$ is not a good measure of total body K$^+$.

(continued)

TABLE 12–1. (*Continued*)

Nutrient	Functions	Factors That Increase Requirements	Deficiency and Clinical Manifestations
Potassium (cont.)			Deficient dietary intake, licorice ingestion Manifestations: Muscular weakness, or paralysis, malaise Anorexia, nausea, vomiting, abdominal distention Apnea, respiratory arrest Irritability, confusion, delirium Serum K^+ low Plasma Cl^- low Plasma bicarbonate high secondary to chloride loss Tachycardia, cardiac arrest, hypotension Digitalis toxicity Paralytic ileus Metabolic alkalosis (for every 0.1 unit rise in blood pH, plasma K^+ decreases 0.6 mEq/L) Polyuria, polydypsia flattening or inversion of T-waves and depression of S-T segment, prolongation of QT interval and prominent U-wave
Chloride	Major anion in extracellular fluid with Na^+. Aids in conservation of K^+. Maintenance of osmotic pressure and acid–base balance. Synthesis of HCl in gastric glands. Chloride shift in RBC to enhance blood carrying of CO_2 to lung. Component of GI secretion and cerebral spinal fluid.	Vomiting Sweating Hypokalemic alkalosis Diuretics	Causes of hypochloremia: Occurs with and indicates alkalosis secondary to increased bicarbonate Persistent vomiting Low sodium diet Heavy and prolonged sweating Manifestations: Metabolic alkalosis, decreased serum chloride
Sulfur (sulfate)	Sulfate is important in fluid–electrolyte and acid–base balance.	Acid–base imbalance	Metabolic alkalosis

Excess and Clinical Manifestations	Requirement	Sources	Other Comments
Intestinal colic Diarrhea, nausea Muscle weakness Plasma K^+ high Bradycardia Apathy, confusion Respiratory paralysis Plasma K^+ rises 0.6 mEq/L for every 0.1 unit decrease in blood pH Paresthesias of face, scalp, tongue, extremities			

Causes of hyperchloremia:
  Routine use of normal saline in nonalkalotic patients
  Acidosis
Manifestations:
  Metabolic acidosis, increased serum chloride
	Usual intake = 3–9 g daily
	Losses are via kidney and skin as NaCl.
	Recommended safe and adequate daily dietary intake for adults = 1700–5100 mg
		Table salt and highly salted foods. Intake parallels Na^+ intake.	Chloride ions can freely pass between cell membranes of extracellular fluid and intracellular fluid.

Metabolic acidosis	Storage is primarily in bone, extracellular fluid, hair, nails.	Protein-containing foods.	

(continued)

TABLE 12–1. (*Continued*)

Nutrient	Functions	Factors That Increase Requirements	Deficiency and Clinical Manifestations
Sulfur (cont.)	Sulfate is formed in metabolism of sulfur-containing amino acids, detoxifying phenols, indoxyls, and other urinary components.		
	As organic forms of sulfur, is part of the protein in every cell, part of methionine, cystine, cysteine, insulin, glutathionine, heparin, thiamin, biotin, lipoic acid, keratin, hair, nails.		
	As sulfate in mucopolysaccharides, chondroitin.		

concentration within cells (ICF). When dehydration occurs because water intake is restricted or because water loss is excessive, the rate of water loss frequently exceeds the rate of electrolyte loss. This causes ECF to become concentrated (hypertonic), and ICF is moved via osmosis into the extracellular space resulting in intracellular dehydration. Although this is probably the most common type of fluid and electrolyte imbalance seen, Snively[1] describes many other types of fluid imbalances. Table 12–3 represents three types of dehydration and their characteristics and treatment with which to be familiar.

In a healthy person, the concentrations (mEq/L) for intracellular and extracellular electrolytes vary only within a narrow range. As can be seen from Figure 12–1, potassium is the major cation and phosphate is the major anion within the cell; ICF is also abundant in protein. The major cation within plasma and interstitial fluid is sodium, and the major anion is chloride. Plasma and interstitial fluids are basically similar with the exception that blood plasma contains a much higher concentration of protein than does the interstitial space. From a therapeutic view-

point, it is important to remember that cells receive and exchange electrolytes and fluid via first the intravascular then the interstitial passageway. Regretfully, routine laboratory tests do not measure intracellular electrolytes but instead measure intravascular compartment electrolytes; therefore, intracellular space content, which may be a major target of therapy, is not readily accessible for content determination but is estimated from monitoring plasma values. The range of normal plasma values of the major electrolytes affecting fluid and electrolyte balance is shown in Table 12-4.

INTERRELATIONSHIPS BETWEEN SODIUM, POTASSIUM, WATER, MALNUTRITION, AND ENERGY REQUIREMENTS

Relationships between starvation and changes in fluid and electrolyte homeostasis (usually manifested as edema) have been recognized for years. The relationship between fluid, electrolytes, and energy needs, however, is only recently becoming understood.

As stated earlier, sodium is the major ECF

Excess and Clinical Manifestations	Requirement	Sources	Other Comments
	Intake is usually adequate if protein intake is adequate.		
	Loss is primarily as urine and feces.		

TABLE 12–2. CONTRIBUTION OF VARIOUS CONSTITUENTS OF NORMAL HUMAN SERUM TO OSMOTIC PRESSURE

Constituent	Valence	Atomic Weight	Mean Concentration (mEq/L)[a]	Osmotic Pressure (mosm/kg Water)[b]	% of Total Osmotic Pressure
Cations					
Sodium	+1	23	142.0	139.0	48.3
Potassium	+1	39	5.0	4.9	1.7
Calcium	+2	40	2.5	1.2	0.4
Magnesium	+2	24	2.0	1.0	0.3
Anions					
Chloride	−1	35.5	102.0	99.8	34.7
Bicarbonate	−1	61	27.0	26.4	9.2
Proteinates	−1	—	16.0	1.0	0.3
Phosphates	−2	95	2.0	1.1	0.4
Sulfates	−2	99	1.0	0.5	0.2
Organic anions	−1	—	3.5	3.4	1.2
Nonelectrolytes					
Urea	—	60	30 (mg%)	5.3	1.8
Glucose	—	180	70 (mg%)	4.1	1.4
Totals				287.7 mosm/kg	99.9
Observed Normal Mean				289.0 mosm/kg	

[a]$mEq/L = \dfrac{mg/100\ ml \times 10 \times valence}{atomic\ weight}$.

[b]Water content of normal serum taken as 94 g/100 ml.

Adapted from Abbott Laboratories: Fluid and Electrolytes, 1974, page 13.

TABLE 12–3. MAJOR CLASSIFICATIONS OF DEHYDRATION

Type	Cause	Results	Recommended Therapy
Loss of water with minimal loss of sodium (Hypertonic dehydration and pure water loss)	Decreased water intake without excess sodium loss.	Decreased intravascular volume Intracellular dehydration Hypernatremia	Administer p.o. pure water, fruit juices, glucose drinks, etc Provide hypotonic IV solutions, or isotonic nonelectrolyte D5W
Sodium and water depletion in isotonic proportions (Isotonic dehydration)	Excess sweating without oral intake. Nausea, vomiting, diarrhea, GI suction, peritonitis, burns, chronic renal failure, osmotic diuresis	No hemoconcentration No change in salt concentration or osmotic pressure of ECF No change in intracellular water	Administer p.o. water with sodium replacement; soups, broth, meat extracts, fruit juices, salty liquids Provide isotonic IV solutions
Sodium loss greater than water loss (Hypotonic dehydration)	Sodium-losing nephrosis, renal failure, severe exercise with water (not salt) replacement, diuretic therapy, adrenal insufficiency, IV infusion of excess electrolyte-free solutions, GI suctioning	Hypotonic ECF Low serum sodium Low serum osmolality Cellular overhydration Hypovolemia	NPO with no fluid intake Treat parenterally with hypertonic IV saline solution

cation and the control of total exchangeable sodium is the predominant physiologic means of controlling extracellular volume (ECV). When dehydration occurs, it most generally means loss of total body sodium as well, because only small changes in ECV can safely occur through changes in water balance alone. In disease conditions including uremia, burns, cancer, severe malnutrition, thyrotoxicosis, and hypertension, intracellular sodium accumulation and intracellular potassium loss often occur. This is suicidal to cells because sodium inhibits many essential enzyme systems (e.g., glycolysis) necessary for cellular life.

The high intracellular potassium and low intracellular sodium concentrations characteristic of human cells are maintained by the sodium pump, which can be equated with the sodium–potassium–ATPase (Na–K–ATPase) pump described in 1965 by Skou[2]. Probably the most important function of the sodium pump is the control of cell volume. If the sodium pump were inactive, the intracellular proteins would allow the cell to become hypertonic with respect to the ECF and the cell volume would swell, bursting the cell membrane. The sodium pump usually catalyzes the exchange of sodium and potassium under physiologic conditions, but it can also exchange sodium for sodium, potassium for potassium, or can pump sodium out of cells without allowing potassium influx. The sodium pump is also necessary to provide for the transmembrane potential difference necessary for activity of excitable tissues and transport of glucose and amino acids (AA) across epithelial membranes.

A potential implication of the sodium pump for nutrition is its energy requirements and the possibility that these requirements may be modified nutritionally. Ac-

TABLE 12–4. NORMAL VALUES FOR MAJOR PLASMA ELECTROLYTES IN HUMAN ADULTS

Cations:
Sodium	135–145 mEq/L
Potassium	3.5–5.0 mEq/L
Magnesium	1.5–2.0 mEq/L
Calcium	8.5–10.5 mg%

Anions:
Chloride	100–106 mEq/L
Inorganic phosphorus	3.0–4.5 mg%
Sulfate	0.5–1.5 mg%
Carbon dioxide	24–30 mEq/L or 20–26 mEq/L in infants as HCO_3^-

From Rieder SV, Ellman L, Kliman B, Bloch KJ: Normal reference laboratory values. N Engl J Med 302:37–48, 1980.

cording to Patrick,[3] acceptance of a reasonable sodium transport via sodium pump for a normal 70-kg man may cost approximately 240 to 400 kcal/day. Edelman[4,5] estimates the energy cost of sodium transport as 30 to 40 percent of basal metabolic rate and 90 percent of thyroid thermogenesis. Exact kilocalorie needs for sodium transport are not known, but it is clear that when membrane permeability to sodium is increased, either intracellular sodium must increase or the sodium pump must increase the rate of sodium transport to maintain normal intracellular sodium values. In so doing, it will expend more energy. Increases in sodium transport probably occur in kwashiorkor and possibly in the flow phase of severe trauma.

Whole body content of sodium, potassium, and water is regulated by the kidney. Malnutrition affects renal function by moderately reducing glomerular filtration rate (GFR), reducing renal blood flow, and reducing concentrating ability and excretion of acid, thereby reducing the kidney's ability overall to handle large changes or loads. Malnutrition with resulting potassium deficiency results in defects in diluting or concentrating urine. Hyponatremia also causes, or is associated with, excretion of highly concentrated urine with excess fluid retention.

Severely malnourished patients are unable to excrete a salt load thus causing impairment in osmolality control and cell volume. Cadaver analysis and organ analysis demonstrate potassium depletion and excess sodium regardless of the presence or absence of edema in malnourished corpses. The most affected organ is the muscle, the impairment primarily due to impairment of the sodium pump. Return to normal total body potassium in malnourished patients often requires up to 3 weeks of potassium therapy.

Malnutrition results in an increase in total body water regardless of the presence or absence of edema. Patrick et al.[6] have studied marasmic nonedematous children with normal total body water (as percent of body weight) before receiving a kilocalorie level supportive of anabolism. With refeeding for the first 2 weeks, a linear increase in total body water as percent body weight can be demonstrated until values similar to those occurring in grossly edematous children are found, followed thereafter by a slow return to normal values. By contrast, edematous children have increased total body water percentage. When given potassium and magnesium supplementation along with a nutritionally adequate diet, diuresis and a return to normal total body water occurs. Patrick et al.[6] also found it was not necessary for the serum albumin to increase for a diuresis to occur and the edema to resolve. These researchers believe the increase in total body water is intracellular because it is not associated with edema despite increases in total body water of more than 10 percent, which is the upper limit for ECF expansion without evidence of edema.

When refeeding malnourished edematous persons with potassium and magnesium supplementation, natriuresis and diuresis occur. Children who are acidotic from severe diarrhea or other causes require potassium supplementation to prevent the development of sodium retention and edema.

Potassium requirements with refeeding are high and unless met can result in disaster. Potassium is required when glycogen and nitrogen are stored. For every gram of glycogen and nitrogen stored, 17.5 mg and 117 gm of potassium will be required and stored respectively.[3] If potassium deficiency is co-existing at the time of refeeding, even more potassium will be required. If potassium is not supplied along with sufficient energy and protein for growth, death from cardiac arrhythmia can occur. Intravenous refeeding of malnourished surgical patients can cause plasma potassium to fall below 2.0 mEq/L in 24 hours resulting in death. Sudden death may occur in children approximately 24 to 48 hours after onset of high energy feeding. Death is often preceded by rapid development of breathlessness, tachycardia, increased venous pressure, liver enlargement, and watery diarrhea. Patrick and Golden[7] have successfully treated these children with digoxin with or without furosemide, which suggests as a possible cause an overactivity of the sodium pump secondary to refeeding. The clinician therefore must be cognizant of potassium needs of patients, goals of therapy, and routinely monitor laboratory electrolytes.

When deficits of potassium occur, replacement is urgently required. IV solutions of potassium may contain high levels, and may be administered fairly quickly; however the patient must constantly be monitored for acute potassium intoxication and hyperkalemia. It is generally recommended that the potassium concentration of peripheral IV solutions not exceed 40 mEq/L, as higher concentrations may promote phlebitis. Concentrations of up to 80 mEq/L can be given through the central vein. As much as 400 mEq may be administered in a 24-hour period. For nonacute patients with moderate potassium depletion and a serum potassium of greater than 2.5 mEq/L, the rate, volume, and concentration of potassium and IV supplementation should generally not exceed 10 mEq/hr in a concentration of 30 mEq/L and not exceed 200 mEq/day.

Rudman et al.[8] have shown that refeeding malnourished adults can result in decreased synthesis of lean muscle mass despite inbolism. As a fast proceeds, the output of am-

creased adipose tissue storage of fat if potassium is removed from the diet. Potassium depletion inhibits insulin and aldosterone synthesis; excess potassium may increase insulin and aldosterone synthesis. With potassium depletion, the effect of insulin on stimulating glycogen synthase synthesis is impaired. Because ouabain, a compound that inhibits the Na–K–ATPase pump, can inhibit the stimulatory effect of insulin on glycogen synthase, it is hypothesized that insulin works via the sodium pump. Potassium depletion, via decreased aldosterone, may be partially responsible for the natriuresis and fluid loss that occurs with fasting. Natriuresis may also occur with fasting as a way to balance metabolically generated anions, e.g., ammonia from protein catamonia increases in parallel with a reduction in sodium loss. Natriuresis can be reversed with a carbohydrate load.

PRINCIPLES OF PARENTERAL FLUID AND ELECTROLYTE THERAPY

When parenteral fluid therapy is required, it is usually for one or both of the following reasons: (1) to maintain a patient's normal fluid and electrolyte balance and (2) to replace fluid and/or electrolyte losses. It is important to remember that general fluid and electrolyte balance values are different from TPN requirements. Basal values for fluid and electrolyte balance do not take into account fluid and electrolyte needs for anabolism, which is often a goal of TPN administration.

Whenever anabolism is a goal of parenteral therapy, the availability of sodium, potassium, phosphorus, calcium, and magnesium must be assessed and adequate amounts given to support anabolism. Nitrogen utilization is adversely affected when any of these nutrients is inadequate. According to Silberman and Eisenberg[9] the retention of 1 g of nitrogen requires the retention of 0.08 g phosphorus, 3.1 mEq potassium, 3.5 mEq sodium, and 2.7 mEq chloride.

Varying recommendations exist for these

minerals with regard to TPN solution formulation. Lee and Hartley[10] recommend a minimum potassium intake of 5 to 6 mEq/g nitrogen via parenteral nutrition support. Sheldon and Kudsk[11] similarly recommend 120 to 160 mEq/day. Sheldon and Kudsk[11] also recommend that 15 to 25 mEq (8 to 14 mmol) of phosphate be provided for each 1000 nonprotein calories administered. This recommendation is based on the observation that phosphorus incorporation into newly synthesized tissues in patients receiving TPN is related to nitrogen retention and therefore calorie intake. Wittine and Freeman[12] cite a minimum daily dose of 5 mg/kg body weight of calcium to achieve calcium equilibrium in normal patients receiving TPN. Although positive calcium balance is not dependent upon nitrogen retention, bone contains phosphorus, sodium, and calcium in a fixed ratio, and simultaneous administration of each appears necessary for bone mineral repletion.[8] Likewise, magnesium plays a role in bone mineralization, protein synthesis, enzyme function, and neuromuscular transmission, and it is essential for normal metabolism of potassium and calcium. Lee and Hartley's work with patients receiving parenteral nutrition formed the basis for recommending a daily magnesium dosage of 2 mEq/g of administered nitrogen.[10] It is important to consider the needs of patients receiving TPN for each of these major elements.

When fluid and electrolyte therapy is provided to patients, it is important to maintain accurate records of total intake and output, including losses such as fistulas or gastrointestinal suction. Daily weights should be recorded, and frequent determinations of plasma electrolytes, urine-specific gravity, and possibly urine electrolytes should be performed. Clinical examination of a patient at the bedside is as important, if not more helpful, than chart values. The clinical findings usually correlate closely with laboratory data and assist in providing therapy.

A patient's baseline fluid need for parenteral administration can be estimated in several ways:

Method I:

1. For adults from ages 18 to 55 years, requirement approximates 35 ml/kg body weight/day.
2. For elderly patients with no major cardiac or renal disease, requirement approximates 30 ml/kg body weight/day.
3. For vigorous young adults with large muscle mass, requirement approximates 40 ml/kg body weight/day.

Method II:

1. For the first 10 kg body weight, add 100 ml/kg/day.
2. For the second 10 kg body weight, add 50 ml/kg/day.
3. For each additional kg, add 20 ml/kg/day if 50 years of age or less, or add 15 ml/kg/day if older than age 50.

To determine a patient's fluid status, intake must be compared to output. Fluid intake parameters include IV or TPN solutions, blood products, tube feedings, beverages, food, and water of oxidation. Fluid output parameters include urine, feces, suction, drainage, vomit, blood loss, sweat, and respiratory losses. To calculate possible water deficit, the following formula is acceptable:

$$\text{calculated water deficit} = (\% \text{ TBW}) \times (\text{BW}) \times [1 - (Na^+pre/Na^+meas)]$$

where (TBW) = total body water
%TBW, normal adult male = 60
%TBW, lean adult male = 70
%TBW, obese adult male = 50
%TBW, normal adult female = 50
%TBW, lean adult female = 60
%TBW, obese adult female = 42
BW = actual body weight in kg
Na^+pre = constant average serum sodium of 140 mEq/L
Na^+meas = patient's actual measured serum sodium

Example: 70-kg man with serum Na^+ of 160 mEq/L

water deficit = (0.6) × (70) ×
[1−(140/160)] = 5.25 liters

To estimate a sodium deficit, a similar calculation is appropriate.

Calculated Na$^+$ deficit = % TBW × BW ×
(Na$^+$pre − NA$^+$meas)

Example: 60-kg woman with serum Na$^+$ of 120 mEq/L

Sodium deficit = 0.5 × 60 × (140 − 120) =
600 mEq

Because 1 liter normal saline contains approximately 150 mEq sodium, 4 liters 0.9 percent saline is needed to replace a 600 mEq sodium deficit. A hypertonic saline solution can be administered if dilutional hyponatremia is due to fluid overload and water restriction is necessary.

Table 12–5 contains a list of common IV solutions used for fluid and electrolyte replacements. The major minerals and their contents in these solutions are also provided. The nutrition support dietitian should find this information useful when deciding upon the solution(s) of choice after a patient's needs have been determined.

Short-Term Parenteral Treatment

Short-term parenteral therapy usually is for less than 5 days and is necessary in patients who are unable to eat or drink. If the initial volume and composition of fluid compartments are normal, then parenteral therapy is needed to replace sweat, insensible losses, and urinary losses. Vanetta and Fogelman[13] estimate that for the average adult with normal body temperature and comfortable environment, sweat and insensible losses are usually 1000 ml/day. Fever or elevated environmental temperature or obesity can double or triple these losses. Vanetta and Fogelman[13] further suggest that urine output be estimated at 1000 to 1500 ml/day unless the clinical history indicates otherwise.

Short-term parenteral replacement can be achieved by admninistering 500 ml of balanced salt solution per day or 1000 ml of 0.45 percent NaCl solution in addition to a total volume of 5 percent D5W to meet the combined daily losses of sweat, insensible losses, and urine loss. Also added should be 60 mEq KCl per day. If a patient on this regimen presents with a high urine specific gravity several times during the day, it is probable that additional D5W is needed. On the other hand, a low specific gravity and/or higher than expected urine output may indicate the need to reduce D5W administration.

Long-Term Parenteral Treatment

Long-term parenteral fluid and electrolyte therapy for more than 5 days involves similar assessment of sweat, insensible and urine losses as described for short-term parenteral therapy. If long-term parenteral therapy is needed, however, losses of magnesium and phosphate become important. The estimated daily requirement of magnesium is 18 to 33 mEq and that of phosphate is 20 millimoles in normal adults. Losses of these and other minerals and vitamins increase with disease, especially chronic diseases with increased calorie needs. When it is determined that long-term parenteral therapy is needed, magnesium and phosphate should be administered immediately. According to Vanetta and Fogelman[13] administering 20 millimoles of sodium or potassium phosphate and 4 ml of 50 percent magnesium sulfate in 1 liter of D5W over an 8-hour period once a day is advisable. Phosphate should not be given faster than this in 40-kg or larger persons, and the rate should be reduced in persons weighing less than 40 kg.

It is important to be cognizant of specific fluid and electrolyte therapies for traumatized or stressed patients (e.g., with burns, sepsis, or undergoing surgery). But, it is also important at this time to acknowledge that physicians are often in disagreement regarding fluid and electrolyte requirements in these different states. Therefore, it is not pos-

TABLE 12–5. COMPOSITION OF COMMON IV SOLUTIONS[a]

Solutions	Sodium (mEq/L)	Potassium (mEq/L)	Calcium (mEq/L)	Chloride (mEq/L)	Bicarbonate (or Precursor) (mEq/L)	Magnesium (mEq/L)	Ammonia (mEq/L)
0.9% saline	154	—	—	154	—	—	—
0.45% saline	77	—	—	77	—	—	—
0.20% saline	29	—	—	29	—	—	—
3.0% saline	513	—	—	513	—	—	—
N/6 Na-Lactate	167	—	—	—	167	—	—
Ringer's Lactate	130	4	3	109	28	—	—
Balanced electrolyte	140	10	5	103	55	3	—
0.9% NH$_4$Cl	—	—	—	170	—	—	170
10% Ca gluconate	—	—	446	—	446	—	—

[a]Approximate water content = 95 to 99 percent.

267

sible at the present time to resolve this problem and provide exact recommendations. The following general guidelines are, however, available.

Parenteral Treatment of Shock Patients.

Shock patients usually possess a low effective blood volume, which is represented by low blood volume, low blood pressure, and poor perfusion of tissues secondary to microcirculatory stasis. In order to restore needed blood flow and ECF, a balanced ECF replacement therapy, often including a low molecular weight dextran to reduce blood viscosity and expand blood volume, is infused. Whole blood or blood components may also be given but a low effective hematocrit of 30 to 35 percent is desired for the purpose of achieving optimum oxygen-carrying capacity. Acidosis following massive hemorrhage that requires blood replacement is treated by sodium bicarbonate administration. Administration of potassium chloride depends upon the level of renal function and the ability of the kidney to excrete K^+.

Parenteral Treatment of Burn Patients.

Severely burned patients require immediate parenteral fluid and electrolyte therapy to preserve adequate circulation. Such therapy must compensate for the sodium and water transferred into the heat-traumatized cells and adjacent tissues. Infused fluid generally should be isotonic with an electrolyte concentration equal to normal ECF concentration. It is important to avoid excessive water administration that could increase the already present peripheral edema. In order to prevent circulatory or renal failure secondary to acidosis, sodium bicarbonate should be administered; addition of bicarbonate may result in a hypertonic alkaline solution that is advantageous to decrease chances of fluid overload. A central venous catheter is a valuable asset in maintaining fluid and electrolyte balance in burn patients and may be used for TPN if necessary after the patient's condition is medically stable. If venipuncture

is impossible, the subcutaneous, intraperitoneal, or intramuscular routes, or application of replacement fluid by hypodermoclysis directly onto the burned tissues, are appropriate modes of administering needed fluid and electrolyte therapy.

Parenteral Treatment of Surgical Patients.

Physicians differ regarding the provision of IV fluids to patients preoperatively. Some physicians recommend providing IV fluids prior to surgery only if the patient is not adequately hydrated. Others recommend insuring hydration and an adequate extracellular fluid volume by administering 1 liter balanced electrolyte solution in D5W the evening prior to surgery. In either case an IV line is usually inserted prior to surgery as an access for use during surgery.

If a patient has reduced ECV prior to surgery, it is likely that the patient may become hypotensive during surgery and anesthesia. Replacement prior to surgery is desired in this case.

During surgery, fluid and electrolyte loss may be significant, the amount lost dependent upon the nature of the surgery and its complications. A simple laparotomy may result in 700 ml ECF loss whereas a colon resection or Whipple procedure may result in 2 to 3 liters of ECF sequestrance in the peritoneal cavity during a 2- to 4-hour surgery. Vanetta and Fogelman[13] recommend the following general guidelines for IV administration during the operative period:

1. Lactated Ringer's is preferable to dextrose in water or sodium chloride solutions.
2. Lactated Ringer's infusion rate should correlate with continuing losses or distributional shifts during surgery.
3. Acidosis and alkalosis should be treated as they develop. It is generally unwise to administer large amounts of potassium, magnesium, or calcium during surgery and anesthesia for fear of overload.

TABLE 12–6. NORMAL DAILY CONTENT OF GASTROINTESTINAL TRACT SECRETIONS

Source	Fluid (Liter)		Sodium (mEq/L)	Potassium (mEq/L)	Chloride (mEq/L)	Bicarbonate (mEq/L)
Saliva	1–1.5	Average	60	20	16	50
Gastric	2–2.5	Average	55	9	100	0–1
		Range	30–90	4–12	50–150	
Upper small bowel		Average	100	5	100	10
		Range	70–130	3.5–6.5	70–130	
	2–3					
Jejunum		Average	148	5.6	138	15
Ileum		Average	120	5.2	95	50
		Range	90–140	3–8	80–130	15–75
Bile	0.5–0.8	Average	145	5.2	100	50
		Range	130–160	4.0–6.3	88–115	30–60
Pancreatic juice	1–1.5	Average	135	5	55	110

From Brobeck JR: Best and Taylor's Physiological Basis of Medical Practice, 10th ed. Baltimore: Williams & Wilkens, 1979;[14] Guyton AC: Textbook of Medical Physiology, 7th ed. Philadelphia: W. B. Saunders, 1981;[15] Harvey AM, et al: The Principles and Practice of Medicine, 20th ed. New York: Appleton-Century-Crofts, 1980.[16]

Postoperatively, fluid and electrolytes should be replaced in amounts equal to losses. Clinical judgment is a better predictor of needs than are predictions of loss by equations and formulas during this period.

Electrolyte Replacement of Gastrointestinal Tract Losses

When patients lose fluid and electrolytes from conditions such as vomiting, suction, and fistulas, these losses must be replaced. Prolonged vomiting, nasogastric suction, or proximal intestinal obstruction, for example, may result in losses of 100 mEq/L of chloride, 10 to 20 mEq/L of potassium, and 50 mEq/L of sodium. In this instance, a replacement of equal volume 0.9 percent NaCl and 40 mEq/L potassium should be given to restore losses. If the patient is achlorhydric, lactated Ringer's solution with the extra KCl added should be used. Prolonged losses of small bowel secretions due to fistulas or prolonged diarrhea should be replaced with lactated Ringer's supplemented by 40 mEq sodium bicarbonate 2 to 3 times daily. Progressive sep-

tic peritonitis may require 6 to 8 liters daily of lactated Ringer's replacement fluid.[13] Table 12–6 provides information on the normal electrolyte content of gastrointestinal tract secretions.

ACID–BASE BALANCE

Regulation of normal hydrogen ion and bicarbonate ion concentration is essential for cellular integrity and life. Cells function within a narrow pH range, the optimum blood range being 7.35 to 7.45. This equilibrium is maintained by elaborate regulatory mechanisms involving blood and tissue buffer systems. The principle buffers in the regulation of acid–base balance are the sodium bicarbonate–carbonic acid system, the phosphate system, the hemoglobin–oxyhemoglobin system, and the blood proteins. Death usually occurs if blood pH is outside the 6.8 to 7.8 range. For buffer systems other than the bicarbonate–carbonic acid system, the reader is referred to a basic physiology text.[14–16]

Bicarbonate Buffer System

Buffering of Acid. From a clinical standpoint, the bicarbonate buffer system is the most important buffer system in the ECF. Normally a ratio of 1 part carbonic acid to 20 parts bicarbonate is present in extracellular fluid. The body cells constantly produce acid upon metabolism, which must be buffered to maintain normal pH within cells. The addition of acid to ECF may be as hydrogen or as nonvolatile acid. The major source of nonvolatile acid is thought to be from metabolism of methionine and cystine in dietary protein to sulfuric acid. Additional sources could include organic acids produced from incomplete combustion of carbohydrates and fats, the metabolism of organic phosphorus-containing compounds that produce inorganic phosphates, and the metabolism of nucleoproteins that produce uric acid. Addition of acid as the end product of any one of these metabolic functions will result in increased carbonic acid (H_2CO_3) synthesis via the sodium bicarbonate–carbonic acid buffer system as follows:

$$H^+ + Cl^- + Na^+ + HCO_3^- \rightarrow NaCl + H_2CO_3$$

This process alters the normal carbonic acid:bicarbonate ratio of 1:20 by decreasing the bicarbonate fraction and increasing the carbonic acid fraction, thereby causing a decrease in blood pH toward the acid side. The synthesized H_2CO_3 is next converted to H_2O plus CO_2, and CO_2 is excreted quickly via the lungs in an attempt to decrease the acid content of the blood. The kidney assists further in correcting the acid pH by acidifying the urine, synthesizing bicarbonate, and excreting chloride, which slowly returns the buffer ratio back to the normal 1:20.

Buffering of Base. If, on the other hand, a base is added to plasma, the bicarbonate–carbonic acid buffer system again is called upon to neutralize the added base. Using so-

dium hydroxide (NaOH) as an example base, NaOH attracts a hydrogen ion from plasma carbonic acid, forming water and a salt of bicarbonate as follows:

$$NaOH + H_2CO_3 \rightarrow H_2O + NaHCO_3$$

Essentially, a strong base (NaOH) combines with a weak acid (H_2CO_3) to form a weak base ($NaHCO_3$). This process alters the normal carbonic acid:bicarbonate ratio of 1:20 by decreasing the carbonic acid fraction and increasing the bicarbonate fraction, thereby increasing the pH of the blood toward the alkaline side. The weak base is next converted to another salt (e.g., NaCl) and bicarbonate (HCO_3^-), both of which are excreted in the urine in an attempt to decrease the alkaline content of the blood. The kidney assists in correcting the alkaline pH by alkalinizing the urine and decreasing synthesis of bicarbonate, which slowly returns the buffer ratio back toward the normal 1:20 ratio.

A few general concepts are appropriate at this time:

1. In general, the carbon dioxide content of plasma is regulated by the respiratory system.
2. Plasma carbonic acid is in equilibrium with plasma CO_2, and the concentration of dissolved carbon dioxide is directly proportional to the partial pressure of the gas CO_2 (pCO_2).
3. Therefore, the concentration of plasma carbonic acid is directly proportional to the partial pressure of CO_2; pCO_2 can be easily measured and monitored whereas plasma carbonic acid is less easily measured.

Acid–Base Imbalances

When conditions result in an accumulation of acid or base in the blood, acid–base imbalances occur. Although there are many types and degrees of acid–base imbalances,

Figure 12–3. Metabolic acidosis.[a]

Causes:
1. Increased acid production (ketoacidosis from uncontrolled diabetes mellitus, alcoholism, low carbohydrate diet, starvation; adrenocortical hyperfunction, anterior pituitary hyperfunction, hyperthyroidism; anesthesia, shock, lactic acidosis secondary to circulatory or respiratory failure; phenformin or fructose or salicylate toxicity)
2. Decreased bicarbonate (loss secondary to intubation, malabsorption or decreased synthesis with renal disease, Addison's disease)
3. Decreased acid excretion (renal failure, hypoaldosteronism, renal tubular acidosis)
4. Parenteral alimentation with excess arginine, lysine, histidine, NaCl

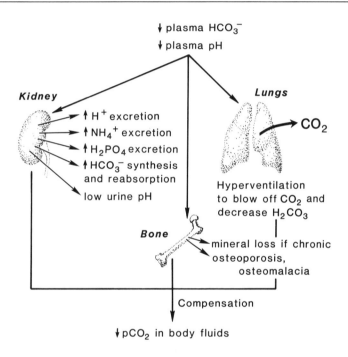

↓ plasma HCO_3^-

↓ plasma pH

Kidney

↑ H^+ excretion

↑ NH_4^+ excretion

↑ H_2PO_4 excretion

↑ HCO_3^- synthesis and reabsorption

low urine pH

Lungs

CO_2

Hyperventilation to blow off CO_2 and decrease H_2CO_3

Bone

mineral loss if chronic osteoporosis, osteomalacia

Compensation

↓ pCO_2 in body fluids

Clinical Observations:
Deep, rapid breathing, SOB
Depression of CNS activity, disorientation, confusion, coma
Weakness, malaise
Nausea, vomiting, abdominal pain
Anorexia

Treatment:
1. Treat underlying disorder
2. Administer bicarbonate, citrate or lactate salts

[a]If the cause of metabolic acidosis is not clearly evident, physicians may calculate the "anion gap" by subtracting the sum of plasma bicarbonate and chloride from plasma sodium concentration; the normal value is 8 to 16 mmol/L with negatively charged albumin making up most of the anion gap. The gap will be increased if metabolic acidosis is due to increased acid production or renal insufficiency because increased ketones, lactate, sulfate, phosphate, or organic acids are produced faster than they can be metabolized or excreted.

Figure 12–4. Metabolic alkalosis.

Causes:
1. Chloride depletion (vomiting, NG suction or drainage)
2. Potassium depletion resulting in bicarbonate retention (diuretic therapy, especially thiazide diuretics; chronic vomiting or diarrhea; some forms of renal tubular dysfunction)
3. Hyperadrenocorticism (Cushing's syndrome, primary aldosteronism, Bartter's syndrome)
4. Excessive alkali intake ($NaHCO_3$ for peptic ulcer disease; milk-alkali syndrome; prolonged hypercalcemia; excessive administration of potassium-free solutions)

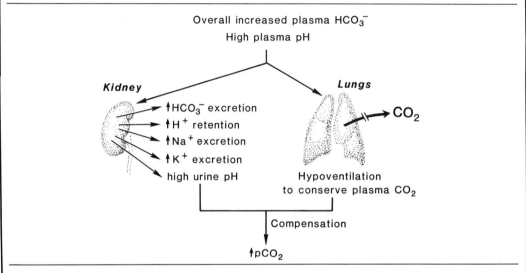

Overall increased plasma HCO_3^-

High plasma pH

Kidney

↑HCO_3^- excretion
↑H^+ retention
↑Na^+ excretion
↑K^+ excretion
high urine pH

Lungs

CO_2

Hypoventilation to conserve plasma CO_2

Compensation

↑pCO_2

Clinical Observations:
Overexcitability of CNS and peripheral nerves, tetany, nervousness, convulsions
Decreased respiratory rate and depth
Muscle hypertonicity

Treatment:
1. Correct underlying disorder
2. Administer KCl if needed

the four major types of imbalance are metabolic acidosis, metabolic alkalosis, respiratory acidosis, and respiratory alkalosis.

The diagnosis of metabolic acidosis or metabolic alkalosis is usually made from alterations in the bicarbonate level in the blood. Normal plasma bicarbonate is 24 to 31 mEq/L. Causes of metabolic acidosis or alkalosis are generally chronic in origin but may result from acute disorders. Renal disease resulting in decreased bicarbonate synthesis or decreased acid excretion is a common cause of chronic metabolic acidosis. Acute metabolic acidosis, on the other hand, may occur secondary to ketosis from uncontrolled diabetes mellitus. Chronic metabolic alkalosis may be due to hyperadrenocorticism whereas acute metabolic alkalosis may be secondary to nasogastric suction or vomiting.

The diagnosis of respiratory acidosis or respiratory alkalosis is primarily made by changes in carbonic acid and represent either hyperventilation or hypoventilation. Normal pCO_2 is 1.2 mmol/L. Respiratory acidosis or alkalosis is almost solely a result of chronic disorders. An increase in respiratory ventilation increases the rate of carbon dioxide elimination from the body, reduces the partial pressure of carbon dioxide and increases

Figure 12–5. Respiratory acidosis.

Causes:
1. Depressed respiratory center activity (cerebral disease, anaesthesia, alcohol, neuromuscular disorders, cardiopulmonary arrest)
2. Inability of lungs to excrete CO_2 (chronic respiratory disease, COPD, pneumonia, asthma, emphysema, bronchitis, pulmonary edema, extreme obesity, poliomyelitis, pulmonary fibrosis)

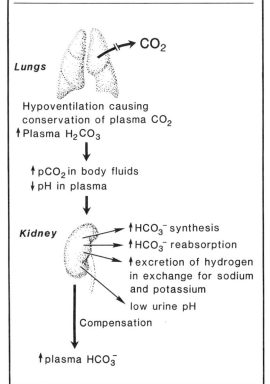

Lungs

Hypoventilation causing conservation of plasma CO_2
↑Plasma H_2CO_3

↑pCO_2 in body fluids
↓pH in plasma

Kidney
↑HCO_3^- synthesis
↑HCO_3^- reabsorption
↑excretion of hydrogen in exchange for sodium and potassium
low urine pH
Compensation

↑plasma HCO_3^-

Clinical Observations:
Slowed respiration
Hypoxia, disorientation, confusion, obtundation, asterixis, coma
Weakness, giddiness

Treatment:
1. Correct underlying disorder
2. Administer bicarbonate or gluconate with cardiopulmonary arrest

Figure 12–6. Respiratory alkalosis.

Causes:
1. Hypoxia (pneumonia, severe asthma, pulmonary edema, pulmonary fibrosis, high altitudes)
2. Respiratory center stimulation (anxiety, fever, salicylate intoxication, cerebral tumor, encephalitis)
3. Other (exercise, sepsis, cirrhosis, pregnancy, hyperthyroidism, cirrhosis, peritonitis, delirium tremens)

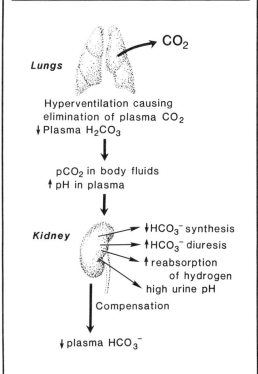

Lungs

Hyperventilation causing elimination of plasma CO_2
↓Plasma H_2CO_3

pCO_2 in body fluids
↑pH in plasma

Kidney
↓HCO_3^- synthesis
↑HCO_3^- diuresis
↑reabsorption of hydrogen
high urine pH
Compensation

↓plasma HCO_3^-

Clinical Observations:
Deep, rapid respirations
Paresthesias, numbness, tingling, tetany
Lightheadedness, confusion, unconsciousness
Increased neuromuscular excitability, sweating
Palpitations, tetany, convulsions, coma

Treatment:
1. Treat underlying disorder
2. Sedation, reassurance
3. Remove drugs
4. Administer NH_4Cl

**TABLE 12–7. COMMON DEVIATIONS IN LABORATORY PARAMETERS WITH MAJOR
ACID–BASE DISORDERS**

Acid–Base Disorders	Plasma pCO$_2$ (nl = 1.2 mmol/L)	Plasma HCO$_3^-$ (nl = 24–31 mEq/L)	Blood pH (nl = 7.35–7.45)	Urine pH (nl = 6.0–7.0)
Metabolic acidosis	Normal with un-compensation Low with compensation	↓↓	↓	↓
Metabolic alkalosis	Normal with un-compensation High with compensation	nl or ↑	↑	↑ Low if due to potassium deficit
Respiratory acidosis	↑↑	Normal if uncompensated High if compensated	↓	↓
Respiratory alkalosis	↓↓	Normal if uncompensated Low if compensated	↑	↑

blood pH toward alkalosis. Conversely, a decrease in respiratory ventilation results in carbon dioxide retention, increased partial pressure of carbon dioxide, and decreased pH toward acidosis.

Figures 12–3 through 12–6 depict these four major acid–base imbalances, their causes, and the compensatory mechanisms of treatment. In treating the patient with acid–base disorders, it is good to remember that simply adding acid or base to the system is not the primary method of treatment, and doing so may even be contraindicated. Treating the underlying disorder as well as the acute condition is of major importance.

In Table 12–7 the typical deviations of blood gases and pH that occur with these imbalances are shown. It is important in nutrition support to understand these conditions and to be able to identify appropriate methods of treating these disorders.

REFERENCES

1. Sniveley WD: Sea Within. Philadelphia: Lippincott, 1960
2. Skou JC: Enzymatic basis for active transport of sodium and potassium across the cell membrane. Physiol Rev 45:596–617, 1965
3. Patrick J: Interrelations between the physiology of sodium, potassium and water, and nutrition. J Hum Nutr 32:405–18, 1978
4. Edelman IS: Thyroid thermogenesis. N Engl J Med 290:1303–08, 1974
5. Edelman IS: Transition from the poikilotherm to the homeotherm: Possible role of sodium transport and thyroid hormone. Fed Proc 35:2180–84, 1976
6. Patrick J, Reeds PJ, Jackson AA, et al.: Total body water in malnutrition: The possible role of energy intake. Brit J Nutr 39:417–24, 1978
7. Patrick J, Golden MH: Leukocyte electrolytes and sodium transport in energy malnutrition. Am J Clin Nutr 30:1478–81, 1977
8. Rudman D, Millikin WS, Richardson TJ, et al.: Elemental balance during intravenous hyperalimentation of underweight adult subjects. J Clin Invest 55:94–104, 1975
9. Silberman H, Eisenberg D: Parenteral and Enteral Nutrition for the Hospitalized Patient. New York: Appleton-Century-Crofts, 1982, p 68
10. Lee HA, Hartley TF: A method of determining daily nitrogen requirements Postgrad Med J 51:441–45, 1975
11. Sheldon GF, Kudsk KA: Electrolyte requirement in total parental nutrition. In Dietel M

(ed): Nutrition in Clinical Surgery. Baltimore: Williams & Wilkins, 1980, pp 103–111

12. Wittine MF, Freeman JB: Calcium requirements during total parenteral nutrition in well-nourished individuals. JPEN 1:152–55, 1977

13. Vanetta JC, Fogelman MJ: Moyer's Fluid Balance, 3rd ed. Chicago: Year Book, 1982

14. Brobeck JR: Best and Taylor's Physiological Basis of Medical Practice, 10th ed. Baltimore: Williams & Wilkins, 1979

15. Guyton AC: Textbook of Medical Physiology, 7th ed. Philadelphia: W.B. Saunders, 1981.

16. Harvey AM, Johns RJ, McKusick VA, et al.: The Principles and Practice of Medicine, 20th ed. New York: Appleton-Century-Crofts, 1980

Part IV. IMPLEMENTING THE ENTERAL NUTRITION CARE PLAN

13. Enteral Nutrition: A Comprehensive Overview

Susanna H. Krey
Grace M. Lockett

Enteral nutrition, the delivery of nutrition to the gastrointestinal (GI) tract via artificial means, is the optimal method of nutrition support for the critically ill patient undergoing severe catabolic stress. This method of nutrition delivery should always be considered first, as with appropriate education it is simple, effective, economical, and safe for all patients either to nutritionally replete or to prevent malnutrition. Its implementation as a feeding system requires a basic understanding of the functional capacity of the patient's GI system, careful evaluation of the patient's condition, assessment of the patient's nutrition requirements with sensitivity to disease-specific needs the patient may have, and a working knowledge of the current formulas and equipment available for optimal patient tolerance, formula administration, and repletion of nutrition status.[1]

In order to best understand enteral nutrition support, this chapter is divided into three main sections. The first section reviews the physiology of the GI tract, as an understanding of its function and role in digestion and absorption is essential in making the appropriate enteral formula selection. The second section reviews the early use of enteral nutrition from an historical perspective and demonstrates how technologic improvements have greatly helped to make the administration of this therapy easier, more efficient, and comfortable for the patient. The third section discusses the rationale, description, and use of enteral formulas as we know the process and use it today. This section focuses on the criteria for patient selection, the sources of enteral nutrients, and the physical characteristics of enteral formulas with regard to osmolality and bacterial contamination. With the explosion of enteral products available today, the various classes of formulas are discussed and organized into functional categories for ease of use and selection. Monitoring techniques are discussed to assure safe and effective delivery of enteral hyperalimentation.

PHYSIOLOGY OF THE GASTROINTESTINAL TRACT: A REVIEW

The principal function of the GI tract is to convert ingested nutrients into simpler, biochemical molecules that can be absorbed, assimilated, and utilized for metabolic processes in the body.[2] In addition, the GI tract serves to detoxify and to eliminate parasites, bacteria, viruses, chemical toxins, drugs, and ingested foodstuffs. In diseased states, normal digestive functions may be affected by many factors, such as emesis, anorexia, inability to swallow, malabsorption, and coma.[3] These factors may also affect substrate availability, utilization, and normal hormone homeostasis in addition to compromising the nutrition status of the patient.

Intravenous, enteral, and tube feeding techniques that bypass the regulatory mechanisms of the upper GI tract and deliver nutrients continously rather than intermittently may also alter the digestive process. This can lead to structural and morphologic changes in the intestines.[4–7] The composition and physical properties of the nutrients in enteral and parenteral formulas will be important determinants of their absorption, and subsequent utilization, in the body.[8]

Thus, an understanding of the physiology and function of the GI tract and the mechanisms responsible for digestion and absorption is essential.

ANATOMY AND PHYSIOLOGY OF DIGESTION

Mouth, Pharynx, and Esophagus

Food is ingested into the mouth, where it is masticated and mixed with salivary secretions before being swallowed. The degree of mastication is dependent upon the texture of the food, the dentition, and the strength of the buccal muscles. The mouth and pharynx are lined with small salivary glands that, in concert with the parotid, submandibular, and sublingual glands, produce ample supplies of saliva. Saliva, a seromucoid liquid containing amylase, lubricates the mouth and food during chewing and deglutition, and also protects the mouth and pharynx. Salivary amylase converts carbohydrates into simpler disaccharides and acts optimally at a pH of 6.5. Upon entry into the stomach, it is inactivated. Its production and secretion are controlled by vision, smell, and taste. Calcitonin, secretin, and pancreozymin also influence the quantity and composition of amylase.[9,10]

The esophagus, a hollow tube of striated and smooth muscle tissue, extends from the posterior portion of the oral cavity to the xiphisternum. It serves to transport food from the mouth into the stomach. The lower esophageal sphincter, at the lower portion of the esophagus, prevents reflux of acidic chyme from the stomach. Gastrin, one of the principal GI hormones, increases pressure at the gastroesophageal junction. It also stimulates the secretion of acid by the stomach and influences the growth of the GI tract mucosa. Secretin, the GI tract hormone that stimulates the excretion of pancreatic juice, lowers pressure. Likewise, cholecystokinin stimulates the production of pancreatic hormones and influences emptying of the gallbladder; whereas glucagon and the prostaglandins decrease pressure. Food composition also influences sphincter tone; proteins and carbohydrates increase it, whereas fats lower it.

Stomach

The stomach has four parts: the fundus, body, antrum, and pylorus. The fundus and body contain the parietal and chief cells, which produce hydrochloric acid and pepsinogen.[2,3] The cells of the antrum and pylorus secrete gastrin. Mucus-secreting cells are distributed throughout the stomach. Secretions by these cells are controlled by three well-defined phases: cephalic, gastric, and intestinal.

In the first, cephalic phase, active secretion of acid, pepsinogen, and gastrin commences before the bolus of food enters the stomach from the esophagus. This phase is controlled by neurogenic factors related to taste, smell, and mastication that are mediated by the vagus nerve.

In the gastric phase, secretion of pepsinogen begins as the bolus enters the stomach (secondary to vagal stimulation) and the direct and indirect actions of secretin and gastrin intervene. Pepsin, activated from pepsinogen in the presence of hydrochloric acid and preexisting volumes of pepsin, converts large proteins into polypeptides. It is optimally active at a pH range of 1 to 3. Gastric juice also contains lipase, which hydrolyzes short and medium chain triglycerides found in milk and dairy products. Hydrochloric acid, the chief gastric factor of digestion, is secreted in response to eating and is mediated by gastrin. A negative feedback system inhibits the production of gastrin as gastric acidity rises. The composition of gastric juice is dependent on the rate of secretion and on gastric blood flow. The latter is increased by cholinergic stimulation, epinephrine, histamine, and gastrin. Gastric blood flow is suppressed by vasopressin, norepinephrine, and secretin. Different foods also stimulate enzyme and acid production at different rates but, in general, maximal rates of secretion occur 45 minutes after ingestion of food and return to basal levels after 3 hours.[2]

The intestinal phase of gastric secretion is initiated by the presence of food in the duodenum and jejunum and is mediated through the vagus nerve gastrin.

The bolus of food, together with the aforementioned secretions of the stomach, form chyme, which is mixed by muscular contractions of the stomach wall, allowing the initial stage of digestion to occur. Gastric emptying of liquid food is more rapid than for solids and occurs as a result of peristalsis of the stomach wall and relaxation of the pyloric sphincter. It is subject to both neurogenic and hormonal control and may be influenced by the chemical composition of foodstuffs.[11,12]

Duodenum

As chyme enters the duodenum, it encounters the combined secretions of the duodenal mucosa, pancreas, liver, and gallbladder. Brunner's glands of the duodenal mucosa produce alkaline secretions (pH ±9) to help neutralize the acidic gastric secretions. The duodenal mucosa also produces some forms of the GI hormones that influence the release of secretions of the organs that empty into the duodenum. These hormones also inhibit gastric secretion and motility. Chyme enters the duodenum at a variable pH, but the endogenous pH and osmolarity controls in the lumen of the duodenum maintain a constant pH of 7 to 9, encouraging optimal digestion and absorption of all nutrients.[13] Luminal acidity is the main stimulus to the production of secretin, whereas fat and the amino acids trytophan and phenylalanine stimulate the production of cholecystokinin.[14]

Pancreas

The pancreas produces both exocrine and endocrine secretions. The exocrine secretions, located in the acinar cells, include enzyme, fluid, and electrolyte secretions. For example, each day the pancreas produces approximately 2 liters of fluids rich in bicarbonate. These alkaline secretions play an important role in neutralizing the acidic chyme delivered from the stomach to the duodenum and help to maintain the neutral pH of the duodenum. The principal pancreatic enzymes are trypsinogen, chymotrypsinogen, amylase, and lipase. Trypsinogen and chymotrypsinogen are converted to their active forms trypsin and chymotrypsin, which are in part responsible for catabolizing proteins into proteases and peptides. Amylase converts starch and glycogen into disaccharides, and lipase is essential for normal fat absorption. The production of these exocrine secretions is stimulated principally by secretin and cholecystokinin, but also by the vagus nerve.[15]

Liver and Gallbladder

The liver plays a central role in substrate and hormonal equilibrium but its role in the production of bile underscores its importance in digestion and absorption. Approximately 1 liter of bile is produced daily in response to GI tract hormone stimulation after food is ingested. Bile, which consists of an independent and dependent fraction, contains water, electrolytes, bile acids, lecithin, and cholesterol. The proportion of these constituents varies whereas the concentration of the bicarbonate ions is constant. The enterohepatic circulation of bile acids, which efficiently controls the reabsorption of the majority of bile acids in the distal small bowel, is an important regulator of the rate of secretion and composition of bile. Bile is concentrated in the gallbladder, which contracts under the influence of hormonal stimulation. The contractions force bile into the duodenum through the ampulla of Vater. The principal stimulant for the contraction of the gallbladder is the presence of fat in the duodenum. This signals the prompt release of cholecystokinin.[17] The chief function of bile is the formation of micelles in fat digestion. Once the biliary and pancreatic secretions mix with the chyme in the duodenum, the intraluminal contents move into the small intestines, where digestion proceeds rapidly.[16]

Small Intestine

The small intestine undergoes extensive growth throughout the life cycle. At birth, its length is approximately 25 percent and its diameter about 13 percent of what it will be at adulthood.[12] The luminal surface of the small bowel is intricate and quite organized. The plicae circulares, a series of folds, are the first most visible anatomic structures. The plicae are covered by a second series of folds or envelopes called villi, which are covered with many epithelial cells called enterocytes. The enterocytes serve as storage vesicles important in the systemic transport of nutrients once digestion and absorption have occurred. Such variables as the type of transport, the physiochemical state of the nutrient, and the molecular weight and osmolarity of the molecule being absorbed are important determinants of absorption in the small intestine.

The absorption of most protein, carbohydrate, and fat in a meal is completed within 45 minutes following ingestion. Absorption of nutrients occurs mainly in the distal duodenum and proximal jejunum. Minimal absorption, except that of fat, takes place in the distal ileum. Contractile activity of the small bowel increases after a meal in response to hormonal and vagal stimulation. In addition, intraluminal contents have a modifying effect on the production of gastric, biliary, and pancreatic secretions. Electrolytes and fluid balance are also regulated by the jejunum and ileum prior to passage of nutrients through the ileocecal valve into the colon.[1]

Colon and Rectum

Large quantities of fluid and electrolytes are also absorbed in the colon, which receives approximately 1.5 liters of fluid daily from the ileum and excretes only 200 milliliters. Movement through the colon is slower than through the small bowel and food residues are exposed to a large number of aerobic and anaerobic bacteria. These bacteria catabolize the residual complex molecules of protein, fat, and carbohydrate from the small intestine. The colon is the endpoint of digestion in the GI tract.

HISTORY OF ENTERAL FEEDING

The use of enteral nutrition dates back to Egypt many centuries before Christ.[18] The goal of enteral feeding then, as it is today, was to achieve and maintain nutrition status and good health.

RECTAL FEEDINGS

The earliest recorded evidence of enteral hyperalimentation was the use of rectal feedings. According to Bliss,[19] the Egyptians were accustomed to using clysters, or nutrient enemas, to treat diarrhea and other related maladies (Fig. 13–1). Wine, whey, milk, barley broth, and various oleaginous substances were the principal ingredients used in these enemas to coat inflamed intestines and to provide nutrients to the nutritionally compromised patient. Many of these same enema components were also used as laxatives.

Providing nutrition by way of rectal feedings was a very popular method of nourishment (Fig. 13–2). In a survey of approximately 400 cases, Bliss[19] reports that eggs, milk, beef, or chicken broth with and without brandy and other stimulants were administered to patients rectally. In an article by Brown-Seguard,[20] a description of rectal feeding in three mentally deficient patients reveals the use of a mixture of pureed beef and bovine pancreas forced into the rectum by means of a wooden syringe twice daily (Fig. 13–2). The rationale for use of the rectal feeding route in these patients was secondary to ther nervous condition, which precluded placement of gastric tubes.

Because bolus injections into the rectum frequently resulted in rectal evacuation, various devices were developed for slow continuous infusion of nutrients. Mackenzie[21] describes a celluloid catheter passed through a thick piece of India rubber tubing and positioned 2 inches into the rectum. The rubber tube had four attached tapes that were passed anteriorly and posteriorly to facilitate placement around the patient's waist. A second rubber tube, approximately 6 feet in length, was attached to the catheter and to a reservoir into which the nutrition formulation was filtered. The rate of flow of this device was adjusted by raising or lowering the reservoir so that the total volume passed into the rectum in about 3 hours. A total volume

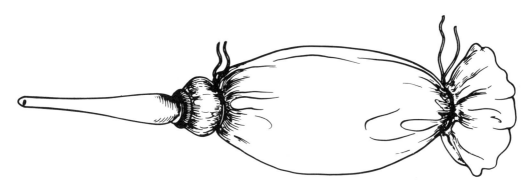

Figure 13–1. An example of a nutrient enema or clyster used during the Egyptian period.

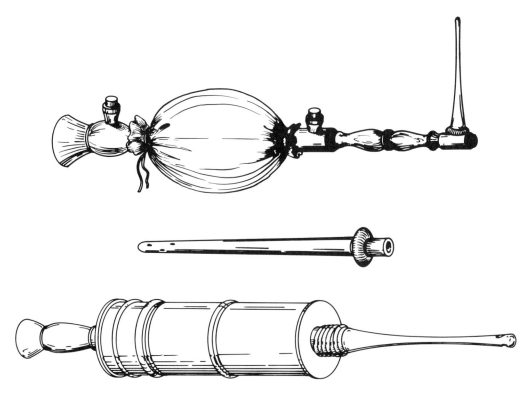

Figure 13–2. Wooden syringes used for rectal feeding.

of 3 pints was delivered daily with rest intervals allowed between feedings.

The objective of rectal feeding, achieving adequate nutrition, was based on the theory of reverse peristalsis. Reflux of the ingredients of the enema into the small bowel would ultimately result in nutrient absorption, storage, and utilization. Concomitantly, hydration of the lower intestinal tract was achieved. In 1913, Myers[22] summarized the status of rectal alimentation. He defined digestion as the catabolism of foods into smaller fundamental subunits that are absorbed by the small intestine with the colon functioning as a reservoir. Crystalline amino acids, glucose, and inorganic salts were shown to be absorbed from the colon in significant concentrations to maintain bedridden patients for considerable periods of time.

The advent of intravenous alimentation, beginning with the protein byproduct absorption studies of Rhoads,[23] led to the eventual decline of rectal feeding during the post-World War II era.

GASTRIC FEEDINGS

Bougies, or sounds, developed for the extraction of foreign matter from the esophagus were the forerunners of feeding tubes used in the upper GI tract. Hemmeter[24] traces the origin of gastric tubes back to the 16th century. Capivacceous of Venice[23,24] was the first to employ a gastric tube for nutrition purposes. The tube he is said to have used was constructed with an animal bladder attached to the upper end as

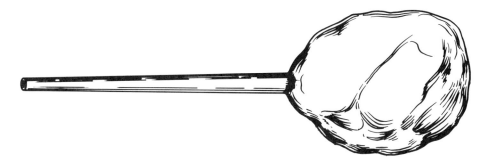

Figure 13–3. Typical animal bladder feeding apparatus.

a reservoir for the nutritious liquids expressed into the esophagus (Fig. 13–3). Around 1617, Fabricius ab Aquapendente used a small silver tube inserted nasally to feed patients afflicted with tetanus. In 1776, Hunter[25] described the use of a syringe with a long hollow bougie or flexible catheter, which would pass into the stomach conveying any substance within it, without affecting the lungs. This "apparatus" was used to feed patients suffering from esophageal paralysis or ulceration and cancer of the esophagus. The tube was fabricated from eelskin covering a flexible whale bone probe with slits at one end to prevent clogging and an attachment to the animal bladder reservoir on the other end for the delivery of foods, liquids, or medication down the tube. The object of this instrument was to provide an artificial feeding modality so that patients could be nourished throughout the course of their disease state in an effort to provide healing or cure.

The use of a pump for emptying the stomach dates back to the beginning of the 19th century. Advances in the manufacturing process of tubing also date back to this period. The inflexible, garden hose type of tubing changed to a more pliable, soft rubber variety. There appears to be little similarity in type of tubing used for gastric feeding in the literature. The earlier types were the source of major complications to gastric feeding. Se-

vere nasal, esophageal, and gastric lacerations and pulmonary aspiration were common side effects resulting from tube placement. The nasal–esophageal–gastric feeding route became a popular alternative to the more direct esophageal–gastric feeding, with the advent of soft rubber tubing.

Indications for the use of gastric feeding and its related counterparts included anorexia, chronic febrility, chronic weight loss or underweightedness, sepsis, and deglutition. Popular gastric feeding ingredients included milk, eggs, pureed meat and meat extracts, especially beef, alcohol (mainly wine and brandy), sugar, and cream. It is obvious from surveying the literature that the provision of adequate intake, including reliable protein, carbohydrate, and fat sources, was the principal goal of the early "clinical nutritionists." It is also clear that these pioneers understood the need for nutrition intervention and support in their critically ill patient populations.

SMALL BOWEL FEEDINGS

Despite the fact that tube feeding into the stomach and the esophagus was well established by the end of the 19th century, little was known about the precise process of digestion in the human small intestine in the early 1900s. Hemmeter[24] invented an intragastric collection device and collected pure pancreatic juice in a patient afflicted with choledocholithiasis. He demonstrated the proteolytic, lipolytic, and starch digestive capacities of human pancreatic juice. In 1910, Einhorn[26] introduced the principal of feeding directly into the duodenum. When nasal, esophageal, and gastric routes were impossible and the rectal route impractical, duodenal feeding became the next viable alternative. Einhorn's feeding protocol included (1) passing a tube into the duodenum, (2) aspirating bile-stained alkali fluid from the duodenum, and (3) slowly administering small volumes of milk, eggs, and/or sucrose. This protocol also included flushing the tubing with small quantities of water or saline to prevent feeding tube obstruction. This practice influenced the hydration and electrolyte status of the patient. Einhorn also varied the rate of delivery of the intraduodenal feedings to prevent epigastric distress, bloating, hyperventilation, and syncope. These symptoms are characterized today as the dumping syndrome. Pilcher[27] modified the rate of delivery of intrajejunal feeding by employing Murphy's drip (slow instillation of feeding) and reported success in patients suffering from bleeding gastric ulcers and severe chronic emesis.

The practice of feeding into the small bowel was refined with the placement of gastroduodenal tubes following surgical gastrostomy. Stengel and Ravdin[28] initiated the practice of bitubal enteral feeding postoperatively. One tube was placed into the jejunum and the other was placed into the stomach to facilitate gastric lavage, decompression, and drainage. Abbott and Rawson[29] introduced a double lumen tube for postoperative nutrition care of patients undergoing gastroenterostomy. The nutrients used in the feedings included casein hydrolysates, peptonized milk, glucose, water, dextrose, salt, vitamins, and minerals.

Several studies reported during the 1930s and 1940s[30-32] demonstrate the effectiveness of the jejunal tube feeding route. Patients receiving chemically defined protein sources in concert with carbohydrate, fat, fluid, vitamin and mineral supplementation were successfully maintained. Positive nitrogen balances and weight gains were reported in the majority of cases. The modification of the former nutrients led to the development of parenteral formulations that significantly advanced the degree of sophistication of nutrition support of critically ill patients.

The type of tubing used to accomplish small bowel feedings underwent several changes throughout the enteral feeding developmental period. Tube diameters were greatly reduced and changes from the use of rubber to other synthetics, like polyvinyl chloride and polyethylene, were made. Tubes were manufactured with fluoroscopic probes to assist in placement. Mechanical pumps were redesigned and were considered essential to assure accurate, continuous delivery and to allow for effective gastric or intestinal drainage.

By the 1950s, the benefits of enteral feeding were well recognized. The development of formulas had advanced to the degree where the roles of the macronutrients and major micronutrients in the digestive and absorptive processes were being seriously addressed. The issues of tube size and type, the use of pump versus gravity administration, hydration, volume, and osmolality were some of the germane points presented in the literature of this period.

ENTEROSTOMY FEEDINGS

Surgical access into the GI tract was the logical extension of nasal, esophageal, gastric, and small bowel feeding techniques. Surgical intervention is indicated in patients who must undergo long-term enteral tube feeding. Refined surgical procedures have been developed to reduce the threats of peritonitis, sepsis, and aspiration. See Chapter 14 for a further discussion of surgical procedures in enteral hyperalimentation.

ENTERAL FORMULAS: AN OVERVIEW

Today, enteral hyperalimentation, whenever feasible, is the preferred route of nutrition support. This method of feeding should not be overlooked because it is proven effective in improving nutrition status of patients, is less costly than its parenteral counterpart, and is safe when delivered and monitored correctly.[1] Enteral nutrition (or tube feeding, as it is defined in this chapter), like the normal process of eating, requires both use and function of the GI tract. As discussed in the physiology section, the GI tract and the liver have important regulatory roles in body protein metabolism, as well as being involved in more than 50 percent of the body's normal daily protein turnover.[1] Evidence is accumulating in support of the role of enteral nutrition in maintaining GI structural integrity. Animal studies demonstrate atrophy of the small intestine and pancreas with the administration of parenteral nutrition alone. The concept of bowel rest with adjunctive parenteral nutrition, though well accepted as a primary treatment for GI disease, may through atrophy reduce GI digestion and absorptive function, making transitional feeding more difficult. It also remains unclear whether parenteral nutrition reduces or stimulates gastric secretions. Nonetheless, more research suggests the importance of continued GI tract stimulation through the use of enteral nutrition to maintain GI tract function. The effects of enteral nutrition, maintaining total mass, protein content, and disaccharidase activity of the GI tract, seem to be a result of direct contact of nutrients and indirect hormonal mechanisms.[33]

PATIENT SELECTION FOR ENTERAL NUTRITION

Enteral nutrition can benefit a wide variety of patients. Function and status of the GI tract are important considerations in identifying candidates for enteral nutrition. It is recognized, however, that a normal well-functioning GI tract is not essential to the use of enteral nutrition. With the advent of predigested elemental formulas and modular tube feeding, much substrate manipulation can be used to nourish the GI tract compromised by trauma, stress, or malnutrition. Adequate nutrition can still be delivered to a reduced functioning segment of small bowel.

There are four main categories of patients who are candidates for enteral nutrition.[18,33-36] These include:

1. Patients who cannot achieve their nutrition intake primarily because of decreased appetite. The most common patient profile in this group is the patient undergoing severe catabolic stress who cannot either qualitatively or quantitatively meet requirements through daily prescribed diet, despite the persistent efforts of the clinical dietition to instruct and creatively supplement the patient's oral diet according to food preferences. These patients typically have normally functioning GI tracts but poor oral intake (typically less than 1000 kcal/day) and, therefore, often benefit from the supplemental use of tube feedings. Such patients often include those with neurologic injury or disease, psychiatric disorders as severe depression or anorexia nervosa, senility, cardiac and pulmonary cachexia, cancer (in particular, those receiving chemotherapy or radiation therapy), minor burns, and trauma.

2. Patients with mechanical problems that interfere with their ability to ingest nutrients. These patients usually

TABLE 13-1. INDICATIONS FOR TUBE FEEDING

Anorexic Disorders	Mechanical GI Tract Dysfunction	Metabolic GI Tract Dysfunction	Hypermetabolic Conditions
Neurologic injury or disease	Face and jaw injuries	Pancreatitis	Major burns
Psychiatric disorders:	Head and neck cancer	Inflammatory bowel disease	Major trauma
Anorexia nervosa	Deglutination impairment	Radiation enteritis	Sepsis
Severe depression	Dysphagia and benign ob-	Blind loop syndrome	Major surgery
Senility	struction of the upper gut	Multiple food allergies	
Cachexia			
Minor burns and trauma			

have normal digestive and absorptive capabilities but with some oral problem or mechanical obstruction that interferes with their ability to eat or digest. The profile includes patients with facial and jaw injuries, head and neck cancer, chewing and swallowing problems, benign obstruction of the upper gut, incomplete or chronic intestinal obstruction, delayed gastric emptying, GI cutaneous fistulas, and short bowel syndrome.

3. Patients with metabolic GI tract dysfunction. Metabolic GI tract dysfunction is the result of impaired digestion and absorption. Examples of malabsorption syndromes that place patients into this category include pancreatitis, inflammatory bowel disease, radiation enteritis, chemotherapy enteritis, blind loop syndrome, and multiple food allergies.

4. Hypermetabolic patients who have an increase in energy and protein requirements secondary to severe stress and catabolism. These patients, because of their increased metabolic demands, often cannot eat sufficient quantities of food despite enhanced caloric density of these foods to meet nutritional requirements. Patients who fall into this category include those with major burns, trauma, and sepsis, as well as major surgery patients. Table 13-1 discusses

the different categories of patients for whom tube feeding is indicated.

Enteral therapy is contraindicated in patients with intractable vomiting, intestinal obstruction, upper GI bleeding, and certain patients who present a severe risk of aspiration. Severe uncontrolled diarrhea, despite the use of antidiarrheal agents, may also be a contraindication for enteral nutrition. Diarrhea, however, is often alleviated through appropriate formula selection and advancement.

PATIENT ASSESSMENT

Many factors need to be considered when a patient is evaluated for enteral therapy. These factors, which help determine the route and appropriate nutrition formula indicated for the patient, include:

- Medical status review. When considering a patient for tube feeding, the level of GI function must be assessed as well as all organ systems to determine what medical constraints the patient may have. Compromised cardiac and renal function may dictate sodium and fluid restrictions. Deteriorating respiratory function may necessitate a shift of energy sources from carbohydrate to fat. Trauma or identification of hepatic disease may require the need for increased branch chain amino acids (BCAA) and so on. A comprehensive medical evaluation of each organ system is essential to the determination of the correct enteral prescription.

• Nutritional requirements. Provision of adequate energy, nitrogen, specific vitamins, minerals, and trace elements, and fluid and electrolyte requirements is fundamental to successful nutrition intervention. Documentation of the patient's oral nutrition intake indicating the patient's inability to meet these requirements via diet alone may establish the need for more aggressive intervention. A 24- to 72-hour eating trial, with nutrient analysis done by the dietition, is a simple method demonstrating whether the patient has the potential to increase oral intake by himself or herself. If the patient is transitioned from parenteral to enteral nutrition, the "eating trial" will often indicate whether the patient can advance directly from parenteral nutrition to an oral diet without the intermediate step of tube feeding. If the patient is not capable of meeting nutrition requirements via oral intake, a tube feeding can still be instituted to provide supplementary nutrition support.

• Risk profile. As discussed in Chapter 15, there are certain complications frequently associated with enteral feeding. The patient should be evaluated to determine whether such risks as aspiration, potential dehydration, and potential dumping syndrome secondary to previous or recent gastric surgery, do exist. If so, certain precautions need to be implemented to assure safe enteral delivery.

• Route of delivery is an important factor to evaluate as it has implications for formula selection and administration. Specifically, the tube type, method of delivery (nasal gastric, duodenal, jejunal, esophagostomy, gastrostomy, or je-

junostomy), and location of the end of the tube need to be determined for appropriate formula selection.

• Discharge plans must be considered before initiating enteral therapy. Clearly understanding the goals and objectives of the therapy, the anticipated length of therapy, and the specific location of discharge, either to the patient's home or an extended care facility, all have significant impact on the decisions made regarding the enteral feeding. Home enteral therapy is best kept as simple as possible to alleviate any additional stress on the patient and family, as discussed in Chapter 16. Many extended care facilities have a very limited selection of enteral formulas. The institution or home caretaker other may not be able to manage small lumen tubes or closely monitor the delivery of the tube feeding. These factors need to be explored and resolved prior to the patient's transition from hospital to extended care facility.

In summary, Table 13–2 reviews the major factors that need to be addressed in developing the appropriate enteral nutrition care plan.

SOURCES OF NUTRIENTS IN ENTERAL FORMULAS

Protein

Protein in enteral formulas is found in four main forms: (1) large molecular weight intact protein, (2) partially hydrolyzed protein, (3) di- and tripeptides, and (4) crystalline free amino acids. The large molecular weight proteins as well as the partially hydrolyzed proteins require further digestion, breaking them down to the most absorbable units, namely di- and tripeptides or amino acids. Amino acids are absorbed via active transport requiring the presence of sodium ions. Di- and tripeptide units are also absorbed by

TABLE 13–2. FACTORS TO DEVELOP ENTERAL NUTRITION CARE PLAN

Medical	Nutritional	Risk Profile
Cardiac function	Traditional assessment	Aspiration
Pulmonary function	Documentation of oral intake	Potential dehydration
Renal function	Energy requirements	Dumping syndrome candidate
Hepatic function	Nitrogen source and amount	
Glucose intolerance	Micronutrient requirements	
	Fluid and electrolyte requirements	

Delivery Route[a]	Goals of Therapy and Discharge Plans

Type of tube/feeding route:
  NG esophagostomy
  ND gastrostomy
  NJ jejunostomy
Position of tube
Delivery method:
  Continuous vs. intermittent
	Rationale of therapy
	Anticipated length of therapy
	Anticipated discharge to:
	  Home
	  Extended care facility

[a]NG, nasogastric; ND, nasoduodenal; NJ, nasojejunal.

active transport but have a separate carrier system that facilitates their rapid absorption.[37] Protein sources in formulas are typically pureed meat, eggs or milk protein, protein isolates from egg white, soybean or casein, or any of the above protein sources hydrolyzed and purified to yield oligopeptides or amino acids (AA).[38]

The quality of the protein source depends upon its essential amino acid (EAA) composition and influences the quantity of protein needed to meet protein requirements. The usual guide for catabolic patients undergoing nutritional repletion is that approximately 40 percent of total AA intake must be from EAA.[37]

Protein quality is determined by its biologic value (BV) which is defined as nitrogen (N) retained divided by nitrogen absorbed.[39] The equation of the calculation follows:

$$BV = \frac{\text{dietary N} - \left(\begin{array}{c}\text{urinary N} \\ + \text{ fecal N}\end{array}\right)}{\text{dietary N} - \text{fecal N}} \times 100$$

Table 13–3 compares the biologic value and therefore protein quality of the most common protein sources used in enteral formulas.

Carbohydrate

Ranging from 40 to 90 percent of total calories, carbohydrates provide the energy source in enteral formulas.[40] Carbohydrate content differs from one formula to another in form and concentration. Carbohydrates vary in complexity from simple sugars, mono- and disaccharides, to the large molecular weight carbohydrate, starch. Overall, the carbohydrate content contributes to three main characteristics of formulas: osmolality, sweetness, and digestibility.

Starch is composed of glucose units linked both by straight and branched chain configurations varying in length from 400 to many thousands of glucose molecules. Because of the large molecular weight of starch, its presence in formulas lowers osmolality and decreases sweetness of the formula. Although starch requires digestion, it is easily

TABLE 13–3. BIOLOGIC VALUE OF PROTEINS FOUND IN COMMERCIAL FORMULAS

Protein Source	Biologic Value
Lactalbumin with methionine	130
Egg, whole	100
Milk, cow	90
Fish	85
Lactalbumin	84
Beef	76
Soybeans	75
Casein	72

From MacBurney MM, Young LS: Formulas. In Rombeau JL, Caldwell MD (eds): Enteral and Tube Feeding. Philadelphia: Saunders, 1984.[37]

digested by most patients and therefore fairly well tolerated. Sources of starch in enteral formulas include hydrolyzed cereal solids, pureed green beans, peas, carrots, modified food starch, and tapioca starch.

Polysaccharides, glucose polymers greater than 10 units, and oligosaccharides, glucose polymers less than 10 units, are carbohydrates that result from the hydrolysis of starch. These shorter glucose chains enhance the solubility of the solution. Because of their reduced molecular weight, they increase osmolality and sweetness. Despite this, they are frequently used in enteral formulas as their molecular weight is approximately 1000 and, when compared to pure glucose (molecular weight 180), they do not contribute as heavily to the osmotic load. They are digested and absorbed with the same ease as pure glucose.[37,41] Sources of glucose polymers include glucose oligosaccharides, glucose polysaccharides, maltodextrins, corn syrup, and corn syrup solids.

The disaccharides found in enteral formulas are sucrose, lactose, maltose, and dextrins. These two-unit glucose chains require the action of disaccharidases located within the brush border of the small intestine to break down into monosaccharides before being absorbed. Digestion of maltose and

sucrose, the disaccharides, occurs rapidly in the small intestine. Lactose, however, is digested much more slowly and its digestion is often compromised by conditions in which there has been some disruption or atrophy of the small bowel mucosa or simply by a decrease in the concentration of lactase, the enzyme which reduces lactose. Difficulty in digesting lactose in critically ill patients is often a result of decreased absorptive surface secondary to short bowel, malnutrition, or increased GI transit time so that the slow lactose digestion process does not occur or lactose concentration in the brush border tissue is decreased. Based on the difficulty frequently encountered in digesting lactose, this disaccharide is absent from almost all enteral formulas currently available on the market. Only the milk-based formulas and one blenderized formula, Compleat-B, still contain lactose. Carbohydrate sources of disaccharides and monosaccharides include sucrose; lactose from milk solids; maltose, a byproduct of starch digestion; glucose; and fructose.

Lipid

Fat, which provides from 1 to 47 percent of total calories, exists in two main forms in enteral formulas—as long chain triglycerides and medium chain triglycerides (MCT). Lipids provide calories, function as a carrier for fat-soluble vitamins, provide a source of essential fatty acids, and enhance flavor and palatability of a formula. The long chain triglycerides in formulas provide the source of essential fatty acids. Three to 4 percent of total calories is the approximate requirement for essential fatty acids. Most formulas easily meet this small amount. The exceptions are very low fat to fat-free elemental diets, low fat modular formulas, and formulas in which the entire fat source is derived from MCT.

MCT, predominantly 8 carbon structures derived from fractionation of coconut oil, are an alternative to long chain fats for patients with fat maldigestion and absorption problems. MCT require little or no pancreatic lipase activity or bile salts for digestion, are transported directly into the blood via the portal system, are more water soluble than long chain fats, and are hydrolyzed within the intestinal lumen much more rapidly than long chain fat. Their rapid hydrolysis can increase osmotic concentration. Side effects of the administration of MCT are nausea, vomiting, abdominal distention, and diarrhea if not delivered gradually. Metabolically, the fatty acids derived from MCT are oxidized into CO_2 and ketone bodies. This may present a problem in cirrhotic patients or in patients with portacaval shunts in which serum octonoate levels increase.[37,42,43] Most commonly, long and medium chain fats are used in combination in enteral formulas. Frequently, the MCT oil component facilitates digestion and absorption of fat while the long chain fat component helps meet the necessary essential fatty acid requirement.

Common sources of fat in enteral formulas include corn, soy, safflower, or sunflower oil, whole milk (in lactose-containing formulas), MCT, lecithin, and mono- and diglycerides.

Vitamins and Minerals

Most nutrition formulas are designed to be nutritionally complete, that is to meet or exceed the National Research Council Recommended Dietary Allowance (RDA) when caloric requirements are met.[44] Each formula has a certain volume that must be attained in order to provide all these essential nutrients. Adequacy of vitamins and minerals is of concern in patients in whom the formula is not being delivered at full strength and full volume. Many of these patients can benefit from the supplement of a liquid vitamin and mineral preparation. Vitamin K is omitted in some formulas. Although deficiency of this vitamin is very rare, a weekly supplementation is indicated. Recently, however, it has also been shown that vitamin K may interfere with the activity of warfarin, a frequently used oral anticoagulant.[45]

Fiber

The early tube feeding formulas used for enteral feeding were frequently high in fiber and overall residue content. Many of these formulas were institutionally prepared from blenderized natural whole foods, such as meat, milk, fruits, vegetables, and other rich sources of natural fiber. The increasing use of enteral formulas for varying disease states resulted in the demand for the development of easier, less time-consuming means for formula preparation and delivery. Thus, ready-to-use formulas for the most part replaced institutionally prepared formulas. In the new ready-to-use formulas, extracts of food sources are often used as macronutrient sources and, therefore, residue/fiber content is minimized. The clinical demand at that time was for low residue formulas. Today, however, there is a resurgence in the question of the use and potential advantageous role of fiber in enteral feeding.

Physiologic Function. Recent research demonstrates the importance of fiber in both the treatment and probable prevention of certain diseases. Studies by Burkitt, Walker, and Painter in 1974 attributed the increased prevalence of certain diseases (appendicitis, colon cancer, diverticular disease, and ischemic heart disease) in the United States, as compared to other countries, to low fiber intake.[46] This effect is primarily due to fiber's main physiologic function, that of regulating or normalizing bowel function. It is hypothesized that either through its water-holding capacity, the osmotic effect of short chain fatty acids, or alterations of the microflora in the large intestine, certain fibers increase stool bulk. Studies have demonstrated that the larger stool bulk decreases intraluminal pressure, prevents constipation, and helps ameliorate secretory diarrhea.

Research has also shown that fiber may affect glucose, protein, and fat metabolism. Anderson and other researchers have demonstrated the ability of fiber to decrease blood insulin levels, resulting in a potential benefit to some diabetic patients.[47-49] It is postulated that fiber may be interfering with glucose absorption, decreasing gastric-emptying rate, or altering the secretion of GI hormones to have this positive effect. Protein metabolism may be affected by stimulating the growth of colonic bacteria and recycling urea nitrogen.[50,51] Certain fiber sources may inhibit lipid absorption and increase the excretion of neutral sterols as cholesterol and bile acids.[49] Certain fibers, through binding, may also decrease absorption of certain minerals (calcium, phosphorus, and magnesium), resulting in increased fecal losses. To evaluate this concern, fiber source, fiber and mineral intake, length of use of fiber, and presence of other mineral-binding agents in the diet are all factors that should be explored.[49]

Dietary fiber is defined as any substance of plant origin, typically the plant's structural and storage components, that passes through the alimentary tract undigested by GI enzymes. The structural and storage components defined as dietary fiber comprise both carbohydrate (polysaccharides) and noncarbohydrate substances. Table 13–4 lists the variety of components of dietary fiber. There

TABLE 13–4. DIETARY FIBER SOURCES

Structural Components (Water Soluble)	Storage Components (Water Soluble)
Lignin[a]	Pectins
Cellulose	Mucilages
Hemicellulose	Gums

[a]Noncarbohydrate source.

are a number of methods for measuring dietary fiber. Each method analyzes certain components of dietary fiber to varying degrees. Therefore, whenever dietary fiber levels are compared, the analytic method or technique should be stated.

Figure 13–4 describes the digestive process of dietary fiber as it passes through the GI tract. Note that dietary fiber is fermented by the bacteria within the large intestine. Lignin, as a noncarbohydrate substance, passes through unchanged; 55 to 85 percent of the hemicellulose, 50 to 80 percent of the cellulose, and about 90 percent of the pectin is digested by bacterial enzymes, resulting in

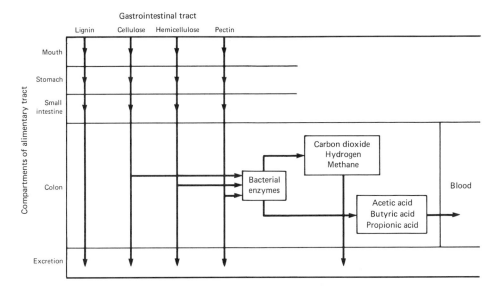

Figure 13–4. The passage of fiber through the gastrointestinal tract. *(Adapted from Ross Laboratories: Enrich, Liquid nutrition with fiber. Columbus, Ohio, June 1984.)*

the production of ammonia, carbon dioxide, hydrogen, and methane in the lower GI tract.

There is no RDA established for fiber, but an intake sufficient to affect bowel function without interfering with absorption of other nutrients is recommended.

PHYSICAL CHARACTERISTICS OF ENTERAL FORMULAS

Aside from the nutrient components, the physical characteristics of an enteral formulation affect the patient's tolerance of the formula. The principal symptoms of tube feeding intolerance are gastric retention, diarrhea, and constipation. Osmolality and microbial competence are the two variables most likely to influence overall tolerance to an enteral feeding.

Osmolality, the physical phenomenon of net permeability resulting in equilibrium across a given cell membrane, is a measure of the concentration of free particles, molecules, or ions in a given solution in water. These particles are electrolytes, minerals, carbohydrates, proteins, and/or amino acids. It is measured by determining the number of particles of solute present per unit weight of water or by the solute per liter other solvent. Osmolality is expressed in units of osmoles or milliosmoles per kg water (one osmole equals one gram molecular weight of a non-dissociated substance) (Table 13–5).[56] It is important biologically because of its role in maintaining a balance between intracellular and extracellular fluids. Osmotic forces within the body are generally kept equivalent by the rapid exchange of water between the body's intracellular and extracellular compartments.

In contrast, osmolarity refers to the degree of depression produced by solute per unit volume of solution. Osmolarity is expressed as osmoles per liter water. For dilute solutions, there is essentially no difference between osmolality and osmolarity, but for concentrated solutions, osmolarity is always less

than osmolality; for example, in a typical 1000 ml volume of a 1 cal/cc enteral formula that contains approximately 20 percent solids and 80 percent water, the osmolarity would be 400 mosm per liter in contrast to an osmolality of 500 osm/kg H_2O.[52]

All nutrients and dietary components, except H_2O, contribute to the osmolality of a solution. Electrolytes, in an enteral formula, have a major effect on osmolality secondary to their size and property of dissociation in solution. Large molecular weight carbohydrates, such as starch and glucose polymers, exhibit less osmotic pressure in a solution than smaller units such as sucrose or glucose. Because carbohydrates are digested more rapidly than other nutrient components, their effect on osmolality is greater. Proteins, which are large molecules, exert little or no effect in solution until they are hydrolyzed. Amino acids, however, contribute greatly to osmotic pressure because of their relatively small size. Fat does not have a profound effect on osmolality because of the manner in which it is digested and transported across the cell membranes. The physical and chemical form, as well as concentration, contributes to fat's effect on osmolality. For instance, MCT are more osmotically active than are neutral normal fats and less active than homogenized ones. In short, the more predigested the nutritive components of a formula are, the higher the osmolality of that formula.[53]

Gastric emptying is slowed by solutions with osmotic pressures greater or less than 200 mosm. The higher the osmolality, the greater the inhibitory effect on the GI tract. For example, if a hypertonic formula (greater than 200 mosm) is fed into the stomach, gastric retention, nausea, and vomiting may ensue. Additionally, hypertonic solutions may cause severe diarrhea, electrolyte depletion, and dehydration.[54,55] The osmotic impact of enteral formulas is mediated by osmoreceptors in the duodenum. To eliminate the symptoms caused by hypertonicity, the water content of a solution can be adjusted so as to

TABLE 13–5. OSMOLALITY CALCULATION

Calculation formula to determine osmolality of an enteral solution:

$$Osm_f = \frac{(H_2O)_{c1}(Osm)_{nc1} + (H_2O)_{c2}(Osm)_{nc2}}{(H_2O)_{c1} + (H_2O)_{c2}}$$

Key:

Osm_f = osmolality of the formula (mosm/kg H_2O)
Osm_{nc1} = osmolality of nutrient component 1 (mosm/kg H_2O)
Osm_{nc2} = osmolality of nutrient component 2 (mosm/kg H_2O)
$H_2O_{c1}{}^a$ = water content of nutrient component 1 (kg)
$H_2O_{c2}{}^a$ = water content of nutrient component 2 (kg)

Example: Osmolality determination of modular formula (Vital + Microlipid)

Step 1: The calculated osmolality of Vital
$y = 902x - 400$ (x = caloric density = 1.2 kcal/ml) (y = osmolality)
$y = 902(1.2) - 400$
$y = 682$ mosm/kg H_2O

Step 2: Since 600 g of H_2O was used to prepare the Vital 1.2 kcal/ml, the H_2O content is approximately 0.6 kg. The moisture content of Microlipid is 42.5% (per Biosearch Medical Products, Inc.)
Therefore the H_2O content is derived by (240 ml $\times$ 42.5 g H_2O/100 ml $\times$ 1 kg/1000 g) or 0.102 kg
The osmolality of Microlipid is 80 mosm/kg

Step 3: Using original equation

$$Osm_f = \frac{(0.6 \text{ kg } H_2O)(682 \text{ mosm/kg } H_2O) + (0.102 \text{ kg } H_2O)(80 \text{ mosm/kg } H_2O)}{(0.6 \text{ kg } H_2O) + (0.102 \text{ kg } H_2O)} = 595 \text{ mosm/kg } H_2O$$

$^a H_2O$ content is determined by multiplying the volume of the component times its moisture content.
Adapted from Ferrett KA, Giudici RA: Osmolality determinations of concentrated enteral nutrition formulas. Nutr Supp Serv 2:6–9, 1982.[56]

create an isotonic environment in the duodenum. Further, the osmolality of an isotonic formula may increase as the intestinal enzymes hydrolyze the formula's components into smaller molecules. In a poorly functioning GI tract or with rapid administration of a hypertonic formula, the body cannot tolerate "hyperosmotic" loads.[53]

Osmolality may affect the solute load and H_2O requirements within the body. The major contributor to total solute load is the protein anabolic product, urea. The electrolytes sodium, potassium, and chloride also contribute to the body's solute load, which is excreted by the kidney. Formulas that yield a large renal solute load can cause clinical dehydration, which is assessed by serum and urine concentrations of electrolytes, blood urea nitrogen, and serum and urine osmolality. Hyperosmolality exists in the extracellular compartments of the body when the concentration of solutes rises above the normal range of 280 to 320 mosm. Conversely, hypoosmolality results when there is too much H_2O per solute in extracellular fluid. With respect to selection of enteral formulas, particle size and osmolality vary according to nutrient composition of the chosen formula and to the number of osmoles that the nutrient contributes. Thus, the osmolality of an elemental product, like those listed in Table 13–12, will vary according to the protein form and concentration of nitrogen present. In short, the osmality of an enteral formula is dependent upon the form and structure of its nutrient components in relation to the total H_2O content of the formula. The degree of hydrolysis contributes to the physical form of the nutrients and greatly influences osmolality.

BACTERIAL CONTAMINATION

In light of the increasing use of enteral formulas in nutrition support, the need to control microbial contamination and its associated sequelae becomes increasingly important. Many studies have demonstrated that enteral feedings must be prepared aseptically and handled properly by food service and nursing personnel in order to avert such clinical complications as septicemia, diarrhea, and GI tract disturbances.[57-60]

Today, many sterilized, premixed, prepackaged formulas are available. All that is required for use of these products is that they be hung using aseptic technique and that they be utilized within a prespecified time period. These prepared enteral formulas are more costly but require less handling by the provider; for example, the enteral preparation facility does not have to open, blenderize, or repackage the formulas. Further, the nursing staff does not have to pour the formula into a feeding bag for delivery. Both of the above interventions enhance the risk of bacterial contamination. The powdered or canned ready-to-use products are by far the most popular, most widely used enteral products.[57] The powdered products require constitution with water whereas canned formulas may require dilution to a concentration that the patient can tolerate. Other nutrient additives or medications may be necessary before packaging for patient use. With this amount of handling, microbial contamination can occur. Inappropriate formula handling and preparation by dietary and nursing personnel can have devastating effects on patient tolerance of enteral formulas as well as on the patient's nutritional utilization and clinical status. Inadequate hand cleansing and formulary equipment sterilization are common dietary sources of bacterial growth in enteral feedings. Improper preparation of tube feeding gavage equipment, in concert with poor hand preparation, is a common cause of microbial contamination. Studies demonstrating the microbial incompetence of ready-to-use enteral formulas using hang time recommended by the manufacturer confirm these sources of contamination in nursing units.[57,60] In both the nursing and dietary departments, thorough planning and training must be implemented in order to reduce the threat of microbial contamination; for instance, there should be adequate space alloted for the preparation, mixing, and dispensing in these departments. The personnel must also be given regular, updated instructions on new techniques of enteral formula preparation. Topics like aseptic technique, accurate measurement, labeling, and formula monitoring, i.e., infection surveillance, are important areas for discussion and training.[62]

Most hospitals have tube feeding protocols for nursing that specify hang time, labeling requirements, residual checks, oral and enteral tube care, formula storage, and patient care. Hang time can be defined as the time the enteral feeding is started to the time it is either emptied or stopped by nursing personnel. The concept of hang time originated among pharmaceutical companies before the advent of modern peristaltic pumps. The rationale for specifying hang time was to control microbial contamination. Given the knowledge of the replication rate of common microbial offenders like *Escherichia coli, Pseudomonas aeruginosa, Enterobacter cloacae,* and *Klebsiella,* the objective was to deliver a prescribed volume before the microbes had the opportunity to replicate to potentially harmful levels.[57]

Labeling is a very important procedure. The label on the enteral infusion bag or bottle should include the patient's name, room and bed number, the rate of administration, the time of preparation, the formula or product content, the caloric content, and nutrient composition. This information is necessary to determine hanging time and to define storage and disposal needs. Residual checks, daily weight, and urine fractional collections are baseline clinical indicators of the patient's formula tolerance. For example, glucose and fluid tolerance can be assessed along with bloating, distention, and cramping, all important variables of formula tolerance by patients. By flushing the enteral tube with continuous jet streams of warm H_2O, clogging is prevented and the threat of microbial contamination from nosocomial passage is reduced.

Manufacturers of enteral products provide guidelines for the use of their products (Table 13–6). Information on formula preparation, stability, and storage requirements as well as clinical trial data should support the hospital's efforts to reduce microbial contamination.[57]

Containers used for storing and delivering enteral formulas to patients are another area of concern when addressing bacterial contamination. The type of material, proper use and handling of containers, and the issue of recyclability are important.[61]

Clinical studies have clearly demonstrated that microbial contamination of enteral formulas is an important issue to consider.[57,58,60]

FORMULA CLASSIFICATION SYSTEM

As any clinician working in nutrition support today recognizes, there is an explosion of enteral products available on the market. Recalling composition and thereby differentiating the use and indications of this myriad of formulas makes formula selection more difficult. The classification system used in this chapter attempts to categorize formulas according to certain criteria and then, within these categories, establish family groupings of products that share similar characteristics. However, many formulas have characteristics shared by more than one grouping, thus making it difficult to assign a formula to one exclusive group.

Table 13–7 demonstrates that basically all formulas can be categorized into three main categories—polymeric, predigested, and modular formulas.

As described by Heymsfield et al.,[38] polymeric formulas contain protein, fat, and carbohydrate in high molecular weight form, thereby requiring complete digestive and ab-

TABLE 13–6. STORAGE AND HANDLING RECOMMENDATIONS FOR ENTERAL FORMULAS

STD Vivonex
Mixed solution may be left at room temperature for up to 8 hours or refrigerated for up to 24 hours.

Vital
Solution to be prepared for 24-hour usage. Refrigerate after preparation.

Travasorb STD
After mixing, may be refrigerated for 24 hours and delivered over 12 hours to the patient.

Precision LR
Use within 4 hours of preparation.

Ensure
Once opened use within 48 hours. During this time unused solution should be covered and refrigerated.

Adapted from Fagerman KE, Paauw JD, McCamish MA, et al.: Effects of time, temperature and preservative on bacterial growth in enteral nutrient solutions. Am J Hosp Pharm 41: 1122–1126, 1984.[57]

sorptive capabilities. These are also complete formulas in that they contain all the necessary macronutrients, as well as vitamins, minerals, and trace elements.

In the predigested category of formulas, one or more of the macronutrients, carbohydrate, protein or fat, has undergone either partial digestion (hydrolysis) or has been predigested to an elemental form ready for absorption. Protein is the nutrient most commonly altered. In these formulas, carbohydrate is typically in the form of glucose; fat exists as long chain triglyceride usually in very small quantities or MCT may be added. Protein, depending upon the formula, exists in varying stages of hydrolyzation—from partially hydrolyzed protein sources to the end product of protein digestion, di- and tripeptides or amino acids. Enteral modules are formulas made up from individual nutrient modules, as listed in Table 13–7. The modules typically consist of one major macronutrient, either carbohydrate, protein, or fat. They may be used to modify an already existing commercial formula or mixed to-

TABLE 13–7. ENTERAL FORMULA CLASSIFICATION

	Polymeric			Predigested	
Milk-Based Formulas	Fiber-Containing Formulas	Routine Standard Formulas	Routine Calorically Dense Formulas	Peptide Formulas	Amino Acid-Based Formulas
Meritene Liquid	Vitaneed	Ensure	Travasorb MCT	Criticare HN	Standard Vivonex
Carnation Instant Breakfast	Compleat-B	Ensure HN	Traumacal	Vital High Nitrogen	High Nitrogen Vivonex
	Compleat-Modified	Osmolite	Ensure Plus	Travasorb STD	Vivonex T.E.N.
	Enrich	Osmolite HN	Ensure Plus HN	Travasorb HN	
		Isocal	Sustacal HC		
		Sustacal	Isocal HCN		
		Precision Isotonic Diet	TwoCal HN		
		Travasorb Liquid	Magnacal		
		Entri-Pak with Entrition			
		Renu			
		Isotein HN			

gether in a de novo synthesis to construct a modular formula tailored to a patient's specific nutrition requirements. Figure 13–5 demonstrates how this categorization of enteral formula relates the choice of formula to the degree of GI function as affected by a GI disorder or by the effect of malnutrition. Malnutrition affects digestive and absorptive function through atrophy of the mucosal lining of the small intestine.[43,63] Based on composition, therefore, polymeric formulas require an intact GI tract, whereas predigested formulas are ideal for patients who have compromised GI tracts. Of course, total GI tract dysfunction requires the intervention of parenteral nutrition.

Predigested			Modular	
Disease-Specific Formulas	Carbohydrate Modules	Protein Modules	Fat Modules	Modular Enteral System
Amin-Aid	Polycose	Pro-Mix	Microlipid	Nutrisource Carbohydrate
Travasorb Renal	Sumacal	Propac	MCT Oil	Nutrisource Protein
Hepatic-Aid 11	Moducal	Casec	Pro-Mix High Fat Supplement	Nutrisource Amino Acids
Travasorb Hepatic	Pro-Mix Pure Carbohydrate Supplement	Citrotein		Nutrisource AA-High Branched Chain
Traum-Aid HBC		Ross SLD		Nutrisource Lipid-LCT
Stresstein				Nutrisource Lipid-MCT
Pulmocare				Nutrisource Minerals for Protein Formulas
				Nutrisource Min. (Protein) Elect. Restricted
				Nutrisource Minerals for Amino Acids
				Nutrisource Min. (AA) Elect. Restr.
				Nutrisource Vitamins

MILK-BASED FORMULAS

The first formulas used for tube feeding were milk-based. However, their lactose content (37 to 96 g per 1000 kcal) renders them difficult for critically ill patients to digest when delivered via tube.[64] These formulas are better suited as meal replacements or enteral supplements. They are sweet, palatable, available in a wide variety of flavors, and contain a full complement of vitamins and minerals, making them extremely useful to patients who cannot meet requirements by meals alone. These products are practical for home use because of their cost and availability. Symptoms of bloating, flatulence, cramp-

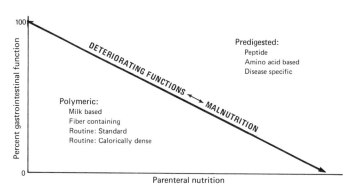

Figure 13–5. Nutrition support as determined by gastrointestinal tract function.

TABLE 13–8. MILK-BASED FORMULAS

	Meritene Liquid	Carnation Instant Breakfast
kcal/cc	1	1
NPC: g N	79:1	88:1
Source: CHO	Lactose, corn syrup, sucrose	Sucrose, corn syrup, lactose
Source: Pro	Skim milk	Milk, sodium caseinate, soy protein isolate
Source: Fat	Corn oil	Whole milk
g/L: CHO	110	135
g/L: Pro	58	58
g/L: Fat	32	31
mEq/L: Na	38	41
mEq/L: K	41	70
Osmolality mosm/kg H$_2$O	505–570	—
Vitamins (cc for 100% U.S. RDA)	1250	1400
Lactose free	NO	NO

ing, and diarrhea are often the first symptoms of the inability to digest lactose, in which case a lactose-free product should be used. Table 13–8 gives the nutrition composition of these products.

To avoid the complication of lactose intolerance, most new enteral formulas produced are lactose free. The milk base in these formulas is replaced by protein that is derived from caseinate salts, soy protein isolates, and/or egg white solids.[54] To contain costs, some hospitals have substituted milk-based formulas as enteral supplements with their own institutionally prepared nourishments or with other tube feeding formulas of similar taste and palatability.

FIBER-CONTAINING FORMULAS

There are two types of available formulas that fall into this formula grouping: those that contain fiber from natural food sources and those to which a fiber source has been added. Blenderized formulas, the common name of the first group, are made from whole foods—meat, milk products, fruits, and vegetables. Commercially produced blenderized enteral solutions are available to replace the institutionally prepared formulas. The commercially prepared formulas are more homogeneous and less viscous, making them easier to flow through small lumen feeding tubes. There is less risk of microbial contamination with commercial blenderized solutions.

A #10 French tube is recommended for

TABLE 13–9. FIBER-CONTAINING FORMULAS

	Vitaneed	Compleat-B	Compleat-Modified	Enrich
kcal/cc	1	1	1	1.1
NPC: g N	154:1	131:1	131:1	173:1
Source: CHO	Maltodextrin, pureed fruit and vegetables	Hydrolyzed cereal solids, pureed foods, nonfat dry milk, maltodextrin	Hydrolyzed cereal solids, fruit and vegetable puree	Hydrolyzed corn starch, soy poly-saccharide
Source: Pro	Beef sodium and calcium casein-ates, vegetables	Beef puree, nonfat dry milk	Beef, calcium caseinate, vege-tables	Na + Ca casein-ates, soy protein
Source: Fat	Soy oil, beef	Corn oil	Corn oil	Corn oil
g/L: CHO	125	128	141	162
g/L: Pro	35	43	43	40
g/L: Fat	40	43	37	37
mEq/L: Na	22	57	29	37
mEq/L: K	32	36	36	40
Osmolality mosm/kg H_2O	310	405	300	480
Vitamins (cc for 100% U.S. RDA)	2000	1500	1500	1391
Lactose free	Yes	No	Yes	Yes

gravity flow and #8 French tube if pump delivered. Based on composition, these nutritionally complete formulas require full digestive capabilities.

Blenderized formulas are frequently indicated in three types of patients: (1) stable long-term tube feeding patients, e.g., nursing home patients, because the long-term use of a whole-food formula may provide trace nutrients as yet unidentified and the fiber helps prevent constipation and impaction; (2) patients who develop an intolerance to other enteral formulas while tolerating a formula made from whole foods; and (3) diabetic patients or other patients demonstrating glucose intolerance. These patients may benefit from the complex carbohydrate starch content of these formulas if sucrose has not been added to these formulas.

The nutritional composition of such formulas is listed in Table 13–9. Only Compleat B contains lactose in this grouping. The fiber content of blenderized formulas varies depending upon the analytic method used to quantitate dietary fiber. The fruit and vegetables used in the processing of these formulas result in moderate amounts of fiber. Because of lack of flavoring, these formulas are recommended for tube feeding only.

Enrich, which is not blenderized, is a new standard enteral formula supplemented by fiber in the form of soy polysaccharide. Each 8 fluid ounce serving of this product contains 5 g of soy polysaccharide, which yields 3.4 g of dietary fiber.[49] This formula provides balanced nutrition and can be used both as a supplement and as a tube feeding. Table 13-9 compares the nutritional composition of this formula with blenderized formulas. For tube feeding, Enrich is best used at room temperature as cooler temperatures increase the viscosity of the product, making it more difficult to infuse. A large-bore tube (#10 French) is necessary if formula is not pump delivered.

Indications for a fiber-supplemented formula may include glucose intolerance, renal failure, hypercatabolism resulting in increased total body urea, and colonic disease states.[50] Both diarrhea and constipation can sometimes be corrected through the use of a fiber-supplemented formula, as the fiber helps maintain normal colonic mucosa and intestinal motility. This formula is contraindicated in any patient who requires a low residue diet.

ROUTINE FORMULAS: STANDARD AND CALORICALLY DENSE

Standard formulas, which are lactose free, typically 1.0 kcal/ml, relatively isotonic, low residue, low in electrolytes, and low in cost, flow through small lumen tubes with ease and are used as routine tube feedings in uncomplicated patients who require enteral hyperalimentation to meet nutrition requirements. Percentages of carbohydrate, protein, and fat composition range from 50 to 55 percent, 10 to 15 percent and 25 to 30 percent, respectively. Table 13-10 compares the nutrition composition of the products in this group.

In general, the standard formulas are com-

posed of intact proteins, oligosaccharides, and long chain triglycerides (a limited number contain some MCT). These formulas require a functional GI tract and can be used both for tube feeding and oral supplementation.

Calorically dense formulas, shown in Table 13-11, have similar nutritional composition, except that they are concentrated to provide more kilocalories in less volume. Table 13-8 compares the nutrition composition of formulas in this grouping. They are indicated for fluid-restricted patients or patients whose tube feeding is cycled during certain time blocks of the day or night, i.e., for patients who need a formula that can meet nutrition requirements in less volume. Fluid balance, glucosuria, blood sugar levels, and body weight changes require close supervision in patients receiving these formulas, because of their high glucose concentration and limited free water content. Patients receiving these formulas can become dehydrated and develop hyperosmolar hyperglycemic nonketotic dehydration syndrome. Close monitoring of fluid requirements, intake and output, and body weight changes can prevent this syndrome from occurring (see Chapter 15).

AMINO ACID-BASED FORMULAS

Definition and Brief History

The elemental diet is a specific enteral formula made up of chemically well-defined elemental components that require minimal digestion in the intestinal tract. The experimentation of Rose in the 1940s led to the discovery that nutritionally balanced AA mixtures, when substituted for intact protein, could maintain positive nitrogen balance in humans and animals.[65] Greenstein and Winitz[66] demonstrated that chemically defined diets containing L-amino acids, glucose, corn oil, minerals, and vitamins could maintain growth, reproduction, and lactation in experimental animals. In 1965, in collaboration with Winitz, NASA Apollo projects developed an elemental diet that would provide adequate nutrition while reducing bulky fecal production during space missions. These objectives were achieved, but the impalatibility of the mixture led to its eventual abandonment.[18]

Winitz, in a study using an elemental diet formula in normal human volunteers, showed that positive nitrogen balance and general well-being could be maintained for up to 6 months. In addition, a reduction in serum cholesterol and fecal output was demonstrated.[67,68] Bounous et al. showed the benefits and effectiveness of the elemental diet in both animal and human models receiving chemotherapy and nuclear therapy.[69] It has since been shown to be effective in maintaining and improving nutrition status in a broad spectrum of clinical disease states.

Formula Profile

Unlike conventional enteral formulas, which contain intact proteins and/or peptides of varying weights, the principal nitrogen source of the elemental diet is the isolated, crystalline L-type AA (Table 13–12). There is controversy in the literature about the value of administering free AA, those found in elemental formulations, over intact proteins. This controversy involves the relative rate of protein utilization or absorption of one protein form over the other. No definitive statement can be made within the context of this presentation. More research is required, however, at the molecular level to obtain a better understanding of the physiology and transport mechanisms within the intestinal lumen and brush border mucosal cells as they relate to digestion, absorption, concentration, and the rate of delivery of hydrolyzed versus nonhydrolyzed protein sources.

The basic carbohydrate source is glucose in the form of oligosaccharides or dissaccharides. A high percentage of simple carbohydrates in an elemental formula increases the osmolality of the formula and is generally problematic for patients with glucose intolerance. Further, diarrhea and the "dumping" syndrome are possible consequences when high carbohydrate concentrations are used.

The lipid source is largely essential fatty acids (chiefly linoleic acid) supplied from vegetable oils. In terms of percent of total composition, however, lipids are a limited calorie source because they require intact pancreatic and bile function to emulsify and hydrolyze long chain triglycerides for absorption. Elemental enteral formulas provide 1 to 4 percent of total calories as essential fatty acids.

Osmolality. As previously mentioned, the osmolality of an elemental formula may influence the patient's tolerance of the formula and affect the nutritional benefit derived from the formula. Gastric emptying is slowed when osmotic pressure is greater than 220 mosm.[70] When a hyperosmotic formula is delivered directly into the small intestines, patients may experience abdominal cramping and discomfort along with diarrhea and consequential dehydration.[106] Over a period of time, secondary to a reduction in fecal mass, constipation may ensue. Therefore, one must consider the clinical status of the patient and the osmolality of a formula before determining the rate of administration. Diluting the initial concentration of the formula may reduce the initial physiologic effects of hyperosmolar formulas.

Fat Content. It has been suggested that the low concentration of long chain triglycerides in many elemental diets may promote essential fatty acid deficiency. However, clinical evidence of long-term clinical signs and symptoms caused by a reduced intake of essential fatty acids appears insufficient to support this conclusion.[71]

Vitamins, Minerals, and Electrolytes. Hypoprothrombinemia can be a consequence of

TABLE 13–10. ROUTINE FORMULAS: STANDARD

	Ensure	Ensure HN	Osmolite	Osmolite HN	Isocal
kcal/cc	1	1	1	1	1
NPC: g N	153:1	124:1	153:1	124:1	167:1
Source: CHO	Hydrolyzed corn starch, sucrose	Hydrolyzed corn starch, sucrose	Hydrolyzed corn starch	Hydrolyzed corn starch	Glucose oligo-saccharides
Source: Pro	Na + Ca caseinates, soy protein isolate	Na + Ca caseinates, soy protein isolate	Ca + Na caseinates, soy protein isolates	Ca + Na caseinates, soy protein isolates	Ca + Na caseinates, soy protein isolates
Source: Fat	Corn oil	Corn oil	MCT oil, corn oil, soy oil	MCT oil, corn oil, soy oil	Soy oil, MCT oil
g/L: CHO	145	141	145	141	133
g/L: Pro	37	44	37	44	34
g/L: Fat	37	36	39	37	44
mEq/L: Na	37	40	24	40	23
mEq/L: K	40	40	26	40	34
Osmolality mosm/kg H_2O	450	460	300	310	300
Vitamins (cc for 100% U.S. RDA)	1887	1321	1887	1321	2000
Lactose free	Yes	Yes	Yes	Yes	Yes

prolonged usage of elemental formula if the vitamin K content is not sufficient. This is a particular concern if the patient is being treated with broad-spectrum antibiotics. Other fat- and water-soluble vitamin deficiencies may arise if exogenous supplementation is not given.[71]

Minerals, such as calcium, iron, phosphorus, and zinc, may be present in lower than recommended levels. Periodic serum evaluations should be included in the nutrition care protocol of patients receiving long-term elemental formulas.[71]

The concentration of electrolytes, sodium and potassium, again varies according to the formula. Care should be taken when choosing an elemental formula for cardiac, renal, or hepatic patients requiring sodium re-

Sustacal	Precision Isotonic Diet	Travasorb Liquid	Entri-Pak with Entrition	Renu	Isotein HN
1	1	1	1	1	1.2
79:1	183:1	154:1	154:1	154:1	86:1
Sucrose, corn syrup	Glucose oligo-saccharides, sucrose	Sucrose, corn syrup solids	Maltodextrin	Maltrodextrin, sucrose	Maltodextrin, fructose, monosaccha-rides
Ca + Na caseinates, soy protein isolate	Egg albumin	Na + Ca caseinates, soy protein isolate	Na + Ca caseinates	Ca + Na caseinates	Delactosed lactalbumin
Soy oil	Soy oil	Corn oil, soy oil	Corn oil	Soy oil	Soy oil, MCT
140	144	145	136	125	156
61	29	37	35	35	68
23	30	37	35	40	34
40	33	32	31	22	27
53	25	32	31	32	27
625	300	450	300	300	300
1080	1560	2000	2000	2000	1770
Yes	Yes	Yes	Yes	Yes	Yes

strictions. Patients with excess losses of electrolytes, GI fistulas, electrolyte-depleting nephropathies, or burns may require electrolyte supplementation.[71]

Trace minerals, e.g., cobalt and chromium, are generally absent from elemental formulations. With extended use of an elemental formula, trace element status and formula supplementation must be considered.[71]

PEPTIDE-BASED FORMULAS

The dietary protein sources in a peptide-based formula are principally di- and tripeptides formed by incomplete hydrolysis of whole protein. The fat source is principally vegetable oil combined with MCT oil. The carbohydrate source is either hydrolyzed corn starch or glucose oligosaccharides.

TABLE 13–11. ROUTINE FORMULAS: CALORICALLY DENSE

	Travasorb MCT	Traumacal	Ensure Plus	Ensure Plus HN	Sustacal HC	Isocal HCN	TwoCal HN	Magnacal
kcal/cc	1	1.5	1.5	1.5	1.5	2	2	2
NPC: g N	100:1	90:1	146:1	125:1	134:1	145:1	150:1	154:1
Source: CHO	Corn syrup solids	Corn syrup sucrose	Hydrolyzed corn starch, sucrose	Hydrolyzed corn starch, sucrose	Corn syrup solids, sugar	Corn syrup	Hydrolyzed corn starch, sucrose	Maltodextrin, sucrose
Source: Pro	Lactalbumin potassium caseinate	Ca and Na caseinates	Na and Ca caseinates, soy protein isolate	Na and Ca caseinates, soy protein isolate	Ca and Na caseinates	Ca and Na caseinates	Na and Ca caseinates	Ca and Na caseinates
Source: Fat	MCT oil, sunflower oil	Soy oil and MCT	Corn oil	Corn oil	Soy oil	Soy oil, MCT oil	Corn oil, MCT oil	Soy oil
g/L: CHO	108	143	200	200	190	225	216	250
g/L: Pro	49	83	55	63	61	75	83	70
g/L: Fat	29	69	53	50	58	91	91	80
mEq/L: Na	15	51	50	52	36	35	46	44
mEq/L: K	26	36	60	47	38	36	59	32
Osmolality mosm/kg H_2O	312	490	600	650	650	690	750	590
Vitamins (cc for 100% U.S. RDA)	2000	2000	1600	947	1800	1500	950	1000
Lactose free	Yes	Yes	Yes	Yes	Yes	Yes	Yes	Yes

TABLE 13–12. PEPTIDE AND AMINO ACID-BASED FORMULAS

	Criticare HN	Vital High Nitrogen	Travasorb STD	Travasorb HN	Standard Vivonex	High Nitrogen Vivonex	Vivonex T.E.N.
kcal/cc	1	1	1	1	1	1	1
NPC: g N	148:1	125:1	202:1	126:1	286:1	127:1	149:1
Source: CHO	Maltodextrin corn starch	Hydrolyzed corn starch, sucrose	Glucose oligo-saccharides	Glucose oligo-saccharides	Glucose oligo-saccharides	Glucose oligo-saccharides	Maltodextrin and modified starch
Source: Pro	Hydrolyzed casein, amino acids	Whey, soy and meat protein, hydrolysates, free amino acids	Hydrolyzed lactalbumin, peptides	Hydrolyzed lactalbumin peptides	L-amino acids	L-amino acids	L-amino acids
Source: Fat	Safflower oil	Safflower oil, MCT oil	MCT oil, sunflower oil	MCT oil, sunflower oil	Safflower oil	Safflower oil	Safflower oil
g/L: CHO	222	185	190	175	231	210	206
g/L: Pro	38	42	30	45	22	44	38
g/L: Fat	3	11	14	14	1	1	3
mEq/L: Na	27	20	40	40	20	23	20
mEq/L: K	34	34	30	30	30	30	20
Osmolality mosm/kg H_2O	650	460	560	560	550	810	630
Vitamins (cc for 100% U.S. RDA)	1892	1500	2000	2000	1800	3000	2000
Lactose free	Yes	Yes	Yes	Yes	Yes	Yes	Yes

With respect to formula composition, the elemental formula differs only in its protein source. (See Table 13–12 for comparison of nutritional composition.) There is substantial controversy as to whether AA-based elemental formulas are a better choice. Evidence does not preclude the possibility that the more complex di- and tripeptides are absorbed as efficiently as the AA-based elemental formulas. Silk et al. propose that there is no significant difference in the maintenance of nitrogen balance in patient populations receiving crystalline AA versus peptide-based enteral formulas.[72,73] Further, there is no definitive evidence on the exact nature of peptide absorption and transport at the intestinal brush border level.[74] Thus, the increased osmolar load of the elemental diet may not offset the physiologic gains of this enteral regime.

In view of this controversy, it behooves the clinician to consider using peptide-based formulas among patients who cannot tolerate the hyperosmotic load presented by elemental formulations.

DISEASE-SPECIFIC FORMULA: RENAL

The selection of an enteral formula for the treatment of a patient with impaired renal function must consider these factors: degree of disease state, i.e., acute or chronic renal disease; dialysis therapy; nutrition status; whole body organ function/status; and degree of physiologic stress present. Formula selection will depend upon the relatively fixed ability of the kidneys to excrete or retain elements such as water, protein, and electrolytes.

As in any other disease state, selection of specific formulations for patients with renal disease begins with the basal energy requirements. Sufficient calories must be provided to promote endogenous protein synthesis.

Protein Requirements

Depending on the degree of loss of renal function, protein requirements will vary from 0.45 to 0.8 to 1.0 g/kg/day in nondialyzed patients and from 1.0 to 1.5 g/kg/day for dialyzed patients. The principal objective is to achieve nitrogen balance by providing high quality protein. This can be achieved by using completely digested protein in the form of L-amino acids. With regard to the specific types of AA required, Steffee asserts that the former essential and nonessential categories be replaced with the terms dispensable and indispensable AA. A third group, conditionally indispensable AA, may or may not be required by renal patients, but it is Steffee's opinion that these AA should be included in their nutrition care regimen. (Fig. 13–6).[75]

Age, degree of stress, and the clinical status of the patient are the principal dictates of AA choice in formula selection. The practitioner must also be cognizant of the "stress" dialysis places on protein status. For example, once dialysis is begun, the requirement for AA delivery is enhanced by the additional losses imposed by the procedure itself.[76] Peptide losses across all membranes, membrane surface area and pore size, duration of dialysis, and whole protein losses associated with peritoneal dialysis are contributing "stress" factors of dialysis.

Carbohydrate and Fat Requirements

In general, the ratio of fat and carbohydrates delivered as nonprotein calories is not of significant importance in renal dysfunction. Therefore, an enteral formula that provides glucose and the essential fatty acids in bioavailable forms should suffice. One should also consider GI tract function and pancreatic status so as to prevent any endocrine imbalances and to avert symptoms of intolerance.

Fluid Requirements

The patient with normal kidney function has the ability to reduce urine volumes to as low as 350 ml up to 22 L daily should fluid intake so demand. The normal excretory volume is approximately 1.5 L. In sharp contrast, the patient with renal dysfunction excretes more urine than normal depending upon renal concentrating ability. The normal patient can produce urine with a concentration as low as 30 and as high as 1500 mosm/L, with an average of 1200 mosm/L. With renal disease, the patient's ability to concentrate ranges from 250 to 300 mosm/L and averages 300 mosm/L. Therefore, it is important to assess the patient's urinary output ability before prescribing an enteral formulation. Formulas that are too concentrated may result in dehydration in the patient. In contrast, too much fluid volume can result in water intoxification. Thus, the need to monitor and assess the patient's fluid balance and electrolyte status routinely throughout their clinical course cannot be overstated.[75]

Electrolyte Requirements

Sodium. The normal kidney can alter sodium excretion to a level as low as 1 mEq/day. It can also adjust excretion based on food intake (2 to 4 g/day). In light of the broad range of normal daily sodium intake, this is astonishing. In renal disease patients, the ability to control excretion is compromised. The average range of sodium excretion is 30 to 50 mEq/day. Thus, it is most often necessary to restrict sodium intake. There is a subset of renal disease patients who have salt-losing nephropathy, in which exogenous sodium losses occur despite adequate sodium intake. Sodium excretion should be monitored continuously and changes to the enteral formulation of choice should be made wherever deemed necessary.

Potassium. Similar to sodium excretion, potassium excretion in healthy individuals is

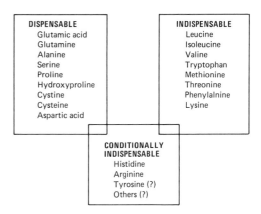

Figure 13–6. Amino acid classification in clinical nutrition.

quite dependent upon intake, ranging from 0 to 125 mEq/day. Renal patients exhibit an increased inability to excrete excess dietary potassium. Potassium imbalances caused by internal dysfunction (such as trauma, abscess, internal bleeding) create significant complications in renal patients. An accurate assessment of nutrition and clinical status must therefore be completed to rule out hyperkalemia, resulting from endogenous disorders and clinical malnutrition. Table 13–13 lists the nutritional composition of renal formulas currently available.

DISEASE-SPECIFIC FORMULA: TRAUMA/STRESS

In the last 10 years, total parenteral nutrition has been the method of choice for nutrition support of the surgical patient. In light of the complications associated with this treatment modality, and given the fact that burn and trauma patients usually have functional GI tracts at the time of injury, the use of enteral formulations specifically designed for the needs of this patient population is clearly reasonable and appropriate. One ma-

TABLE 13–13. DISEASE-SPECIFIC FORMULAS

	Amin-Aid	Travasorb Renal	Hepatic-Aid 11	Travasorb Hepatic	Traum-Aid HBC	Stresstein	Pulmocare
kcal/cc	2	1.35	1.1	1.1	1.0	1.2	1.5
NPC: g N	838:1	362:1	148:1	218:1	102:1	97:1	150:1
Source: CHO	Maltodextrin, sucrose	Glucose oligo-saccharides, sucrose	Maltodextrin, sucrose	Glucose oligo-saccharides, sucrose	Maltodextrins	Maltodextrins	Hydrolyzed corn starch, sucrose
Source: Pro	Crystalline amino acids	Crystalline L-amino acids	Crystalline amino acids	Crystalline L-amino acids	Crystalline amino acids	L-amino acids, glycine	Na + Ca caseinates
Source: Fat	Soy oil, lecithin, mono- and diglycerides	MCT oil, sun-flower oil	Soy oil, lecithin, mono- and diglycerides	MCT oil, sun-flower oil	Soybean oil, lecithin, mono- and diglycerides, MCT	MCT, soybean oil	Corn oil
g/L: CHO	366	271	169	209	166	171	106
g/L: Pro	19	23	44	29	56	69	63
g/L: Fat	46	18	36	14	12	27	92
mEq/L: Na	<15	—	<15	10	23	29	57
mEq/L: K	<6	—	<6	22	30	28	49
Osmolality mosm/kg H_2O	1095	590	560	690	675	910	490
Vitamins (cc for 100% U.S. RDA)	—	2100	—	2100	3000	2000	1000
Lactose free	Yes	Yes	Yes	Yes	Yes	Yes	Yes

jor limitation in the prescription of an "ideal" enteral formula for this patient group is the lack of original research on the nutrient requirements of the traumatized patient. Though not directly related, the application of TPN prescription criteria is the model from which current enteral formulas for trauma/stress were developed.

Review of the Physiologic Response to Injury

Physiologic trauma can be divided into two phases.[77] The initial response is called the "ebb" phase. This period is brief—lasting a few hours in minor trauma and a few days in the burn patient. Increased knowledge and improvements in fluid replacement therapy and emergency medicine have allowed more patients to reach the "flow" phase of their injuries. This period is characterized by a period of marked hypermetabolism lasting anywhere from a few days to several months. Aggressive nutrition intervention is required during this period of hypermetabolism, which is the focus of this discussion on enteral formulation in the traumatized or stressed patient population.

Hypermetabolism and Energy Prerequisites

The main physiologic response to injury is an increase in metabolic rate. The magnitude of increase is directly related to the nature of the trauma. Burn patients manifest the greatest degree of hypermetabolism whereas lesser responses are found in other injuries,[78,79] More specifically, increases of 100 to 150 percent in metabolic rate have been reported in burn patients,[80,81] whereas uncomplicated elective surgical cases demonstrate temporary increases that may be within normal basal energy requirements. Other variables such as age, pretrauma health status, mental disposition, and adequate medication influence energy utilization. Heat loss through radiation, conduction, convection, or evaporation and wound openings are significant variables in metabolic rate.

Given all of these factors, the typical treatment decision is to provide surplus calories to the traumatized patient. Great care should be taken, however, to closely approximate the "actual" caloric requirements of the patient in order to avoid such conditions as fatty liver and acute respiratory distress. The calorie prescription for the enteral formula can be derived either through indirect calorimetry or by estimating the basal metabolic requirement (BMR) using one of the equations developed for that purpose and multiplying BMR by a predefined stress factor (see Chapter 10, Protein and Energy Requirements).

Nutrient Metabolism: A Brief Review

Carbohydrate. Gluconeogenesis is the most dramatic change in carbohydrate metabolism in traumatized patients. Supplying an adequate level of carbohydrates in the enteral formula minimizes the degradation of AA that would be oxidized to gluconeogenic precursor or utilized as a physiologic energy source. Excessively high carbohydrate concentrations in enteral formulas for the treatment of trauma impair liver function. Fatty liver, one example of such an impairment, results from glucose interference in hepatic and adipose tissue lipid mobilization secondary to chronic hyperinsulinemia from continuously infused glucose. Excess carbohydrate concentration may also affect pulmonary function. Fatty liver can interfere with diaphragmatic exhalation, requiring an increase in energy expenditure. Further, excess carbohydrate intake places an increased demand upon the respiratory system secondary to removal of CO_2 produced during the synthesis of triglycerides.

Protein. Trauma causes the body to catabolize protein and to excrete it as urea from the kidneys. During periods of extreme stress, the body alters its protein priorities from storage in peripheral compartments (muscle) to utilization in visceral compartments (organs and tissue repair). Thus, the enteral prescription for stress and trauma patients must provide an adequate quantity of high quality protein. Branch chain amino acid (BCAA) formulas should be used to fulfill this requirement. Research indicates that the inclusion of BCAA in the enteral formula results in improved nitrogen retention, reduced muscle protein catabolism, and increased protein synthesis. Studies also demonstrate that other nutrients such as potassium, phosphorus, and sodium must be available for optimal utilization of exogenously supplied protein sources.[82,83]

Fat. There is positive evidence that fats are the body's major source of energy in burns, trauma, and sepsis.[84,85] Over one-fourth of the CO_2 production is related to fat oxidation. It is important to include fat in trauma/stress enteral formulas in order to (1) minimize protein catabolism of existing protein stores and (2) prevent fatty acid deficiency. Table 13–13 lists the nutritional composition of trauma formulas available.

DISEASE-SPECIFIC FORMULA: PULMONARY

There is definitive evidence that patients with chronic obstructive pulmonary disease and acute respiratory failure suffer from malnutrition.[86] For example, more than 50 percent of patients afflicted with the former conditions experience weight loss as a result of (1) inadequate caloric intake caused by anorexia, apnoxia, and GI tract distress; (2) increased energy requirements secondary to increased energy expenditure; (3) lean body mass catabolism; (4) systemic infections secondary to pulmonary disease; and (5) long-term respirator dependency. It is important that aggressive nutrition intervention be employed to improve the nutrition status of this patient population.

Carbohydrate. The goal of the pulmonary enteral regimen is to decrease the level of

CO_2 in the blood. Administration of an enteral formula with an increased proportion of fat calories and decreased carbohydrate calories can decrease CO_2 production and the respiratory quotient (RQ), the ratio of CO_2 produced to oxygen consumed. In turn, reduction of the RQ and of CO_2 production diminishes ventilatory requirements. Studies have demonstrated that high carbohydrate diets result in increased CO_2 production, O_2 consumption, and respiratory quotient.[87,88] Further, these diets can precipitate respiratory failure and impair the ability to wean from artificial ventilation.

Protein. It is important to provide sufficient protein for anabolism, while avoiding protein overfeeding. Protein intake has little effect on CO_2 production, but it has been demonstrated to augment the physical mechanics of respiration. In a study by Askanazi et al.,[89] it was shown that the ventilatory drive mechanics significantly improved following the feeding of a high protein parenteral regimen. It should be noted, however, that high protein diets benefit patients with residual alveolar reserves but may prove detrimental to patients without alveolar reserves.

Fat. The presence of fat in the diet reduces CO_2 production and decreases ventilation requirements. A study by Askanazi et al.[90] demonstrated that a balance of carbohydrate to fat nonprotein calories resulted in decreased CO_2 production and improved ventilatory requirements. A high carbohydrate regime resulted in an increase in CO_2 production along with an increase in RQ greater than 1. An RQ of 1 or more is suggestive of lipogenesis. Lipogenesis, the conversion of glucose to triglycerides or fat, dramatically increases CO_2 production. Table 13–13 lists the nutritional composition of Pulmocare, a relatively new product designed for respiratory patients.

DISEASE-SPECIFIC FORMULA: HEPATIC

The goal of nutrition therapy in patients afflicted with liver disease is (1) to maintain adequate nutrition; (2) to facilitate organ regeneration and recovery, and (3) to prevent or improve hepatic encephalopathy whenever possible.[91] Provision of sufficient protein and calories is essential to maintain nitrogen balance and to support the liver metabolically and biochemically.

The liver is the principal site of protein synthesis, detoxification, and drug excretion. It also plays an important role in the storage and utilization of many vitamins. The liver is composed of more than one cell type, with the principal site of metabolic activity being the hepatocyte.

Under normal physiologic conditions, exogenous nutrition sources are absorbed by way of the intestinal epithelium and transported into the portal circulation. They are further modified by the liver prior to their deposit into the systemic circulation. Ingested protein, carbohydrates and fats reach the portal circulation in the form of free AA, monosaccharides, and short and medium chain fatty acids. Additionally, the liver receives endogenously generated substrates, including free fatty acids released by adipose tissue stores and AA and lactate derived from tissue catabolism. It is quite apparent that the liver is a regulatory center for the complex processes of carbohydrate, protein, and fat metabolism.

Normal Hepatic Metabolism

Carbohydrate. Dietary carbohydrate sources, most commonly absorbed as hexose polymers, i.e., galactose and fructose, are converted into glucose, the major circulating sugar and energy source in the body. The liver is a key organ in this conversion process. The enzymes hexokinase, glucose-6-phosphatase, and glucokinase ultimately convert endogenous carbohydrate sources to glucose. The specific mechanisms of (1) the hexose monophosphate shunt and (2) the Embden-Meyerhof pathway (an aerobic reaction) convert glucose in the liver into glycogen.

Protein. Protein derived from exogenous and internal sources undergoes a continuous process of hydrolysis and resynthesis at variable rates. In addition, there is a constant interchange between AA (derived from amination, transamination, and deamination processes) and nonprotein byproducts of fat and carbohydrate metabolism. The end results of these reactions are urea, ammonia, acetyl CoA, ketone bodies, and adenosine triphosphate.

The rate of AA turnover and catabolism by the liver is variable and is affected by endogenous digestive hormones. For example, a study by Elwyn[92] in an animal model demonstrated that more than half of a given quantity of ingested AA were converted to urea, 20 percent were incorporated into plasma and hepatic proteins, and a little more than 20 percent were deposited into the AA pool. Hormonal changes, e.g., an increase in plasma insulin, can result in an increase in the uptake of BCAA into muscle and adipose tissue. In contrast, a decrease in insulin concentration and an increase in glucagon levels can result in an increase in circulating AA concentration. Again it is clear that the liver's production of AA can be used for protein synthesis or for catabolic states.

Fat. The liver has a principal role in the metabolism of endogenous and dietary lipids (triglycerides and phospholipids). Lipids circulate through the blood bound to hepatic proteins and sterols. Medium and short chain fatty acids, in concert with triglycerides released from adipose tissue sites, can be converted to acetyl CoA by the liver. Glycerol, an end product of fatty acids cleared from triglycerides, can be transformed into glucose by the liver. Under prolonged starvation, the liver can spare the degradation of protein muscle stores to support gluconeogenesis by mobilizing free fatty acids as an energy substrate from adipose tissue and lipid oxidation. The end result is a temporary production of ketone bodies that can be metabolized by body tissues, including the brain, in lieu of glucose.

Altered Hepatic Metabolism

Carbohydrate. Liver disease alters carbohydrate metabolism. Abnormal glucose tolerance is most common although hypoglycemia can also ensue.[93] Hyperglycemia is postulated to result from (1) a decrease in the number of insulin receptors; (2) a shifting of insulin away from the liver; and (3) a decrease in the number of parenchymal cells thereby reducing the number of hepatic insulin-binding sites. Other external factors such as the circulating levels of growth hormone, glucagon, corticosteroids, and sex hormones, as well as potassium deficiency and organ dysfunction, i.e., pancreatitis, can influence a diabetogenic state and glucose intolerance.

Fat. Cholesterol production is altered in hepatic disease secondary to a decreased rate of synthesis or a decreased synthesis of apolipoproteins by the liver.[96] Steatorrhea is a common clinical indication of lipid malabsorption in cirrhotic liver disease and one- to two-thirds of patients will manifest fat malabsorption.[94]

Fatty infiltration in liver disease can be caused by a number of biochemical factors acting singularly or in concert with each other. Fatty liver may result secondary to the pharmacologic effects of certain drugs such as ethanol, which mobilizes lipids from adipose tissue. It can result from increased synthesis of fatty acids or a decreased level of fatty acid oxidation. Hepatic triglyceride release is dependent upon lipoprotein formation. Thus, a reduction in apoprotein synthesis can result in hepatic triglyceride anabolism. Finally, impaired lipoprotein synthesis or secretion can result in hepatic metamorphoses.[96]

Protein. There are two basic theories explaining the alteration of protein metabolism in hepatic disease. The first focuses on the physiologic changes in the liver that result in liver encephalopathy. Ammonia was be-

lieved to be the specific neurotoxin that accumulated as a result of AA deamination, protein catabolism, and GI tract fermentation. The increased levels of ammonia supposedly caused localized encephalopathy as well as peripheral damage to the central nervous system.[95] The relationship between ammonia and hepatic encephalopathy is not well grounded. Several drugs have been shown to decrease blood ammonia levels while increasing the severity of the encephalopathy.

The second theory involves the aminergic system of the central nervous system.[95] Alteration of this neurotransmission system results in complex metabolic processes and changes in hormonal homeostasis as well as brain function.[99] This shift in hormonal equilibrium involves a variety of endocrine and GI hormones. The end results are decreased production of glucose, ketone, and BCAA (valine, leucine, and isoleucine), and increased plasma concentrations of aromatic AA (phenylalanine, tyrosine, tryptophan, and methionine).

Nutrition Therapy

As stated earlier, the objective of nutrition intervention is (1) to improve liver function and (2) to avoid aggravating the condition. The medical care team should carefully monitor the patient's use of pharmacologic agents and alcohol and should be aware of preexisting medical conditions and sepsis. Fluid and sodium restriction may be indicated to prevent or enhance formation of ascitic fluid. Adequate protein and caloric intake must be required in order to achieve nitrogen balance and assist organ recovery. Vitamin replacement therapy may be necessary to replete deficiencies of folic acid, B_6, and thiamine. Protein restriction is not indicated in the treatment of hepatic disease. Studies of protein metabolism in acute and chronic liver disease demonstrate that protein restriction does not alter serum or hepatic AA levels.[97] In fact, severe protein restrictions in this patient population have deleterious effects.[98] Delivery of sufficient protein to diseased patients will decrease gluconeogenesis, inhibit catabolism, and enhance protein synthesis.[99] Glucose and AA therapy can effect hepatic regeneration.[96]

Use of BCAA is indicated in critically ill patients who develop symptoms of hepatic encephalopathy on diet or commercial enteral formulas. BCAA, in concert with other AA and hypertonic glucose, may ameliorate encephalopathy and support the previous nutrition objectives.[96] It is important to note that the content of the BCAA is paramount to its beneficial effects. For example, by decreasing the amount of ammonia-generating AA, like glycine, and by increasing the arginine level, one can effect positive results. Oral, defined formula enteral products (see Table 13–13), enriched in BCAA, are commercially available and are efficacious in improving encephalopathy.

MODULAR FORMULAS

As knowledge of nutrition requirements in various disease states expands, the need to make modifications to already existing enteral formulas is frequently necessary to meet the metabolic demands of the critically ill patient. Freed et al. conducted a retrospective study that attempted to determine the frequency and need of modifying fixed enteral formulas in 83 patients on a metabolic support service.[100] Forty-three percent of the 83 patients studied required modification of one or more of the macronutrient requirements, which was met through the addition of one or more enteral modules to the formula. Some of the clinical situations that required modifying the formula included organ dysfunction, vitamin deficiencies, electrolyte imbalances, and essential fatty acid deficiencies.[100] This author and others conducted a study (data in publication) to further define the percentage of patients who require modulation. This study was part of a larger study in which all enteral tube feeding orders for patients who were re-

ferred to a nutrition support service were written daily, according to a generic nutrition prescription, i.e., according to nutrition requirements on a standard order sheet as is done for the prescribing of parenteral nutrition. As in parenteral nutrition, certain guidelines were established for physician ordering, which biased the study to allow for as frequent use of fixed ready-to-use formulas as possible. Additionally, a clinical justification, e.g., fluid overload, or electrolyte restriction had to be present to make a prescription change. Out of 335 daily prescriptions (40 patients), 106 prescriptions were new formulas modified from the existing day's formula. In reviewing these formulas, 13.2 percent of these prescriptions could be met by a fixed standard enteral formula; 5.6 percent required the addition of one nutrient module; 60.5 percent required the addition of two or more modules to modify the formula; 20.7 percent of the prescriptions could not be met by any combination of 34 available standard enteral products from which the dietitian was selecting.[101] Using a modular enteral system (MES), a totally modular formula (Nutrisource), the prescriptions previously not filled could be formulated. As in Freed's study, these data suggest that when nutrition requirements are clearly specified and tailored to a patient's clinical status, standard enteral fixed formulas may not always meet clinical demands, necessitating the need for formula modulation.

As described above, there are two types of modular formulas. The first involves the addition of a nutrient module to a base formula. Table 13–14 lists the nutritional composition of most carbohydrate, protein, and fat modules available to modify existing enteral formulas. These modules can be used either to increase total caloric content of the formula or to modify one constituent nutrient without affecting other nutrients.[102] Smith et al. discuss the flexibility and usefulness of adding nutrient modules both to enteral formulas as well as to oral nourishments.[103] The complexities of designing, mixing, and feeding many of these spe-

TABLE 13–14. CARBOHYDRATE, PROTEIN, AND FAT MODULES

	Polycose		Sumacal	Moducal	Pro-Mix Pure Carbohydrate Supplement	Pro-Mix
kcal/cc	3.8/g	2/cc	3.8/g	4/g	4/g	4/g
NPC: g N	—	—	—	—	—	—
Source: CHO	Hydrolysis of corn starch		Maltodextrin	Maltodextrin	Glucose polymers	—
Source: Pro	—	—	—	—	—	Whey protein
Source: Fat	—	—	—	—	—	—
g/L: CHO	—	500	—	—	96.5/100 g	—
g/L: Pro	—	—	—	—	—	9/11.8 g
g/L: Fat	—	—	—	—	—	—
mEq/L: Na	—	30	4/100 g	3/100 g	.65/100 g	7/100 g
mEq/L: K	—	2	<1/100 g	<1/100 g	Trace	41/100 g
Osmolality mosm/kg H_2O	—	850	—	—	131 (diluted)	—
Vitamins (cc for 100% U.S. RDA)	—	—	—	—	—	—
Lactose free	Yes		Yes	Yes	Yes	Yes

cialized diets are discussed. One constraint of these modules is the frequency with which they may exist in combination with other macronutrients or contain some amount of electrolytes or vitamins, making simple calculation of their addition to a formula difficult.[104] Additionally, because many of these modules were not designed to be mixed together, some potential formula incompatabilities, precipitation, or layering of solution can occur, potentially interfering with the delivery of the tube feeding. Another disadvantage of these formulas is their construction from a base formula, which prevents the reduction of any ingredients below what levels exist in the base formula.

The second modular formula is a system of nutrient modules, carbohydrate, protein, fat, vitamins, and minerals, designed to be mixed together to construct a patient-specific formula. Nutrisource MES, as this author and others refer to them, is a family of nu-

Propac	Casec	Citrotein	Ross SLD	Microlipid	MCT oil	Pro-Mix High Fat Supplement
4/g	4/g	.66	.7	4.5	7.7	6/g
—	—	78:1	117:1	—	—	—
—	—	Sucrose, malto-dextrin	Sucrose, hy-drolyzed corn starch	—	—	Corn syrup, sugar
Whey protein	Calcium caseinate	Egg albumin	Egg white solids	—	—	Sodium caseinate
—	—	Soy oil	—	Safflower oil	Fractionated coconut oil	Coconut oil, mono- and diglyce-rides, leci-thin
—	—	122	137	—	—	40.5/100 g
15/19.5 g	—	41	38	—	—	5/100 g
—	—	2	.5	500	933	47.5/100 g
10/100 g	7/100 g	30	36	—	—	7.8/100 g
13/100 g	3/100 g	18	21	—	—	Trace
—	—	480–515	545	80	Negligible	109 (diluted)
—	—	1152	1200	—	—	—
Yes	Yes	Yes	Yes	Yes	Yes	Yes

trient modules including macro- and micro-nutrient modules that are designed to be mixed together in any combination to form a de novo synthesis of an enteral formula. Currently, there is only one such system available. This capability, which up until now has only existed in parenteral nutrition, allows for maximum flexibility in constructing a formula specifically tailored to a patient's ever-changing clinical course. This flexibility allows the use of such a formula as an alternative to parenteral nutrition because changing fluid, electrolyte, and other nutrition requirements can be met on a daily basis without changing from one new formula to another.

An MES is indicated for cardiac, hepatic, renal, trauma, pulmonary, and diabetic patients. Each of these medical conditions requires manipulation of the substrates delivered and therefore requires formulas tailored to these specific nutrition require-

TABLE 13–15. INDICATIONS FOR A MODULAR ENTERAL SYSTEM

Types of Patients	Medical Conditions
Cardiac failure	Fluid imbalance
Renal failure	Electrolyte imbalance
Hepatic failure	Acid–base disorders
Respiratory failure	Glucose intolerance
Multiorgan system failure	Hypermetabolic
Trauma	Malabsorption
Diabetes	Multiple nutrient restrictions

ments. Other important MES candidates are patients with fluid and electrolyte imbalances, acid–base disorders, malabsorption conditions, or multiorgan system failure. Patient indications are summarized in Table 13–15.

The Nutrisource MES complete with carbohydrate, protein, fat, minerals, and vitamins offers the precise nutrient control previously available only through parenteral nutrition. Figure 13–7 lists the nutrient components of this system. Currently, there

are three choices of nitrogen source: intact protein, AA, and high branch chain AA. In this MES the nitrogen source, intact protein or AA, determines which mineral supplement to use. Although there is great flexibility among the macronutrient modules, there is limited flexibility in the vitamin and mineral modules. The two mineral supplement choices are dependent upon selection of nitrogen source. This is based on the fact that the intact protein modules contain some trace minerals not present in the AA module.

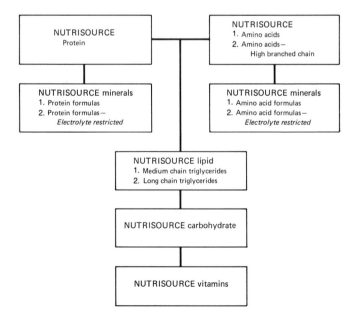

Figure 13–7. Overview of Nutrisource modular enteral system components. *(From Nutrisource Technical Information Manual. Minneapolis: Doyle Pharmaceutical Co., 1982.)*

The two choices of mineral supplements for each nitrogen source differ in that one provides a complete profile of electrolytes, other minerals, and trace elements to meet the RDA, and the other mineral component restricts sodium, potassium, and chloride, which have been removed from the module. This is helpful except when it is clinically desired to begin supplementing back quantities of these electrolytes. In that case, an alternate electrolyte supplement must be used to meet requirements. All vitamins are combined in one module to meet the RDA. This again works as both an advantage and a disadvantage. The advantage is the ability to meet the RDA regardless of the volume delivered. The disadvantage is that only multiples of the existing module can be supplemented for additional vitamins. Specific vitamin supplements from other sources need to be used. Table 13–16 lists the nutritional composition of the modules in this system.

Implementation Strategy

As this is a relatively new system, its new approach and complexities have challenged the clinician to safely and effectively prepare and administer this type of formula. There are four main concerns that must be addressed in order to safely deliver an MES formula: (1) the need for the development of a standardized MES order sheet to facilitate the prescription process, (2) the requirement of a calculation system either manually through the use of work sheets or through the use of computer support, (3) the need for an adequate preparation facility, and (4) the need for appropriate administration protocols to safely deliver this formula.

Prescription Development

As when parenteral nutrition was introduced, standardized order sheets streamline the ordering and delivery process. Because of the complexity of ordering an MES, it is helpful as well to have a standardized order sheet specifying all the necessary elements that must be determined to complete a prescription. Otherwise, prescriptions will not be complete, and much time will have to be spent tracking down the appropriate physician to determine the unprescribed requirements. Therefore, standard order sheets specifying the nutritional composition, concentration, and delivery rates are most efficient. Table 13–17 lists information requiring specification on an MES order sheet. Concentration advancement is usually determined by osmolality of the formula. Unless there is a clinical laboratory to test the osmolality on an aliquot of the formula, in most cases it is necessary to rely on the osmolality graphs provided in the Doyle Technical Manual.[105]

Prescription Calculation

When this system was first introduced, calculation time in clinical trials conducted by this author ranged from approximately 20 to 45 minutes per formula. With the use of work sheets (available from Sandoz Nutrition), the time required for the clinical dietitian or other nutrition support service member to do calculations has been greatly reduced to under 10 minutes per formula. This author participated in the development of the use of a handheld computer to further expedite the calculations. These computer support software packages greatly ease the calculation process by allowing the prescription to be entered, calculating the formula, and printing out the prescribed nutritional composition. If the formula is accepted, the computer will then print the ingredient listing, preparation instructions, and a sample label to be used for the formula. The advantage of computer support is that it reduces the calculation time to under 3 minutes or less plus minimizes mistakes in calculation, especially when the user does these calculations infrequently. Figures 13–8 and 13–9 are printouts of prescriptions and recipe from a handheld computer.

TABLE 13–16. A MODULAR ENTERAL SYSTEM: NUTRISOURCE

	Carbohydrate	Protein	Amino Acids	Amino Acids-High Branch Chain	Lipid-LCT
kcal/cc	3.2	4/g	3.9/g	3.9/g	2.2
NPC g N	—	—	—	—	—
Source: CHO	Deionized corn syrup solids	Polysorbate 80	—	—	—
Source: Pro	—	Delactosed lactalbumin, egg white solids	L-amino acids	L-amino acids	—
Source: Fat	—	Mono- + di-glycerides	—	—	Soybean oil, polyglycerol, fatty acids
g/L: CHO	800	8.5/100 g	0	0	0
g/L: Pro	0	76/100 g	97/100 g	97/100 g	0
g/L: Fat	0	7.1/100 g	0	0	240
mEq/L: Na	0	11.7/100 g	0	0	0
mEq/L: K	0	14.6/100 g	0	0	0
Osmolality mosm/kg H$_2$O	—	—	—	—	—
Vitamins (cc for 100% U.S. RDA)	—	—	—	—	—
Lactose free	Yes	Yes	Yes	Yes	Yes

Preparation

Each hospital needs to evaluate its strengths to determine the appropriate location for preparation of these formulas. Preparation responsibility will therefore vary from institution to institution. In many hospitals, the dietetics department is responsible for all preparation and dispensing of enteral for-

mulas. If such departments assume the responsibility for preparing MES formulas, quality control measures not currently used in practice because of widespread use of ready-to-use formulas may have to be reestablished. In preparing MES formulas, the central concerns are accuracy in the measurement of the actual product ingredients. This requires the ability to read meniscus

Lipid-MCT	Minerals for Protein Formulas	Minerals for Protein Form.: Elect. Restr.	Minerals for Amino Acid Formulas	Minerals for Amino Acid Elect. Restr.	Vitamins
2	—	—	—	—	—
—	—	—	—	—	—
—	Maltodextrin	Maltodextrin	Maltodextrin	Maltodextrin	Maltodextrin
—	—	—	—	—	—
MCT, poly-glycerol fatty acids, lecithin	—	—	—	—	—
0	6/24 g	13/24 g	3/24 g	12/24 g	9/10 g
0	0	0	0	0	0
240	0	0	0	0	0
0	44	0	57	0	0
0	45	0	56	0	0
—	—	—	—	—	—
—	24 g for 100% RDA minerals	24 g for 100% RDA minerals	24 g for 100% RDA minerals	24 g for 100% RDA minerals	24 g for 100% RDA vitamins
Yes	Yes	Yes	Yes	Yes	Yes

levels on graduated cylinders and to utilize appropriate weighing techniques for dry ingredients. Secondly, as these products require a fair amount of handling for preparation, clean aseptic techniques need to be employed to minimize bacterial contamination. A laminar flow hood, though very useful to help control bacterial contamination, does not appear essential for preparation. As an aid to the technician preparing these formulas, clear and bold recipe forms help to minimize any errors that may be made through possible misreading of the ingredient quantities. This author describes the development of an enteral preparation facility elsewhere in the literature.[62] Lastly, because every MES formula varies in composition relative to each patient's specific

TABLE 13–17. SPECIFICATIONS FOR MODULAR ENTERAL SYSTEM ORDER SHEET

Prescription ordering
_____ Initial Enteral Order
_____ No Change,
　　　　　　　　 Use Last Order
_____ Prescription Change

Formula composition

Amount/day	Nutrient
_____ kcal	Kilocalories
	Protein
_____ g	Amino Acids
_____ g	Amino Acids-BCAA
_____ g	Intact Protein
_____ %	% Carbohydrate
_____ %	% Fat-LCT
_____ %	% Fat-MCT
_____ mEq	Sodium
_____ mEq	Potassium
_____ ml	Fluid
_____ %	Concentration
_____ ml	Delivery Rate

needs, as in parenteral nutrition, clear concise labels must list the nutritional and electrolyte composition of the formula. Without patient's name, date, and composition, informed decisions as to controlling electrolyte imbalances cannot be made. There is no ability to look these formulas up on a chart to find composition. Figure 13–10 demonstrates a sample MES label.

Administration

The administration of an MES is essentially no different than the delivery of any other enteral solution. Communication among all members of the patient care team is necessary for effective implementation. Nursing needs to be informed to monitor delivery and to note any delivery concerns that might develop through use of the formula. Nursing should also have an established mechanism so that when the formula is delivered to the patient floor, the nurse can easily check the formula label against the order to determine whether it is the correct formula. The clinical

```
  *   PRESCRIPTION   *
For:
Smith, J
CASE: 33-9945-01
Rm 415

--------------------

1. PROTEIN SOURCE
   AMINO ACIDS
2. FAT SOURCE
   MCT LIPID
3. TOTAL CALORIES
   2300 Cal
4. PRO = 57 g

5. % TOT CAL AS FAT
   30 %
6. MINERAL PACKS = 1
7. VITAMINS
   200 % of RDA
8. ELECTROLYTES
   Na = 35 mEq
   K = 34 mEq
   Cl = 34 mEq
   P = 77 mEq
   Ca = 50 mEq
9. TOTAL VOLUME
   1900 ml
10. STRENGTH:  HALF
```

Figure 13–8. A modular enteral system formula prescription generated through use of computer support.

dietitian needs to be fully informed of how prescription changes are made so that the appropriate calculation changes can be made and that these prescription changes are carried through to the preparation facility, either the dietetics department or the pharmacy. In many situations, the clinical pharmacist may be the clinician responsible for carrying out these changes.

Daily clinical monitoring is also critical while patients are receiving an MES formula. Such monitoring is essentially no different from what is currently done for parenteral nutrition support. A sample clinical monitoring protocol is shown in Table 13–18.

```
    *     RECIPE     *
For:
Smith, J
CASE: 33-9945-01
Rm 415

-------------------

-NUTRISOURCE MODS--
Amino Acids
   -> 30 g
Carbohydrate
   -> 197 ml
MCT Lipid
   -> 148 ml
Restricted Minerals
For Amino Acids
   -> 1 pkg
Vitamins
   -> 2 pkg
-----ADDITIVES-----
Potassium Cloride
   -> 45 ml
Sodium Bi-Carbonate
   -> 46 g
Calcium Carbonate
   -> 13 g
-------WATER-------
Start with 1494 ml
Add to make 1900 ml
-------------------
   Prepare as directed,
in NUTRISOURCE
Technical Manual.
```

Figure 13–9. A modular enteral system recipe generated through use of computer support.

N.I.T. Modular Tube Feeding Solution

Name _____ Room _____

Date mixed _____ Time _____ AM/PM

Do not use after 2PM on _____

Mixed by _____

Formula Composition
(per 1000 cc)

_____	Calories/cc
_____	Pro (g)
_____	CHO (g)
_____	Fat (g)
_____	Na (mEq)
_____	K (mEq)
_____	Cl (mEq)
_____	Ca (mEq)
_____	P (mEq)

Shake before using

Please keep container tightly closed

Save unused formula

Keep refrigerated

Figure 13–10. Modular enteral system label for tube feeding container.

TABLE 13–18. SAMPLE CLINICAL MONITORING PROTOCOL FOR MODULAR ENTERAL SYSTEM PATIENTS

Daily	Twice Weekly	Weekly	Monthly
Electrolytes	Phosphorus	Total protein	Serum B_{12}
Glucose	Calcium	Albumin	Folate
BUN	Magnesium	Triglycerides	Zinc
Creatinine		Liver function tests	Iron
Urine fractionals		TIBC	Trace minerals as indicated
Fluid balance			
Body weight			
Nutrition intake			

REFERENCES

1. Homsy FN, Blackburn GL: Modern parenteral and enteral nutrition in critical care. J Am Coll Nutr 2:75–95, 1983
2. Rowlands BJ, Miller TA: The physiology of eating. In Rombeau JL, Caldwell MD (eds): Enteral and Tube Feeding (Vol 1). Philadelphia: Saunders, 1984, pp 10–19
3. Mayes PA: Digestion and absorption from the gastrointestinal tract. In Harper HA et al. (eds): Review of Physiological Chemistry, ed 17. Los Altos: Lange Medical Publications, 1979, pp 245–259
4. Lickley HLA et al.: Metabolic responses to enteral and parenteral nutrition. Am J Surg 135:172–176, 1978
5. McArdle AH et al.: A rationale for enteral feeding as the preferable route of hyperalimentation. Surgery 90:616–623, 1981
6. Gimmon Z et al.: The effect of parenteral and enteral nutrition on portal and systemic immunoreactivities of gastrin, glucagon and vasoactive intestinal polypeptide (VIP). Ann Surg 196:571–575, 1982
7. Johnson LR et al.: Structural and hormonal alterations in the gastrointestinal tract of parenterally fed rats. Gastroenterology 68:1177–1183, 1975
8. Young EA et al.: Gastrointestinal response to nutrient variation of defined formula diets. JPEN 5:478–484, 1981
9. Drack GT et al.: Human calcitonin stimulates salivary amylase concentration in man. Gut 17:620–623, 1976
10. Mulcahy AH et al.: Secretin and pancreozymin effect on salivary amylase concentration in man. Gut 13:850, 1972
11. Grossman MI: Control of gastric secretion. In Sleisenger MH, Fordtran JS (eds): Gastrointestinal Disease—Pathophysiology, Diagnosis and Management, ed 2. Philadelphia: Saunders, 1978, pp. 640–659
12. Moran JR, Greene HL: Digestion and absorption. In Rombeau JL, Caldwell MD (eds): Enteral and Tubefeeding (Vol 1). Philadelphia: Saunders, 1984, pp 21–43
13. Cooke AR: Control of gastric emptying and motility. Gastroenterology 68:804–816, 1975
14. Miller LJ et al.: Postprandial duodenal function in man. Gut 19:699–706, 1978
15. Wheeler HO: Bile formation and physiology of the biliary tract. In Sleisenger MH, Fordtran JS (eds): Gastrointestinal Disease—Pathophysiology, Diagnosis and Management,

ed 2. Philadelphia: Saunders, 1978, pp. 1279–1284
16. Meyer JH: Pancreatic physiology. In Sleisenger MH, Fordtran JS (eds): Gastrointestinal Disease—Pathophysiology, Diagnosis and Management, ed 2. Philadelphia: Saunders, 1978, pp 1398–1408
17. Banfield WJ: Physiology of the gallbladder. Gastroenterology 69:770–777, 1975
18. Randall HT: Enteral nutrition: Tube feeding in acute and chronic illness. JPEN 8:113–136, 1984
19. Bliss DW: Feeding per rectum. Med Rec 22:64–67, 1882
20. Brown-Seguard CE: Feeding per rectum in nervous affections. Lancet 1:144, 1878
21. Mackenzie DJ: Continuous rectal alimentation; an artificial stomach. Br Med J 1:1161, 1886
22. Myers VC: The present status of rectal and duodenal alimentation. Post-Graduate 28:987–995, 1913
23. Rhoads JE et al.: The absorption of protein split products from chronic isolated colon loops. Am J Physiol 125:707–712, 1939
24. Hemmeter JC: Gastric lavage with a continuous current. N Y Med J 62:819–824, 1895
25. Hunter J: Proposals for the recovery of persons apparently drowned. In The Works of John Hunter. Philadelphia: Haswall, Barrington and Haswell, 1840, pp 185–194
26. Einhorn M: A practical method of obtaining the duodenal contents in man. Med Rec 77:98–101, 1910
27. Pilcher JT: Enteric feeding: Its practicability and indications. Long Island Med J 8:205–232, 1914
28. Stengel A Jr, Ravdin I: Maintenance of nutrition in surgical patients with description of orojejunal method of feeding. Surgery 6:511–519, 1939
29. Abbott WO, Rawson AJ: A tube for use in the postoperative care of gastroenterostomy patients—a correction. JAMA 112:2414, 1939
30. Elinan R, Weiner DO: Intravenous alimentation—with special reference to protein (amino acid) metabolism. JAMA 112:796–802, 1939
31. Co Tui et al.: Studies on surgical convalescence. Ann Surg 120:99–122, 1944
32. Riegel C et al.: The nutritional requirements for nitrogen balance in surgical patients during the early postoperative period. J Clin Invest 26:18–23, 1947

33. Imbembo AL, Walter JZ: Enteral alimentation. In Walser M, Imbembo AL (eds): Nutritional Management: The Johns Hopkins Handbook. Philadelphia: Saunders, 1984, pp 69–83

34. Torosian MH, Rombeau JL: Feeding by tube enterostomy. Surg Gynecol Obstet 150:918–927, 1980

35. Cerra FB: Pocket Manual of Surgical Nutrition. St. Louis: Mosby, 1984

36. DelRio D, Williams K, Esvelt BM: Handbook of Enteral Nutrition. El Segundo, CA: Medical Specifics, 1982

37. MacBurney MM, Young LS: Enteral formulas. In Rombeau JL, Caldwell MD (eds): Enteral and Tube Feeding (Vol 1). Philadelphia: Saunders, 1984, pp 171–198

38. Heymsfield SB, Horowitz J, Lawson DH: Enteral hyperalimentation. In Berk EJ (ed): Developments in Digestive Diseases. Philadelphia: Lea and Febiger, 1980, pp 59–83

39. Mitchell HH: A method of determining the biological value of protein. J Biol Chem 58:873–903, 1924

40. Gordon AM: Enteral nutritional support: Guidelines for feeding product selection. Postgrad Med 72:72–82, 1982

41. Shils ME, Bloch AS, Chernoff R: Liquid formulas for oral and tube feeding. Clinical Bulletin 6, A publication of Memorial Sloan-Kettering Cancer Center, No. 4:151–158, 1976

42. Shils ME, Bloch RS, Chernoff R: Liquid formulas for oral and tube feeding. Clinical Bulletin, A publication of Memorial Sloan-Kettering Cancer Center, pp 1–10, 1979

43. Steffee WP, Krey SH: Enteral hyperalimentation. In Newell GR, Ellison NM (eds): Nutrition and Cancer: Etiology and Treatment. New York: Raven Press, 1981, pp 367–391

44. Food and Nutrition Board, National Research Council: Recommended Dietary Allowances. Natl. Acad. Sci., Washington, D.C., 1984

45. Michaelson R, Kempin SJ, Naria B, et al.: Inhibition of the hypoprothrombinemic effect of warfarin (Coumadin®) by Ensure Plus, a dietary supplement. Clinical Bulletin 10 No 4:171–172, 1980

46. Burkitt DP, Walker ARP, Painter NS: Dietary fiber and disease. JAMA 229:1068–1074, 1974

47. Anderson JW: Dietary fiber and diabetes. In Vahouny GV, Kritchevsky D (eds): Dietary Fiber in Health and Disease. New York: Plenum Press, 1982, pp 151–167

48. Cummings JH: Nutritional implications of dietary fiber. Am J Clin Nutr 31:S21–S29, 1978

49. Ross Laboratories: Enrich, liquid nutrition with fiber. Ross Laboratories, Columbus, OH: June, 1984

50. Rolandell R: Role of dietary fiber in enteral nutrition. In ASPEN 8th Clinical Congress: Advances in Enteral Feeding. Las Vegas: ASPEN Publication, 1984, pp 8–20

51. Jackson AA: Amino Acids: Essential and non-essential. Lancet May 7:1034–1037, 1983

52. Ross Laboratories: Water and electrolytes in enteral nutrition. Ross Laboratories, Columbus, OH: April, 1983, pp 1–25

53. Randall HT: Osmolality and its relationship to GI tolerance. In Norwich Eaton Pharmaceuticals: Current Concepts in Nutritional Support, Monograph 1. New York: Biomedical Information, 1983, pp 5–8

54. Niewiec PW, Vanderveen TW, Morrison JL, et al.: Gastrointestinal disorders caused by medication and electrolyte solution osmolality during enteral nutrition. JPEN 7(4):387–389, 1983

55. Mirtallo JM, Fabri PJ: Concurrent therapy for complications of enteral nutrition support. Hosp Form 7:945–953, 1982

56. Ferrett KA, Giudici RA: Osmolality determinations of concentrated enteral nutrition formulas: Nutr Supp Serv 2(12):6–9, 1982

57. Fagerman KE, Paauw JD, McCamish MA, et al.: Effects of time, temperature, and preservative on bacterial growth in enteral nutrient solutions. Am J Hosp Pharm 41:112–6, 1984

58. Bastow MD, Greaves P, Allison SP: Microbial contamination of enteral feeds. Human Nutr Appl Nutr 36A:213–217, 1982

59. Schroeder P: Tube feeding contamination: Considerations for the community hospital. Nutr Supp Serv 1:23–24, 1981

60. Anderton A: Microbiological aspects of the preparation and administration of naso-gastric and naso-enteric tube feeds in hospitals—a review. Hum Nutr Appl Nutr 37A:426–440, 1983

61. Groschel DMH: Disposable enteral feeding bags should not be reused. (Questions and Answers) JAMA 248(19):2536, 1982

62. Krey SH, Porcelli KA, Lockett GM: Enhanc-

ing enteral nutrition delivery: Development of an enteral preparation facility. J Am Diet Assoc 85(6):693–697, 1985

63. Suskind RM: Gastrointestinal changes in the malnourished child. Pediatr Clin North Am 22:873–883, 1975

64. Chernoff R: Nutritional Support: Formulas and delivery of enteral feeding. J Am Diet Assoc 79:426–432, 1981

65. Rose WC: Amino acid requirements of man. Fed Proc 8:546–552, 1949

66. Greenstein JP, Birnbaum SM, Winitz M, et al.: Quantitative nutritional studies with water soluble chemically defined diets. I. Growth, reproduction, and lactation in rats. Arch Biochem Biophys 72:396–416, 1957

67. Winitz M, Seedman DA, Graff J: Studies in metabolic nutrition employing chemically defined diets. I. Extended feeding of normal human adult males. Am J Clin Nutr 23:525–545, 1970

68. Winitz M, Adams RF, Seedman DA, et al.: Studies in metabolic nutrition employing chemically defined diets. II. Effects on gut microflora populations. Am J Clin Nutr 23:546–559, 1970

69. Bounous G, Gentile JM, Hugon J: Elemental diet in the management of the intestinal lesion produced by 5-fluorouracil in man. Can J Surg 14:312–324, 1971

70. Davenport HW: Physiology of the Digestive Tract, Edition 4. Chicago: Year Book Medical Publishers, 1977

71. Young EA, Heuter N, Russell P, et al.: Comparative nutritional analysis of chemically defined diets. Gastroenterology 69:1338–1345, 1975

72. Silk DB, Chung YC, Berger KL, et al.: Comparison of oral feeding of peptide and amino acid meals to normal human subjects. Gut 20:291–299, 1979

73. Jones BJ, Lees R, Andrews J, et al.: Comparison of an elemental and polymeric enteral diet in patients with normal gastrointestinal function. Gut 24:78–84, 1983

74. Professional Products Group: Peptides versus amino acids utilization. Norwich Eaton Pharmaceuticals, 1979

75. Steffee WP, Anderson CF: Enteral nutrition and renal disease. In Rombeau JL, Caldwell MD (eds): Enteral and Tube feeding, Vol 1. Philadelphia: Saunders, 1984, pp 363–374

76. Teschan PE, Baster CR, O'Brien TF, et al.: Prophylactic hemodialysis in the treatment

of acute renal failure. Ann Intern Med 53:992, 1960

77. Molnar JA, Bell SJ, Goodenough RD, et al.: Enteral nutrition in patients with burns or trauma. In Rombeau JL, Caldwell MD (eds): Enteral and Tube Feeding, Vol 1. Philadelphia: Saunders, 1984, pp 412–433

78. Long CL: Energy balance and carbohydrate metabolism in infection and sepsis. Am J Clin Nutr 30:1301–1310, 1977

79. Gump FE, Martin P, Kenney JM: Oxygen consumption and caloric expenditure in surgical patients. Surg Gynecol Obstet 137:449–513, 1973

80. Bartlett RH, Allyn PA, Medley T, et al.: Nutritional therapy based on positive caloric balance in burn patients. Arch Surg 112:974–980, 1977

81. Wilmore DW, Long JM, Mason AD Jr, et al.: Catecholamines: Mediator of the hypermetabolic response to thermal injury. Ann Surg 180:653–688, 1974

82. Elwyn DH: Nutritional requirements of adult surgical patients. Crit Care Med 8:9–20, 1980

83. Rudman D, Millikan WJ, Richardson TJ, et al.: Elemental balances during intravenous hyperalimentation of underweight adult subjects. J Clin Invest 55:94–104, 1975

84. Askanazi J, Carpenter YA, Elwyn DH, et al.: Influence of total parenteral nutrition on fuel utilization in injury and sepsis. Ann Surg 191:40–46, 1980

85. Birkhahn RH, Calvin LL, Fitkin DL, et al.: A comparison of the effects of skeletal trauma and surgery on the ketosis of starvation in man. J Trauma 21:513–519, 1981

86. Brown SE, Light RW: What is now known about protein-energy depletion. When COPD patients are malnourished. J Respir Dis 5:36–50, 1983

87. Saltzman HA, Salzano JV: Effects of carbohydrate metabolism upon respiratory gas exchange in normal men. J Appl Physiol 30:228–231, 1971

88. Gieseke T, Gurushanthaiah G, Glauser FL: Effects of carbohydrates on carbon dioxide excretion in patients with airway disease. Chest 71:55–58, 1977

89. Askanazi J, Weissman C, La Sala PA, et al.: Effect of protein intake on ventilatory drive. Anesthesiology 60:106–110, 1984

90. Askanazi J, Nordenstrom J, Rosenbaum SH, et al.: Nutrition for the patient with respira-

tory failure: Glucose vs fat. Anesthesiology 54:373–377, 1981

91. Fischer JE, Bower RH: Nutritional support in liver disease. Surg Clin North Am 6:653–660, 1981

92. Elwyn DH: The role of the liver in the regulation of amino acid and metabolism. In Munro NH (ed): Mammalian Protein Metabolism. New York: Academic Press, 1970, pp 523–571

93. Johnston DC, Alberti KGM: Carbohydrate metabolism in liver disease. Clin Endocrinol Metab 5:675–702, 1976

94. Mezey E: Liver disease and nutrition. Gastroenterology 74:770–783, 1978

95. Freund HR, Fischer JE: Hepatic failure. In Hill GL (ed): Nutrition and the Surgical Patient, Vol 2, Clinical Surgery International. New York: Churchill Livingstone, 1981, pp 201–212

96. Jacobs DO, Boraas MC, Rombeau JL: Enteral nutrition and liver disease. In Rombeau JL, Caldwell MD (eds): Enteral and Tube Feeding, Vol 1. Philadelphia: Saunders, 1984, pp 376–402

97. O'Keefe SJD, Abraham RR, Davis R, Williams R: Protein turnover in acute and chronic liver disease. Acta Chir Scand (suppl) 507:91–101, 1981

98. Silk DBA: Malnutrition in liver disease and its relationship to hepatic encephalopathy. Acta Chir Scand (suppl) 507:106–111, 1981

99. Fischer JE, Fishman AP: Panel report on nutritional support of patients with liver, renal and cardiopulmonary disease. Am J Clin Nutr 34:1235–1245, 1981

100. Freed BA, Hsia B, Smith HP, Kaminski MV: Enteral nutrition: Frequency of formula modification. JPEN 5(1):40–45, 1981

101. Krey SH, Porcelli KA, Crocker KS, Steffee WP: The use of generic prescriptions in enteral hyperalimentation. Unpublished data, Cleveland, Ohio, 1984

102. MacBurney MM, Jacobs DO, Apelgren KN, et al.: Modular feeding. In Rombeau JL, Caldwell MD (eds). Enteral and Tube Feeding, Vol 1. Philadelphia: Saunders, 1984, pp 199–211

103. Smith JL, Heymsfield SB: Enteral nutrition support: Formula preparation from modular ingredients. JPEN 7(3):280–288, 1983

104. Materese LE: Enteral alimentation: Oral and tube feedings, Part 1. Nutr Supp Serv 1(8):41–42, 1981

105. Doyle Pharmaceutical Company: Nutrisource Technical Information Manual. Minneapolis: Doyle Pharmaceutical, 1982, pp 1–34

106. Koretz RL, Meyer JH: Elemental diets—facts and fantasies. Gastroenterology 78:393–410, 1980

14. The Mechanics of Delivery
Lucinda K. Lysen

FEEDING TUBES

Selecting a method of tube feeding should largely be determined by (1) the functional status of the patient's gastrointestinal (GI) tract, (2) the types of medical or surgical intervention the patient requires, (3) the estimated length of time required to be tube fed, and (4) the severity of malnutrition (Tables 14–1 and 14–2). Routes of tube feeding delivery include the nasogastric, nasoduodenal, and nasojejunal feeding routes, and the surgically performed esophagostomy, gastrostomy, and jejunostomy methods of feeding (Fig. 14–1*).

Nasoenteral

Nasoenteral feeding tubes, which encompass nasogastric, nasoduodenal, and nasojejunal tubes, are most appropriate for those patients in whom oropharyngeal and esophageal functioning are not impaired, and in whom long-term feedings are not required. They can safely be inserted through the nares at the patient's bedside and be assessed for proper placement by ausculation or x-ray (Fig. 14–2). Nasogastric tubes are ideal for the alert, unrestrained patient with an intact gag reflex and adequate stomach functioning to tolerate a high osmotic load.

Nasoduodenal and nasojejunal feedings are implemented when the risk of feeding formula aspiration is high, and in cases where nutrient breakdown and absorption are impaired and a simpler formula may be required. A tube is placed via the nares through the GI tract transpylorically either into the duodenum or jejunum.

Surgically Inserted Feeding Tubes

Cervical Esophagostomy. The esophagostomy is an opening created surgically under a local or general anesthetic at the lower border of the neck to slightly below the cervical esophagus.[1] A permanent stoma can be designed to allow for intermittent catheterization at feeding times. The esophagostomy is particularly useful in conjunction with head and neck surgery, and when long-term nutritional therapy is necessary. As with nasogastric feedings, the chance for pulmonary aspiration with this method of access is relatively high.

Gastrostomy. The feeding gastrostomy is useful when oropharyngeal or esophageal trauma or malfunctioning exists. This procedure is performed during general surgery or under a local anesthetic. Extra sedation is often required during surgical insertion of the gastrostomy tube when a local anesthetic is used. This should be kept in mind so that

---

* All figures are grouped at end of chapter.

TABLE 14-1. INDICATIONS FOR ENTERAL
FEEDING ADMINISTRATION

**TABLE 14-1. INDICATIONS FOR ENTERAL
FEEDING ADMINISTRATION**

Neurologic/Psychiatric
  Central nervous system disorders
  Cerebral vascular accidents
  Neoplasms
  Trauma
  Inflammation
  Demyelinating diseases
  Severe depression
  Anorexia nervosa
Oropharyngeal/Esophageal
  Neoplasms
  Inflammation
  Trauma
Gastrointestinal
  Pancreatitis
  Inflammatory bowel disease
  Short bowel syndrome
  Neonatal intestinal diseases
  Malabsorption
  Preoperative bowel preparation
  Fistulas
Burns
Chemotherapy/Radiation Therapy

Reprinted with permission from Rombeau JL, Barot LR: Enteral nutrition therapy. Surg Clin North Am 61(3):607, 1981.

respiratory monitoring equipment can be made available in surgery if needed. Two types of surgical gastrostomies commonly performed are the Stamm and Janeway procedures.[2] The Stamm procedure involves the suturing of the stomach to the anterior abdominal wall and the insertion of a catheter that is sutured into place.[2] A disadvantage to this procedure is that if the catheter is accidentally removed, the tract will close rapidly.[2] As a result, the Stamm procedure[3] is frequently referred to as a temporary gastrostomy.[4] The Janeway procedure[5] is a permanent type of gastrostomy.[4] A piece of mucosa is taken from the stomach leading to the skin, and is sutured. A valve is created at the base of the tube to prevent fluid from refluxing out of the stomach. A catheter can intermittently or permanently be left in

place without concern for tract closure if the tube is removed.[2] The feeding tube can be placed and removed with intermittent types of feeding regimens.

Nonsurgical endoscopic placement of a permanent feeding gastrostomy has been recently implemented at the Mayo Clinic.[6] Using this method, a gastroscope is introduced into the stomach. A local anesthetic is infiltrated through the abdominal wall where a stab wound is made. A catheter is then introduced into the stomach lumen.

The gastrostomy is ideal for those patients in whom there is no malfunctioning of the gut, who are in good nutritional status and can tolerate substances such as intact proteins, fat, and blenderized diets, but cannot adequately ingest the necessary amount of nutrients for tissue repletion to occur. As with other discussed methods of tube feeding, the disadvantage associated with this method of feeding is the unavoidable danger of feeding aspiration in high-risk patients.[7]

Jejunostomy. The jejunostomy provides a route of access for nutrient infusion directly into the jejunum through the peritoneum, and eliminates the risk of aspiration. Feedings can be implemented immediately postoperatively if the small bowel is normal at operation,[8] and require less pancreatic stimulation than gastric and nasoduodenal diets. This technique of feeding can be initiated during general surgery or under a local anesthetic, and is highly beneficial to patients with proximal diseases or obstruction. Elemental formulas like Vivonex HN[9] and the chemically defined formula Vital HN[10] have been used quite successfully as jejunostomy feedings. The use of intact proteins, however, has been of concern, as the efficacy of nutrient absorption in the jejunum is questionable because of poor mixing of bile salts and pancreatic juices with intrajejunal nutrient formulas.[7,11]

As described by Del Rio et al.,[2] the technique for insertion of a jejunostomy tube requires that:

TABLE 14–2. SOME COMMERCIALLY AVAILABLE FEEDING TUBES

Nasoenteral Feeding Tubes

Name of Tube	Manufacturer	Specifications
Flexiflo	Ross	8 Fr, 45″, 12 Fr, 36″; One 8 Fr with Teflon-coated 3 wire braided stylet, one without; C-Flex material; radiopaque
Corpak	Corpak	5, 6, 8, 10 Fr; 15″, 22″, 36″; stylet; tungsten tip; radiopaque
Keofeed	IVAC	5, 7.3, 9.6 Fr; 43″ length silicone; mercury weight; radiopaque available
Entriflex	Biosearch	8 Fr; 36″ and 43″ lengths; polyurethane; mercury-weighted
Dobbhoff	Biosearch	8 Fr; 43″ polyurethane; mercury tip
Duotube	Argyle	5, 6, 8 Fr; 40″ length silicone; silicone- or mercury-weighted tip; radiopaque
Vivonex Tungsten Tip	Norwich-Eaton	8 Fr; 43″ length; polyurethane material; tungsten-weighted tip
Vivonex Moss	Norwich-Eaton	20 Fr; 44″ Nasoesophagogastric decompression tube with duodenal feeding tube

Jejunostomy Tubes

K-Tube	Midwest Metabolic Support Group	8 Fr; silicone
Vivonex	Norwich-Eaton	5 Fr; polyurethane
Arrow	Arrow	5 Fr; polyurethane
Surgifeed	IVAC	7.3 Fr; silicone

Gastrostomy Tubes

Rombeau	IVAC	Combined silicone mercury-weighted jejunal tube and mushroom-tip gastrostomy tube
Foley	Bard Dover Argyle	8 Fr with 3-cc balloon; 10–28 Fr with 5-cc balloon; 12–30 Fr with 30-cc balloon; latex with silicone coating
Pezar	Bard	8–32 Fr; latex
Malecot	Bard	12–36 Fr; latex

a section of the jejunum not attached to the mesentery be selected so that bowel manipulation is allowed if needed. If the bowel is not being resected, the Ligament of Treitz is commonly used. A needle is inserted into the lumen of the jejunum through the subserosa and a catheter is inserted through the needle and threaded into the jejunum. The needle is removed after the catheter is sutured into place. Sutures are applied to attach the jejunum to the abdominal wall after a second needle functions to pass the other end of the catheter to the outside of the abdomen.

Lastly, sutures are placed around the catheter at the exit to prevent accidental removal.[2]

Gastrostomy and jejunostomy tubes are more frequently being used today in long-term nutritional therapy because they are more acceptable to patients who are at home leading active work and social lives. They have reduced some of the psychological problems associated with the dehumanizing appearance of nasoenteral feeding tubes. Table 14–2 lists the commonly available gastrostomy and jejunostomy feeding tubes. The K-tube feeding jejunostomy tube is pictured in Figure 14–3.

Physical Characteristics

The market of tube feeding delivery systems has developed tremendously over the past several years. An array of feeding tubes is now available, varying in construction, length, and diameter[7] (Table 14–2). Plastic tubes of the "garden hose" variety, like the red rubber Robnel tube, have been replaced by polyurethane and silicone tubes that are more resilient and less reactive with body tissue.[7] Feeding tube selection should be based on the formula required by the patient. The large bore feeding tubes, 10 to 14 French, are necessary when a blenderized "house" diet or viscous formula such as Compleat Modified is used. Commercially prepared formulas generally flow well through the smaller bore—8 French or less—tubes[7] (Fig. 14–4).

Nasoenteral tubes—nasogastric, nasojejunal, and nasoduodenal tubes—range in length from the short 76.2-cm (30-inch) size, which is intended for gastric feedings, to the long 109.2-cm (43-inch) size used for nasoduodenal and nasojejunal feedings. Many of the tubes have radiopaque, mercury-weighted tips to assist in tube introduction and to maintain the tube in proper position. Other tubes have tungsten and silicone tips. Mercury tips create a problem because they release toxic vapors and must be clipped and boxed properly for disposal after tube feeding use. The tungsten tip found in the new Corpak, Entriflex, and Flexiflo tubes (Figs. 14–4, 14–5) provides more weight and eliminates this concern. Silicone-weighted tips are also popular but are lighter than the tungsten or mercury tips and are not as effective in preventing tube dislodgement. A comparison of different types of 9 French tube weights is illustrated in Figure 14–5.

Most tubes now have distal feeding ports or "exit eyelets," which vary in size and number and allow for smoother infusion of feeding formulas without clogging (Fig. 14–5). They also reduce the amount of solution stasis considerably.

The softness and pliability of newer tubes necessitate the use of guidewires and stylets for ease of insertion. Most of these guidewires are steel and come preassembled in a number of tubes. The Corpak, Biosearch, and Pharmaseal stylets pictured (Fig. 14–6) all have features that distinguish them from one another. The Duotube manfactured by Argyle (not illustrated) is unique in that it is ensheathed in a removable plastic tube that acts as a guide.

Guidewires must be used only upon initial feeding tube insertion. Reinsertion of the guidewire after a tube has been inserted may cause perforation of the feeding tube or slippage through an exit eyelet into the GI tract.

Lubricants, such as the hydromer coating found on the Entriflex and Dobbhoff tubes and Keolube found on the Keofeed tube, facilitate tube passage. Directions for activation of prelubricated coatings are included in the particular tube feeding guides. Water-soluble jelly may also be recommended for ease of insertion.

Insertion Techniques

Patient Preparation. In alert cooperative patients, nasoenteric tube insertion can be performed at the patient's bedside with the patient in a semi-Fowler's position. Unconscious or uncooperative patients require facilitation of nasogastric feeding tube insertion with the use of a guidewire.

Prior to tube insertion, a full explanation of the insertion procedure should be provided to the patient. It is helpful to show the patient the feeding tube, and allow him to feel and examine it, especially if he is anxious or has had previous unfortunate tube feeding experiences. This will increase his confidence in the staff members and gain his cooperation during the insertion procedure.

Preparation of Materials. Before insertion, all appropriate materials should be gathered and placed on a tray table at the patient's bedside. These materials should include the feeding tube, a glass of water, a 50-ml syringe, hypoallergenic tape, a towel, water-soluble lubricant, a stethoscope, and an emesis basin. To determine the amount of tube to be inserted, the tube should be measured from the nose to the ear to the xyphoid process (Fig. 14–7). This will provide an estimate of the distance to the stomach.[12] Twenty to 30 cm should be added for nasoduodenal and jejunal feeding tubes. Most feeding tubes are premarked at designated lengths for a measure of depth of tube insertion.

Actual Insertion Procedure. Following the preparation of the appropriate materials for feeding tube insertion, the following list of guidelines is recommended to assist in the actual insertion procedure:

1. Elevate the head of the patient's bed to at least 30 degrees or have the patient sit at the bedside with his feet dangling.
2. Assess the nasal passages for obstruction.
3. Select the more patent nostril for insertion.
4. Assess the tube and stylet for defects.
5. Lubricate the tube as needed.
6. Determine the length of the tube required for insertion.
7. Begin passing the tube through the nares to the back of the throat while encouraging the patient to swallow.

Water may be required to stimulate the swallowing reflex.

8. If the tube meets strong resistance, pull it back and pass it again. The tube should never be forced.

Verification of Feeding Tube Position. It is always advisable that feeding tube position be verified by x-ray before the feeding is initiated. Aspiration of gastric contents with a syringe or injecting air and listening for bubbles in the left upper quadrant of the stomach are the only evidence of proper tube placement. Smaller tubes can easily be inserted into the trachea, where lung aspirate may be obtained, instead of into the stomach. Litmus paper should be used to check for acid pH, which would correlate with the pH of stomach secretions.

For intraduodenal or jejunal feedings, the additional 20 to 30 cm of tubing left extending from the nose should be passed transpylorically at a rate of approximately 5 cm/hour. Placement of the patient in the right lateral decubitus position will facilitate spontaneous peristaltic advancement of the feeding tube[7] (Fig. 14–8). X-ray confirmation of tube placement again is required.

Postinsertion Management. When the tube is in proper position, it should be taped to the cheek or forehead without tension, using hypoallergenic tape. Improper taping can cause tissue irritation and facial disfigurement (Fig. 14–9).

BAGS AND PUMPS

Manufacturers of feeding tubes have now designed complementary feeding bags and pumps to create a total delivery system. The Competitive Enteral Pump Quick Reference (Table 14–3) summarizes a number of the delivery systems available and provides a detailed description of their characteristics. Ideally, characteristics of an enteral feeding system should include adaptability to a vari-

TABLE 14–3. COMPETITIVE ENTERAL PUMP QUICK REFERENCE[a]

Pump Supplier	Corpak	IVAC Corp.	Chesebrough-Ponds	
Pump model	VTR 300	Keofeed 3000	Kangaroo 220	Kangaroo 330
Flow range	1–299 ml/hr	1–300 ml/hr	5–295 ml/hr	1–295 ml/hr
Flow setting increments	1 ml/hr	1 ml/hr	5 ml/hr	1 ml (1–50 ml) 5 ml (50–295 ml)
Pumping mechanism	Delta	Rotary Peristaltic	Delta	Delta
Accuracy— selected flow	± 10%	± 8%	± 10%	± 10%
Battery life	3 hr @ 125 ml	5 hr @ 125 ml	3 hr @ 125 ml	3 hr @ 125 ml
Pressure maximum	12 psi	18 psi	12 psi	12 psi
Weight	8 lb	8 lb	5.5 lb	5 lb
Functional test— automatic	Yes	Yes	No	
Alarms—audio visual				
Occlusion/empty bag	Audio visual	Audio	Audio visual	Audio visual
Door open	n/a	Audio	n/a	n/a
Rate change	n/a	Audio	Audio visual	No
Low battery	Audio visual	Audio visual	Audio visual	Audio visual
Features				
Rate display	LED	LED	Yes, no light	LED
Volume infused display	LED, constant display	LED, not continuous	No	LED not counting
Memory retention (rate, vol, time)	Yes	Yes	No	Yes
Elapsed time recall	Yes	Yes	No	Yes
RUN/STOP switch for pump	Yes	Yes	No	Yes (hold)
Rate setting mechanism	Touch control, pressure sensitive	Touch control, pressure sensitive	Push up or down	Touch control
Product available	Pump Single pump set (fits Kangaroo 220) Pump set w/500 or 1000 ml bags Single 500 & 1000 ml bags Adult, Pedi, Neonatal polyurethane tubes	Pump Single pump set Pump set w/500 or 1500 ml bag Adult silicone feeding tubes	Pump Single pump set Pump set w/500, 1000, 1200 ml bags Single bag—1200 ml	Same CP Kangaroo 220
Suggested Price	$675–710	$600	$550–575	$575–600 Trade-in policy

[a]Prepared by Corpak Company, Wheeling, Illinois.

Ross Labs		Biosearch		Travenol
Flexiflo	Flexiflo II	14–7000	14–7005	Flo Gard 2000
50, 75, 100, 150, 175, 200 ml/hr	20, 30, 40, 50, 60, 75, 100, 125, 150, 175, 200, 250 ml/hr	20–100 ml/hr or 100–250 ml/hr	5–30 ml/hr	
25 ml/hr		10 ml/hr or 25 ml/hr	5 ml/hr	
Delta	Delta	Delta	Rotary Peristaltic	Delta
		± 10%	± 10%	± 10%
	8 hr	8–10 hr		6 hr
12 psi	12 psi	12 psi	12 psi	12 psi
2 lb		4.5 lb		
No	No	No	No	Yes
No A/V alarms	Audio visual	Audio visual	Audio visual	Audio visual
n/a	n/a	n/a	n/a	
No	No	No		
No	Audio visual	No	Visual	
Yes, no light	Yes, no light	Yes, no light	Yes, LED	LED
No	No	No	No	LED
No	No	No	No	Yes
No	No	No	No	No
No	No	No	No	Yes
Stretch tube		Turn dial		Touch control, pressure sensitive
Pump		Pump		Pump
Foods		Prefilled container		Foods
Pump set w/cap 1000, 1500 ml rigid containers		Single pump set Pump set w/old side fill bag not preattached Adult, Pedi urethane tubes		Pump set 1300 ml bag
$350	$500	$500	$600	$550–600

ety of feeding tubes, adaptability to a variety of enteral feeding products of differing viscosities, unbreakable leakproof containers, a container volume of 1000 ml on a durable hanger with volumetric markings, a wide opening easy for one person to fill, and a roller clamp.

Containers should be designed to minimize the risk of bacterial contamination. Many containers are disposable, which reduces the potential for cross-patient contamination. In addition, most containers are sterilely packaged. Rigid bags are easier to open and fill and lend themselves to less contamination. The Ross Flexitainer is an example of this

(Fig. 14–10). Other commonly used feeding bags pictured (Figs. 14–11 through 14–14) are manufactured by Biosearch, Corpak, IVAC, and Travenol. See feeding bag table for explanation (Table 14–4).

Feeding bags and containers are susceptible to airborne bacterial contamination. Most of the feeding bags and containers do provide an airtight seal, and they should be closed and sealed during use to avoid such contamination. In addition to closing the bags tightly, formulas should never be hung for more than 4 to 8 hours at a time.

The necessity of a feeding pump should be determined by prior feeding intake, feeding

TABLE 14–4. FEEDING CONTAINER QUICK REFERENCE

Feeding Container	Manufacturer	Features
Vitafeed	Pharmaseal	Supplied with or without tubing. Has luer adaptor. Universal port. Will accept any standard IV-type tubing. Refillable while hanging. 1200-ml capacity.
Keofeed	IVAC	Supplied with or without tubing. Tube adaptor can be used with all sizes of Keofeed tubes and most other feeding tube systems. Will accept any standard IV-type tubing. Refillable while hanging. 500- and 1500-ml capacities.
Flexitainer	Ross	Screw-cap type tubing. Tubing supplied has catheter tip. Narrow opening. Cannot refill while hanging. 1000-ml capacity.
Travasorb	Travenol	Supplied with or without tubing. Universal port. Will accept any standard IV-type tubing. Narrow opening. Difficult to refill while hanging. 1300-ml capacity.
Dobbhoff	Biosearch	Without tubing. Universal port. Will accept any standard IV-type tubing. 1000-ml capacity.
Ethox–Barron	Ethox	Two types of tubing. Designed to fit Barron pump. Narrow opening. Fillable while hanging. 1000-ml capacity.
Kangaroo easy-cap	Chesebrough-Ponds	With or without tubing. Tubing with universal luer adaptor. Fillable while hanging. 1200-ml capacity.
Kangaroo	Chesebrough-Ponds	Tubing with universal luer adaptor. Difficult to fill while hanging. Narrow opening. 500-ml and 1000-ml bags.
Irrigation container	McGaw	Prefilled with sterile water. Special McGaw tubing needed. Narrow opening. Not fillable while hanging. 500-ml capacity.
Monitor	Corpak	Tubing with universal luer adaptor. Fillable while hanging. 500-ml and 1000-ml capacities. 1000-ml bag has burette chamber holding 250 ml. 500-ml bag has burette chamber holding 125 ml.
Enteral feeding bag	Corpak	Tubing with universal luer adaptor. Fillable while hanging. 500-ml and 1000-ml capacities.
Acutrol	Norwich-Eaton	Universal luer adaptor. Side burette chamber without clamping system. 1000-ml capacity.

site, formula selection, and present medical status. Gravity drip is acceptable when a large volume of solution is being infused, the viscosity of the solution is low, or the radius of the tubing is wide, and when the patient has adequate absorptive capacity to tolerate inconsistent formula flow. Gravity feeding can be continuous or intermittent, over a 20- to 30-minute time period. The Ross and Mead–Johnson delivery sets have roller clamps to control their flow rate and are used frequently for gravity drip feedings (Fig. 14–15).

Bolus feedings are administered using a syringe or bulb. The feedings are administered rapidly and the volume usually ranges from 300 to 400 ml at one feeding with 4 to 6 feedings daily. As with gravity drip feedings, the tolerance of bolus feedings largely depends upon the functional ability of the gut. Both gravity and bolus feedings can lead to many GI and metabolic complications.

Pumps allow for a continuous infusion at low pressure. They provide a more consistent flow of formula at a regular rate and thus enhance formula absorption. There are a number of pumps on the market now, and selection of the appropriate pump will largely depend upon the type of tubing used at the institution and the cost of the pump (Figs. 14–16 through 14–21, see Table 14–3).

Pumps are either volumetric or peristaltic. Volumetric pumps measure infusion by volume, as compared to peristaltic pumps which rely on the number of drops infused per minute. Most enteral feeding pumps measure infusion by volume, which makes them more accurate since drop size will depend upon solution viscosity, and will vary from formula to formula. With enteral feeding pumps, delta or rotary peristaltic mechanisms act to pump or force the solution through the tubing, while also preventing backflow. The major disadvantage of the peristaltic pump is that drop size varies with the viscosity of the solution and rate of administration, yielding a variance, from time to time, in volume infused. Standard intravenous infusion or peristaltic pumps can be adapted to enteral feed-

ing infusion but are expensive and can be cumbersome because of their weight.

The most attractive pump will be one that is volumetric, easy to use, equipped with batteries, and portable and lightweight for ambulatory patients. It should have a rate range and increment changes for necessary adjustments and an alarm system to indicate mechanical problems.

CONCLUSIONS

Employing the following safety measures will reduce the risk of tube feeding delivery complications:

1. Assess all tubing and pump equipment throughout the day for cleanness and proper functioning.
2. Clearly label feeding containers with the patient's name and room number, the name of the feeding solution, the time and date the feeding was hung, and the time at which the tubing was last changed.
3. To avoid bacterial contamination, hang only a 4- to 8-hour supply of feeding formula at one time.
4. Change bags and tubing every 24 hours.
5. If a continuous feeding is turned off for any reason, flush it with 30 to 50 ml of water before reinitiating tube feeding delivery.
6. With intermittent feeding, regularly assess the consistency of flow to avoid clogging or stasis and flush the system with 30 to 50 ml of water after each feeding.
7. After each use, rinse and dry irrigation tubing thoroughly.
8. Clip mercury-tipped tubes after using and dispose of them appropriately in a covered container.

These measures should reduce delivery problems considerably and will protect the patient from potential delivery-induced complications.

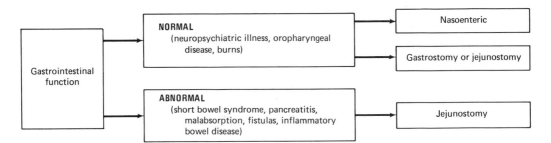

Figure 14–1. Routes of tube feeding delivery. *(Adapted from Rombeau JL, Barot LR: Enteral nutrition therapy.* Surg Clin North Am *61(3):614, 1961.)*

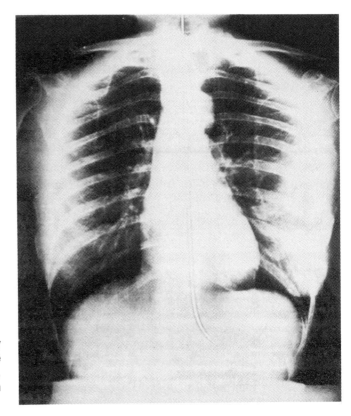

Figure 14–2. X-ray of a properly inserted nasogastric feeding tube in left upper quadrant of stomach. The outline of the tube has been enhanced by a medical artist.

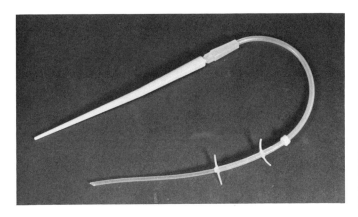

Figure 14–3. The K-Tube modified feeding jejunostomy tube used in long-term nutrition support therapy.

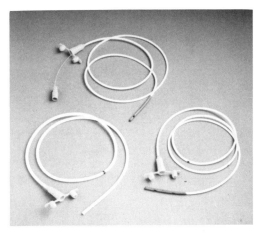

Figure 14–4. The new Ross Flexiflo Enteral Feeding tubes come in 8 French (top and left tubes) and in 12 French (lower right tube). The 8 French sizes are both tungsten-tipped. One 8 French tube comes with a Teflon-coated, 3-wire-braided stylet. *(Photograph courtesy of Ross Laboratories, Columbus, Ohio.)*

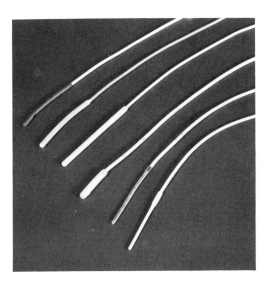

Figure 14–5. An 8 French tube comparison. *From left to right:* (**1**) Corpak smooth tip urethane tube with tungsten. Exit eyelets in bolus. (**2**) Entriflex tube (Biosearch) with tungsten-filled urethane tip. Exit eyelets in tube. (**3**) Mercury-tipped Keofeed (IVAC) silicone feeding tube. Exit eyelets in tube. (**4**) Travenol tungsten-tipped tube. Exit eyelets in bolus. (**5**) Superior silicone tube with exit eyelet in end of tube. Metal spring weight. (**6**) Ross C-Flex Tube with exit holes in pliable bolus.

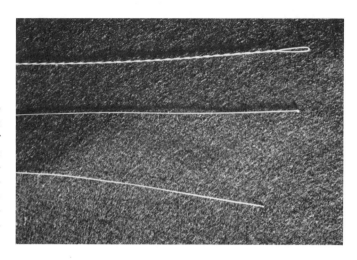

Figure 14–6. Stylet types. *Top to bottom:* (**1**) Corpak Flow-Through Stylet. Braided with end loop for friction reduction and elimination of inadvertent stylet exit. (**2**) Single-wire Biosearch with ball-bearing end. Flow-through feature. (**3**) Braided Pharmaseal with ball-bearing end. Flow-through feature.

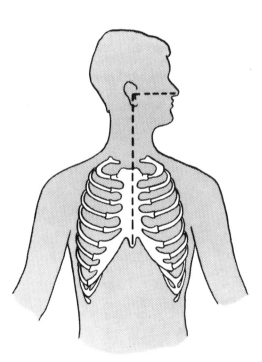

Figure 14–7. Estimation of distance for feeding tube insertion.

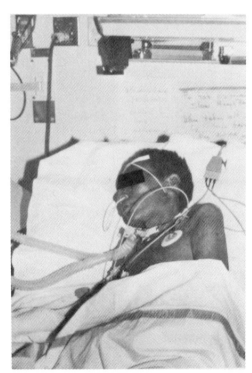

Figure 14–8. Patient positioned in the right lateral decubitus position for ease of transpyloric feeding tube passage.

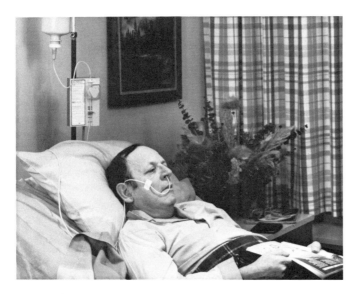

Figure 14–9. Feeding tube taped to cheek with minimal tension. *(Photograph courtesy of Ross Laboratories, Columbus, Ohio.)*

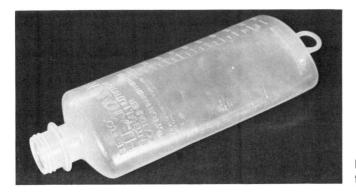

Figure 14–10. The Ross Flexi-tainer.

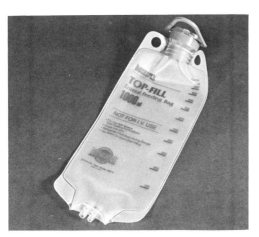

Figure 14–11. The Biosearch Top-Fill Enteral Feeding Bag.

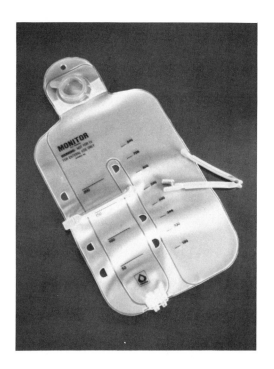

Figure 14–12. The Corpak Monitor Feeding Bag.

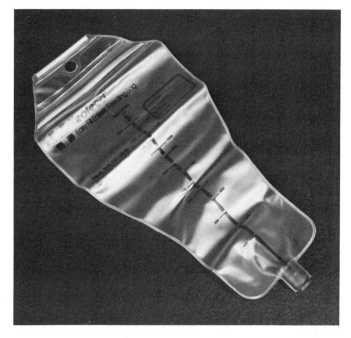

Figure 14–13. The Keofeed (IVAC) Easy Fill Enteric Feeding Bag.

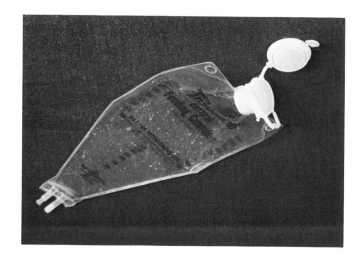

Figure 14–14. The Travenol Enteral Feeding Container.

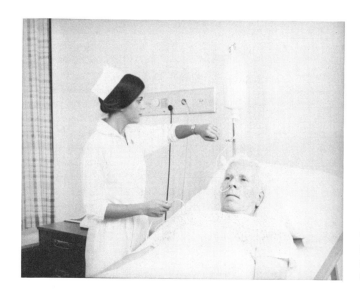

Figure 14–15. The Ross Delivery Set. A roller clamp regulates gravity infusion. *(Photograph courtesy of Ross Laboratories, Columbus, Ohio.)*

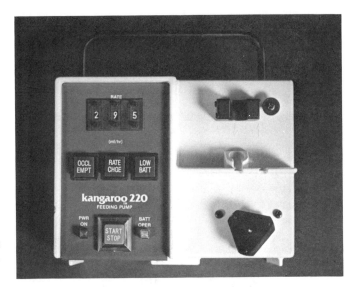

Figure 14–16. The Kangaroo 220 Feeding Pump by Chesebrough Ponds.

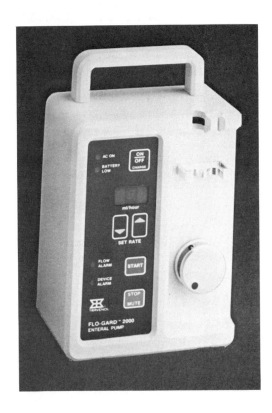

Figure 14–17. The Flo-Gard 2000 Enteral Pump by Travenol.

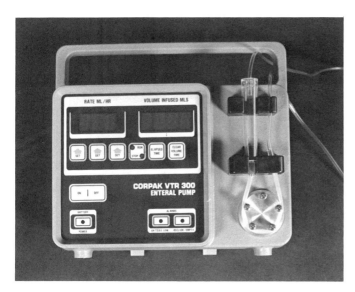

Figure 14–18. The Corpak VTR 300 Enteral Pump.

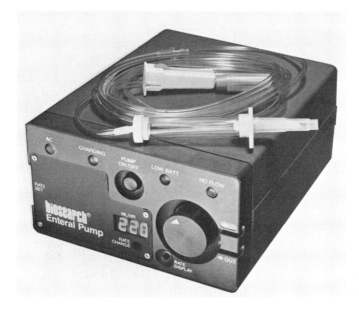

Figure 14–19. The Biosearch Enteral Pump.

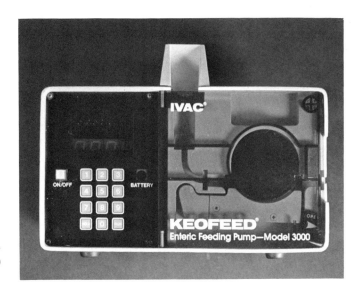

Figure 14–20. The Keofeed Enteric Feeding Pump Model 3000 by IVAC.

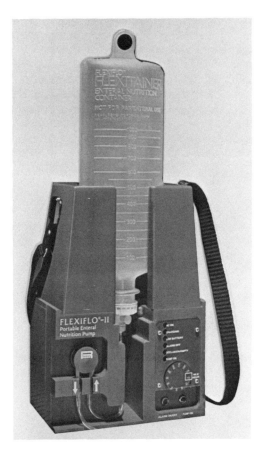

Figure 14–21. The Ross Flexiflo-II Portable Enteral Nutrition Pump.

ACKNOWLEDGMENTS

The author wishes to gratefully acknowledge Mr. David Quinn, President, Corpak Company, for his technical assistance, and Mr. Bruce Freed, R.D., M.S., for his assistance in the organization of this manuscript.

REFERENCES

1. Acquarell MJ: Cervical esophagostomy. An improved technique for alimentation of the debilitated patient. Arch Otolaryng 96:453–465, 1972

2. Del Rio D, Williams K, Esvelt BM: Handbook of Enteral Nutrition: A Practical Guide to Tube Feeding. El Segundo, Calif: Medical Specifics, 1982

3. Stamm M: Gastrostomy: A new method. Medical News 65:324–326, 1894

4. Deitel M: Nutrition in Clinical Surgery. Baltimore, Md: Williams & Wilkins, 1980, pp 43–52

5. Janeway HH: Eine neue Gastrostomie-methode. Muench Med Wochensehr 60:1705–1707, 1913

6. Larson DE, Fleming RC, Ott BJ, Schroeder KW: Percutaneous endoscopic gastrostomy. Mayo Clin Proc 58:103–106, 1983

7. Silberman H, Eisenberg D: Parenteral and Enteral Nutrition for the Hospitalized Patient. Norwalk, Conn: Appleton-Century-Crofts, 1982, pp 78–114

8. Vazquez RM: A Manual of Nutritional Support. Chicago: Travenol Laboratories, 1982, pp 65–77

9. Hoover HC, Ryan JA, Anderson EJ, Fischer JE: Nutritional benefits of immediate post-operative jejunal feeding of an elemental diet. Am J Surg 139:153–159, 1980

10. Riley KH, White JL, Jarrett PA, et al.: Immediate post-operative enteral nutrition. Surg Forum 31:103–105, 1980

11. Shils M, Randall HT: Modern Nutrition in Health and Disease, 6th ed. Philadelphia: Lea & Febiger, 1980, pp 1082–1124

12. Hanson RL: Predictive criteria of nasogastric tube insertion for tube feeding. JPEN 3:160–163, 1979

15. Metabolic Complications During Enteral Nutrition Support

Lucinda K. Lysen

Complications of enteral nutrition support can be divided into four categories: metabolic, pulmonary, gastrointestinal (GI), and mechanical. These complications can be minimized by close patient monitoring and evaluation, astute clinical management, and careful preventative measures throughout the course of enteral feeding. Selected complications of enteral nutrition support and their frequencies are shown in Table 15–1.

METABOLIC COMPLICATIONS

Fluid and Electrolytes

An increase or decrease in electrolytes may be due to the concentration of the formula, excessive bodily losses, insufficient excretion, or water depletion or excess.[1] Among more commonly observed electrolyte changes are hyponatremia, hypernatremia, and hypokalemia. Individual needs in terms of fluids and electrolytes should be determined before fluid and electrolyte supplementation is undertaken. Fluid and electrolyte supplementation may be provided by the addition of electrolytes to the enteral formula, or by peripheral intravenous infusion. If electrolyte values are dilutional, diuretic therapy may be indicated; higher than needed amounts of fluids may require that the formula be changed to a more concentrated one. If electrolyte values are elevated, a formula that is lower in electrolyte content or higher in water may be necessary.

Monitoring fluid status involves assessing intake (I) and output (O) on every shift, checking daily weights and urine-specific gravity, and assessing skin turgor. Carefully measured I and O is the best index of fluid balance.

Laboratory indices of fluid status include hematocrit, serum sodium, and blood urea nitrogen. These values will rise with dehydration and fall with overhydration. They should be evaluated at least one to two times weekly or more as necessary.

Hyperglycemia

Hyperglycemia and its resultant glycosuria can lead to hyperglycemic, nonketotic dehydration, coma, and death. This condition is most prevalent in patients who are receiving high carbohydrate-containing formulas, who are diabetic and receiving inadequate in-

349

TABLE 15–1. SELECTED COMPLICATIONS OF ENTERAL NUTRITION SUPPORT AND THEIR FREQUENCIES OF OCCURRENCE

Complication	Frequency (%)
Edema	20–25
Diarrhea and cramping	10–20
Vomiting/distention	10–15
Hyperglycemia and glucosuria	10–15
Clogged lumen	<10
Hypernatremia	<5
Pulmonary aspiration of gastric contents	<1
Hyperosmolar coma	<1

Adapted from Heymsfield SB, Bethel RA, Ansley JD, et al: Enteral hyperalimentation: An alternative to central venous hyperalimentation. Ann Intern Med 90:69, 1979, and Fundamentals of Nutritional Support. Deerfield, Ill: Travenol Laboratories, Inc, 1981, p 116.

sulin, who are on steroid therapy, who are otherwise stressed and intolerant of glucose, or who are receiving excessive calories, particularly carbohydrates in excess of needs.[1,2] Hyperglycemia is usually managed with insulin on a sliding scale and assessed every 4 hours by testing the urine for sugar. In addition, some institutions perform daily blood sugars for more accurate management. A change to a lower carbohydrate-containing formula, or a decrease in caloric intake that provides adequate nutrients for repletion but not in excess of needs, also may reduce blood sugar levels.

Essential Fatty Acid Deficiency/Vitamin Deficiency

Patients receiving elemental diets that contain minimal amounts of fat may develop a deficiency of fat-soluble vitamins and essential fatty acids (EFA) after prolonged periods of treatment.[3–7] This problem can be resolved by administration of additional vitamin supplementation and linoleic acid supplementation.

An inadequate volume of formula and increased nutrient requirements as a result of stress may also increase the need for vitamins and minerals. Vitamin/mineral supplementation is possible via liquid multivitamin preparations or individual vitamin and trace element tablets crushed and added to the enteral formulation, depending upon the size of the tubing. Linoleic acid may be administered enterally in the form of Microlipid or safflower oil, or via IV administration of a fat emulsion. Malabsorptive states may require the intravenous infusion of vitamins and minerals.

Liver Abnormalities

Hyperammonemia and hepatic encephalopathy are common metabolic complications, particularly in patients with liver dysfunction. Recent literature provides evidence that the use of higher branch chain amino acid (BCAA) formulations will increase protein tolerance and improve the condition of the patient with chronic hepatic encephalopathy.[8] Protein intake should be restricted in these patients, with the emphasis on higher BCAA products. (See enteral feeding formulas in Chapter 13.)

Fat Intolerance

Patients who lack pancreatic enzymes in sufficient quantities or who have diminished bile production or secretion will have an intolerance to dietary fat. This will most likely present itself in the form of steatorrhea. A formulation low in fat will resolve the problem, with provision of EFA over a long period of time via intravenous infusion. Pancreatic enzyme replacements, such as Pancrease—one capsule four times per day orally—or dissolved Cotazym tablets bolused through the nasogastric or jejunal tube, can also be administered to digest fat when appropriate. Stool consistency should be assessed daily, particularly when there is evidence of fat intolerance.

Medium chain triglycerides are useful in a number of conditions (Table 15–2). They undergo rapid lipolysis, are not dependent on bile acid availability for degradation, and will be absorbed adequately even when the intestinal absorptive area is reduced.[9] They do not provide EFA, but do provide a source of energy for those patients in whom other fats are not tolerated.

Prerenal Azotemia

Inadequate hydration, excessive protein administration, or insufficient nonprotein calorie provision can cause prerenal azotemia. This can be corrected by changing the enteral formulation to one lower in protein or by providing additional nonprotein hydration to the formulation being used.

Respiratory Complications

Excess calories, particularly carbohydrate calories, can produce excess CO_2 and further impede respiratory status in previously respiratory-compromised patients. These patients require enteral formulations of lower carbohydrate and higher fat content. Chapter 13 specifically discusses enteral formulations used for respiratory-compromised patients.

Inadequate Nutritional Repletion

Protein synthesis and a positive nitrogen balance are indicative of an optimal nutrition response to nutrition support therapy. These are evidenced by increased serum transferrin and albumin, along with weight gain in those patients who are underweight. Activity enhances nutritional repletion and should be encouraged on a daily basis.

In those patients who do not achieve a positive response to enteral nutrition support, reevaluation of the patient's requirements is needed and adjuvant parenteral intervention or a change in enteral intervention may be required to avert the development of deficiencies.

TABLE 15–2. CLINICAL INDICATIONS FOR USE OF MEDIUM CHAIN TRIGLYCERIDES

Impaired fat hydrolysis
   Pancreatic insufficiency
   Cystic fibrosis
   Biliary obstruction
Impaired fat absorption
   Sprue
   Steatorrhea
   Intestinal resection
   Blind loop syndrome
   Type V hyperlipidemia
   Abetalipoproteinemia
Impaired transport of lipid
   Lymphangiectasia
   Chylothorax
   Chyluria
   Chylous ascites
   Exudative enteropathy

From Dietel, M: Nutrition in Clinical Surgery. Baltimore, Md: Williams & Wilkins, 1980, p 31.

PULMONARY COMPLICATIONS

Aspiration

Aspiration of enteral feeding formulation is life threatening. If the potential for this complication is apparent, i.e., if the patient has an altered gag reflex or is comatose, frequently the use of parenteral nutrition should be considered as an alternative until the risk subsides.

With patients who are at risk for aspiration, it is advisable to select a feeding tube that is designed to be placed distal to the pylorus and that has a weighted tip. Jejunostomy tubes are frequently used for the purpose of avoiding aspiration because they are inserted directly into the jejunum, where the potential for gastric reflux is mimimized. A problem with nasoduodenal and nasojejunal tubes is that they do not always promptly pass the pylorus and, therefore, they can remain in the stomach for several days. Facilitation of transpyloric passage of these tubes may require that the patient rest on his right side for a period of time, which can be quite uncomfortable, or passage may require insertion with the aid of fluoroscopy.

X-ray confirmation is frequently recommended to verify the position of any non-surgically placed feeding tube before initiating a feeding. Thereafter, feeding tube placement is typically assessed every 4 to 8 hours with continuous feedings, and before each feeding with intermittent feedings, by injecting air through the tube while listening with a stethoscope over the epigastric area.

Vazquez[10] recommends that with continuous nasogastric or nasoduodenal feedings, gastric residual be checked every 6 hours for the first 24 hours and then as clinically indicated. Other centers recommend checking gastric residuals continually on a routine schedule, as every 4 or 6 hours. Patients on bolus nasoenteral feedings and bolus gastrostomy feedings are typically assessed for gastric residuals prior to each feeding. In most cases, a residual of greater than 100 ml shows clinical evidence of poor gastric emptying and the feeding should be held.[10] If gastric emptying cannot be augmented, the enteral feeding should be decreased to a rate that the patient can tolerate, the formula re-evaluated, or parenteral support considered.[10] If an anatomic obstruction of the stomach seems unlikely, metaclopramide may be given to the patient to stimulate gastric motility. When the risk of aspiration is high, a continuous infusion is preferable to a bolus feeding of formula to assure meeting nutrition requirements. Small continuous amounts of infusion minimize solution accumulation in the stomach and the potential for regurgitation. In addressing these issues, close attention particularly should be paid to comatose patients.

With either method of delivery, bolus or continuous, the patient should be positioned with the head of his bed at 30 degrees or more, while feeding and in the immediate postprandial period. If this position is impos-sible, the patient should be placed on his right side.[1] Feedings should be stopped during treatments requiring a supine or head-down position such as postural drainage or insertion of a subclavian catheter.[1]

GASTROINTESTINAL COMPLICATIONS

Diarrhea

Diarrhea is commonly associated with tube feeding administration and has a number of etiologies. Atrophied intestinal villi secondary to malnutrition or cancer chemotherapy impede absorption of nutrients and can cause diarrhea. Malabsorption, secondary to pancreatitis, small bowel disease, and Crohn's disease, also causes diarrhea. A defined formula diet consisting of di- and tri-peptides and/or free amino acids, such as Criticare HN or Vivonex HN, requires minimal digestion and frequently remedies this complication, especially if administered slowly and continuously.

Dumping syndrome occurs after gastric surgery and is mostly due to the presence of hyperosmolar solutions in the intestinal lumen. The resultant diffusion of water from the villous capillaries causes shortness of breath, restlessness, weakness, palpitations, distention, pain, and diarrhea.[10] A solution of lesser hypertonicity like Isocal or Osmolite should be utilized when possible, or the available solution should be diluted with water to half strength.

Another cause of diarrhea is lactose intolerance. Lactose intolerance results from a deficiency in the enzyme lactase, which commonly occurs in the black and Oriental populations and in patients who are malnourished and therefore have diminished lactase production. Lactose intolerance requires a change from a milk-based enteral formula, if being used, to a lactose-free formula.

Another contributing factor to diarrhea is

hypoalbuminemia, which creates a decrease in oncotic pressure. This can be managed by either parenteral nutrition, or the IV administration of albumin, which is costly but effective in improving intestinal absorptive capacity. It is important to keep in mind that the IV administration of albumin does not contribute to the amino acid pool but will elevate the serum albumin considerably.

Broad-spectrum antibiotics may allow the overgrowth of *Clostridium difficile* and other organisms, causing enteritis and its resultant diarrhea, curable only by bowel rest or by administration of *Lactobacillus* to replenish GI flora.[2] Administration of antidiarrheal agents, such as paregoric, Kaopectate, and Lomotil should be reserved for those patients without a viral or bacterial enteritis.[10]

Contaminated formula or equipment can contribute to diarrhea. Many hospitals require feeding formula to be hung for no longer than 8 hours. New formula is often not allowed to be added to the existing formula. Formulas should be refrigerated after opening and discarded after 24 hours, if not used. The feeding container and tubing should be changed daily using clean technique, and the container should close properly to prevent bacterial contamination.

If formula is started and/or advanced too rapidly, diarrhea may occur. The rate and/or concentration should be advanced slowly until tolerance is achieved. Continuous infusion is advocated over bolus or intermittent feedings to avoid the potential for diarrhea which commonly occurs with high volumes of feeding given over a short time period.

Lastly, diarrhea or "liquid stool" may be a sign of fecal impaction. This complication must be assessed and diagnosed by rectal examination and then treated appropriately.

Nausea/Vomiting/Cramps/Abdominal Distention

Nausea, vomiting, cramps, and/or abdominal distention may also occur in tube feeding delivery. This is particularly true with rapid administration of solution, and can be avoided by slowing the administration rate. These symptoms can also be a result of intolerance to formula concentration. In this instance, a decrease to the most recently tolerated concentration or a change of formula is indicated. A cold formula may initiate nausea and vomiting. Enteral formulas, therefore, should be infused at room temperature. Finally, lactose intolerance will often cause nausea and vomiting, which, as was stated earlier, will require a change in formula to a lactose-free one. (See Chapter 13 for discussion of lactose-free formulas.)

Gastric Retention

Positioning the patient in a semi-Fowler's position or in the right lateral decubitus position may be beneficial to gastric emptying.[3] Gastric residual may be used to monitor the severity of fluid retention. If less than 100 ml of residual is obtained, either gastric emptying is adequate or the retained gastric contents are not being adequately sampled. Metachlopramide can be used to enhance GI motility and gastric emptying. With a feeding into the duodenum or jejunum, a decompression tube may be required until the patient can protect his airway from aspiration, or until pyloric function returns. GI obstruction will cause gastric retention, and tube feeding in obstructed patients is contraindicated. Bolus and intermittent feeding of formulations can cause gastric retention. The rapidity or amount of infusion should be decreased, or the formula changed to a continuous infusion.

Constipation

Constipation is often a result of immobility and decreased GI motility, a change in diet, lack of dietary fiber, poor fluid intake, fecal impaction, or drug therapy (particularly narcotics). Treatment typically includes increasing free water intake or changing the drug therapy. Determination of the appropriate method of treatment depends on the particular patient. Stool consistency should be monitored on a daily basis to assess for constipation and overall tolerance of enteral regime.

MECHANICAL COMPLICATIONS

Pulmonary Aspiration

A deflated tracheostomy cuff can cause feeding aspiration. It is therefore recommended that the tracheostomy cuff be inflated before feeding and be maintained for 1 hour afterwards.[2] This, however, will not guarantee protection against aspiration. As was mentioned earlier, a long nasoenteral feeding tube or a jejunostomy tube can prevent this problem.

A displaced feeding tube can also cause aspiration. The anchoring effect of tungsten, silicone, and mercury tips virtually prevents normal displacement. Slippage can occur, however, as a result of undue tension on the tube and tubing. A sufficient length of tubing should prevent tension. If the tube is displaced, the etiology should be determined. A patient who pulls at his tube may require mitts and should have his tube taped out of reach. If the tube has been causing him irritation or pain, these problems should be corrected. Frequent tube pulling may indicate the need for a gastrostomy or jejunostomy, and the patient should not be restrained if at all possible. Coughing can dislodge the tube and may require the placement of a larger, softer tube. If endotracheal suctioning is necessary, suctioning in the region of the feeding tube should be avoided to prevent displacement of the tube.

Feeding Tube Obstruction

The most common cause of feeding tube obstruction is failure to irrigate the tube. If a feeding is interrupted for any length of time, the feeding tube should be irrigated with at least 20 ml of water. Liquid medications should be used whenever possible and crushed medications must be thoroughly dissolved before bolused. All medications and thick formulas require that the tube be flushed with 50 to 150 ml of water immediately after administration. Viscous formulas should be mixed well to avoid separation and clogging. A continuous infusion of formula provides constant tube flushing and is encouraged when possible. The use of a guidewire to clear a plug or clogged tube should never be undertaken. Patency can usually be restored by irrigation with a 20-ml syringe of water or air.[1] If this is not successful, the tube may need replacement.

Irritation/Discomfort

This can be caused by the use of a large-bore polyvinyl chloride tube that is left in place for a long period of time. Smaller-bore, softer tubes have, for the most part, replaced these tubes and should be used whenever possible. If used, polyvinyl chloride should be repositioned daily and tape should be changed on a daily basis. Other tubes require tape to be changed as needed. Alcohol should be used to clean tape from the nose because acetone may cause feeding tube erosion.

Routine care of the patient requires that the nose, teeth, and oral cavity be cleaned and moistened several times daily and that the tube be assessed for pressure points.

ADMINISTRATION GUIDELINES

Infusion of Solution

Enteral hyperalimentation administered intermittently or around the clock by continuous drip can normally be started at 50 ml/hour full strength. Bolus nasoenteral and gastrostomy feedings, however, may initially require a half-strength dilution.

Voided specimens should be assessed for

glucosuria. If two consecutive specimens are negative for glucose and no loose stools are observed, the rate can be increased to 75 ml/hour.[11] Management should be continued this way with an increase in rate of 25 ml/hour until the desired rate of infusion is achieved. When full strength solutions are not tolerated, dilution to one-half or one-third strength is suggested. The infusion rate should be increased as tolerated to meet the patient's fluid requirements.

Addition of crushed medications to feeding tubes can cause clogging and is discouraged, but may be necessary in some cases as has been discussed in the text. Crushed tablets should never be placed in a needle catheter jejunostomy tube[10] or in other small bore tubes.

For diarrhea, the feeding should be decreased to the most recently tolerated rate, and Kaopectate 30 ml (only through large-bore tubes) and paregoric 5 ml as a bolus should be given.[10] Two to 5 cc paregoric per liter of solution may be necessary to control persistent diarrhea,[10] but an assessment of feeding formula intolerance must be made if this management is unsuccessful.

Monitoring Techniques

The optimal goal in enteral nutritional support is to provide adequate nutrition with minimal complications. This should be achieved if the following are assessed regularly:

1. Intake and output every shift.
2. Urine fractionals every 6 hours.
3. Daily weights.
4. Stool consistency.
5. Tube placement.
   a. Prior to initiation of the first feeding via x-ray.
   b. Before each bolus or intermittent feeding.
   c. Every 4 to 8 hours with continuous feedings by injecting 5 to 10 ml of air into the tube and listening with a stethoscope over the abdomen.

6. Residual. 100 ml or less is acceptable every 6 hours with continuous feedings or during the first 24 hours after the feeding is initiated, or prior to intermittent or bolus feedings, unless there is suspicion of poor sampling. Gastric residuals are usually obtainable in small-bore feeding tubes.
7. Oral hygiene. Perform at least two times daily.
8. Tape. Change as needed and clean area with alcohol daily.
9. Head of bed. Should be at 30 degrees or greater during and for 1 hour after feedings.
10. Patency of tube. Flush with 20 ml of water if feeding is stopped and before and after intermittent or bolus feedings.
11. Changes in formula color and consistency after hanging that might indicate contamination or formula separation. Hang no more than a 4- to 8-hour supply of formula.
12. Nausea, vomiting, diarrhea, cramping, and distention.
13. Serum electrolytes, blood count, and glucose level weekly.
14. Nutrition indices such as albumin, transferrin, and nitrogen balance weekly.
15. Ambulation/activity. Encourage whenever possible.

A chart depicting the complications frequently associated with enteral nutrition support has been provided (Table 15–3). Its intent is to act as a summary to the chapter and a reference for those individuals needing quick access to enteral tube feeding guidelines. As it has been emphasized, the patient receiving enteral nutrition requires constant reassessment. Close monitoring and evaluation, alert clinical management, and adherence to specific treatment of complications should optimize patient care and minimize the hazards involved with enteral nutrition support.

TABLE 15–3. COMPLICATIONS ASSOCIATED WITH TUBE FEEDING

Complication	Causes/Contributing Factors	How to Treat/Prevent
Mechanical		
Aspiration	Deflated tracheostomy cuff	Inflate trach cuff before feeding and keep inflated for 1 hour after feeding
		Consider long, small-bore feeding tube or surgically placed tube for long-term feeding or persistent aspiration
	Displaced feeding tube	Reinsert tube and check placement
		Check residuals every 4 to 8 hours
		Administer gastric stimulant
		Select tube with weighted tip
		Assess for tension on tubing
	Coma	Raise head of bed more than 30 degrees
Irritation/discomfort	Reduced gastric motility	Place feeding tube in small bowel
	Large-bore, polyvinyl chloride tube for long periods in same position	Reposition tube every day and change tape
		Consider smaller-bore feeding tube
		Make sure tube is positioned without pressure
		Moisten mouth and nose several times a day
		Use alcohol to clean tape from nose (acetone, if used, may cause erosion of tube)
Tube obstruction	Poorly crushed medications	Use liquid medications whenever possible
		Crush medications thoroughly and dissolve in water if possible
	Inadequate flushing after medications or thick formula	Flush feeding tube with 50 to 150 ml of water after instilling medications or thick formula
	Poorly dissolved formula	Use a blender to mix formulas if necessary (check manufacturer's guidelines)
		Never try to clear plug by forcing guidewire stylet into tube
Essential fatty acid deficiency	Elemental formulations	Intravenous provision of fat containing linoleic acid
		Addition of safflower oil to feeding
		Use of enteral fat formulations
Vitamin deficiency	Infusion of nutrients below requirements	Liquid multivitamin supplementation
		Crushed vitamins/minerals bolused through tube
	Malabsorption	Intravenous infusion of vitamins and minerals
Liver abnormalities: hyperammonemia and hepatic encephalopathy	Liver dysfunction	Reduced protein intake with emphasis on high branch chain amino acid formulations
Fat intolerance	Reduced pancreatic enzymes	Provision of pancreatic enzymes, i.e., Pancrease or Cotazym
	Diminished bile production	Use of an elemental diet
		Use of MCT oil
Gastrointestinal		
Diarrhea	Atrophied villi in GI tract	Use a chemically defined or free amino acid formula until nutritional status improves

TABLE 15–3. (*Continued*)

Complication	Causes/Contributing Factors	How to Treat/Prevent
	Low serum albumin	Provide intravenous albumin to increase oncotic pressure
	Hypertonic formula	Dilute the strength
	Formula started and/or advanced too rapidly	Reduce rate and/or concentration temporarily
		Consider continuous drip if patient on intermittent regimen
	Dumping syndrome	Decrease rate
		Dilute the strength
		Select less hypertonic formula
	Lactose intolerance	Change to lactose-free formula
	Drug therapy (e.g., antibiotics)	Administer *Lactobacillus* to replenish GI flora
		Administer antidiarrheal such as Lomotil, paregoric, or Kaopectate
	Contaminated formula	Hang fresh feeding every 4 to 8 hours
		Do not add new formula to remaining formula
		Change feeding container and tubing every day, using clean technique
		Avoid unnecessary manipulation of feeding system
		Discard opened formula after 24 hours
Nausea, vomiting, cramping, distention	Too rapid administration	Slow rate
	Intolerance to concentration	Dilute strength and/or decrease volume temporarily
	Formula too cold	Bring to room temperature before administering
	Gastric retention	Raise head of bed to 30 degrees or greater
		Check gastric residuals
		Consider medication to increase gastric motility (e.g. metachlopramide/Reglan)
		Pass feeding tube into small bowel
	Lactose intolerance	Use Lactose-free formula
High gastric residuals (gastric retention)	Reduced gastric motility	Hold feedings until residuals decrease
	Inactivity (e.g., bedrest)	Administer gastric stimulant to increase motility (e.g., metachlopramide/Reglan)
		Pass feeding tube beyond pylorus into small intestine
		Raise head of bed to 30 degrees or greater
Constipation	Inadequate water intake	Increase free water intake
	Inadequate bulk	Offer prune juice, if allowed
	Fecal impaction	Administer stool softener
	Drug therapy (e.g., narcotics)	Consider high-fiber formula
	Reduced GI motility	Encourage ambulation
Metabolic Hyperglycemia; glycosuria (can lead to hyperglycemic nonketotic dehydration, coma, or death)	Stress response	Monitor urine sugar and acetone every 4 hours
	High-carbohydrate formula (particularly the defined and free amino acid formulas)	Administer insulin as ordered
		Daily blood sugar

(*continued*)

TABLE 15–3. (*Continued*)

Complication	Causes/Contributing Factors	How to Treat/Prevent
	Diabetes mellitus with inadequate coverage	Lower calorie level
	Drug therapy (e.g., steroids)	
Excess carbon dioxide production (respiratory compromise)	Stress	Monitor respiratory status of acutely ill patients or those who have chronic obstructive lung disease
	Excess calories, especially carbohydrate calories	Decrease caloric intake, especially carbohydrate calories
Hyponatremia	Dilutional states (e.g., fluid overload)	Administer diuretics
		Restrict fluids—decrease formula
		Add table salt to formula (1 tsp = 2 g Na or 90 mEq)
	Excess GI losses	Replace GI losses
Hypernatremia	Dehydration	Monitor I&O carefully; weigh free fluid intake
Hypokalemia	Dilutional states	Administer diuretics
	Diuretic therapy	Administer potassium
	Large-dose insulin therapy	
	Excessive dietary protein	Select lower protein-containing formula
Prerenal azotemia	Insufficient nonprotein calorie provision	Addition of nonprotein calories to formula
	Excessive GI losses	Replace GI losses
	Inadequate hydration	Increase water
Respiratory compromise	Excess calories, particularly carbohydrate calories	Reduce carbohydrate content and increase fat content
Inadequate nutrition repletion	Requirements above estimated needs	Increase administration of feeding formulation
		Initiate a more calorically dense formula
		Add intravenous hyperalimentation to therapy regimen
		Check serum albumin, transferrin, nitrogen balance weekly
Pulmonary Aspiration	Altered gag reflex	Stop feeding if patient aspirates and suction trachea
	Coma	Elevate head of bed 30 degrees during and for 1 hour after feeding
		Place on right side during feeding when possible
		Check gastric residuals every 4 to 8 hours
		Observe for residual > 100 ml
		Consider metachlopramide for increase in gastric motility
		Check tube placement prior to feeding .
		Place feeding tube beyond pylorus

Adapted from Konstantinides NN, Shronts E: Tube feeding: Managing the basics. Am J Nurs 83:1319–1320, 1983.

REFERENCES

1. Del Rio D, Williams K, Esvelt BM: Handbook of Enteral Nutrition: A Practical Guide to Tube Feeding. El Segundo, California: Medical Specifics, 1982, pp 112–117
2. Konstantinides NN, Shronts E: Tube feeding: Managing the basics. Am J Nurs 83:1312–1320, 1983
3. Silberman H, Eisenberg D: Parenteral and Enteral Nutrition for the Hospitalized Patient. Norwalk, Conn: Appleton-Century-Crofts, 1982, pp 78–112
4. Freeman JB, Egan MC, Millis BJ: The elemental diet. Surg Gynecol Obstet 142:925–932, 1976
5. Farthing MJG, Jarrett EB, Williams G, Crawford MA: Essential fatty acid deficiency after prolonged treatment with elemental diet. Lancet 2:1088–1089, 1980
6. Dodge JA, Salter DG, Yassa JG: Essential fatty acid deficiency due to artificial diet in cystic fibrosis. Brit Med J 2:192–193, 1975
7. Dodge JA, Yassa JG: Essential fatty acid deficiency after prolonged treatment with elemental diet. Lancet 2:1256–1257, 1980
8. Fischer JE, Bower RH: Nutritional support in liver disease. Surg Clin North Am 61(3):653–660, 1981
9. Deitel M: Nutrition in Clinical Surgery. Baltimore, Md: Williams & Wilkins, 1980, pp 30–33
10. Vazquez RM: A Manual of Nutritional Support. Chicago: Travenol Laboratories, 1982, pp 55–88
11. Kaminski MV, Freed BA: Enteral hyperalimentation: Prevention and treatment of complications. Nutr Supp Serv 1(4):29–35, 40, 1981

16. Home Enteral Nutrition

Karen A. Porcelli
Susanna H. Krey

RATIONALE FOR HOME TUBE FEEDING

Home enteral nutrition for long-term nutrition support will increase dramatically in the future, especially with the current emphasis on cost containment moving to the outpatient arena. Home enteral nutrition has been used in chronically ill patients who are unable to consume adequate food to meet nutritional requirements. It is also indicated in those individuals who are unable to consume any food items, e.g., the patient with dysphagia or an obstruction such as head or neck cancer. These feedings can be used for an intermediate length of time, as in the individual with dysphagia caused by a cerebral vascular accident who with continued therapy may learn to swallow again. An indefinite period of home enteral nutrition may be indicated in cases when the patient will not be able to consume enough foods to meet requirements, such as in cases of head or neck cancer. The successful use of home enteral nutrition has been documented in both pediatric and adult populations.[1-3]

Patients and health care institutions can receive benefits from the use of home enteral nutrition. Table 16–1 lists some of these benefits.

To provide for patient safety and the suc-

cess of a home enteral program, a comprehensive program of selection, education, and follow-up is essential. The following specifies the essential components of a home enteral nutrition program:

- Identification of home enteral nutrition patients
- Selection of formula and equipment
- Seeking third-party reimbursement and a home care agency
- Instructing the patient and significant others
- Documentation
- Follow-up and transitional feeding

IDENTIFICATION OF HOME ENTERAL NUTRITION PATIENTS

Defining criteria for patient selection may result in the long-term success of a home program. Criteria should be defined by each multidisciplinary nutrition support team based on its experiences. Table 16–2 lists some examples.

The patient or a significant other must be able to learn to carry through the home enteral nutrition plan. Early involvement of a discharge coordinator or social worker should assist the nutrition support team in

TABLE 16–1. BENEFITS OF HOME ENTERAL NUTRITION

I. Patient
   A. Metabolic/Nutrition
      1. Allows for long-term repletion of nutrition status
   B. Psychosocial
      1. Patient can return to home setting among family and friends
      2. Patient can participate in home or work activities
      3. Patient can gain sense of self-confidence/independence by leaving hospital setting
   C. Economic
      1. Reduced health care costs
II. Health Care Institution
   A. Economic
      1. Reduces length of stay by allowing patient nutritional rehabilitation at home once otherwise medically stable
      2. Reduces complications when compared to home parenteral nutrition, which should reduce need for readmission
      3. Reduces time for education and preparation for discharge as compared to home parenteral nutrition
   B. Development
      1. Provides growth potential as referral program for institution
      2. Collaborative agreements are available with many home care companies

TABLE 16–2. SAMPLE CRITERIA FOR PATIENT SELECTION

Inability to consume foods to meet nutritional requirements on short-term basis (greater than 3 weeks)

Ability to digest and/or absorb nutrients so as to tolerate enteral formulas

Extended hospitalization for medical/surgical condition not warranted

Patient and significant others interested and able to learn how to continue tube feeding at home

Appropriate support (either family, significant other, or home care agency) available if patient cannot provide care independently

No metabolic or anamtomical complications that would be difficult to control or monitor closely as an outpatient

From Folk CC, Courtney ME: Nutr Supp Serv 2:18, 1982;[4] Adams MM, Wirsching RG: J Am Diet Assoc 84:68, 1984.[5]

Home enteral nutrition support affects a patient's life in ways other than the correction of malnutrition. Table 16–3 lists important questions that should be addressed in the selection of candidates.

TABLE 16–3. ISSUES OF CONCERN IN THE SELECTION OF HOME ENTERAL PATIENTS

Social/Psychological: How motivated and willing is the candidate in continuing with home enteral nutrition? Will patient's quality of life improve?

Financial: Can third party reimbursement be obtained? Can the patient or significant other handle economic situation?

Educational: Can the patient or significant other comply with minimal required standards for safety?

Medical: Will medical or physiologic condition benefit from long-term enteral nutrition?

Nutritional: Will nutrition status improve or maintain with long-term nutrition support?

Physical: Are there any physical limitations that prevent patient or significant other from safely and effectively dealing with long-term nutrition support?

Additional concerns

the proper identification and selection of candidates.

The route of delivery should be considered during patient selection. If home enteral nutrition is to be of intermediate duration (less than 3 months), a nasogastric or nasoduodenal route of delivery may be used. Patients who will require a long-term or permanent feeding tube would benefit from a gastrostomy or jejunostomy. The patient who is trying to return to an independent lifestyle or who is extremely self-conscious of the feeding tube may also benefit from a gastrostomy or jejunostomy. Another option is to instruct the patient on daily reinsertion of a nasogastric tube.

SELECTION OF FORMULA AND EQUIPMENT

Once a candidate has been selected and the route of delivery determined, the formula and equipment can be selected. Formula selection must consider the degree of digestive and absorptive ability, formula composition, and the ability to meet nutritional requirements in a defined volume and concentration. In selecting the formula for home use, convenience of preparation and cost must also be considered. Will the patient be able to mix a powdered formula? Does he or she have a food preparation area? Is there refrigerated storage if a formula needs to be mixed and then refrigerated? Does the patient have storage space for canned formulas?

The formula and equipment selected should conform to the patient's lifestyle. Daytime or nighttime cycles can be used instead of 24-hour continuous feedings to promote ambulation. If transitional feeding is to occur, nighttime cycling of feedings or bolus feedings may be preferred. Calorically dense formulas can meet nutritional requirements in smaller volumes. Lifestyle and patient needs should be considered in conjunction with equipment needs. If the patient is not always alert or requires supervision, an enteral infusion device with appropriate alarms should be selected. If the patient

TABLE 16–4. AN EXAMPLE OF A STANDARD NASOENTERAL TUBE FEEDING SUPPLY LIST

Saint Vincent Charity Hospital & Health Center, Cleveland Ohio
Nutrition Intervention Team Home Nutrition Support

Name _____

Address _____

Telephone _____

Date order called in to NECCI _____ Delivery date _____

Days/Week of infusion _____

1. **Formula**

   Brand: _____

   Daily Amount: (In mls or cans) _____

2. **Ancillary Supplies**

Item	Usage (indicate day/week/month)
Entriflex, 8 Fr., 36" feeding tube with stylet	One/week
Coverlets nose bandaid	Three/week
60 ml syringes, luer lock	Two/week
1200 ml Kangaroo, Easy Cap Administration Bag w/tubing	One/infusion
1" Micropore Tape	One/month
Kangaroo Enteral Pump 220	One—first order only
IV Pole, light weight	One—first order only

3. **Options**

Stethoscope	One—first order only
Dobbhoff 8 Fr., 43" enteric feeding tube w/stylet	would be in place of Entriflex, if specified

Note: The number of feeding tubes/coverlets as defined above is for patient not scheduled for routine reinsertion of feeding tube. If reinsertion on a regular basis is ordered, the weekly amounts of these two items will be defined.

TABLE 16–5. AN EXAMPLE OF A STANDARD GASTROSTOMY/JEJUNOSTOMY TUBE FEEDING SUPPLY LIST

Saint Vincent Charity Hospital & Health Center, Cleveland Ohio
Nutrition Intervention Team Home Nutrition Support

Name _____

Address _____

Telephone _____

Date order called in to NECCI _____ Delivery date _____

Days/Week of infusion _____

1. **Formula**

   Brand: _____

   Daily Amount: (In mls or cans) _____

2. **Ancillary Supplies**

Item	Usage (indicate day/week/month)
Foley Catheter Plug	Two/week
60 ml syringes, catheter tip	Two/week
1200 ml Kangaroo, Easy Cap Administration Bag w/tubing	One/infusion
Gauze 4×4 sponges (split)	Two/day
1" Micropore Tape	One/week
Kangaroo Enteral Pump 220	One—first order only
IV Pole, light weight	One—first order only

plans on taking enteral feedings away from home on a routine basis, bolus or intermittent feedings may be preferred because equipment need not be transported.

Based on the multidisciplinary team's needs, a standard supply list should be developed for routine formula and equipment needs. This list can then be individualized according to a patient's specific needs. Table 16–4 is an example of a standard nasoenteral feeding supply list; Table 16–5 is an example of a standard gastrostomy/jejunostomy supply list.

SEEKING THIRD PARTY REIMBURSEMENT AND A HOME CARE AGENCY

Prior to instructing the patient, the area of reimbursement or the use of a home care company should be explored. Although the cost of home enteral nutrition is relatively inexpensive when compared to home parenteral nutrition, the use of specialty or elemental formulas can increase the daily cost. The importance of exploring reimbursement prior to patient instruction is that: (1) if a patient is concerned about the financial aspects, he or she may not be "ready" to learn the operation, and (2) necessary changes in the use or elimination of equipment, formulas, or supplies can be made without confusing the patient once instructions have begun. Conferring with a social worker or discharge coordinator may be of great assistance in unraveling the reimbursement issues.

The use of home enteral nutrition support is not generally reimbursed by third party providers despite the obvious fact that it is cost effective over long periods of time. Table

16–6 highlights the major third party groups and their general stands on such reimbursement.

If a patient is to be discharged on more than one therapy, a social worker can often help arrange the delivery of medical supplies. If possible, home supplies should come from only one or two sources so as not to confuse or overwhelm the patient and family. The home supply agency, once given the patient's insurance information, can pursue reimbursement from third party providers. After the decision to use a home supply agency has been made, criteria should be followed to choose the agency that can best provide service. Table 16–7 gives sample criteria for selecting the appropriate home supply agency.

To facilitate communication among the nutrition support team, home care agency,

TABLE 16–6. THIRD PARTY PROVIDERS AND THE MAJOR STAND OF EACH ON HOME ENTERAL NUTRITION

Third Party Provider	Definition of Home Enteral Nutrition Services	Coverage Based Upon
Medicare (National)	Enteral nutrition defined as "reasonable and necessary for a patient with a functional gastrointestinal tract who, due to pathology to or nonfunction of structures that normally permit food to reach the digestive tract, cannot maintain weight and strength commensurate with his or her general condition. Enteral therapy may be given by nasogastric, jejunostomy or gastrostomy tubes, and can be provided safely and effectively in the home by non-professional persons who have undergone special training."[6]	1. Patient's attending physician must document medical necessity in view of patient's condition. This must be in form of written order or prescription as well as medical documentation. 2. Recertification of patient's need for home nutrition support every 90 days.
Medicaid (Varies state to state)	Since it varies from state to state, there are no set criteria or standards developed for home enteral nutrition. State Medicaid plans for those defined as poor and in specific categories of need (categorically needy) must specify services for home health, whereas those defined as near-poor (medically needy) have much more flexibility in the plans the state devises. Thus within a certain state the categorically needy may be covered for home enteral nutrition whereas the medically needy may not be covered.[6]	1. Prior authorization is generally necessary for all supplies and products. 2. Medical necessity criteria usually required.
Blue Cross/Blue Shield	From the 1981 Uniform Medical Policy Manual, "Enteral nutrition is appropriate when there is an anatomical inability to swallow or when adequate alimentation cannot be obtained by the normal route."[6]	1. Prior approval of each individual case.
Commercial Carriers	Many carriers do not have specified definitions of home enteral nutrition. The extent of coverage depends on the individual policy.	1. Statement of medical necessity. 2. Circumstances of each individual case.

TABLE 16-7. EXAMPLES OF CRITERIA TO CONSIDER IN SELECTING A HOME SUPPLY AGENCY

1. Standards of Care: What is the philosophy of the agency? Review the policies and procedures of the agency. How does the agency determine quality control and quality assurance?

2. Expertise of Personnel: What are the qualifications of the personnel? Does the staff have experience with all forms of enteral nutrition that the institution or nutrition support service uses? What is the role of personnel in patient care? What continuing education is required by the agency for its personnel?

3. Equipment and Supplies: Does the agency have access to all equipment used by the nutrition support service? How will the use of substitutions be determined? How does the agency assist the patient with inventory control? Do they routinely check equipment function in the home and replace malfunctioning equipment?

4. Communication: What type and frequency of follow-up will be made to the nutrition support service regarding patient care? How easily can a patient contact the agency personnel? How will the agency be notified of changes in therapies or methods ordered by the nutrition support service? How quickly can the agency implement these changes?

5. Reimbursement: How quickly will the agency notify nutrition support service or patient that insurance coverage has been approved? How are patients with either partial or no coverage handled?

6. Instructions: Is the nutrition support service or agency personnel going to instruct patient and/or family? Can the patient receive further instruction once he/she is at home? Will the agency use the methods and instructions the nutrition support service has used so as to ease communication?

7. Home Care: What type and extent of services does the agency provide the patient after discharge? Will supplies and equipment be delivered to the patient's home if necessary? Is communication maintained with the patient or significant other in the home? Can the agency provide skilled care for in-home patient monitoring?

and patient, a checklist can be designed to enable quick assessment of how the home enteral nutrition program is progressing. This form can be adapted to record how much time is spent preparing a patient for discharge. An example is found in Table 16–8.

INSTRUCTING THE PATIENT AND SIGNIFICANT OTHERS

Although circumstances vary, instruction in home enteral nutrition can usually be completed in three sessions. During these sessions verbal and written instructions should be used. Demonstrations of the system should be given with confirming demonstrations made by all parties who will at one time or another be involved with the home enteral program. Repetition of the instructions should occur until both the nutrition support team and patient/significant other feel comfortable that the program can be handled safely at home.

The first step in the instruction is to teach the location and purpose of the feeding tube. Using models, diagrams, and samples of feeding tubes gives the patient an opportunity to make a mental picture of where the feeding tube goes and why it is needed. Next, the method of feeding (e.g., bolus, intermittent, continuous, cyclic) should be explained. If the patient's condition permits, allow flexibility as to the hours of feeding or method based on lifestyle, work schedules, times that someone is available to assist, and so on. This gives the patient a sense of control in the situation. Also, adapting the times of delivery to meet the patient's lifestyle will assure greater compliance once the patient is back in his or her environment.

After these initial steps have been covered, the actual demonstration and return demonstrations should follow. A thorough instruction should cover the topics listed in Table 16–9.

The demonstrations will indicate any problems in comprehension or learning as well as manual dexterity before the patient

TABLE 16–8. AN EXAMPLE OF A HOME TUBE FEEDING CHECKLIST

Name _____

Date of Home Tube Feeding Initiation _____

Prior to Instructions	Date	Time	Initials
1. Insurance information gathered			
2. Insurance information called to home supply agency			
3. Discharge Planning notified of home tube feeding			
4. Patient/family contacted to explain need for home tube feeding			
5. Insurance approval obtained			
Instructions	**Date**	**Time**	**Initials**
1. Minimum of 3 dates/times identified for instructions			

2. Education sessions
  a. System demonstration
  b. Patient/family demonstration with supervision
  c. Patient/family demonstration with minimal supervision			

3. Supplies called in to home supply agency			
4. Delivery date/time tentatively defined with family/patient			
5. Written instructions provided			
Upon Discharge	**Date**	**Time**	**Initials**
1. Home supply agency notified of discharge			
2. Home tube feeding chart compiled for patient			
3. Follow-up appointment made with NSS			
4. 24 hrs after discharge, patient/family contacted to assess situation			

is discharged. It is important to use the same type of equipment the patient will receive at home so that potential problems will surface and necessary adjustments can be made.[7]

Written material is essential as an additional resource in the instruction. This material should highlight the important components of the tube feeding program, such as the feeding schedule, as well as provide phone numbers of team members or the home care agency for follow-up. Booklets, instruction sheets, diagrams, and so on can be used to provide this information. The key factor is individualizing the material to meet the concerns and issues of each patient. If a general booklet is used to describe home en-

Clean technique
Position during feedings
Checking for residuals
Formula preparation and storage
Care of the feeding tube
Use and care of the equipment (including infusion device)
Potential complications and actions to take
Administration of medications through feeding tube

teral nutrition, the location of the feeding tube and purpose, the feeding schedule, and formula, a patient may still need step-by-step instructions. Table 16–10 gives an example of supplemental directions for a home tube feeding.

DOCUMENTATION AND MONITORING

As length of hospital stay continues to decrease, there will be more and more instances when a patient discharged on a home enteral nutrition program will require the feeding schedule to be adjusted at home. In order for a home enteral nutrition program to be successful, very close follow-up and documentation of the patient's progress must be done.

Physical signs of patient intolerance include aspiration, poor gastric emptying, nausea, vomiting, and diarrhea. It is important that the patient or home assistant understands the potential intolerance and why certain items need to be monitored during the feeding process. While instructing the patient, reinforcement should be continuously given as to why certain procedures are done.

Preparing patient for feeding:

1. Check tube location to prevent aspiration.
2. Gastric residuals are checked routinely to monitor for gastric emptying.

3. Head of bed is elevated to prevent aspiration.

Setting up pump and formula:

1. If a pump is used, close monitoring of rate of delivery is necessary to avoid aspiration, abdominal distention, etc.
2. If no pump is used, a limited amount of formula is hung at one time to avoid runaway infusions.
3. Rate or length of feeding should be decreased if nausea, abdominal distention, or cramping occurs. If vomiting occurs, feeding should be stopped.

It may be necessary to devise a daily checklist so that monitoring is documented and potential problems can be spotted easily during follow-up. Table 16–11 gives an example of a checklist that can be used.

FOLLOW-UP AND TRANSITIONAL FEEDING

To assure compliance, follow-up is necessary. It may be necessary to involve a home care agency so that frequent home visits are made for monitoring and for education. If a home supply agency is used, it will be necessary to explore how much home follow-up is provided, if any. Also, the nutrition support team or at least the instructor should ensure adequate access to the patient for follow-up. Patients should be encouraged to call as problems or questions arise. All parties involved should have copies of all written materials received by the patient.

The frequency of outpatient visits will need to be determined on an individual basis in consultation with the attending physician. The frequency of outpatient visits may be reduced for those patients without transportation, who live far from the hospital or institution, and who are terminally ill. In all these cases, it may be necessary to use an outside agency.

If the patient will be able to consume foods

TABLE 16–10. DIRECTIONS FOR HOME TUBE FEEDING—AN EXAMPLE

Steps to set up continuous tube feeding using a Kangaroo Enteral Pump

A. Gather all supplies:
   Formula
1 feeding bag with tubing	1 cup with lukewarm water
1 60 ml syringe	1 empty cup
1 roll paper tape	Kangaroo Pump and IV Pole

B. Preparing for the feeding:
   1. Check tube for any changes from previous day.
   2. Connect syringe to feeding tube and pull back to see amount of stomach *residual.* Pull out stomach residual until you are unable to pull anymore (this is usually when you meet resistance in the syringe). Then if gastric residual is:
      a. Less than one syringe (60 ml), proceed to step 3.
      b. Less than two syringes (120 ml), proceed to step 3.
      c. Greater than two (2) syringes (over 120 ml), feed *only* two syringes of residual back into the feeding tube. Flush the tube with 30 ml of water and hold the feeding for one hour. At the end of the hour, recheck residual. If less than two syringes (120 ml), proceed to step 3. If greater than 2 syringes (over 120 ml), call member of the Nutrition Intervention Team.
   3. Take syringe and draw up 30 ml of water. Gently flush through tube to make sure feeding tube is clean and open.
   4. Make sure head of bed is elevated to 30–45° during the time of feeding.

C. Setting up pump and formula:
   1. To fill feeding bag:
      a. Roll clamp down to closed position.
      b. Pour 5 cans of formula into the bag.
      c. Snap the bag closed and lock.
   2. Fill tubing:
      a. Take off cap and put the end of tubing into empty cup.
      b. Roll clamp to open position.
      c. Allow tubing to fill and drip into cup. Only 5 or 6 drops are necessary.
      d. Roll clamp down to closed position and recap tubing.
   3. Threading the pump:
      a. Place drip chamber in black sensor and let it sit on ledge.
      b. Stretch silastic tubing around the rotor and place disc on second ledge.
      c. Check that pump is set at the correct rate.

D. Connecting bag with tubing to feeding tube:
   1. Take end of tubing from bag, remove cap, and connect to feeding tube.
   2. Tape the connection.
   3. Press green start button on pump.
   4. Roll clamp to open position.
   5. Add additional can(s) of formula as bag starts to empty.

E. To disconnect from feeding:
   1. Turn pump off at end of 24-hour period.
   2. Roll clamp down to closed position.
   3. Disconnect tubing from feeding tube.
   4. Flush approximately 30 ml of water through feeding tube to make sure tube is clean and open. Cap tube.
   5. Unthread tubing from pump and throw away old bag.

Follow-up Care:
Should you have any questions or difficulty with the tube feeding, call any member of the Nutrition Intervention Team. We will be making arrangements with you for follow-up, either by phone or appointment.

TABLE 16–11. AN EXAMPLE OF A CHECKLIST FOR HOME TUBE FEEDING MONITORING

		5/1	5/2	5/3
A.	Preparation for Feeding			
	1. Location of tube	√	√	
	2. Gastric residuals	<100	<50	
	3. HOB elevated	√	√	
	4. Feeding tube flushed	√	√	
B.	Setting Up Formula/Pump			
	1. Pump at correct rate	√	√	
	2. Correct amt. formula hung	√	√	
C.	Miscellaneous (note time)			
	1. Nausea	N	N	
	2. Vomiting	N	N	
	3. Diarrhea	N	Y × 1	
	4. Constipation	N	N	
	5. Other			
D.	Thirst	N	Y	
E.	Weight	100.0	99.8	
F.	Urine S/As	N/N	N/N	

TABLE 16–12. FOOD INTAKE RECORD

Name _____

Dietitian _____

Your food intake record is an important monitor in your home nutrition care. It helps to determine what nutrients you are getting through the foods you eat or may show certain patterns or habits that affect your body's nutrition. Try to be as accurate as possible in describing both solids and liquids you consume.

Directions: 1. Record the time of day or night you consume the food or beverage.
2. Describe the food item and/or how it was prepared.
3. Record the amount consumed to the nearest household measure (i.e., ½ cup, 1 cup, etc.).
4. If physical signs or symptoms are to be recorded, the time and description of signs/symptoms should be given (ex: 3 a.m.—abdominal cramping)

Sample Food Intake Record:

Time	Food Item	Amount	Physical Sign/ Symptom
7:00 a.m.	Orange juice, unsw.	½ cup	
	Rye toast	½ slice	
	Margarine	1 teaspoon	
10:00 a.m.	Eggnog with Polycose	¾ cup–2 T	
10:30 a.m.			Abdominal cramping
noon	Chicken noodle soup	1 cup	
	Saltine crackers	3	

at some time, it will be important to closely monitor the amount of food consumed daily. As the amount of food increases and stabilizes, the tube feeding rate can be adjusted to avoid overfeeding. A sample food intake record is found in Table 16–12.

In transitional feeding, it is important not to discontinue one form of nutrition therapy before nutritional requirements can completely be met by the other form. In this instance, it is important that a stable oral intake of food is occurring daily before the tube feeding is decreased and eventually discontinued. Some sources state that when two-thirds of a patient's requirements can be met by one form of nutritional therapy, then the former method can be discontinued.[8]

Transitional feeding in the home is challenging because food intake, although recorded daily by the patient, is usually analyzed on a weekly or bimonthly schedule by the dietitian. If food intake is stable on a weekly basis, there are three options for the home patient:

1. Decrease rate of feeding.
2. Decrease time of feeding (e.g., if on a 24-hour feeding, decrease to a 16-hour nighttime cycle)
3. Decrease the number of days on the feeding (e.g., if patient receives tube feeding seven days a week, give the patient an entire day off the feeding so patient takes feeding only six days per week)

If possible, allow the patient some say in the selection of the transitional feeding schedule.

The use of home enteral nutrition is expected to increase in the future. Developing a systematic approach to the identification of home enteral patients, selection of formulas and equipment, reimbursement, instructions, documentation, and follow-up will enable one to provide thorough and successful treatment.

ACKNOWLEDGMENT

The authors wish to thank Kathy Crocker, R.N., M.S.N., for assistance in the development of home enteral nutrition forms and instruction material.

REFERENCES

1. Chrsomilides SA, Kaminski MV: Home enteral and parenteral nutritional support: A comparison. Am J Clin Nutr 34:2271, 1981
2. Greene HL, Helinek GL, Folk CC, et al.: Nasogastric tube feeding at home: A method for adjunctive nutritional support of malnourished patients. Am J Clin Nutr 34:1131, 1981
3. Newmark SR, Simpson S, Beskitt P, et al.: Home tube feeding for long-term nutritional support. JPEN 5:76, 1981
4. Folk CC, Courtney ME: Home tube feedings: General guidelines and specific patient instructions. Nutr Supp Serv 2:18, 1982
5. Adams MM, Wirsching RG: Guidelines for planning home enteral feedings. J Am Diet Assoc 84:68, 1984
6. Parver A: Reimbursement for Parenteral and Enteral Nutrition. Washington, DC: American Society for Parenteral and Enteral Nutrition, 1985
7. Bayer LM, School DE, Ford EG: Tube feeding at home. Am J Nurs 83:1321, 1983
8. Skipper A: Transitional feeding and the dietitian. Nutr Supp Serv 2:45, 1982

Part V. IMPLEMENTING THE PARENTERAL NUTRITION CARE PLAN

17. Principles of Parenteral Nutrition: Indications, Administration, and Monitoring

Lorraine See Young

Parenteral nutrition (PN) is the administration of varying concentrations of carbohydrate, protein, fat, vitamins, and minerals into the circulation of individuals who are unable to assimilate nutrients via the gastrointestinal tract because of some degree of gut dysfunction. The use of PN in patients to provide nutrition support is a relatively new technique. Intravenous (IV) feedings were first used in the mid-19th century, when the French physiologist Claude Bernard infused sugar solutions into animals. The use of IV glucose and physiologic saline did not gain wide acceptance in the medical community until the early 1930s, however, because of the high incidence of sepsis and complications with their use before this time. The concentrations of glucose were limited to 5 and 10 percent as stronger glucose solutions were found to sclerose and thrombose peripheral veins. In 1936, Dr. Robert Elman was the first to successfully infuse a protein hydrolysate and glucose solution peripherally into humans and demonstrate positive nitrogen (N) balance and decreased morbidity.[1]

The technique of subclavian vein catheterization was perfected in 1952 by Aubaniac, a French surgeon. His work with war casualties in Vietnam necessitated quick, easy access to the central venous system for the rapid administration of fluid and blood products. In the 1960s, Dudrick et al., at the University of Pennsylvania, utilized PN solutions infused via central catheters to feed beagle puppies and demonstrated that total parenteral nutrition (TPN) alone could sustain growth and development.[2] Shortly thereafter, the first human infant successfully received TPN as her sole source of nutrition and also demonstrated normal growth and development.[3] These classic investigations marked the beginning of an era in PN therapy that continues to advance toward the optimal nutrition care of patients who require intravenous nutrition support.

The use of the terms "TPN," "hyperalimentation," and "PN" is frequently confused in clinical practice, as each term confers a different meaning. TPN can mean many things, with definitions differing from institution to institution, and hyperalimentation can refer to parenteral or enteral feedings. Therefore, the term PN will be employed in this chapter to encompass all aspects of IV feedings. Central and peripheral vein PN will be designated as such.

INDICATIONS FOR PN

The purpose of PN is to supply the essential nutrients (carbohydrates, proteins, fats, vitamins, minerals, and fluids) necessary to maintain body functions and N balance in those patients who cannot receive adequate nutrition enterally. Medical conditions that interfere with the intake of an adequate enteral diet are many, and candidates for PN may include patients who will not eat (i.e., anorexia nervosa); those who cannot eat (i.e., gastrointestinal [GI] tract obstruction); those who should not eat (i.e., upper GI tract fistulas); or those who cannot eat enough (i.e., the anorexia caused by cancer chemotherapeutic agents). All attempts should be made, however, to nourish patients enterally if possible, as enteral feedings are more physiologic and cost-effective.

The specific indications for PN can be broken into two categories: (1) those in which PN is considered primary therapy and in which its positive effect on patient outcome is established, and (2) those in which PN provides nutrition support as an adjunct to the total care plan of the patient, but in which effect on patient outcome is variable.

PN as Primary Therapy

PN is considered primary therapy in adult patients who would otherwise develop malnutrition secondary to severe nonmalignant intestinal disease. Clinical examples of the need for such therapy include short bowel syndrome, upper gastrointestinal tract fistulas, or enterocutaneous fistulas secondary to operation or injury and pancreatic pseudocyst.[4] In these instances, PN provides metabolic support and maintenance, or re-

pletion of lean body mass, in addition to allowing the intestinal tract time for repair and adaptation.

PN as Adjunctive Therapy

In specific diseases, it is clear that PN does not affect disease outcome, but it may be necessary for patients undergoing aggressive medical–surgical treatment to provide maintenance nutrition support or to correct existing malnutrition. Table 17–1 lists some of the categories of patients in which it is appropriate to consider PN as adjuvant therapy. A few of these are discussed in greater detail below.

Acute Renal Failure. The use of PN in the acute renal failure (ARF) patient is a much debated topic. Whether PN influences the overall morbidity and mortality of this patient population or whether it hastens recovery of renal function and regeneration of renal tissue still remains to be answered. In 1973 Abel et al.[5] performed the first randomized, double-blind clinical trial comparing hypertonic dextrose with dextrose plus essential amino acids (EAA) in a highly selective group of ARF patients. The patients receiving the EAA plus glucose mix had a higher incidence of recovery of renal func-

TABLE 17–1. PN AS ADJUNCT TO MEDICAL CARE

Acute renal failure

Inflammatory bowel disease

Radiation enteritis

Acute gastrointestinal tract effects of chemotherapeutic agents

Anorexia nervosa

Acute pancreatitis

PN pre- and postmajor surgery

Respiratory failure

Prolonged ileus; intestinal obstruction

Hepatic failure

tion, but mortality was not significantly improved. Patients with serious complications or more severe renal failure fared better with the EAA mix than with glucose alone.[5] Despite these findings, more recent clinical trials have failed to observe similar feeding effects.[6,7] Thus, the influence of PN on morbidity and mortality rates, and on recovery of renal function and regeneration of renal tissue, remains unclear. PN should be considered when dialysis is necessary for the resolution of the metabolic abnormalities and septic complications frequently present in ARF and when the patient does not have a functional GI tract.

Perioperative PN. Studley[8] reported in 1936 that patients with peptic ulcer disease who exhibited a loss of 20 percent of their usual body weight prior to surgery experienced a 33 percent mortality, while those with no weight loss had only a 3.5 percent operative mortality. Since that time, the relationship between a patient's nutrition status and surgical outcome has received a great deal of attention.

Abel et al.[9] conducted a prospective randomized evaluation of early postoperative PN in 44 malnourished patients. Twenty-four patients were used as controls; 20 received immediate postoperative PN at rates approximating 2200 kcals and 7.65 grams nitrogen daily. Five days of postoperative nutrition therapy had no notable effect on overall morbidity and mortality experienced by the malnourished patients when compared to controls receiving 5 percent dextrose in water. Five days of PN postoperatively had no effect on parameters such as sepsis, renal failure, pneumonia, time patient required ventilatory assistance, or total hospital stay.[9] This trial is criticized, however, because of the short time, 5 days, the patients were fed postoperatively.

Heatley et al.[10] studied 74 patients with stomach and esophageal cancer and randomly allocated them to receive either 7 to 10 days of preoperative PN or a soft or liquid diet during this time. PN had a significant effect on postoperative wound infections when compared to control patients, but only in those patients deemed most malnourished by low serum albumin levels (<3.5 g/liter). This clinical benefit was not associated with measurable improvement in immune parameters, weight change, or total length of time the patients were in the hospital.[10]

A more recent clinical trial examined the influence of 10 days of preoperative PN in GI cancer patients. Fifty-nine patients served as controls receiving the regular hospital diet, and 66 received PN. The rates of major complications—including intraabdominal abscesses, peritonitis, and anastomotic leakage—and mortality were significantly lower in the PN group. This clinical benefit was further supported by improvement in protein status and humoral and cellular immunocompetence in the PN group. This study suggests that in this select group of patients, preoperative PN for at least 10 days may positively affect the surgical outcome of patients.[11]

Preoperative nutrition support, if administered for 10 days or more, may have a beneficial effect on outcome in select patient populations. Short-term preoperative PN (3 to 5 days) will serve to restore liver glycogen stores, which may buffer the effects of anesthesia, operation, and infection.[12]

The major objective of postoperative feeding is to curtail loss of lean body mass and to help maintain metabolic homeostasis. This becomes very important in hypermetabolic or depleted patients. Thus, implementing postoperative nutrition support in these groups of patients should begin as soon as the patient is hemodynamically stable.

Inflammatory Bowel Disease. The use of PN in inflammatory bowel disease (IBD) is also an area where outcome is not specifically improved in all patients. PN provides nutrition support during an acute exacerbation of IBD, reverses weight loss, and prevents malnutrition. Its effect on clinical outcome, however, is not proven. In a nonrandomized prospective study undertaken in 30 patients with

IBD refractory to medical therapy (20 with Crohn's disease and 10 with ulcerative colitis), weight gain was accomplished in all but 1 patient; however, clinical improvement was variable and unpredictable after an average of 21 days of PN.[13]

A more recent retrospective review of 33 patients who underwent surgery for IBD was completed by Rombeau et al.[14] These patients were divided into two groups: those who received no PN during the 5-day preoperative period, and those who received at least 5 days of preoperative PN, at levels averaging 43.8 kcal/kg and 0.2 g N/kg body weight. The group of patients who received preoperative PN had fewer postoperative complications than the group that did not receive PN. Therefore, these authors recommended at least 5 days of preoperative PN in patients with IBD who have severe protein depletion based on serum albumin and transferrin levels. It is clear that PN will prevent or ameliorate weight loss and malnutrition in this group of patients; however, PN significantly affects the outcome of only those surgical candidates who are protein malnourished.

Multisystem Organ Failure. In a retrospective review of surgical intensive care patients with multisystem organ failure, PN was shown to act as an adjuvant to medical–surgical therapy only. In spite of safe and adequate nutrition support, outcome was determined by the underlying disease processes.[15] In this group of critically ill patients, however, the nutritional goal should be the safe provision of nutrients rather than attempting repletion and weight gain, as the number and degree of complications tend to increase with more vigorous feeding.[16,17]

Cancer. The use of PN in cancer patients has not been proven unequivocally efficacious. It is used as adjunctive therapy in cancer patients receiving therapeutic chemo- or radiation therapy or undergoing surgical cytoreduction so that they can withstand therapy and possibly experience a greater sense of well-being. Questions remain regarding the stimulation of tumor growth at the expense of the host when concomitant antitumor therapy is withheld. The evidence in animal studies to date suggests that amino acids (AA) alone or with glucose promote tumor proliferation, whereas provision of nonprotein calories as fat promotes host maintenance without tumor stimulation.[18,19] In tumor-bearing rats not receiving antineoplastic therapy, increasing ratios of tumor weight to total body weight correlated positively with increasing levels of calorie intake.[20] Therefore, it is not recommended that PN be used in terminal cancer patients who are not receiving simultaneous antitumor therapy.

Liver Failure. Another area of PN use that requires further critical evaluation is the administration of branch chain amino acid (BCAA)-enriched, low aromatic AA solutions to patients with hepatic encephalopathy.[21] The results of a few clinical trials support the use of BCAA-enriched AA solutions to promote nitrogen equilibrium and favorably modulate the metabolic stress response in noncirrhotic surgical patients.[22,23] In patients with hepatic insufficiency, these solutions were shown to cause no worsening of or improvement in hepatic encephalopathy; in addition, they enhanced N equilibrium.[21]

Recently, however, infusion of a BCAA-enriched, low aromatic AA solution in three patients with cirrhosis and subclinical encephalopathy revealed AA imbalances, specifically hypotyrosinemia and hypocystinemia, without improvement in encephalopathy.[24] Moreover, studies using the enteral product Hepatic Aid in cirrhotic, encepahlopathic patients show that there is no amelioration of encephalopathy using this solution.[25] These specialized solutions should not be used in patients with any degree of hepatic dysfunction, or in standard postoperative or traumatized patients without a complete understanding of how these formulas and solutions will affect whole body AA metabolism and economy.

Criteria for Patient Selection

This review of the indications for use of PN would not be complete without a brief discussion of situations in which PN would be contraindicated. Topping the list of contraindications, and most obvious, would be a functional GI tract in patients who can tolerate adequate amounts of oral supplements and/or enteral tube feedings. Patients with either irreparable central nervous system damage or terminal disease and from whom other aggressive treatment modalities are withdrawn also should not begin PN.

Once a patient is deemed a candidate for PN, it is the responsibility of the dietitian/nutritionist to make an accurate assessment of the patient's nutrition requirements and to monitor the patient's nutrition status while on PN (see Part II, Identifying the Patient at Nutrition Risk and Part III, Determining the Nutrition Care Plan).

CHOOSING THE PN MIXTURE

There are two major types of PN solutions available for administration. Hypertonic mixtures are administered by a central venous catheter, while isotonic or slightly hypertonic mixtures are administered by peripheral vein. The decision to provide central versus peripheral PN is related to the following factors:

1. The duration of therapy planned
2. The energy requirements of the patient
3. The overall goal of therapy (minimize weight loss, achieve weight maintenance, and/or weight gain)
4. The available routes of administration

Table 17–2 lists various factors to consider in choosing peripheral versus central PN. For example, peripheral PN is indicated when a patient without weight loss has had surgery and is unable to tolerate an oral or tube feeding intake 5 or more days postoperatively; or when a patient without weight loss is to receive an extensive GI work-up

TABLE 17–2. INDICATIONS FOR USING PERIPHERAL VERSUS CENTRAL VEIN FEEDINGS

Peripheral Vein Feedings
1. Enteral intake interrupted, but enteral feeding expected to resume within 5–7 days
2. Supplementation to enteral feedings or as transitional phase until enteral feedings meet needs
3. Mild to moderate malnutrition, necessitating intervention in order to prevent further depletion
4. Normal or mildly elevated metabolic rate
5. No organ failure

Central Vein Feedings
1. Unable to tolerate enteral intake for greater than 7 days
2. Moderately to severely elevated metabolic rate
3. Moderate to severe malnutrition, not correctable with enteral feedings
4. Cardiac, renal, hepatic failure, or other conditions necessitating fluid restriction
5. Limited access to peripheral veins
6. Able to access central vein

preventing adequate oral intake prior to surgery. Peripheral PN is sometimes necessary when central veins are inaccessible or thrombosed, or when the central venous catheter is questioned as a source of bacterial contamination. Peripheral vein feedings are generally hypocaloric, but can usually meet protein, vitamin, mineral, and fluid requirements. At best, maintenance calories can be provided with fat emulsion serving as the major calorie source. Peripheral PN minimizes weight loss or sustains weight maintenance in stable patients, but is usually not recommended for prolonged periods of time.

Any patient who is hypermetabolic, has sustained a greater than 10 percent weight loss, and has a nonfunctioning GI tract is generally a candidate for central vein feedings. For example, a patient with short bowel syndrome may sustain a substantial weight loss prior to surgery because of underlying bowel disease, thus requiring central vein PN for a prolonged period. Central vein PN is hyperosmolar and therefore destructive to peripheral veins. Infusion into a high flow

TABLE 17–3. CHARACTERISTICS OF PN REGIMES

	Central Feedings	Peripheral Feedings
Osmolality	≥1800	650–900
Route of administration	Central venous catheter	Nonocclusive catheter in large peripheral vein
Usual daily caloric intake	2000–3000	700–1800
Parenteral lipid emulsion	Minor caloric source; provides essential fatty acids	Major caloric source
Overall objectives	Weight maintenance; weight gain	Minimize weight loss; weight maintenance
Duration of therapy	≥7 days	5–7 days

central blood vessel rapidly dilutes the solution. However, it provides enough calories, primarily as glucose, for weight maintenance or gain. Central vein PN is used when access to peripheral IV sites is limited or difficult to maintain and when PN needs to be continued for more than 1 week (Table 17–3).

SOLUTION ORDERING AND PREPARATION

When the decision is made regarding solution prescription for each individual patient, the next steps are to initiate ordering and organize administration of the solutions. A sample order form is shown in Figure 17–1.

The PN orders then reach the intravenous pharmacy where they are mixed under sterile conditions. Laminar flow hoods are generally used with a 0.22 micron membrane filter. These hoods will filter any particles greater than 0.3 microns in size with a 99.99 percent efficiency. On a daily basis, an aliquot of parenteral solution is placed in a microbiologic medium (thiroglycolate or soy broth) and sent for bacteriologic testing. PN solutions must be refrigerated at 4°C until the time of administration.

The PN solution is carefully inspected in the pharmacy for precipitates and discolora-

tion. It is then labeled with the exact contents of the solution, the expiration date and time, the patient's name, unit number, and date, and, where necessary, a statement in bold letters "for central venous catheter use only." Nothing should be added to PN solutions once they leave the pharmacy, and tamper-proof closures should cover the additive port. Certain medications are compatible with PN solutions. Any additive or medication that is not a standard component of PN should be checked for compatibility with the solution and cleared with those persons responsible for PN in each institution before administering it via the PN solution. (See Chapter 18, Formulation of Parenteral Solutions, for an indepth discussion of the design, mixing procedures, storage, and additive compatibility of PN solutions.)

ADMINISTRATION OF PN

Intravenous Central Catheter Placement

For use of hypertonic solutions, a central vein catheter must be inserted by a qualified physician. Figure 17–2 illustrates the most common access sites used to cannulate the superior vena cava. Subclavian catheter insertion via an infraclavicular venipuncture is the preferred method of cannulation, pri-

ADULT PARENTERAL NUTRITIONAL ORDERS

CHECK DESIRED SOLUTION:

☐ 1. **Standard Central Vein (CV) Solution**

Each liter bag contains:

Crystalline Amino Acids	(4.25%) 42.5 g		
Dextrose	(25%) 250 g		
Sodium	35 mEq	Nitrogen	= 7.15 g
Potassium	30 mEq	Cal/N	= 119
Magnesium	5 mEq	Total Cals	= 1029
Calcium	4.7 mEq	mOsm	= 1970
Phosphate	15 mM		
Acetate	67.5 mEq		
Chloride	35 mEq		

Vitamins (Daily):

Thiamine	3 mg	Ascorbic Acid	100	mg
Riboflavin	3.6 mg	Folate	400	mcg
B6	4 mg	B12	5	mcg
Niacin	40 mg	Vitamin A	3300	IU
Dexpanthenol	15 mg	Vitamin D	200	IU
Biotin	60 mcg	Vitamin E	10	IU

Vitamins (Weekly):

Vitamin K   10 mg (Contraindicated in patients receiving Warfarin)

☐ 2. **Modified Central Vein (CV) Solution**

Same as above <u>EXCEPT</u>

		Range
Total Na⁺ _____	mEq/L	(20-150)
Total K⁺ _____	mEq/L	(0-80)
Total Mg⁺⁺ _____	mEq/L	(0-15)
Total PO₄ _____	mM/L	(0-20)

☐ Add salts as chloride

☐ Add salts as acetate.

LABORATORY – WEEKLY ORDERS

1. SMAC-20 Mg and TRIG every Monday
2. Cl, CO₂, K, Na, Ca₂, PO₄, glu, BUN, alb, cre, Alk Phos, LDH, GOT, Bili T, Bili D every Thursday

NURSING

1. Daily weights with same scale.
2. Urine for Sugar and Acetone every six hours.
3. Central TPN catheter is inviolate.
4. If TPN is not available, substitute D-10-W at the same rate.

CALL/DELIVER TO IV PHARMACY BY 11 A.M. DAILY

☐ 3. **Standard Peripheral Vein (PV) Solution**

Each liter bag contains:

Crystalline Amino Acids	(2.75%) 4.63 g		
Dextrose	(5%) 50 g		
Sodium	30 mEq	Nitrogen	= 4.63 g
Potassium	30 mEq	Cal/N	= 37
Magnesium	5 mEq	Total Cals	= 286
Calcium	4.7 mEq	mOsm	= 655
Phosphate	5 mM		
Acetate	48 mEq		
Chloride	34 mEq		

Vitamins: Same as CV #1.

☐ 4. **Modified Peripheral Vein (PV) Solution:**

Same as above <u>EXCEPT</u>

		Range
Total Na⁺ _____	mEq/L	(20-150)
Total K⁺ _____	mEq/L	(0-80)
Total Mg⁺⁺ _____	mEq/L	(0-15)
Total PO₄ _____	mM/L	(0-20)

☐ Add salts as chloride

☐ Add salts as acetate.

COMPLETE IF REQUIRED: (Check)

_____ 10% FAT EMULSION (500 ml/u) ____1 Unit; ____2 Units

_____ 20% FAT EMULSION (500 ml/u) 1 Unit only.
FREQUENCY _____

_____ TRACE ELEMENTS DAILY.

_____ μ REGULAR INSULIN PER LITER.

SPECIAL INSTRUCTIONS TO PHARMACY:

_____ Liters per 24 hours _____ Date

_____ M.D.
Physician's Signature

Figure 17–1. Sample physician's order form for parenteral nutrition.

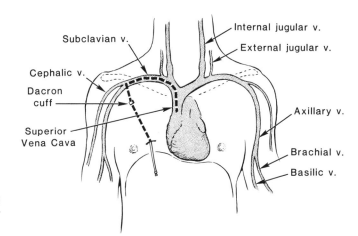

Figure 17–2. Venous access sites from which the superior vena cava may be cannulated.

marily because it provides a flat, relatively immobile area on the chest to maintain a clean dressing. According to Silberman and Eisenberg,[31] subclavian catheter insertion is contraindicated when any of the following occur at the proposed site of insertion: infection, hematoma, recent or anticipated surgery, radiation therapy, fistulas, drainages, extensive tumors or burns. The same authors[31] note that deformities of the neck and spine may increase risk of pneumothorax from subclavian catheterization and that purulent secretions from tracheostomy sites or radical head and neck resections may contaminate the catheter and dressings. In both of these cases, alternate sites of catheter insertion need to be considered.

Other common sites for central catheter insertion include internal jugular vein, peripherally inserted long lines with centrally located catheter tips, and arteriovenous shunts and fistulas. Each has advantages and disadvantages. Internal jugular central lines are uncomfortable for the patient and difficult to keep clean because of their location on the neck and because motions of the neck and, in men, beard growth disrupt the sterile occlusive dressing. Peripherally inserted long lines are also not ideal for PN administration. A 24-inch catheter is inserted into the superior vena cava through the

basilic or cephalic vein. X-ray confirmation of the catheter tip location is imperative before beginning PN to ensure that the solution is not infused into a smaller vessel and that the vein was not thrombosed or punctured in attempting to pass the catheter. The incidence of thrombophlebitis is higher with peripherally placed central catheters because of irritation to the peripheral blood vessels by the catheter. Use of silicone elastomer catheters minimizes irritation to the peripheral vein and prolongs the time that the catheter can remain in place. Arteriovenous shunts and fistulas, commonly used for hemodialysis, are sometimes indicated for long-term PN patients in whom subclavian vein catheterization is not possible. Arteriovenous shunts and fistulas are not central lines. A final concentration of no greater than 15 percent dextrose should be infused via these vessels. Clotting and infection are frequent complications of shunts and fistulas. Use of the femoral vein or artery for placement of the shunt is contraindicated because of the difficulty in keeping the groin area clean. Hickman or Broviac-type catheters can also be used for central PN infusion. These catheters are indicated in patients requiring prolonged PN support or home PN support. They need to be inserted in the operating room (see Chapter 21).

All central catheters must remain inviolate, i.e., they are reserved only for the nutrient solution in order to minimize the risk of becoming contaminated. Infusion of blood products and medications, or blood drawing, must be made via other access. If the central catheter has more than one lumen, one should be reserved for PN infusion only. The other lumen(s) can be used for blood products, medications, and so forth.

Techniques of Solution Infusion and Equipment

Once central line placement is verified by a chest x-ray, the hypertonic nutrient solution can then be infused, beginning with 1 liter over 24 hours on the first day. Before the chest x-ray is done, D5W should be infused at a "keep open" rate. The superior vena cava and the innominate veins are the only acceptable vessels for location of the catheter tip.[26]

When central PN is first started, the patient should be observed for hypersensitivity reactions or complications with catheter placement. Central vein solution should be administered with the aid of an IV regulator, ideally a volumetric infusion pump.

There are two major types of IV regulators: controllers and pumps. Controllers are essentially electronic flow clamps in which gravity provides the fluid pressure necessary to overcome the patient's normal venous pressure.[27] They may present difficulties in the administration of viscous solutions such as blood or oral alimentation.[28] Although controllers have been used for PN, they are not the ideal infusion apparatus. Nonvolumetric pumps infuse at a drop rate (GTT/minute).[27] The controlling mechanism is a peristaltic device that moves fluid by intermittently squeezing the IV tubing.[27,28] In administering PN with a controller, the rate should be regulated with two regulator clamps. The nurse should calculate the drop rate (GTT/minute) from the total amount of fluid in the bag. The bag should be time-taped and checked hourly to ensure accurate infusion of the solution.

Volumetric infusion pumps generate their own pressure to overcome the resistance of the patient's pressure. The volumetric pump is calibrated to infuse a specific volume of fluid over a specific time period (ml/hour). The controlling mechanism is a piston-cylinder with a refillable chamber calibrated to deliver a set volume. The piston produces pressure within this chamber sufficient to expel fluid from it.[27,28]

In purchasing pumps, there are certain features that should be assessed. These include cost, ease of maintenance, ease of use, portability, degree of accuracy of delivery, alarm system, and minimal and maximal rate settings. After evaluating each of these features, a decision can be made as to which pump is best for the particular institution.

Central vein PN infusions should be initiated and terminated gradually to allow adjustment of endogenous insulin production to altered glucose infusions. If central PN solutions are at any time unavailable, D10W or D20W should be substituted and administered at the same rate until central PN solution is obtained.[26]

Catheter Maintenance

The catheter insertion site is maintained with a dry, sterile, air-occlusive dressing that is changed every 48 hours and as necessary. The procedure consists of alcohol/acetone, povidone–iodine scrub, povidone–iodine ointment, gauze, and a covering such as Elastoplast. Waterproof dressings should be applied to insertion sites located near a draining wound or tracheostomy. When the dressing is changed, the surrounding area of skin and insertion site should be inspected and cultures taken if there is any drainage from the area.[29]

Administration sets and tubing are changed daily to prevent contamination, preferably with the first bag of the day. To prevent against air emboli during this procedure, the patient lies supine in bed and performs the Valsalva maneuver when the catheter is open to the air.[29]

Catheter Complications

Central catheter-related problems are either mechanical or septic in nature. Table 17–4 lists some of these complications, their causes, and possible solutions. The majority of the mechanical complications that occur are associated with catheter insertion. Some of these complications include pneumothorax, where the pleura is nicked during catheter insertion, hemothorax, a result of excessive bleeding, and hydrothorax, caused by catheterization of the pleural space with subsequent infusion of solution. Laceration of the subclavian artery can also occur. Plac-

ing direct pressure on the artery for 10 minutes can usually stop the bleeding if the patient's clotting parameters are normal. Malposition of the catheter occurs when the catheter tip is placed too far, reaching the right atrium, or not far enough, staying in the subclavian vein rather than the superior vena cava. In such cases the catheter must be replaced.

The majority of these complications can be prevented, however, by strict adherence to a written protocol, by adequate patient teaching prior to insertion of the catheter, and by having an experienced operator place the catheter.

TABLE 17–4. CATHETER-RELATED COMPLICATIONS

Problem	Possible Causes	Solutions
I. Mechanical		
A. Catheter Insertion		
1. Pneumo-, hydro-, hemo-, chylothorax	Improper catheter insertion	Strict adherence to protocol
2. Brachial plexus injury	Inexperienced operator	Experience operator with good knowledge of anatomy
3. Subclavian artery puncture	Nonadherence to catheter insertion protocol	Adequate patient teaching and preparation
4. Subclavian vein thrombosis	Injury to wall of vessel during catheterization	Ensure placement of catheter tip in SVC
5. Air embolus		Appropriate suturing of catheter
6. Malposition of catheter		
7. Catheter embolus		
B. Delivery System		
1. Increased or decreased infusion rates	Catheter occlusion	Inspect catheter
	Pump failure	Check pump every 30 minutes
	Tubing separation	Check battery
		Tape tubing connections
II. Septic		
A. Catheter		
1. Primary	Contamination and infection at catheter site due to improper catheter care	Sterile dressing changes; remove catheter immediately if catheter sepsis is suspected and culture; rotate site of catheter
2. Secondary	Catheter "seeding" from distant site of infection	Remove catheter
B. Solution	Improper mixing/handling/administration of solutions	Adherence to protocols for preparation and administration

Inadvertent increase or decrease in the rate of infusion of the solution results from pump failure, catheter occlusion, or tubing separation. Most of these problems can be prevented if the catheter, tubing, and pump apparatus are inspected at least once every 30 minutes by the nursing staff.

Another very serious catheter-related complication is catheter sepsis. The patient receiving PN is at an increased risk of sepsis for three main reasons: the PN solution is a perfect medium for growth of bacteria and fungi; patients receiving PN are often immunologically compromised either by underlying medical conditions and therapies or by their nutritionally depleted state; and the primary barrier to infection, the skin, is no longer intact.[24] Catheter sepsis can be due to contamination at the insertion site because of improper catheter care or to catheter "seeding" from a distant site of infection. The PN solutions themselves can be contaminated as a result of improper mixing and administration. Because of these potential problems, adherence to a strict protocol of catheter care is imperative. Prominent signs of sepsis are fever, chills, tachycardia, and glucose intolerance. Temperature, vital signs, and urine levels for sugar and acetone are monitored every 6 hours. If a fever develops, a complete work-up should be initiated to delineate the source of possible infection. If no other source is found, the catheter should be removed and the tip cultured.

It is not necessary to replace subclavian catheters routinely to prevent catheter-related sepsis. However, burn patients should have their central catheters changed every 3 to 5 days at least, especially if the catheter was introduced through burned tissue, to avoid contamination of the catheter, and thus catheter sepsis.

Peripheral Vein Feedings

Peripheral vein PN is accomplished by infusing the isoosmolar or slightly hyperosmolar solution through a cannula inserted into a large-bore peripheral vein. The catheter is placed and maintained in most institutions by either the staff nurses, house staff, or intravenous nursing team. Peripheral catheters should be changed every 72 hours to prevent thrombophlebitis.

The catheter insertion site and surrounding tissue should be checked frequently for signs of phlebitis or infiltration and the catheter should be removed immediately if any of these symptoms occur. Peripheral vein solution can be safely administered by gravity drip, but the use of two regulator clamps is recommended. Only parenteral lipid emulsion may run simultaneously with the peripheral PN, and this should be done through a Y-connector placed as close to the insertion site as possible (Fig. 17–3). If the peripheral line is needed for the administration of other medications or blood products, the solution

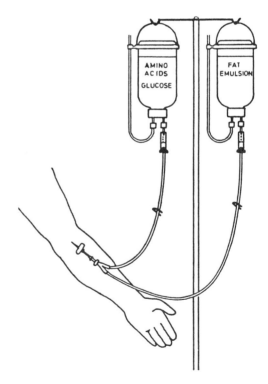

Figure 17–3. Illustration of technique for infusing peripheral parenteral nutrition with fat emulsion. *(From Fischer, JE (ed): Total Parenteral Nutrition. Boston: Little, Brown and Co., 1976, p 348, Fig 18–1.)*

may be temporarily discontinued. The line, however, must be flushed with normal saline before and after the administration of solutions other than peripheral PN.[26] As peripheral PN is nearly isotonic, it is not necessary to start infusions slowly or taper solutions when terminating therapy.

Peripheral PN contains constituents similar to central PN, i.e., water, dextrose, AA, electrolytes, minerals, vitamins, and trace minerals; however, the amounts of these ingredients are usually less than in central PN. The final concentration of dextrose should not exceed 10 percent; AA concentration may vary between 3.5 and 5.5 percent; electrolyte concentrations are usually similar to central PN; however, other mineral (calcium, phosphorus, magnesium) concentrations may be less than in central PN, since anabolism is not occurring at as fast a rate. Many institutions will not routinely add trace minerals to peripheral PN, as it is usually a temporary feeding regime. If the time of peripheral PN with no enteral intake exceeds a week, trace minerals should be added.

Parenteral Lipid

Parenteral lipid emulsions are designed for use as an energy source and as a source of EFA. They are used as an energy source primarily with peripheral PN, but in certain instances may be necessary on a daily basis with central PN (when carbohydrate intake needs to be decreased, i.e., respiratory failure). As a source of EFA, one bottle (500 ml) of 10 percent fat emulsion every 3 days will prevent deficiencies. However, daily infusions are necessary to treat an essential fatty acid deficiency.

To avoid the risk of infection, it is recommended that the fat emulsion be infused into a peripheral vein past the location of the intravenous filter, either via a Y-connector, as shown in Figure 17–3, or via a separate peripheral vein. Parenteral lipid emulsion may be run centrally, although manipulation of the line may increase the risk of infection. Adequate training of nurses in central line

and catheter care, and strict adherence to protocols, should prevent this problem from occurring.

There are two major types of parenteral lipid emulsion, 10 percent and 20 percent. The fat source and fatty acid composition will vary depending on the brand used (see Chapter 18, Formulation of Parenteral Solutions). Ten percent fat emulsion is 1.1 kcal/cc and 20 percent is 2 kcal/cc. Up to 2.5 g fat/kg/day may be infused, and it should not greatly exceed 60 percent of the total calories. After running the first bottle (500 ml) of 10 or 20 percent emulsion, the patient should be checked for signs of intolerance before continuing the lipid infusion. The infusion should not exceed 125 ml/hour, thus 500 ml over 4 hours for 10 percent fat emulsion, or 60 ml per hour, thus 500 ml over 8 hours for 20 percent fat emulsion. Neither solution should be left hanging for more than 24 hours.

Caution must be taken when infusing parenteral lipid emulsion in patients with hyperlipemia, pancreatitis, severe liver damage, pulmonary disease, anemia, or blood coagulation disorders. Specific monitoring parameters should be checked before the infusion begins, and at least 6 hours after the infusion ends, to assess the patient's baseline status and capacity to clear the lipid from the bloodstream. Monitoring will be discussed in the next section. The patient should be watched closely during the first 30 minutes of infusion to assess for signs of fat intolerance, i.e., dyspnea, cyanosis, allergic reactions, nausea, vomiting, headache, increase in temperature, or pain in the chest or back. Delayed adverse reactions can include hepatomegaly, jaundice, thrombocytopenia, or fat overload syndrome (fever, leukocytosis, splenomegaly, and shock).

MONITORING

The major purpose of monitoring during PN is to avoid complications. But monitoring is also used for assessing nutrition status, assessing the appropriateness of nutrient regimes, correcting or preventing nutrient deficiencies, preventing metabolic complications associated with longer term PN, and evaluating special considerations for specific diseases.[30] Monitoring falls into three major categories: clinical, biochemical, and bacteriologic.

Clinical monitoring includes daily visitations to assess the patient's appearance and tolerance to PN. This is particularly important to detect adverse reactions when the infusion first begins, and to assess for clinical signs of nutrient deficiencies or excesses when the patient is receiving PN over the long term. For example, skin integrity, hair color and texture, status of mucous membranes, and appearance of nail beds are all evaluated on a regular basis (clinical assessment is discussed in greater detail in Chapter 4). Weighing the patient is also part of clinical monitoring; the patient should be weighed before PN begins and daily thereafter throughout PN.

Biochemical monitoring can be broken down into baseline studies that are done before PN begins and ongoing monitoring that is performed on a regular basis throughout therapy. Table 17–5 lists the parameters that must be checked, and recommended times for their assessment (see Chapter 5, Laboratory Values and Their Interpretation.

Frequent evaluation of energy and nitrogen balance is necessary to assess the adequacy of the feeding regime (see Chapter 10 for a discussion of methods). This should be done before PN begins and weekly thereafter.

Urine urea nitrogen, although only an approximation of N balance, is the simplest, quickest, and least costly method available to assess N economy. This test is not necessary for all uncomplicated patients receiving PN, but should be reserved for those cases in which there is a question concerning feeding adequacy or patient tolerance.

Baseline laboratory studies are performed primarily to monitor fluid and electrolyte balance and to rule out liver or kidney dysfunction, which would preclude high dose AA

TABLE 17–5. MONITORING PARAMETERS FOR PN

Baseline Laboratory Evaluation:
  SMA-20: Serum electrolytes and pH
              Serum Ca^{++}, inorganic phosphorus
              Blood urea nitrogen (BUN)
              Serum creatinine
              Liver function tests
              Total protein/albumin
              Serum glucose
              CO_2
  PT, PTT
  Serum magnesium
  Complete blood count (CBC) with differential
  Serum iron, total iron-binding capacity
  Serum triglycerides (if fat emulsion is used)
  Urine analysis
  Serum and urine osmolarity
  Additional tests for central vein infusions: serum levels of B$_{12}$, folate, trace elements (Mn, Cu, Zn)

Ongoing Monitoring Procedures:
  Every 4 to 6 hours: vital signs; urine glucose and ketones
  Daily: serum electrolytes, BUN, CO_2, serum glucose, pH, fluid intake and output, weight
  Twice per week: SMA-20, CBC with differential (when the patient is stable, these may be ordered weekly)
  Weekly: serum magnesium, serum and urine osmolarity, urine analysis, serum triglycerides (until fat emulsion is discontinued), other serum vitamin and mineral levels as needed

infusions. Before a central line is inserted, clotting parameters must be checked to prevent unnecessary bleeding and its related insertion complications. Also, a baseline triglyceride level should be checked to rule out hyperlipidemia prior to infusing the fat emulsion, especially in patients with pancreatitis, liver dysfunction, or a history of hyperlipidemia. A subsequent level should be checked at least 6 hours after the infusion is completed to assess clearance.

Ongoing studies are important to evaluate tolerance to PN and to prevent complications. A SMA-20 battery (see Table 17–5) should be checked twice weekly. If the patient is taking nothing by mouth, magnesium level should be checked weekly and more frequently if necessary, i.e., in renal failure. Triglyceride levels should be checked weekly, and more often if they are elevated or if the patient has a history of hyperlipidemia. Other tests may be requested as necessary to monitor the patient's nutrition care. These may include mineral balances or trace element and vitamin determinations.

The patient must also be monitored for signs of infection and changes in hydration status, cardiac function, and respiratory function. The patient's vital signs and fluid intake and output are followed daily. Catheter insertion sites are also regularly checked. If the site becomes reddened or there is drainage of any kind, cultures should be taken and the patient monitored for other signs or symptoms of infection.

Peripheral catheters should also be checked on a regular basis if being used for PN to prevent phlebitis. Infusing solutions with greater than 10 percent dextrose may irritate the vein, and some patients have reported burning or irritation with fat emulsion infusion. By paying careful attention to the above monitoring details and procedures, many of the potential complications associated with PN can be avoided.

CONCLUSIONS

PN can be a successful, life-saving support system for patients who are unable to tolerate nutrients enterally. The use of PN varies from providing primary therapy in the treatment of a specific disease, to adjuvant therapy in which the underlying disease is treated separately.

The two major types of PN therapy, peripheral and central, have specific indications. It is essential that strict protocols are followed as to how solutions are ordered, mixed, and administered to eliminate error and complications. Central catheters require particularly strict care and attention to minimize infectious or mechanical complications. All patients receiving PN should be carefully monitored for intolerances and adverse reac-

tions to the solutions, in addition to being assessed for adequate provision of nutrients. If these guidelines are followed carefully, with particular emphasis on administering the solutions safely, the use of PN can be successful in any institution.

REFERENCES

1. Elman R, Weiner DO: Intravenous alimentation with special reference to protein (amino acid) metabolism. JAMA 122:796, 1939
2. Dudrick SJ, Vars HM, Ravonsley HM, Rhoads JE: Total intravenous feeding and growth in puppies. Fed Proc 25:481, 1966
3. Dudrick SJ, Wilmore DW, Vars HM, Rhoads JE: Can intravenous feeding as a sole means of nutrition support growth in the child and restore weight loss in an adult? An affirmative answer. Ann Surg 169:974, 1969
4. MacBurney M, Wilmore DW: Rational decision-making in nutritional care. Surg Clin North Am 61:571, 1981
5. Abel RM, Beck CH, Abbott WM, et al.: Improved survival from acute renal failure after treatment with intravenous essential α-amino acids and glucose. N Engl J Med 288:695, 1973
6. Feinstein EI, Blumenkrantz MJ, Healy H, et al.: Clinical and metabolic responses to parenteral nutrition in acute renal failure. A controlled double-blind study. Medicine 60:124, 1981
7. Leonard CD, Luke RG, Siegel RR: Parenteral essential amino acids in acute renal failure. Urology 6:154, 1975
8. Studley HO: Percentage of weight loss; a basic indication of surgical risk in patients with chronic peptic ulcer. JAMA 106:458, 1936
9. Abel RM, Fischer JE, Mortimer JB, et al.: Malnutrition in cardiac surgical patients. Results of a prospective, randomized evaluation of early postoperative parenteral nutrition. Arch Surg 111:45, 1976
10. Heatley RV, Williams RHP, Lewis MH: Preoperative intravenous feeding—a controlled trial. Postgrad Med J 55:541, 1979
11. Muller JM, Dienst C, Brenner U, Pichlmaier H: Preoperative parenteral feeding in patients with gastrointestinal carcinoma. Lancet 1:68, 1982
12. Thomas RJS: The modifying effect of nutritional intake on posttraumatic depletion in hepatic glycogen in rats. Surgery 87:539, 1980

13. Elson CO, Layden TJ, Nemchausky BA, et al.: An evaluation of total parenteral nutrition in the management of inflammatory bowel disease. Dig Dis Sci 25:42, 1980

14. Rombeau JL, Barot LR, Williamson CE, Mullen JL: Preoperative total parenteral nutrition and surgical outcome in patients with inflammatory bowel disease. Am J Surg 143:139, 1982

15. Malloy DF, Young LS, MacBurney MM, Wilmore DW: The influence of multi-organ system failure on survival rate in patients receiving nutritional support (abstract). JPEN 5:578, 1981

16. Askanazi J, Rosenbaum SH, Hyman AI, et al.: Respiratory changes induced by the large glucose loads of total parenteral nutrition. JAMA 243:1444, 1980

17. Lowry SF, Brennan MF: Abnormal liver function during parenteral nutrition: relation to infusion excess. J Surg Res 26:300, 1979

18. Steiger E, Oram-Smith J, Muller E, et al.: Effects of nutrition on tumor growth and tolerance to chemotherapy. J Surg Res 18:455, 1975

19. Buzby GP, Mullen JL, Stein P, et al.: Host–tumor interaction and nutrient supply. Cancer 45:2940, 1980

20. Popp MB, Wagner SF, Brito OJ: Host and tumor responses to increasing levels of intravenous nutritional support (abstract). Soc Univ Surg, February 1983

21. Freund H, Dienstag J, Lehrich J, et al.: Infusion of branched chain enriched amino acid solution in patients with hepatic encephalopa-

thy. Ann Surg 196:209, 1982

22. Kern KA, Bower RH, Atamian S, et al.: The effect of a new branched chain-enriched amino acid solution on postoperative catabolism. Surgery 92:780, 1982

23. Cerra FB, Upson D, Angelico R, et al.: Branched chains support postoperative protein synthesis. Surgery 92:192, 1982

24. Millikan WJ, Henderson JM, Warren WD, et al.: Total parenteral nutrition with FO80® in cirrhotics with subclinical encephalopathy. Ann Surg 197:294, 1983

25. McGhee A, Henderson M, Millikan WJ, et al.: Comparison of the effects of Hepatic Aid and a casein modular diet on encephalopathy, plasma amino acids, and nitrogen balance in cirrhotic patients. Ann Surg 197:288, 1983

26. Brigham and Women's Hospital, Adult Parenteral Nutrition Protocol, 1979

27. Huey FL: What's on the market? A nurse's guide. Am J Nurs 83:902, 1983

28. Turco SJ: Inaccuracies in I.V. flow rates and the use of pumps and controllers. J Parent Drug Assoc 32:242, 1978

29. Appleby L: Initiation, maintenance, and termination of total parenteral nutrition. Nat Intraven Ther Assoc 6:31, 1983

30. Lee HA: Monitoring intravenous feeding. In Karran SJ, Alberti KGMM (eds): Practical Nutritional Support. Kent, England: Pitman Medical, 1980

31. Silberman H, Eisenberg D: Parenteral and Enteral Nutrition for the Hospitalized Patient. Norwalk, Conn: Appleton-Century-Crofts, 1982

18. Formulation of Parenteral Solutions

Mary Rajala

Parenteral nutrition (PN) solutions contain a nitrogen (N) source, energy sources, electrolytes, vitamins, minerals, and a source of essential fatty acids (EFA). Research is refining the existing knowledge regarding nitrogen balance, preferred fuels during stress and in various conditions, as well as vitamin and mineral requirements. As a result, solutions can be tailored to suit individual patient's needs.

PROTEIN SOURCES

Hydrolysates

The first N sources available for parenteral use were protein hydrolysates of casein (milk) and fibrin (beef blood). Enzymatic or mineral acid hydrolysis is an inexact and incomplete process resulting in batch-to-batch variations of amino acid (AA) content. Hydrolysates contained approximately 60 percent free AA, 50 percent dipeptides and tripeptides.[1] Although positive N balance could be achieved with protein hydrolysates, better results were obtained when hydrolysates were given orally rather than intravenously (IV)[2] because of the ability of the intestine to split small peptides into AA.

Questions exist concerning the bioavailability of peptides administered IV.[2,3] Small peptides may be metabolized by the liver,[4] while some are degraded into free AA in the glomerular filtrate and either reabsorbed into the blood for utilization or excreted into the urine.

When compared to crystalline AA, the quantity of utilizable N from hydrolysates is relatively small. Long[1] reported 0.7 g of N per 100 ml of fibrin protein hydrolysate, as compared to 1.30 g of N per 100 ml of crystalline AA via Kjeldahl technique. Casein hydrolysate was found to have lower N utilization than fibrin, and a relative deficiency of sulfur-containing and aromatic AA, plus an excess of valine and lysine.[2,3]

In addition to providing less N than crystalline AA, experience with hydrolysates indicated intrinsic problems. Frequent metabolic acidosis occurred because of the net cationic residue.[5] High free ammonia content (20,000 to 40,000 micromoles free ammonia or ammonium ion/100 ml) in hydrolysates led to hyperammonemia in premature infants and individuals with liver disease.[6] This required treatment using arginine and ornithine.

Protein hydrolysates served as sources of electrolytes and trace minerals. Fibrin contains significant quantities of sodium and potassium,[7] while casein has a more complete profile of electrolytes and generally less potassium and magnesium. By comparison, crystalline AA solutions contain few electrolytes as contaminants of water,[8] although some solutions are available with maintenance electrolytes already added. Hydrolysates were also found to support bacterial growth and were associated with an increased risk of contamination.[9]

Hydrolysates were a less expensive product than crystalline AA. Competition and increased availability have decreased the cost of crystalline AA, which in turn decreased the demand for hydrolysates. Recently, the last hydrolysates were removed from the market.

Crystalline Amino Acids

Crystalline AA were developed after protein hydrolysates. Originally, only racemic mixtures of L and D forms existed.[10] A racemic mixture contains equivalent amounts of mirror image molecules.[11,12] When a beam of plane-polarized light encounters the mixture, rotation of the plane does not occur because of the cancelling out caused by exact mirror reflections.[13]

Now, solutions containing only the metabolically active L form are available. Acetates of AA, rather than chloride salts, are used to prevent the metabolic acidosis experienced when hydrolysates were in common use.[8] Products are available in concentrations of 3.5, 5, 5.5, 7, 8.5, 10, and 11.4 percent crystalline amino acids.

Formulating crystalline AA mixtures allows the manufacturer to determine the quantity of specific amino acids and the ratio of essential to nonessential amino acids. Unlike hydrolysis, there is no variation in composition between batches. As more knowledge is acquired regarding requirements of specific AA for specific metabolic aberrations, solutions will be tailored to specific conditions.[14] Solutions for liver and renal diseases are currently available. Several manufacturers have recently released condition-specific solutions: a high branch chain

formula for patients severely stressed as a result of trauma, burns or sepsis (FreAmine HBC); a solution for neonates based on the amino acid profile of breast milk (Neopham); and maintenance solutions with more complete AA profiles. Use of specialized solutions is discussed in Chapter 19.

ESSENTIAL AMINO ACIDS

There are several maintenance solutions containing different AA concentrations currently available. Generally, the lower concentrations may be used for nonstressed individuals whose protein requirements are not excessive, in uremia where it is desirable to limit protein, or to limit osmotic load as in peripheral hyperalimentation. No controlled studies indicate if similar concentrations of these different AA solutions are therapeutically equivalent. Comparisons have been made using the FAO/WHO standard for protein comparison, whole egg.[15] The liver normally functions as an intermediary in AA metabolism through the portal venous system.[16] In PN, however, the portal venous system is bypassed. Therefore, the evaluation of plasma AA profiles and the ability of various parenteral solutions to maintain normal plasma ranges may be a more valid approach to evaluate differences as opposed to making comparisons using dietary standards.[17] This recommended approach has been used in formulating branch chain-enriched solutions with low aromatic AA for liver disease, and is also being used to formulate branch chain-enriched solutions for hypermetabolic patients.

When evaluating parenteral maintenance solutions, all nine essential amino acids (EAA) should be present. Table 18–1 lists general requirements of EAA taken orally. Although the total N needs for parenteral nutrition do not differ from those for enteral,[18] the requirement for EAA increases from 19 percent of the total N intake for a normal person, to approximately 40 percent for repleting lean body mass in debilitated patients.[8]

TABLE 18-1. ESSENTIAL AMINO ACID REQUIREMENTS OF ADULTS

	Adult Men		Adult Women[c]	Calculated Percent of Total Protein	Adult[d]	AA Pattern for High Quality Proteins, mg/g of Protein[d]
	Rose[a]	Inoue[b]				
Histidine	—	—	—	—	?	17
Isoleucine	10	11	10	2.4	12	42
Leucine	11	14	13	3.0	16	70
Lysine	9	12	10	2.4	12	51
Methionine and cystine	14	11	13	3.0	10	26
Phenylalanine and tyrosine	14	14	13	3.2	16	73
Threonine	6	6	7	1.5	8	35
Tryptophan	3	3	3	0.7	3	11
Valine	14	14	11	3.0	14	48
Total essential amino acids	81	87	80	—	91	—
Average total protein needs	425	425	425	—	—	—
Essential amino acids as percent of protein	19%	20%	19%	19%	—	—

Note: Requirement is mg/kg of body weight.
[a]Rose, W.D., Lambert, C.F., Coon, M.J.: J. Biol. Chem. 211:815, 1954.
[b]Inoue, G., Fujita, Y., Nii yama, Y.: unpublished results, 1971.
[c]Hegsted, D.M.: Federation Proceedings 22: 1424, 1963.
[d]RDA, 9 ed., p. 43.

Any metabolic aberration occurring with a disease may alter serum levels of AA, rendering a specific ratio of essential to nonessential amino acids (NEAA) invalid.[17] In specific situations, NEAA may become essential. EAA and NEAA are listed in Table 18-2. Practitioners should be aware of this and look critically at AA profiles of available parenteral formulations. (Refer to Table 18-3 for comparisons of existing AA formulations.)

During periods of growth (infancy, wound

TABLE 18-2. ESSENTIAL AND NONESSENTIAL AMINO ACIDS

Essential (Must Be Supplied)	May Become Essential in Specific Conditions	Nonessential (May Be Synthesized)
Histidine	Alanine—Infancy	Asparagine
Isoleucine	Arginine—Stress, growth,	Aspartic acid
Leucine	↑ urea cycle activity	Glutamic acid
Lysine	Cysteine—Premature infancy	Glutamine
Methionine	Cystine—Stress	Glycine (aminoacetic acid)
Phenylalanine	Proline—Infancy	Hydroxylysine
Threonine	Taurine—Infancy	Hydroxyproline
Tryptophan	Tyrosine—Premature infancy	Serine
Valine		

TABLE 18–3. AMINO ACID FORMULATIONS

	Aminosyn 10%[a]	FreAmine III 10%[b]	Travasol 10%[c]	VeinAmine 8%[d]	Novamine 11.4%[e]
Essential Amino Acids (mg/100ml)					
L-isoleucine	720	690	600	493	570
L-leucine	940	910	730	347	790
L-lysine	720	725	580	535	900
L-methionine	400	530	400	427	570
L-phenylalanine	440	560	560	400	790
L-threonine	520	400	420	160	570
L-tryptophan	160	150	180	80	190
L-valine	800	660	580	253	730
Total essential amino acids (mg/100ml)	4700	4625	4050	2695	5110
Nonessential Amino Acids (mg/100ml)					
L-alanine	1280	710	2070	—	1590
L-arginine	980	950	1150	749	1120
L-aspartic acid	—	—	—	400	330
L-glutamic acid	—	—	—	426	570
L-histidine	300	280	480	237	680
L-proline	860	1120	680	107	680
L-serine	420	590	500	—	450

L-tyrosine	44	—	40	—	30
Aminoacetic acid (glycine)	1280	1400	1030	3387	790
L-cysteine	—	<24	—	—	<60
Total nonessential amino acids (mg/100ml)	5164	5074	5950	5306	6300
Total amino acids (mg/100ml)	9864	9699	10,000	8001	11,410
Essential: Total	0.48	0.48	0.41	0.32	0.45
BCAA (mg/100ml)	2460	2260	1910	1093	2660
Total nitrogen (g/L)	15.72	15.3	16.84	13.3	18.0
Protein Equivalents (g/L)	100	95.6	103.3	80.0	112.5
Electrolytes (mEq/L)					
Sodium	—	10	—	40	—
Potassium	5.4	—	—	30	—
Magnesium	—	—	—	6	—
Phosphate	—	20	—	—	—
Chloride	—	<2	40	50	—
Acetate	148	88	87	50	—
pH (approximate)	5.3	6.5	6.0	6.2–6.6	5.6
Calculated osmolarity (mosm/L)	1000	950	1000	950	1049

[a]Abbott Laboratories. Also available without electrolytes in 3.5, 5, 5, 7, or 8.5%; with electrolytes in 7 or 8.5%; or with maintenance electrolytes in 3.5%M.
[b]American McGaw. Also available in 8.5 or 3% with electrolytes.
[c]Travenol Laboratories, Inc. Also available with or without electrolytes in 5.5 or 8.5%.
[d]Cutter Laboratories, Inc.
[e]Also available in 8.5% concentration.

TABLE 18–4. SPECIAL AMINO ACID FORMULATIONS

	HepatAmine 8%[a]	Aminosyn-RF 5.2%[b]	RenAmin 6.5%[c]	NephrAmine 5.8%[a]	FreAmine HBC 69%[a]	ProcalAmine (3% Amino Acid and 3% Glycerin with Electrolytes)[a,d]	Neopham[e]
Essential Amino Acids (mg/100ml)							
Isoleucine	900	462	600	560	760	210	310
Leucine	1100	726	500	880	1370	270	700
Lysine	610	535	450	900[f]	410	310[g]	560
Methionine	100	726	500	880	250	160	130
Phenylalanine	100	726	490	880	320	170	270
Threonine	450	330	380	400	200	120	360
Tryptophan	66	165	160	200	90	46	140
Valine	840	528	800	640	880	200	360
Branch chain amino acids (BCAA)	36%				45%		
BCAA: Aromatic amino acids (AAA)	17:1				7.3:1		
Nonessential Amino Acids (mg/100ml)							
Alanine	770	—	560		400	210	630
Arginine	600	600	630		580	290	410
Histidine	240	429	420	250	160	85	210

	1	2	3	4	5	6	7
Proline	800	—	350		630	340	560
Serine	500	—	300		330	180	380
Aminoacetic acid (glycine)	900	—	300		330	420	210
Cysteine	<20	—	—	<20	<20	<20	100
Tyrosine	—	—	40				50
Total nitrogen (g/L)		7.87	10	6.5			
Protein equivalents (g/L)		52	65				9.27
Electrolytes							
Sodium (mEq/L)	10	—	3	6	10	35	
Potassium (mEq/L)	—	5.4	—		—	24	
Phosphate (mmole/L)	10	—	—		—	7	
Chloride (mEq/L)	<3	—	31		<3	41	
Acetate (mEq/L)	~62	—	60	44	57	47	
Osmolarity (calculated) (mosm/L)	785	475	600	440	620	735	519
pH (approximate)	6.5	5.2	6	6.5	6.5	6.8	5.3

[a] American McGaw.
[b] Abbott Laboratories.
[c] Travenol Laboratories.
[d] Also contains 5 mEq magnesium/L, 3 mEq calcium/L.
[e] Cutter Laboratories.
[f] As lysine acetate (640 mg free base).
[g] As lysine acetate (220 mg free base).

healing, pregnancy, body building) and in uremia, histidine is an EAA.[18-23] In the ninth revised edition of the Recommended Dietary Allowances (RDA), histidine was added to the original eight EAA.[24]

Methionine is the precursor of cystine. During stress, the requirement for cystine increases. At the same time, the ability to convert methionine to cystine may become limited, thereby making cystine essential.[25]

In infants, several AA are essential, including proline, alanine, and taurine.[26] In premature infants, tyrosine and cysteine are essential since the liver cannot form them.[18,26] Since cysteine oxidizes to cystine and becomes insoluble, it cannot be added at the time of manufacture.[26,27] Cysteine can be added just before dispensing from the pharmacy, however, since the reaction is not immediate.

Studies have been conducted on the N requirements of patients with chronic and acute renal failure. When patients undergoing dialysis require nutriton support for maintenance, parenteral support can be used. There is controversy, however, regarding the approach to the nondialyzed patient. Some clinicians recommend that all N be given as EAA, based on evidence that excess urea N will then be recycled to form NEAA, reducing uremia.[28,29] Other clinicians believe that it is adequate to limit total protein and provide both EAA and NEAA. Several available products provide limited protein in the form of EAA for renal patients who have potentially reversible acute renal failure, who are unable to eat, and whose access to dialysis is limited (See Aminosyn RF, Ren-Amin, and NephrAmine in Table 18–4. These solutions contain all nine EAA and arginine.[21-23]

Arginine plays a role in ammonia metabolism[20,21,30] and in preventing hyperammonemia. When protein hydrolysates were used widely, hyperammonemia was observed in infants and in patients with liver disease.[6] During stress, when urea cycle activity is accelerated, the requirements for arginine are high. Though not an EAA, it should be in-cluded in the AA profile. Aspartic acid, glutamic acid, and ornithine deficiencies may also be related to the development of this condition.

Branch Chain Amino Acids

Isoleucine, leucine, and valine are nonpolar, neutral EAA classified as aliphatic because of the chemical nature of the radical group (R).[31] These three are also known as branch chain amino acids (BCAA) to specify their molecular structure. (See Table 18–5 for the structures.) In a normal person deriving protein from an oral diet, the liver metabolizes EAA except the BCAA, which are metabolized by muscle, kidney, brain, and adipose tissue.[16] All three of these AA serve as alternate fuels for muscle tissue when the external supply is inadequate.[32] After being processed by the liver, the concentration of BCAA and the ratio of BCAA to non-BCAA released to the peripheral tissue is higher than before entering the hepatic portal venous system because of the liver action on non-BCAA. Parenteral solutions therefore should be higher in branch chains to offset the bypassed intermediate effect of the liver during parenteral alimentation.

Studies with branch chain-enriched formulas have reported success in reversing encephalopathy in patients with advanced liver disease and in hypermetabolic patients. A solution specific for the treatment of hepatic encephalopathy from cirrhosis or hepatitis, HepatAmine, has recently become available (Table 18–4). A branch chain-enriched formula, FreAmine HBC, containing 35 to 45 percent of the AA as branch chains has been produced for patients with sepsis, trauma, or multiple organ failure. Although it appears there are several applications of BCAA, one should not interchange solutions intended to treat liver failure for those intended to treat trauma, and vice versa. This is because the need for other AA, such as the aromatic AA and sulfur-containing AA, differs between these conditions. As seen in Table 18–4, the AA profiles are different in these solutions.

TABLE 18–5. AMINO ACID STRUCTURES

1. General structure of amino acids:

NH₂
|
COOH—C—R
|
H

Note: Radical group (R) differs for each amino acid.

2. Branch chain amino acids (BCAA):

NH₂   NH₂   NH₂
| | |
COOH—C—CHCH₃   COOH—C—CH₂CHCH₃   COOH—C—CHCH₂CH₃
| | | | | |
H   CH₃   H   CH₃   H   CH₃

Valine   Leucine   Isoleucine

3. Aromatic amino acids (AAA):

NH₂   NH₂
| |
COOH—C—CH₂—⬡   COOH—C—CH₂—[indole ring]
| |
H   H

Phenylalanine   Tryptophan

(See Chapter 19 for more details on utilizing AA formulations for specific diseases.)

Aromatic Amino Acids

The aromatic AA include phenylalanine and tryptophan. These are also nonpolar, neutral EAA.[31] They are classified as aromatic because of the ring structures replacing the radical group (R) of the general structure of an AA. (Refer to the structures shown in Table 18–5.) Normally, the liver converts phenylalanine to tyrosine.[25,33] In liver disease, high quantities of phenylalanine, tryptophan, and tyrosine accumulate and are thought to cause hepatic coma by decreasing competition at the blood–brain barrier.[34] The solution for liver disease, therefore, is low in aromatic AA. Methionine is also provided in low concentrations to allow glutamine synthetase production and further ammonia clearance from plasma.

NONESSENTIAL AMINO ACIDS

NEAA are required AA that can be synthesized endogenously without provision by an external source. They still have important functions. The NEAA provided in parenteral solutions contribute to the overall N content of the solution. Although NEAA can be synthesized from precursors, N balance is improved when a combination of several NEAA, though not necessarily all, are supplied. (Refer to Table 18–2 for a list of NEAA.)

Low levels of glycine in parenteral solutions have been associated with improved N balance.[18,35–39] Glycine is sometimes used in excessive amounts as filler because it is an inexpensive source of nitrogen. For this reason, one should look critically at the level of glycine in various solutions. According to Munro,[18,40] high levels of glycine should be avoided.

Alanine, glutamic acid, and leucine enhance protein-sparing effects.[41,42] Because alanine functions as the major form of amino N transport between tissues[38,39] and is available to the liver for gluconeogenesis,[16] it should be a major NEAA in the solution.

As mentioned in a previous section, arginine is needed to prevent hyperammonemia and is used in instances where urea cycle activity is high.

Inborn Errors of Metabolism

In phenylketonuria, phenylalanine cannot be metabolized and formulas containing this AA should not be administered. Approximately 2 percent of the population is heterozygous for this disease, and thus has decreased levels of the enzyme needed to convert phenylalanine. The recommendation has therefore been made that some of the required phenylalanine be given as tyrosine to compensate for lower enzyme levels.[18]

Maple syrup urine disease and isovaleric acidemia are disorders involving BCAA metabolism for which available parenteral solutions cannot be used. In cases in which metabolic errors exist, it is possible to formulate a total solution that eliminates or substitutes the necessary AA. This requires knowledge of AA requirements and careful monitoring of the patient. To avoid accidentally omitting individual AA, use of a manufactured solution is preferable except in extreme and special cases.

Ketoanalogs

The substitution of nitrogen-free alpha-keto analogs for corresponding AA is an intriguing area of current research that has little clinical application at this time.[43,44] To decrease protein degradation,[45] it is being investigated in patients with diseases of protein intolerance or N retention,[43] in renal failure,[46–49] in Duchenne muscular dystrophy,[45] and in children with disorders of urea cycle enzymes. The original rationale for the success of experimental treatments was that urea N was recycled, but this theory has been discredited.[45] Studies have shown that in renal patients given ketoanalogs, blood urea nitrogen usually decreases, while N balance improves.[48] More work is needed to clarify the nutritional benefits of alpha ketoanalogs, to clarify the metabolic effects, and to derive optimum proportions of ketoanalogs needed in place of AA.

ENERGY SOURCES

Although several calorie sources have been used in parenteral alimentation, the major sources used are dextrose and fat emulsion.

Dextrose

Dextrose is by far the least expensive calorie source. (See Table 18–6 for its chemical structure.) It is available in concentrations in water from 5 to 70 percent. Most frequently, a 50 percent solution is used in central venous hyperalimentation, and a 10 percent solution is used peripherally. A lower dextrose concentration may be used centrally in patients who do not tolerate high carbohydrate loads because of diabetes mellitus or peripheral insulin resistance, or in patients whose fluid requirements are high and to whom it is undesirable to feed excess calories. In patients whose volume intake is restricted, a 70 percent dextrose solution may be used to maximize the calories provided in limited volume. This concept is presented in more detail under Mixing Procedures later in this chapter.

Each gram of dextrose in the monohydrated form provides 3.4 kilocalories. This is different from the value of 4.1 kcal/g from the oxidation of orally ingested carbohydrate. (See Table 18–7 for a sample calculation of kilocalories and protein from a parenteral solution.)

Lipid Emulsions

Fat emulsion has been significantly more expensive than dextrose as a source of calories, even though competition has caused decreasing prices. Its caloric density (1.1 to 2.0

TABLE 18–6. CARBOHYDRATE STRUCTURES

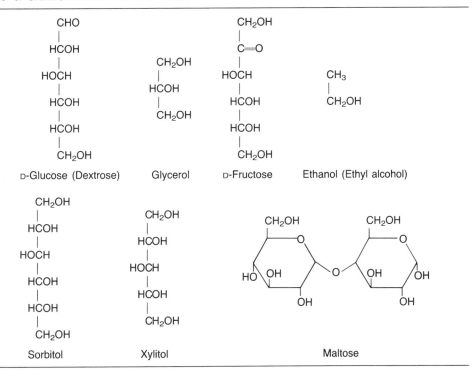

kcal/ml) is higher, thus allowing the practitioner to provide more calories, as compared to dextrose, when the volume allowance is restricted in a patient. Fat emulsions contain long chain triacylglycerols (triglycerides) of 12 to 26 carbons that are the size of chylomicrons (0.4 to 0.5 microns). As with chylomicrons, they are hydrolyzed in the capillary spaces by lipoprotein lipase to free fatty acids and glycerol. They are then either taken up in the tissues or circulated in the plasma bound to albumin. Currently, research is being done to explore medium chain triglycerides, those with 6 to 12 carbons, as a viable intravenous calorie source[32,50–53] Although the review article by Birkahn and Border[32] presents a convincing rationale, published studies are conflicting.

TABLE 18–7. CALCULATION OF CALORIES AND PROTEIN IN PARENTERAL SOLUTIONS

To calculate carbohydrate, protein, and calories:

_____ cc solution × _____% final concentration amino acids = _____ g (amino acids) × 4.0 cal/g = _____ calories

_____ cc solution × _____% final concentration dextrose = _____ g (dextrose) × 3.4 cal/g = _____ calories

_____ cc 10% fat emulsion × 1.1 cal/cc = _____ calories

_____ cc 20% fat emulsion × 2.0 cal/cc = _____ calories

Sum calories from carbohydrate and fat to obtain nonprotein calories. Include protein calories to arrive at total calories.

LONG CHAIN TRIGLYCERIDES

Currently available fat emulsions are composed of a source of fat (soybean or safflower oil), an emulsifier (1.2 percent egg yolk phospholipids), and an agent to adjust the osmolarity of the emulsion (2.5 percent glycerol) to that of blood, since fat is osmotically neutral. All three components provide calories. The fat and phospholipid provide 9 kcal/g, while the glycerol provides 4.3 kcal/g. The final caloric content of fat emulsions is 1.1 kcal/ml for 10 percent fat emulsion (1 kcal from fat, 0.1 from glycerol) and 2 kcal/ml for 20 percent solutions (1.9 kcal from fat, 0.1 from glycerol).[54] Because the concentration of fat in solution is low, more free water is provided by fat mixtures than by AA and dextrose mixtures. Less water retention occurs with fat administration than with glucose.[55]

Different sources of fat are used for various emulsions. These emulsions have their own characteristic fatty acid profiles based on the origin of the fat. (Refer to Table 18–8 for the fatty acid composition of the available solutions.) Nomenclature and structures of the primary fatty acids constituting available lipid emulsions are shown in Table 18–9.[13,56]

Essential Fatty Acid Deficiency

Fat emulsion is given to prevent EFA deficiency in depleted patients and in patients receiving continuous infusions of high dextrose concentrations. Although recommendations vary somewhat, it is generally agreed that providing 2 to 4 percent of calories as linoleic acid will prevent fatty acid deficiency.[8,57–59] To correct an existing deficiency, at least 4 percent of the calories should be given as linoleic acid, i.e., 8 percent of calories as 10 percent soybean oil, 6 percent as 10 percent safflower oil. This can be achieved by administering 500 ml of 10 percent fat emulsion one to three times per week. If parent-

TABLE 18-8. COMPOSITION OF LIPID EMULSIONS

	10% Intralipid[a] (20%)[b]	10% Liposyn[c] (20%)	10% Travamulsion[d]
Source of fat	Soybean	Safflower	Soybean
Linoleic acid (%)	50–54	77	56
Oleic acid (%)	26	13	23
Palmitic acid (%)	10	7	11
Linolenic acid (%)	8–9	0.1	6
Stearic acid (%)	2.5	2.5	?
Egg phospholipid (%)	1.2	1.2	1.2
Glycerol (%)	2.25	2.5	2.25
Kilocalories per cc	1.1 (2.0)	1.1 (2.0)[e]	1.1
Vitamin E activity (mg/L)[f]	15	20	41
Osmolarity (mosm/L)	280 (330)	300 (340)	270
pH	5.5–9.0	8.0 (8.3)	5.5–9.0
Particle size (microns)	0.5	0.4	0.4

[a]Cutter Laboratories.
[b]Parentheses indicate differences for 20% emulsions.
[c]Abbott Laboratories.
[d]Travenol Laboratories.
[e]0.7 kcal/ml as linoleic acid in 10% emulsion, 1.4 kcal/ml as linoleic acid in 20% emulsion.
[f]Batch-to-batch variations exist for vitamin E content of oils.

TABLE 18–9. NOMENCLATURE AND STRUCTURES OF LONG CHAIN TRIGLYCERIDES

Trivial Name (IUPAC[a])	Molecular Formula (Numerical Formula)[b]	Structure
Linoleic acid (9,12-Octadecadienoic acid)	$C_{18}H_{32}O_2$ (18:2ω6)	$H_3C-CH_2-CH_2-CH_2-CH_2-CH=CH-CH_2-CH=CH-CH_2-CH_2-CH_2-CH_2-CH_2-CH_2-CH_2-COOH$
Oleic acid (9-Octadecenoic acid)	$C_{18}H_{34}O_2$ (18:1ω9)	$H_3C-CH_2-CH_2-CH_2-CH_2-CH_2-CH_2-CH=CH-CH_2-CH_2-CH_2-CH_2-CH_2-CH_2-CH_2-COOH$
Palmitic acid (Hexadecenoic acid)	$C_{16}H_{32}O_2$ (16:0)	$H_3C-CH_2-CH_2-CH_2-CH_2-CH_2-CH_2-CH_2-CH_2-CH_2-CH_2-CH_2-CH_2-CH_2-COOH$
Linolenic acid (2 forms: 6,9,12-Octadecatrienoic acid 9,12,15-Octadecatrienoic acid)	(18:3ω3 18:3ω6)	$H_3C-CH_2-CH_2-CH=CH-CH_2-CH=CH-CH_2-CH=CH-CH_2-CH_2-CH_2-CH_2-CH_2-COOH$
Stearic acid (Octadecanoic acid)	$C_{18}H_{36}O_2$ (18:0)	$H_3C-CH_2-CH_2-CH_2-CH_2-CH_2-CH_2-CH_2-CH_2-CH_2-CH_2-CH_2-CH_2-CH_2-CH_2-CH_2-COOH$

[a]IUPAC = International Union of Pure and Applied Chemists. Formal system of nomenclature.
[b]Holman numerical system of nomenclature. Notes carbon length, the number of double bonds, and the position of the first occurring double bond with respect to the end containing the methyl group.

403

eral alimentation continues for more than 2 weeks, fat should be incorporated into the regimen.[55]

Several researchers have reported successful treatment of flaky dermatitis from EFA deficiency with topical application of fat.[60] Recent evidence indicates that though physical symptoms may disappear, biochemical levels of EFA are not corrected by this method.[61]

Arachidonic acid was formerly considered an EFA, in part because of its role as a precursor of prostaglandins, thromboxane, and prostacyclins. It has been shown, however, to be synthesized by humans.

There has been recent concern over the possible occurrence of linolenic acid deficiency if insufficient quantities are provided in the fat source, implicating safflower oil emulsion as inadequate. One case was reported in the literature.[62,63] While gamma linolenic acid (18:3ω6) can be synthesized from linoleic acid, alpha linolenic acid (18:3ω3) follows a separate metabolic pathway, and may play a role in antithrombotic activity and platelet regulation. Its essentiality to humans, however, has not been clearly established in clinical studies.[24,57,64,65]

OTHER COMPONENTS

Fat emulsions provide alpha tocopherol as a source of vitamin E. The concentration, however, is variable among batches according to soil conditions and harvest times for crops. Vitamin E requirements are related to the intake of polyunsaturated fats.[66] High intakes create high requirements and can tax the body's antioxidant capacity. Since fat emulsions comprise polyunsaturated fats, the naturally occurring vitamin E is necessary to protect the fatty acids from oxidation and, therefore, does not obviate the need for vitamin E supplementation during parenteral alimentation.

Fat emulsions also contain significant quantities of phosphate as phospholipid. Ap-

proximately 15 mmol of phosphate (14.8 mmol = 456 mg phosphorus in Intralipid, 13.9 mmol = 432 mg phosphorus in Liposyn) are contained in each liter.[67] This may need to be considered when treating renal patients.

Metabolic Effects

Researchers continue to debate which calorie source maintains the most favorable protein-sparing effect. Jeejeebhoy et al.[68] reported that the effects of fat emulsions on protein sparing in patients with gastrointestinal disorders were approximately as efficient as those of glucose. It has been postulated that the nitrogen-sparing effect of fat emulsion may be attributable to the glycerol content of the emulsion.[69] In studying thermal injuries and postoperative patients, glucose has been found to be superior to fat in N retention.[70,71] Cerra,[72] however, states that in low stress and early sepsis there is an increased demand for fat that diminishes in late sepsis. Wolfe et al.[73] found no statistical difference between N balance when comparing a regimen of fat emulsion and AA to one of glucose and AA. The protein-sparing effect of fat in hypermetabolic, late septic, and burned patients, and on tissues dependent on anaerobic glycolysis, appears limited.[72,73] It is possible that the extent of stress accompanying a particular disorder may affect which substrate or combination of substrates supports optimum N retention. What is needed is a prospective study comparing isocaloric regimens utilizing lipid and glucose at various stress levels for long enough periods to allow for any adjustment needed.

A common practice is to provide the basal metabolic requirement with dextrose calories, and the remainder of caloric needs with fat. Another method is to supply the nonprotein calories as half glucose and half fat. One should keep in mind that the maximum rate of glucose metabolism ranges from 0.4 to 1.2 g/kg/hr (0.5 g/kg/hr) in average adults,[6,74,75] and that to maximize nutrient utilization the type of substrates supplied should be tailored to the individual's stress-induced metabolic response.[72] At least 100 to 150 g of dextrose are needed to meet requirements of tissues that are obligate glucose users.

Fat emulsions can be used to provide calories in excess of the basal metabolic rate and to allow weight gain. Fat combined with glucose may be more effective as an energy source in patients with low metabolic rates or when alternate metabolic pathways exist.[55,76–79] The ability of the individual patient to clear lipids and the triglyceride level can be used to evaluate the effectiveness of fat as a calorie source, since ability to clear infused lipid varies with clinical conditions.[72] According to manufacturers' guidelines, administered fat should not exceed 60 percent of the total calories or 2.5 to 3.0 g/kg/day in adults, although some clinicians advocate up to 80 percent of calories as fat in peripheral hyperalimentation.[80]

Recent work has pointed to the benefits of fat emulsion in weaning patients from respirators.[81–83] The administration of fat reduces the respiratory quotient and carbon dioxide, in turn lessening the work of breathing. For purposes of weaning, it is recommended that dextrose provide less than 60 percent of calories.

Fat calories may be substituted for glucose calories in patients with impaired glucose tolerance, as in diabetes mellitus, hyperglycemia, hypoinsulinemia, and in patients receiving corticosteroids. In hypersomolar syndromes, where high glucose concentrations lead to excess water losses in urine and hemoconcentration, fat emulsion can be used to provide considerable free water, and to lower the osmolarity of administered fluid. Fat emulsion is a useful component when giving peripheral hyperalimentation because it is isotonic and is a concentrated source of calories.

Fat should be used cautiously in patients with pancreatitis when it is accompanied by hyperlipidemia. Intravenous fat emulsions have been used successfully in acute pancreatitis.[84–86] Triglyceride levels should be checked before and after infusion to assess underlying disorders of lipid metabolism.[87] Lipoprotein lipase in peripheral tissues should be adequate to clear administered fat. To improve fat clearance, concomitant low dose heparin has been used.[57,87,88] However, its efficacy is debatable.[89,90] In patients with hemorrhagic pancreatitis, one must weigh the risks of possible bleeding with the unproven effect of heparin on fat clearance.

The use of fat emulsion is contraindicated in acute pancreatitis if accompanied by hyperlipidemia, hyperchylomicronemia, lipid nephrosis, egg allergy, or bleeding diathesis.

Occasionally, toxic or allergic reactions have occurred in response to fat emulsions. When fat emulsions were composed of cottonseed oil, hepatic, hematologic, and general systemic reactions were reported.[91,92]

Soybean and safflower oils have replaced cottonseed oil in modern emulsions. Occasionally patients report minor phlebitis at the site of the infusion. Febrile reactions have been reported to occur, particularly after initial infusions of emulsions containing phospholipids.[93] Hematologic changes have included mild decreases in platelet count,[94] platelet adhesiveness,[95] and hypercoagulability.[96] Mild elevations in liver function tests[97] and deposition of fat in Kupffer cells[94] commonly occur. Marked hepatic dysfunction may contraindicate lipid infusion.[67] Diminished pulmonary diffusing capacity has been observed.[98] Previously unidentified lipoproteins have been detected after long-term infusion in adults.[99] Elevations in cholesterol, ketone bodies, free fatty acids, and triglycerides have been reported[68] when patients received more than 80 percent of their energy calories as lipids. After therapy was discontinued, however, values returned to normal, and no ill effects were observed.

ALTERNATE ENERGY SOURCES

Although dextrose and fat continue to be the preferred substrates, alternate calorie sources have been used. Nonglucose carbohydrates such as fructose, sorbitol, and xylitol have been used in German medical centers.[74,100] Their structures are shown in Table 18–6. They are converted gradually to glucose in the liver, without dependence on insulin and without blocking lipolysis as does glucose. Because low turnover limits the quantities of nonglucose carbohydrates that can be oxidized, some work has been done using combinations with glucose.[101] Results have shown lower plasma glucose and decreased need for exogenous insulin.

Glycerol

There has been some interest in glycerol as an alternate source of energy calories. The metabolism of each gram produces 4.32 kilocalories. Tissues including the brain, leukocytes, liver, lungs, kidney, and spermatozoa can metabolize glycerol.[102] Although not a carbohydrate, its metabolism is closely linked to that of glucose and fat.[102,103] (See Table 18–6 for its structure.) It is readily convertible into a three-carbon sugar for entry into glycolysis and subsequently to the Krebs cycle, or can be utilized for its gluconeogenic properties, thereby sparing the use of amino acids for this purpose. It serves as an electron carrier from the cytoplasm to mitochondria for oxidative phosphorylation in the production of energy. It also forms the backbone structure for triglycerides. It does not require the presence of insulin for transport across the cell membrane,[103] and at doses of 1 g/kg does not seem to increase insulin secretion, although at higher doses it may, thereby resulting in fatty acid mobilization.

Although it has been used as a pharmacologic agent, only recently has it been investigated as a nutrient source.[104–107] One available product, ProcalAmine, uses glycerol as its energy source. It is listed in Table 18–4.

The manufacturer claims the advantages of this product are that (1) it is more protein sparing than traditional regimens and since glycerol metabolism is independent of insulin, it may be of benefit to patients who cannot utilize glucose; (2) it only requires admixing of multivitamins and trace minerals; (3) 3 liters contain maintenance electrolyte needs; and (4) since glycerol is nonreducing it does not undergo the Maillard reaction, is stable when combined with AA, and can be autoclaved. Although the osmolarity is approximately 735 mosm/liter, the product is designed to be given peripherally because of the protective effect glycerol offers the vessels. Adverse reactions including hemolysis, hemoglobinuria, renal failure, and fatty liver have been reported, but are generally associated with much higher doses of glycerol. In addition, they seem to be associated with subcutaneous and intraperitoneal administration,[103] and have not been reported in clinical trials of ProcalAmine.

Fructose

Fructose has been investigated in liver disease, diabetes mellitus, and postoperative stress. It has protein-sparing effects and its metabolism is partially insulin independent. Because it must first be converted to glucose for utilization by most tissues, because there are limits in the quantities the liver can metabolize, and because it is costly, many have concluded that there is no apparent advantage in its use. If administered rapidly, fructose can lead to acidosis from increased blood lactate levels.[108] It has also been reported to decrease phosphate levels and increase uric acid and bilirubin.[8,74] If used at all, it has been recommended that fructose be given with glucose, since it is not well utilized by the brain.[74]

Sorbitol and Xylitol

Sorbitol and xylitol are sugar alcohols partially dependent on insulin that are metabolized in the liver. They have the same caloric value as monohydrated glucose. Because sorbitol is metabolized to fructose in an intermediate step, and both molecules must be converted to glucose for tissue utilization, they have the same disadvantages as fructose. Adverse effects, possibly caused by osmotic effects on the brain leading to cerebral edema, coma, and death, have been associated with sorbitol when it was used in peritoneal dialysis.[74] Xylitol has been associated with serious changes in liver function.[74]

Ethanol

The metabolism of ethyl alcohol produces 7.1 kcal/g, but it is toxic to liver, brain, and muscle. It is a strong sedative causing inebriation and, therefore, is not recommended for use in parenteral nutrition, especially in patients with cirrhosis, pancreatitis, or pulmonary disease.[7,8,74]

Maltose

IV maltose, which is metabolized, has been used only experimentally in PN. Because serum does not contain maltase, the enzyme that splits maltose into two glucose molecules, it theoretically can be given at high concentrations that avoid the osmotic effects of monosaccharides and at the same time provide double the calories for the same concentration. The use of maltose is undergoing further investigation.

Other disaccharides and polysaccharides are not metabolized.

Medium Chain Triglycerides

As mentioned previously, preliminary work is being done in the area of IV medium chain triglycerides as an alternative to available fat emulsions.[32,51–53] Animal studies have indicated that in periods of high metabolic stress, alterations of fat metabolism occur, increasing the oxidation of short and medium chain triglycerides, which are carnitine independent.[32,109] The medium chain triglyceride emulsions are rapidly cleared from the blood, but do not provide EFA. Although the work is intriguing, it is still limited to animals. Compare the structure of medium chain triglycerides in Table 18–10 to those in Table 18–9. Perhaps a future emulsion will

TABLE 18–10. STRUCTURAL FORMULAS OF MEDIUM CHAIN TRIGLYCERIDES

Name	Number of Carbons	Structural Formula
Caproic acid	6	$CH_3(CH_2)_4COOH$
Caprylic acid	8	$CH_3(CH_2)_6COOH$
Capric acid	10	$CH_3(CH_2)_8COOH$
Lauric acid	12	$CH_3(CH_2)_{10}COOH$

be a combination of medium and long chain triglycerides, containing a balance of both linoleic and linolenic acids, or triglycerides modified to contain both medium and long chain fatty acids.

ELECTROLYTES

Requirements

The six major electrolytes include sodium, potassium, chloride, calcium, phosphate (not phosphorus), and magnesium. When considering electrolyte needs of individuals, one can look at ranges that will approximate basal needs (Table 18–11) or base daily needs on laboratory values (Table 18–12). Requirements for fluid and electrolytes are discussed in detail in Chapter 12.

Sodium is the main extracellular cation and the principal electrolyte of PN. Sodium status parallels fluid status. Variations from normal requirements may occur in bowel, pancreatic, or biliary fistulas, diarrhea, vomiting, fever, or in renal, liver, and cardiac failure. Potassium is the major intracellular cation. Increased potassium is required during anabolism, refeeding, in instances of high insulin levels, and when urinary conservation of potassium is poor. The major anion is chloride. In the normal situation where acidosis is not present, chloride is added in a 1:1 ratio with sodium.[54]

Calcium and phosphate are included, often in a 1:2 ratio.[30] Phosphate is required for energy transport and bone formation. Conser-

TABLE 18–11. NORMAL RANGE OF DAILY ELECTROLYTE REQUIREMENTS FOR ADULTS

Electrolyte	RDA[a]	Parsa[b]	Shils[c]	Grant[d]	Silberman, Eisenberg[e]	Halberg[f] (Moderate allowance per kilogram body weight)
Sodium, mEq	45–145	125	≥60	60–150	100–300 (typical)	2–3 mg
Potassium, mEq	45–145	100	≥60	70–150	50–150 (typical) 120–160[g] 5–6/g nitrogen[h]	2 mg
Chloride, mEq	45–145	209–229	—	Equal to sodium	100–300 (typical)	2–3 mg
Calcium, mEq	40 (800 mg)	4–6	200–400 mg	0.2–0.3/kg	0.25 (5 mg)/kg[i]	0.15 mg
Phosphate, mmol	25.5 (800 mg)	40–60/mEq	300–400 mg	7–10/1000 kcal	8–14 (15–25 mEq)/1000 kcal[i]	0.4 mg
Magnesium, mEq	Males: 29 (350 mg) Females: 25 (300 mg)	10	8–10	0.35–0.45/kg	2/g nitrogen[h]	0.15–0.2 mg
Acetate, mEq	—	25	—	—	—	—
Gluconate, mEq	—	4–6	—	As calcium gluconate	—	—
Sulfate, mEq	—	10	As methionine	As magnesium sulfate	—	
Iron, mg	Males: 10 Menstruating females: 18	—	Males: 1 Menstruating females: 2			1 µg

[a]RDA, 9 ed. Washington, D.C.: National Academy of Sciences, 1980.[24]

[b]Parsa, M. H. et al: Nutrition in the superior vena cava with a solution of crystalline L-amino acids and hypertonic dextrose. Scientific exhibit presented at the Annual Convention of the Medical Society of the State of New York, February, 1971.

[c]Shils, M. E.: Parenteral Nutrition. In Goodhart, R.S. (eds): Modern Nutrition in Health and Disease, 6 ed. Philadelphia: Lea & Febiger, 1980, p. 1141.[8]

[d]Grant, J. P.: Handbook of Total Parenteral Nutrition. Philadelphia: W.B. Saunders, 1980, p. 98.[110]

[e]Silberman, H., Eisenberg, D. Parenteral and Enteral Nutrition for the Hospitalized Patient, Norwalk, Conn., Appleton-Century-Crofts, 1983, pp. 68–71.[67]

[f]Data from Halberg, D.: Nutr. Supp. Serv. 2(7): 15–23, 1982.

[g]Data from Sheldon, G. F., Kudsk, K. A.: Electrolyte requirements in total parenteral nutrition, In Deitel, M. (ed): Nutrition in Clinical Surgery. Baltimore, Williams & Wilkins, 1980, pp. 103–111.

[h]Data from Lee, H. A., Hartley, T. F.: Postgrad. Med. J. 51:441–445, 1975.

[i]Data from Wittine, M. F., Freeman, J. B.: JPEN 1:152–155, 1977.

[j]Data from Sheldon, G. F., Grzyb, S.: Ann. Surg. 182:683–689, 1975.

TABLE 18–12. SCHEDULE OF ADDITIVES TO THE AMINO ACID SOLUTION[a]

Lab Values	For 1 Bottle Daily	For 2 Bottles Daily	For 3 Bottles Daily
Potassium			
Below 3.5	80 mEq/bottle	40 mEq/bottle	30 mEq/bottle
3.5–3.9	40 mEq/bottle	20 mEq/bottle	Same as Above
4.0–4.8	20 mEq/bottle	10 mEq/bottle	10 mEq/bottle
Above 4.8	None	None	None
Sodium			
Below 136	50–100 mEq/bottle	25–50 mEq/bottle	25–50 mEq/bottle
136–142	25–50 mEq/bottle	15–25 mEq/bottle	15–25 mEq/bottle
Above 142	None	None	None
Chloride			
Below 98	90–100 mEq/bottle	40–50 mEq/bottle	40–50 mEq/bottle
98–100	40–50 mEq/bottle	20–25 mEq/bottle	20–25 mEq/bottle
101–104	20–25 mEq/bottle	10–15 mEq/bottle	10–15 mEq/bottle
Above 104	None	None	None
Calcium			
(Calcium gluconate 1 amp = 4.5 mEq)			
7.0–7.9	9 mEq/bottle	6.75 mEq/bottle	4.5 mEq/bottle
8.0–10.5	4.5 mEq/bottle	4.5 mEq/bottle	4.5 mEq/bottle
Above 10.5	None	None	None
Phosphorus			
Below 2.5	15–30 mm/bottle	15–22.5 mm/bottle	15 mm/bottle
2.5–3.5	15 mm/bottle	7.5–15 mm/bottle	7.5 mm/bottle
Above 3.5	None	None	None
Glucose			
Below 280	None	None	None
	(Unless it stays close to 280 for 2 days; then add 10 U/bottle)		
280–349	10 U reg Ins/bottle	10 U reg Ins/bottle	10 U reg Ins/bottle
Above 350	15 U reg Ins/bottle	15 U reg Ins/bottle	15 U reg Ins/bottle
Magnesium sulfate	8.1 mEq every day		
Iron	2 mg daily		

[a]After The American Journal of Intravenous Therapy and Clinical Nutrition 6(4):25, 1979.

vation of phosphate is generally efficient, but losses of calcium and phosphate in diarrhea can be large. Large calcium losses result in additional phosphate losses via a secondary hyperparathyroidism.

Magnesium is necessary for normal neuromuscular and central nervous activity. Deficits cause symptoms similar to those associated with hypocalcemia. The major pathway for excretion is the feces and the remainder is excreted through the urine, although the kidneys are able to conserve magnesium.

Electrolyte Stability

Sodium, potassium, and chloride appear to be compatible with AA and dextrose at all concentrations and are stable 1 month after preparation. Sodium and potassium are frequently provided as chloride salts although they are available as phosphates or acetates. Sodium lactate or bicarbonate should not be used. Sodium requirements are based on maintenance needs, presence of deficits, and ongoing losses,[7] and are closely related to fluid status and fluid needs. To avoid acid–base disturbances, the ratio of sodium to chloride is usually kept at approximately 1:1.[54]

Potassium, phosphate, and magnesium requirements are closely related to nitrogen and calorie needs. Potassium requirements parallel glucose administration and anabolism, which create intracellular shifts in potassium, phosphate, and magnesium. When high concentrations of dextrose are used, and in refeeding malnourished patients, needs of these electrolytes are increased and extracellular fluid deficiencies are not uncommon.

When chloride load is excessive and hyperchloremic acidosis results,[6] the acid component, chloride, is usually reduced or eliminated, and replaced by a buffer such as acetate. In liver disease, it may be necessary to avoid giving acetates and lactates.[110]

Although bicarbonate is a buffer, it is not used in parenteral solutions because it may liberate carbon dioxide gas in a volatile reaction and may lead to the precipitation of calcium or magnesium carbonates.[8,111,112] Instead, the precursor of bicarbonate, acetate, is given.

Both calcium and phosphate should be provided in hyperalimentation solutions, since phosphate given without calcium can lead to tetany.[6] The presence of both ions, however, can create a precipitate. Curves for the precipitate have been published.[113] No precipitate of calcium phosphate occurs at 4.7 mEq/L, and the concentration of calcium may be as high as 15 mEq with up to 10 mmol of phosphate per liter without exceeding solubility.[110] By adding calcium to the phosphate slowly, mixing in proper order, and adding strong reagents last (i.e., phosphate should be added to the solution prior to the calcium and mixed thoroughly before

adding calcium), one can avoid generating the precipitate.[110] Calcium should be well diluted before mixing. Both AA and dextrose lower the pH and result in greater calcium phosphate solubility. Since dissociation of calcium salts increases at higher temperatures, more calcium phosphate forms and precipitates. This problem can be avoided by following the above recommendations; by adding the calcium to the glucose, and the phosphate to the AA components, before mixing the glucose with the AA; or by adding daily dosages to separate containers.[112]

Calcium is generally given as gluconate, gluceptate, glucoheptonate, or chloride. Because the chloride salt dissociates readily, liberating more calcium ion for the undesirable reaction with phosphate, it is a less desirable form of calcium to use in parenteral solutions. Typical maintenance requirements of calcium have not been difficult to administer. For cases in which calcium needs are increased, careful adjustment of the prescription is needed.[112]

Phosphate may be given as potassium or sodium phosphate. Since inorganic phosphorus is lethal, phosphorus is always provided as organic phosphate. Phosphate requirements are increased during anabolism. Because phosphate is not accurately represented in terms of milliequivalents, it is quantified in millimoles.

Magnesium sulfate may be given IV or intramuscularly. It is compatible in concentrations up to 12 mEq/L, but if present with calcium as a chloride salt, calcium sulfate may precipitate.[110]

Numerous maintenance electrolyte preparations are available to decrease the time a pharmacist spends mixing the parenteral solution. Several AA solutions containing maintenance electrolytes are now available. These may be of benefit in a setting where the volume of parenteral solutions required is low, where facilities or staff available for admixing solutions are limited, or in instances where a patient's electrolyte requirements have stabilized.

MICRONUTRIENTS

Requirements

Micronutrients, which include trace minerals and vitamins, are discussed in detail in Chapter 11. (See Tables 18–13 and 18–14 for requirements of each respective group.) Ranges of recommended daily dosages for trace minerals (Table 18–13) and vitamins (Table 18–14) have been published by the Nutrition Advisory Group of the American Medical Association (AMA).[114,115] Parenteral and enteral needs for vitamins and minerals are not identical. In cases of inefficient intestinal absorption, as with minerals such as calcium and iron, the parenteral requirement is lower. This is because the IV route bypasses the gut, and will therefore be more efficient. In other cases, intestinal absorption may be the more efficient. If water-soluble vitamins are administered rapidly, they may be lost through renal excretion.[116] For this reason, and because hypermetabolic and anabolic states may cause increased demands for vitamins, recommendations are increased for water-soluble vitamins.

In many cases there is a lack of medical knowledge regarding IV requirements, so the recommended daily parenteral requirement is projected based on the Recommended Dietary Allowances (RDA)[24] with an allowance for safety factors.[100] It should be remembered that the RDA are guidelines for dietary intakes of populations comprised of normal individuals, and the needs of malnourished and hypermetabolic individuals may be different. Until more data are available on the needs of special groups of individuals, the AMA recommendations should serve as a guideline.

Trace Minerals

Supplementation of iron is highly controversial because critically ill patients may not respond to iron supplementation, and because high serum levels of iron may increase susceptibility to and severity of infection.[67] Iron is generally given to stable patients as iron dextran and is compatible with parenteral solutions. Although other electrolytes are stable in dextrose and AA for up to 1

TABLE 18–13. INTRAVENOUS TRACE MINERAL PREPARATIONS

	Daily Intravenous Requirements for Adults[a]	Patramin 6-A (1 ml)[b]	IMS[c]	M.T.E.-4 (3 ml)[d]	M.T.E.-Concentrated (1 ml)[d]	Trace Metals Additive (5 ml)[e]
Zinc (mg/d)	2.5–4.0[f]	1.5	4.0	1.0	5.0	4.0
Copper (mg/d)	0.5–1.5	0.5	1.0	0.4	1.0	1.0
Chromium (μg/d)	10–15	5.0	10.0	4.0	10.0	10.0
Manganese (mg/d)	0.15–0.8	0.2	0.5	0.1	0.5	0.8
Selenium (μg/d)	—	25.0	—	—	—	—
Iodide (μg/d)	—	28.0	—	—	—	—

[a]AMA Department of Foods and Nutrition, 1979.
[b]Pent Cal, Inc., Allston, MA.
[c]International Medication Systems, South El Monte, CA.
[d]Lypho-Med, Inc.
[e]Abbott Laboratories.
[f]Add 2.0 mg for catabolism, 12.2 mg/L small bowel fluid loss, 17.1 mg/kg stool loss.

TABLE 18–14. INTRAVENOUS MULTIVITAMIN PREPARATIONS

	AMA/NAG Guidelines for Daily Requirements[a]	Ascot MVC Plus[b]	Berocca-C[c]	Berocca-PN[c]	Multivitamin Concentrate[d]	M.V.C. 9 + 3[d]	MVI[e]	MVI-12[e]	Solu-B-Forte[f]
Ascorbic acid (mg)	100	100	100	100	500	100	500	100	100
Vitamin A (I.U.)	3300	3300	—	3300	10,000	3300	10,000	3300	—
Vitamin D (I.U.)	200	200	—	200	1000	200	1000	200	—
Thiamin (B$_1$) (mg)	3	3	10	3	50	3	50	3	250
Riboflavin (B$_2$) (mg)	3.6	3.6	10	3.6	10	3.6	10	3.6	50
Pyridoxine (B$_6$) (mg)	4	4	20	4	15	4	15	4	50
Niacin (mg)	40	40	80	40	100	40	100	40	1250
Pantothenic acid (mg)	15	15	20	15	25	15	25	15	500
Vitamin E (I.U.)	10	10	—	10	5	10	5	10	—
d-Biotin (µg)	60	60	2000	60	—	60	—	60	—
Folic acid (µg)	400	400	—	400	—	400	—	400	—
Cyanocobalamin (B$_{12}$) (µg)	5	5	—	5	—	5	—	5	—

[a] AMA Department of Foods and Nutrition Multivitamins for Parenteral Use. A Statement by the Nutrition Advisory Group. JAMA 3(4): 258–262, 1979.
[b] Ascot Pharmaceuticals, Inc.
[c] Roche Laboratories.
[d] Lypho-Med, Inc.
[e] USV Laboratories.
[f] The Upjohn Company.

month, iron is generally added no more than 48 hours before use.

Several multiple and single dose trace minerals are available. Several trace minerals are now available as single doses of separate elements. Dosages are generally based on the AMA guidelines.[114] (See Table 18–13 for comparisons of available products and recommended dosages.) The most convenient form to use is a multiple trace metal mixture containing zinc, chromium, copper, and manganese. These mixtures contain fixed dosages, however, and in certain conditions additional trace metals may be needed to offset deficits or losses, as in the case of GI fistulas and zinc. Here the individual doses may be useful. Experience with home parenteral nutrition has elicited information regarding other trace mineral deficiencies. As a result of this work, selenium and molybdenum are now available as individual agents for patients on long-term parenteral therapy. A new mixture containing selenium has just become available and is included in Table 18–13.

Vitamins

To avoid accidental omission of a single vitamin, maintenance doses of parenteral vitamins should be based on the AMA Nutrition Advisory Group statement on IV multivitamin requirements.[115,116] As with trace minerals, IV requirements may differ from enteral requirements. Because of the heavy reliance on glucose for energy in parenteral nutrition, thiamine requirements are high.[116] Since the guidelines were published, several multivitamin preparations that conform to the recommendations have become available. (Refer to Table 18–14.) In addition, individual vitamins may be increased as needed through the use of single doses of separate vitamins.

Specific vitamins are frequently left out of preparations. These are biotin, folate, B_{12}, and K. Normally, biotin is produced by bacteria in the GI tract. When the intestine is not utilized or when normal flora is altered as in

the case of drug therapy, or is diseased or shortened, there may be a need for biotin supplementation.[116] The vitamin supplements that conform to the AMA guidelines contain biotin, folate, and B_{12}. Controversy exists, however, regarding the addition of vitamin K to parenteral solutions. Manufacturers state that some vitamins may react with vitamin K bisulfite. Allergic reactions involving hives, itching, and cardiac effects including palpitations and blood pressure changes have been reported after IV infusion of vitamin K. To prevent complications of therapy, it should not be given to patients receiving anticoagulation from coumadin-type drugs. Instead, vitamin K is typically given intramuscularly on a specified schedule; usually 2 to 4 mg once weekly will maintain a normal prothrombin,[116] although some institutions allow water-soluble phytonadione to be added to parenteral mixtures.

Stability

Dextrose in water is a stable solution. When amino acids are added the mixture is stable, if not exposed to light or heat, for 6 months. When electrolytes and minerals are added the solution is stable for 3 weeks, but it should be refrigerated at 3 to 4°C up to 48 hours before use.

Vitamins lose potency once added to parenteral solutions and, therefore, should be added no more than 48 hours prior to anticipated use. To minimize loss of potency, solutions should be stored at 4°C once multivitamins are added, and exposure to light minimized. Vitamins A and C are lost on exposure to light and room temperature. Riboflavin, thiamine, and vitamin D are also light sensitive. The presence of calcium may reduce the availability of folate by causing it to precipitate.

Vitamin C, an antioxidant, may form a precipitate with minerals when it is present in large quantities. Some of the trace minerals, such as iron, copper, and selenium, exist in several oxidation states. The presence of an oxidizing agent such as ascorbic acid may result in a precipitate if the concentrations of the ascorbate are high, causing a low pH. This can be avoided by ordering electrolytes, minerals, and vitamins specified as total amounts needed daily rather than amounts per liter. This allows the pharmacist to avoid mixing incompatible substances in the same bottle.

Vitamin C may inactivate vitamins B_{12} and K. Vitamins B_{12} and K may inactivate one another and, therefore, these vitamins are given in separate infusions. Vitamin K is usually given intramuscularly, although some institutions add phytonadione (water-soluble vitamin K) to the parenteral solution once or twice weekly.

OTHER ADDITIVES

Insulin

Additions other than nutrients are occasionally made to hyperalimentation solutions. Regular insulin may be needed by diabetic or highly stressed individuals. Regular insulin is used rather than long-acting insulin to avoid complications should the dextrose infusion be interrupted. Acute rises in blood sugar can be treated by IV or intramuscular insulin, but once maintenance insulin needs are defined, insulin can be admixed with the solution in the pharmacy. It is practical to begin with a sliding scale. When insulin requirements are stable, the insulin can then be added to the nutrient mixture. It is preferable to add the insulin to the solution rather than to hang a concomitant drip so that any deviation from a constant infusion rate will affect both the dextrose and insulin components.

Heparin

Heparin is frequently added to parenteral nutrition solutions to prevent fibrin sheath formation on the catheter, which may lead to venous thrombosis, or to facilitate the clearance of fat from the bloodstream during the infusion of lipid. One study found that 1000 units per liter did not eradicate formation of the fibrin sleeve.[117] Another recommendation is that 6000 U/day be divided evenly among the patient's bottles.[26,118] (Refer to the previous discussion on the effect of heparin on fat clearance under Metabolic Effects.)

ADDITIVE COMPATIBILITIES OF TPN

Physical Versus Chemical Compatibility

In formulating solutions consideration must be given to compatibility of each component. Incompatibilities may be classified as either physical or chemical. Those reactions considered physical include formation of precipitates, gas, or turbidity. They can be observed by examining the solution against a dark or light background. Solutions that are physically compatible may not be chemically compatible. Detection of chemical compatibilities may necessitate special instrumentation to assess solubility,[119] as opposed to the simple observation required to assess physical compatibility. For example, chromatography is often used to test chemical compatibility. Physical incompatibilities indicate instability while chemical incompatibilities indicate alterations in potency and possibly the production of toxins.[119] Factors that influence compatibility include temperature, pH, acid–base characteristics of additives, oxidation–reduction potentials, concentrations of additives (including dextrose and amino acids), order of mixing, and exposure to light.

The variety of nutrients and drugs in parenteral solutions creates the potential for multiple incompatibilities. Caution must be exercised when composing solutions.

Nutrient–Nutrient Compatibility

Electrolyte and Trace Mineral Compatibility. Refer to the general discussion regarding oxidation states and precipitates under Stability. Calcium and phosphate deserve special consideration. Problems with these ions have been discussed earlier in this chapter under Electrolytes. The lower the pH of the solution, the more calcium and phosphate can be added. Some AA solutions have a high pH, limiting the amount of these ions that can be admixed. (Refer to Tables 18–3 and 18–4 for pH differences in presently available solutions.)

Bicarbonate is omitted from parenteral solutions to avoid evolution of carbon dioxide gas and possible infusion of air embolus. Instead, when a patient becomes acidotic, chlorides and phosphates are limited and replaced with corresponding acetates.

Vitamin Compatibility. The vitamins that may create compatibility problems include A, C, B_{12}, K, and folate. Please refer to the previous section on Micronutrients for a discussion.

Fat Emulsion Compatibility. Fat emulsions are generally infused by piggybacking or through a Y-connector just above the infusion site but below the filter. This is to avoid disturbing the stability of the emulsion and to minimize the exposure of electrolytes, divalent cations, and nutrients.[113] The diameter of particles in fat emulsions is approximately 0.4 to 0.5 microns. Most filters screen particles larger than 0.22 microns. The larger size of the fat particles would clog the filter, so lipids should not be filtered. Acidic solutions are most likely to crack the fat emulsion causing fat globules to aggregate, which if infused, could cause fat embolus. Fat has been shown to support microbial growth more quickly than other parenteral nutrients, making maintenance of sterility an important factor.[120,121] One study found no difference between the fat source of the emulsion or the concentration of fat in ability to support growth[122] of five gram-negative, four gram-positive, or one yeast-type, for up to 48 hours.

The only drug that is currently approved for addition directly to fat emulsion is heparin. Heparin is thought to potentiate the clearance of fat from the bloodstream.[57,88] According to a manufacturer, 2 units of heparin is stable in fat emulsion for 48 hours both at room temperature and at 4°C.

Calcium gluconate is incompatible with fat emulsions in levels greater than 2 mg. Manufacturers do not recommend the addition of multivitamins. Ascorbate has been found to be incompatible after 48 hours at room temperature. Nondextrose carbohydrates appear to be stable in fat emulsions.[123]

Three-in-One Mixtures

Preliminary research is being conducted to study the stability of fat, amino acids, and dextrose when mixed together. Equal volumes of 50 percent dextrose and 8.5 percent AA have been found to be stable for 48 hours both at room temperature and at 4°C when added to fat emulsion.[112]

Several manufacturers are marketing 2- and 3-liter containers for the purpose of combining all three components, but many questions of compatibility and stability still exist. At the time of this writing two manufacturers are marketing this product in the United States, although mixing all three components has been a more common practice in Europe.[124–126] As more experience is gained, and stability improves, this will likely change. The product has particular advantages for home patients. Manufacturers currently advise which lipids and which amino acids are compatible in which containers.

Although the interactions that occur are complex and poorly understood, early studies indicated that when dextrose was added to fat emulsion the pH decreased, causing the lecithin emulsion to deteriorate.[127,128] The result was the formation of coalesced oil globules. One group has recommended that fat be added last to prevent this aggregation of fat.[129] When AA were added to the dextrose-lipid combination, a buffering effect was noted, allowing the emulsion to remain stable for a longer period. Observations also noted that divalent cations such as calcium and magnesium caused immediate flocculation of the lipid, and that this effect was delayed by the presence of AA. Monovalent cations were noted to increase the rate of globule coalescence, but small amounts could be added, and their effect predicted based on regression analysis. Small numbers of clinical applications, all successful, have been reported in the United States.[124,130–132] Not all products appear to be compatible with the lipids.[133] This may be due to the low pH of certain AA solutions, electrolytes, or the interaction of the entire system, causing an oiling out or droplet coalescence. According to manufacturers, three-in-one solutions should be used within 24 hours after mixing.

Drug–Nutrient Compatibility

In patients with limited access or fluid restriction, questions are often raised as to the admixing of drugs with the parenteral solutions. Except for certain drugs, protocols generally do not allow this practice. Protocols generally discourage piggybacking technique as this is considered a line violation that increases the likelihood of infection. Occasionally the situation is avoided by placing a triple lumen catheter. This may not be a viable alternative, however, when infusing incompatible substances.

Insulin. Regular insulin is frequently added to TPN solutions. However, it demonstrates nonspecific surface binding to glass, polyvinyl chloride, and inline filters[134,135] as well as to albumin and AA,[136] making it difficult to determine the quantity of the insulin available to the patient. Adsorption is greater at lower concentrations of insulin,[137] which may be related to saturation of adsorption sites. More insulin is lost after the addition of electrolytes, minerals, and vitamins.[138] The amount of insulin available has been reported to be 53 to 100 percent.[138,139] Because of this large variability, possibly caused by dose-dependent adsorption to binding sites, it may be necessary to provide extra insulin. Good mixing of the TPN solution is necessary to prevent physical separation of insulin from the solution.[112] The quantity of IV insulin to deliver is determined by the serum glucose, while additional subcutaneous requirements are based on fractional urines every 4 to 6 hours.[8] Insulin is not stable in the presence of sodium bicarbonate.[138–140]

Heparin. Heparin may be added to parenteral solutions to enhance lipid clearance[57,88] and to prevent fibrin sheath formation on the catheter.[118] As with insulin, heparin adheres to tubing and glass and can be inactivated by ascorbate or vitamins K and B_{12}.[112,136]

Cimetidine. Cimetidine is compatible with parenteral solutions and is frequently given to postsurgical patients.[111,141,142] Crystalline AA stimulate gastric acid secretion particularly when PN is initiated,[67] creating another potential use for cimetidine. Circulating lipid seems to inhibit this secretory response.

Albumin. Albumin seems to be stable and effective for 24 hours[140] when added in limited quantities to hyperalimentation solutions.[110] It is usually added to maintain colloid pressure so that amino acids will be utilized for tissue protein synthesis rather than albumin synthesis.[64] Suggested dosages based on compatibility are 50 ml of 25 percent albumin in 1 liter of 25 percent dextrose and 3.5 percent amino acids[113] or up to 35.5 g of albumin per liter of hyperalimentation solution.[110] Albumin can pass through a 0.2-micron filter, but other particulate matter can clog filters, making an infusion pump necessary.[26] Albumin may decrease adherence of insulin to plastic, but the cost of albumin precludes it as a common additive to parenteral solutions. Although albumin contains trace elements, the amounts are negligible,[143] and it should not be considered a source of protein or trace minerals.

Hydrocortisone. Sodium hydrocortisone is physically and chemically stable in AA solutions.[110,112,119] It is often added to parenteral solutions of patients who require bowel rest because of exacerbation of inflammatory bowel disease.

Antibiotics. Because of the potential for chemical and physical incompatibilities between various antibiotics and parenteral mixtures, it is wise to avoid admixing. An antibiotic may interact in multiple ways depending on its family. Antibiotics may bind with proteins or form insoluble salts with calcium and magnesium. Penicillins are degraded by nonprotonated N fractions in the AA solution.[112] Tetracycline, by contrast, is not affected by N, but may form insoluble complexes with calcium and magnesium ions at neutral pH.[112] Sodium cefazolin and sodium cephalothin are incompatible with multivitamins in parenteral solutions.

When problems of allowed fluid volume and limited access make it difficult to avoid admixing, one should look at literature specifying the compatibility of individual drugs with TPN solutions. Several resources are available including *Handbook on Injectable Drugs*[111] and *Guide to Parenteral Admixtures,*[113] in addition to several journal articles.[119,144,145]

Chemotherapeutic Agents. Recently published research has shown the chemotherapeutic agent 5-fluorcuracil to be compatible with TPN solutions.[146] No precipitates, color changes, or pH changes have been noted. This allows the delivery of chemotherapy without interruption of IV nutrition support. Some practitioners who work with cancer patients have expressed enthusiasm for concomitant nutrition and chemotherapy. A double or triple lumen catheter is the typical means used in this situation to prevent mixing of the drug and nutrient solution before delivery into the bloodstream, where rapid dilution occurs. More research remains to be completed in this area. As with other drugs, evaluation of both physical and chemical compatibility with TPN solutions must be studied with individual drugs. This should be done as a trial prior to delivering the mixture to the patient.

COMPATIBILITY EFFECTS OF THE INFUSION SYSTEM

The infusion system consists of a glass or plastic container and plastic tubing. The material chosen for delivery of parenteral solutions affects the availability of nutrients. Glass containers are impervious to air and gas and provide a truly closed system. Glass containers may be associated with more particulate matter, however, particularly in shipping and agitation.[147] They also have greater mass and are more easily broken than is plastic.

Plastic bags have been associated with both higher and lower frequency of contamination[135] than glass, perhaps because of the technique of admixing and the separate entry port that houses the administration set in a closed compartment. Plastic, whether polyvinyl chloride or polypropylene, provides a tight seal, but it is not hermetically closed as it is permeable to moisture.[148] Because plastic is not rigid, there is an increased potential for bacterial entry when the wall of the container is accidentally punctured during admixture.

The diffusion of toxic stabilizers and plasticizers such as di-2-ethylhexylphthalate (DEHP) into parenteral solutions has been investigated.[135] Much of the literature concerns blood and hemodialysis equipment and, therefore, does not directly apply to parenteral nutrition. However, polyvinyl chloride (PVC) IV tubing does contain DEHP, which is somewhat lipid soluble. Fat-soluble vitamins are known to act as surfactants and leach out DEHP. Vitamin A readily adsorbs to polysorbate 80, a stabilizer added to various components of the nutrient solution.[149] DEHP has been detected in the serum of patients who received blood that was stored in PVC bags and in dialysis patients who were dialyzed utilizing PVC tubing.[67] The long-term use of PN by home patients is cause for concern because of problems potentially caused by DEHP. IV tubing not containing DEHP is available through Cutter Laboratories for use with Intralipid.

The potential risks and benefits of plastic versus glass containers need to be weighed by the clinician. Justifications can be made for either case. Glass containers that come in 1-liter volumes are frequently preferred for hospital use, whereas plastic bags that come in 2- and 3-liter volumes are often selected for convenience of the home patient who may receive a cycled infusion at night.

COMPOSING THE TPN ORDER

Peripheral Versus Central TPN

The composition of the parenteral solution will depend on whether it is to be delivered via central or peripheral routes. The anticipated length of therapy, the assessment of fluid requirements, caloric and protein requirements, and nonprotein calorie to nitrogen ratio for optimal nitrogen utilization, and the decision to provide energy calories primarily as dextrose or fat are all factors that will influence the route chosen.

Osmolarity and potassium concentration of the solution, as well as the condition of the patient's veins, are limiting factors in peripheral hyperalimentation. Osmolarity is a useful clinical concept described by Deardorff.[150] Osmolarity, the number of small particles which contribute an osmotic load, should not exceed 600 mosm/L in peripheral parenteral solutions.[151] Hypertonic solutions, those with greater than 300 mosm/L of solution, are irritating to vessels and contribute to phlebitis. Potassium is an extremely caustic agent and its concentration therefore should not exceed 60 mEq/L.[26,151] AA, dextrose, electrolytes, trace minerals, and vitamins are osmotically active, with AA and glucose contributing the most to the final osmolarity of the solution. For this reason peripheral solutions are composed of 3.5 to 5 percent AA and 5 to 10 percent dextrose. To compensate for a low dextrose concentration, and therefore for fewer calories, lipid is frequently incorporated, forming what is called the lipid system. Lipid is isotonic and can be given peripherally.

Osmolarity and osmolality are frequently confused terms.[150] As mentioned above, osmolarity is a clinical tool, and is based on osmotically active particles per unit volume of solution. It is possible to estimate the osmolarity of a parenteral solution by following the method in Table 18–15. Osmolality is a more precise term that is based on osmotically active particles per mass of solution. Osmolality takes into account freezing point depression, boiling point elevation, and

---

TABLE 18–15. APPROXIMATING OSMOLARITY

To calculate osmolarity:
1. Sum total mEq/L of all electrolytes (Na, K) excluding those not prescribed in mEq (i.e., trace minerals):   _____ mEq × 2 = _____ mosm
   Multiply by 2 to account for anions (i.e., Cl^-, $PO_4^=$, acetate).
2. Calculate grams dextrose in each liter: _____ g × 5 = _____ mosm
   _____% dextrose × 1000 cc/L = _____ g dextrose.
   Multiply by 5.
3. Calculate grams amino acids in each liter: _____ g × 10 = _____ mosm
   _____% amino acids × 1000 cc/L = _____ g amino acids.
   Multiply by 10.
4. Sum steps 1–3 to arrive at total mosm/L.   Total = _____ mosm

intermolecular forces, i.e., phenomena that must be measured in a laboratory. Osmolality, therefore, is of little practical use for the clinician.

Fat emulsions, since they provide free water and are isotonic, may be infused through a Y-connector or piggybacked to decrease the osmolarity of the infusion.

In central hyperalimentation, osmolarity is not of concern. Solutions can be infused into the superior vena cava with concentrations much greater than the osmolarity of serum, because the rate of blood flow causes rapid dilution.[30] Final dextrose concentrations of the parenteral nutrient solution may approach 45 percent in renal failure and liver failure when allowed infusion volume is restricted. With AA and electrolytes, total osmolarity approaches 2500 mosm/L. More common dextrose concentrations range from 15 to 25 percent per liter.

Fluid Replacement

In composing the TPN order, one should first take into account the fluid requirement or restriction.[152-156] The calorie and protein needs are then calculated as percent solution in the allowed fluid. There are different ways to calculate an individual's fluid needs, as discussed in Chapter 12, but an average estimate of daily water requirements for an adult is 35 ml/kg.[30] It may be wise to start with 1 to 2 liters in the first 24 hours, limiting the solution to a 10 or 15 percent dextrose concentration. Maintaining a constant rate of delivery is essential to prevent drastic changes in blood glucose. The dextrose concentration may be increased daily as monitoring shows tolerance, allowing 3 to 5 days for the patient to achieve nutrient requirements. If the infusion is interrupted suddenly, i.e., in the event a bottle breaks or a patient is taken to surgery, 10 percent dextrose in water should be infused to prevent hypoglycemia and insulin shock. At the conclusion of parenteral nutrition therapy, dextrose load should be decreased or tapered gradually over several days as a precaution.

In home patients, the approach differs as the dextrose load is decreased quite rapidly by slowing the rate over the last 1 to 2 hours of the infusion.

Electrolyte Replacement

Electrolytes can be ordered one of two ways, either on a per day basis or on a per volume (per liter) basis. When ordered on a per day basis, the pharmacist has flexibility to separate into different bottles those additives that are not compatible. An example would be calcium and phosphate, as discussed previously in this chapter. Refer to the TPN order sheet in Chapter 17 and to the previous discussions of stability and additive compatibility.

Administering Fat Emulsion

Fat emulsions are usually infused over 6 to 10 hours. The infusion rate should be less than 1 g of fat per kg per 4 hours. Too rapid an infusion can result in fluid or fat overload, leading to decreased electrolyte concentrations, congestion, pulmonary edema, decreased diffusion, or metabolic acidosis. Unlike the glucose component, lipid infusion may be stopped without tapering, with no ill effects. As mentioned, fat should not contribute more than 60 percent of the total calories.

MIXING PROCEDURES

Although mixing is generally of concern for the pharmacist, it is helpful for other members of the nutrition support team to understand some basic considerations in mixing and to appreciate the contribution the pharmacist makes.

Pharmacist Role

Whatever method of compounding is used, it is necessary to have personnel trained in aseptic technique who have expertise in physical and chemical compatibility, incompatibility potentials of components, proper storage and handling of solutions, and sta-

TABLE 18–16. DERIVING FINAL CONCENTRATIONS OF PARENTERAL SOLUTIONS

Graphically	Mathematically

A. Original Concentrations:	A. 1. Calculate total grams amino acids and dextrose:
	   a. 500 cc × 10% amino acid concentration = 50 g amino acids
	   b. 500 cc × 50% dextrose concentration = 250 g dextrose
	  2. Calculate volume of final solution (neglect additives):
	   500 cc amino acids + 500 cc dextrose = 1000 cc
	  3. Calculate final concentrations amino acids and dextrose:
	   a. 50 g amino acids ÷ 1000 cc = .05 g/cc = 5%
	   b. 250 g dextrose ÷ 1000 cc = .25 g/cc = 25%

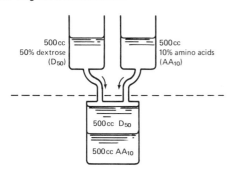

Final Concentration: 1000 cc D_{25} AA_5

Graphically	Mathematically

B. Original Concentrations:	B. 1. Total grams amino acids and dextrose:
	   a. 300 cc × 5% amino acids = 15 g amino acids
	   b. 500 cc × 70% dextrose = 350 g dextrose
	  2. Final volume of solution:
	   300 cc amino acids + 500 cc dextrose = 800 cc
	  3. Final concentrations amino acids and dextrose:
	   a. 15 g amino acids ÷ 800 cc = .019 g/cc = 1.9% amino acids
	   b. 350 g dextrose ÷ 800 cc = 0.438 g/cc = 44% dextrose

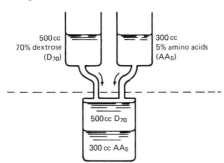

Final Concentration: D_{44} $AA_{1.9}$

Graphically	Mathematically

C. Original Concentrations:	C. 1. Total grams amino acids and dextrose:
	   a. 750 cc × 6.9% amino acids = 51.75 g amino acids
	   b. 250 cc × 75% dextrose = 187.5 g dextrose
	  2. Final volume of solution:
	   750 cc amino acids + 250 cc dextrose = 1000 cc
	  3. Final concentrations amino acids and dextrose:
	   a. 51.75 g amino acids ÷ 1000 cc = .052 g/cc = 5.2% amino acids
	   b. 187.5 g dextrose ÷ 1000 cc = .188 g/cc = 19% dextrose

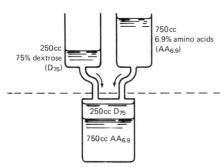

Final Concentration: D_{19} $AA_{5.2}$

bility of the final product when properly stored. The goal is to avoid potential contamination by maintaining a closed system once the solution is prepared and attached to the tubing.[67] For this reason additions should not be made to the solution except under laminar flow. No compounding should be allowed in patient areas.[140] No blood products, insulin, or other drugs, with the exception of lipids, should be administered or piggybacked through the parenteral infusion apparatus.

A number of available publications explain proper methods for compounding parenteral solutions, guidelines for quality assurance, testing for contamination, and problem-solving techniques.[157-160]

Mixing Dextrose with Amino Acids

Compounding frequently involves equal parts of AA and dextrose. Five hundred milliliters of dextrose mixed with an equal volume of AA, will result in final concentrations of dextrose and AA that are half the original concentrations. For example, 500 ml of 50 percent dextrose, added to 500 ml of 10 percent AA becomes 1 liter of 25 percent dextrose and 5 percent AA. Renal failure solutions are supplied in 300 ml volumes, to which 500 ml of dextrose are added. Another method involves the use of varied volumes of the two components, and possibly the addition of water. This method is used with automatic formulators, described later in this chapter. (See Table 18-16 outlining the method for deriving final concentrations of solutions.)

Mixing Methods

There are two basic methods of mixing: batch or bulk, and individual or single unit. In batch mixing, large quantities of solutions and chemicals are mixed simultaneously in vats and then measured into containers for infusion. Large volume filtration, sterilization, and bottling are employed when batch mixing is used. Solutions should be filtered through a 0.22- or 0.45-micron filter prior to infusion since the procedure is not sterile. A 0.45-micron filter will block all fungi and bacteria except *Pseudomonas* and some aberrant bacteria,[67] whereas a 0.22-micron filter will screen all bacteria. The smaller pore size, 0.22 microns, will necessitate a pump to overcome the flow resistance created by the filter. Both filters block particulate matter, air emboli, and bacteria, but not endotoxin. Many hospitals filter the solution a second time as it is being administered to screen out all particulate matter between the extension tubing and the IV tubing.

Up to 30 days' worth of solution may be mixed if the solution is maintained at 3°C. Once the vitamins are added, however, expiration is within 48 hours. Batch mixing is frequently used in large institutions in which many patients receive parenteral solutions each day, and by home care companies when mixing for stable patients at home. Patients usually learn to admix their own multivitamins and trace elements to prolong stability and allow less frequent delivery of solutions to the home.

Individual mixing is done under a laminar flow hood. This method utilizes a sterile solution and sterile additives under sterile conditions. It is used when patients' prescriptions are changed frequently, and in pharmacies that mix a small number of parenteral solutions, as in hospitals.

In standard solutions, glucose and AA are mixed together, along with electrolytes, trace minerals, and multivitamins. This is the usual procedure in both batch and individual mixing.

An alternate method for individual mixing involves purchase of a premixed glucose and AA solution to which additives are added by the pharmacy, or an AA solution with or without premixed electrolytes to which dextrose, vitamins, and trace minerals are added. This requires less pharmacist time, and might benefit a hospital where the need for PN is limited, or where laminar flow conditions are unavailable.

There are a number of variations in products available for compounding. For instance, empty 1-liter containers of glass or plastic may be used to transfer the two 500-ml containers of dextrose and AA. Alternatively, 1-liter partial fill, partial vacuum glass bottles or plastic bags that contain dextrose may be used to contain the final solution after transferring 500 ml of amino acids. The transfers may be made by gravity through a transfer set and a 0.22-micron filter, hanging the container to be filled below the container used to fill, or by using a vacuum pump.

In three-in-one solutions, lipid emulsion is included in the same container in addition to the items mentioned above. As with individual mixing, the transfer is carried out under aseptic techniques afforded by the laminar flow hood.

Questions regarding the stability of this mixture were raised in the section discussing compatibility of the fat emulsion. At the present time, manufacturers specify which fat emulsions and which AA solutions are compatible in their container. Strict guidelines for ratios of AA to dextrose to lipid are provided and should be followed.[161]

Rather than ordering on a per liter basis, electrolytes, dextrose, and AA are ordered on a per 24-hour basis.

Advantages of this system include availability of non-DEHP plastic bags, which may be of importance to the long-term patient. Because all components are contained in one bag, only one pump and one set of tubing are needed, which, in conjunction with a single flow rate, alleviate problems of lipid backing up into the main tubing. Within product guidelines, any amount of lipid can be given in this system. Opacity of the system protects light-sensitive vitamins. Total infusion time may be decreased.

Disadvantages of this sytem include a short shelf-life, necessitating frequent mixing. The solution cannot be filtered because it contains lipid, so it must be sterile. This makes it difficult for a home patient to use,

for admixing trace minerals and multivitamins would break sterility. Because the fat is opaque, the presence of precipitate cannot be assessed against light and dark backgrounds, although the solution should be examined for integrity of the emulsion (presence of oily droplets). It is a different system and, therefore, requires that different protocols be adhered to. This method can be used with automatic formulators described below.

Another method of mixing that incorporates principles of both batch and individual methods, and that is currently used in hospitals that mix a large number of parenteral solutions each day, requires the use of a formulator. A formulator is an instrument that provides a mechanical means of preparing a solution. Separate channels within the apparatus control the flow of 10 percent AA, 70 percent dextrose, and sterile water so that any final concentration and volume of nutrient solution can be prepared. This system allows individual tailoring of a variety of solutions while minimizing the quantity and variety of solutions a pharmacy must stock. Various compounding methods are compared in detail elsewhere.[162] After mixing the components of the solution, it must be inspected against light and dark backgrounds for precipitates or other irregularities that were discussed under Additive Compatibilities of TPN.

Storage and Handling

Dextrose and amino acid mixtures containing electrolytes are stable for hours at 4°C. Once multivitamins and trace minerals are added, however, the solution should be used within 48 hours. The final solution should be refrigerated to prevent reduction reactions between the glucose and AA (Maillard reaction), and to prevent loss of potency of vitamins and possible contamination.

Fat emulsions should not be stored above 30°C and should be protected from freezing. Fat emulsions are stable for 18 to 24 months at 25°C, or 24 months under refrigeration.

The 3-liter bags that contain complete mixtures of dextrose, AA, lipids, electrolytes, multivitamins, and trace minerals should be used within 24 hours.[161] Some studies have shown longer stability times,[127] but 24 hours is recommended to ensure a margin of safety.

REFERENCES

1. Long DL, Zikria BA, Kinney JM, Geiger JW: Comparison of fibrin hydrolysates and crystalline amino acid solutions in parenteral nutrition. Am J Clin Nutr 27: 163–174, 1974
2. Patel D, Anderson GH, Jeejeebhoy KN: Amino acid adequacy of parenteral casein hydrolysate and oral cottage cheese in patients with gastrointestinal disease as measured by nitrogen balance and blood aminogram. Gastroenterology 65(3):427–437, 1973
3. Jeejeebhoy KN: Total parenteral nutrition. Ann R. Coll Phys Surg Can 9:287–300, 1976
4. Wochner RD, Strober W, Waldmann TA: Role of the kidney in the catabolism of Bence Jones proteins and immunoglobulin fragments. J Exp Med 126:207–221, 1966
5. Heird WC, Dell RB, Driscoll JM, et al.: Metabolic acidosis resulting from intravenous alimentation mixtures containing synthetic amino acids. N Engl J Med 287:943–948, 1972
6. Dudrick SJ, MacFayden BV, Van Buren CT, et al.: Parenteral hyperalimentation. Metabolic problems and solutions. Ann Surg 176(3):259–264, 1972
7. Fundamentals of Nutrition Support. Deerfield, Ill: Travenol Laboratories, 1981
8. Shils ME: Parenteral nutrition. In Goodhart RS, Shils ME (eds): Modern Nutrition in Health and Disease, 6 ed. Philadelphia: Lea & Febiger, 1980, pp 1125–1152.
9. Goldman DA, Mak DG: Infection control in total parenteral nutrition. JAMA 233:1360–1364, 1973
10. Peaston MJT: A comparison of hydrolyzed L- and synthesized DL-amino acids for complete parenteral nutrition. Clin Pharmacol Ther 9(1):61–66, 1968
11. Lehninger AL: Biochemistry. New York: Worth, 1970, p 78
12. Harper HA, Rodwell VW, Mayes PA: Review of Physiological Chemistry, 16 ed. Los Altos,

Calif: Lange Medical Publications, 1977, pp 5,94
13. Solomons TWG: Organic Chemistry. New York: John Wiley, 1978, p 249
14. Tweedle DEF: Intravenous amino acid solutions. Br J Hosp Med 13:81–85, 1975
15. Rusho W, Standish R, Bair J: A comparison of crystalline amino acid solutions for total parenteral nutrition. Hospital Formulary, January:29–33, 1981
16. Munro H: Metabolic integration of organs in health and disease. JPEN 6(4):271–280, 1982
17. Phillips GD, Odgers CL: Parenteral and enteral nutrition. A practical guide. The Flinders Univ. of So. Australia, 1980
18. Munro H: Protein hydrolysates and amino acids. In White PL, Nagy ME, Fletcher DC (eds): Total Parenteral Nutrition. Acton, Mass: Publishing Sciences Group, 1974, pp 59–79
19. Holt LE, Snyderman SE: Protein and amino acid requirements of infants and children. Nutr Abst Rev 35:1–13, 1965
20. Swendseid ME, Kopple JD, Panigua M: Effect of essential amino acid diets on nitrogen balance and amino acid levels in chronic uremia (abstract). Am Soc Nephrol 5:79, 1971
21. Bergström J, Bucht H, Fürst P, et al.: Intravenous nutrition with amino acid solutions in patients with chronic uremia. Acta Med Scand 191:359–367, 1972
22. Kopple JD, Swendseid ME: Evidence that histidine is an essential amino acid in normal and chronically uremic man. J Clin Invest 55:881–891, 1975
23. Bergström J, Fürst P, Josephson B, Norée LO: Improvement of nitrogen balance in a uremic patient by the addition of histidine to essential amino acid solutions given intravenously. Life Sci 9:787–794, 1970
24. Recommended Dietary Allowances, 9 ed. Washington, D.C.: National Academy of Sciences, 1980
25. Dale G, Young G, Latner AL, et al.: The effect of surgical operation on venous plasma free amino acids. Surgery 81:295–301, 1977
26. Griffin RE, Williams SK: Product selection and parenteral nutrition solution preparation. In Kaminski MV (ed): Textbook of Contemporary Clinical Nutrition. New York: Marcel Dekker, in press
27. Snyderman S: The protein and amino acid

requirements of the premature infant. In Jonxis JH, Troelstra JA (eds): Metabolic Processes in the Foetus and Newborn Infant. Baltimore: Williams and Wilkins, 1971, p 128

28. Giordano C: Use of exogenous and endogenous urea for protein synthesis in normal and uremic subjects. J Lab Clin Med 62:231–246, 1963

29. Rose WC, Dekker EE: Urea as a source of nitrogen for the biosynthesis of amino acids. J Biol Chem 223:107–121, 1956

30. Paul G: Total parenteral nutrition: A guide for its use. Am J Gastroenterol 72(2):186–192, 1979

31. Bohinski RC: Modern Concepts in Biochemistry, 3 ed. Boston: Allyn and Bacon, 1979

32. Birkham RH, Border JR: Alternate or supplemental energy sources. JPEN 5(1):24–31, 1981

33. Groves AC, Woolf LI, Allardyce DB, Hasinoff C: Arterial plasma amino acids in patients receiving elemental diet. Surg Forum 25:54–56, 1976

34. Fischer JE, Fishman AF: Panel report on nutritional support of patients with liver, renal, and cardiopulmonary diseases. Am J Clin Nutr 34:1235–1245, 1981

35. Tweedle DEF: In Wilkinson A (ed): Parenteral Nutrition. London: Balliere, 1972

36. Steginck LD: Amino acid metabolism. In Winters RN, Hasselmeyer EG (eds): Intravenous Nutrition in the High Risk Infant. New York: John Wiley, 1975, pp 181–203

37. Steginck LD: Studies of normal adults receiving amino acids as the nitrogen component of total parenteral nutrition. Abbott-Ross Conference on Current Approaches to Nutrition of the Hospitalized Patient, North Chicago, Illinois, 1977

38. Tuttle SG, Swendseid ME, Mulcare D, et al.: Essential amino acid requirements of older men in relation to total nitrogen intake. Metabolism 8:61–72, 1959

39. Johnston IDA, Tweedle D, Spivey J: Intravenous feeding after surgical operations. In Wilkinson AW (ed): Parenteral Nutrition. Baltimore: Williams & Wilkins, 1972, pp 189–197

40. Munro HN: Basic concepts in the use of amino acids and protein hydrolysis for parenteral nutrition. AMA Symposium on Total Parenteral Nutrition, Nashville, Tennessee, January 17–19, 1972, pp 7–35

41. Buse MG, Reid SS: Leucine. A possible regulator of protein turnover in muscle. J Clin Invest 56:1250–1261, 1975

42. Dolif D, Jurgens P: Die bedentung der nicht-essentiellen Amino-sauren bei der parenteralen ernahrung. In Berg G (ed): Advances in Parenteral Nutrition. Symposium of the International Society of Parenteral Nutrition. Stuttgart: George Thieme Verlag, 1969

43. Mitch W: Metabolism and metabolic effects of keto acids. Am J Clin Nutr 33:1642–1648, 1980

44. Giordano C: Amino acids and keto acids—advantages and pitfalls. Am J. Clin Nutr 33:1649–1653, 1980

45. Walser M: Rationale and indications for the use of alpha-keto analogues. JPEN 8(1):37–42, 1984

46. Alvestrand A, Ahlberg M, Fürst P, Bergström J: Clinical experience with amino acid and keto acid diets. Am J Clin Nutr 33:1654–1659, 1980

47. Schauder P, Matthei D, Hennig HV, et al.: Blood levels of branched chain amino acids and alpha-ketoacids in uremic patients given keto analogues of essential amino acids. Am J Clin Nutr 33:1660–1666, 1980

48. Frohling PT, Schmicher R, Vetter K, et al.: Conservative treatment with keto acid and amino acid supplemented low protein diets in chronic renal failure. Am J Clin Nutr 33:1667–1672, 1980

49. Kampf D, Fisher H, Kessel M: Efficacy of an unselected protein diet with minor oral supply of essential amino acids and keto analogues with selective protein diet in chronic renal failure. Am J Clin Nutr 33:1673–1677, 1980

50. Sailer D, Muller M: Medium chain triglycerides in parenteral nutrition. JPEN 5(2):115–120, 1981

51. Stein TP, Presti ME, Torosian ME, et al.: Comparison of calorie sources in parenterally nourished rats. JPEN 6(6):581A, 1982

52. Yamazaki K, Maiz A, Sobrado J, et al.: Effect of various lipid emulsions on amino acid kinetics in injured rats receiving hypocaloric feedings. JPEN 6(6):581A, 1982

53. Maiz A, Yamazaki K, Sobrado J. et al.: Protein dynamics using dextrose and different lipid emulsions in burned rats. JPEN 6(6):592A, 1982

54. Shatsky F: Substrates available for intra-

venous nutrition. Nutr Supp Serv 1(7):27–30, 1981

55. Macfie J, Smith R, Hill G: Glucose or fat as a nonprotein energy source? A controlled clinical trial in gastrointestinal patients requiring intravenous nutrition. Gastroenterology 80:103–107, 1981

56. Food fats and oils. Technical Committee of Shortening and Edible Oils, Inc. Institute of Shortening and Edible Oils, Inc., November, 1982

57. Pelham LD: Rational use of intravenous fat emulsions. Am J Hosp Pharm 38:198–208, 1981

58. Caldwell M: Human essential fatty acid deficiency: A review. In Meng HC, Wilmore DW (eds): Fat Emulsions in Parenteral Nutrition. Chicago: AMA, 1976, pp 24–29

59. Riella MC, Broviac JW, Wells M, Scribner BH: Essential fatty acid deficiency in human adults during total parenteral nutrition. Ann Intern Med 83:786–789, 1975

60. Press M, Hartop PJ, Prottey C: Correction of essential fatty acid deficiency in man by cutaneous application of sunflower seed oil. Lancet 1:597–598, 1974

61. O'Neill JA: Essential fatty acid deficiency. Clin Nutr Newsletter, October 1982, pp 1–4

62. Holman RT, Johnson SB, Hatch T: A case of linolenic acid deficiency involving neurological abnormalities. Am J Clin Nutr 35:617–623, 1982

63. Holman RT: Linolenic acid deficiency in man. Nutr Rev 40:144–147, 1982

64. Bivins BA, Bell RM, Rapp RP, Griffen WO: Linoleic acid versus linolenic acid: What is essential? JPEN 7(5):373–379, 1983

65. Linolenic Acid—An Update. Berkeley, Calif: Cutter Medical, Division of Cutter Labs, Inc.

66. Alfin-Slater RB: Vitamin E. In Meng HC, Wilmore DW (eds): Fat Emulsions in Parenteral Nutrition. Chicago, AMA, 1976, pp 85–90

67. Silberman H, Eisenberg D (eds): Parenteral and Enteral Nutrition for the Hospitalized Patient. Norwalk, Conn, Appleton-Century-Crofts, 1983

68. Jeejeebhoy KN, Anderson GH, Nakhooda AF, et al.: Metabolic studies of total parenteral nutrition with lipid in man: Comparison with glucose. J Clin Invest 57:125–136, 1976

69. Brennan MF, Fitzpatrick GF, Cohen KH, Moore FD: Glycerol: Major contributor to the short term protein sparing effect of fat emul-

sions in normal man. Ann Surg 182(4):386–394, 1975

70. Long JM, Wilmore DW, Mason AD, et al.: Fat-carbohydrate interaction: Effects of nitrogen-sparing in total intravenous feeding. Surg Forum 25:61–63, 1974

71. McDougal WS, Wilmore DW, Pruitt BA: Effect of intravenous near isosmotic nutrient infusions on nitrogen balance in critically ill injured patients. Surg Gynecol Obstet 145:408–414, 1977

72. Cerra FB: Profiles in Nutritional Management: The Trauma Patient. Chicago, Ill: Abbott Laboratories, 1982

73. Wolfe BM, Culebras JM, Sim AJW, et al.: Substrate interaction in intravenous feeding. Comparative effects of carbohydrate and fat on amino acid utilization in fasting man. Ann Surg 186:518–540, 1977

74. Digest of Colloquium: Carbohydrates. In White PL, Nagy ME, Fletcher DC (eds): Total Parenteral Nutrition. Acton, Mass: Publishing Sciences Group, 1974, pp 235–237

75. Wolfe RR, O'Donnell TF, Stone MD, et al.: Investigation of factors determining optimal glucose infusion rate in total parenteral nutrition. Metabolism 29:892–900, 1980

76. Blackburn GL: Nitrogen conservation using fat as a non-protein calorie source. In Meng HC, Wilmore DW (eds): Fat Emulsions in Parenteral Nutrition. Chicago, AMA, 1976, pp 65–66

77. Kinney JM: Energy flow—a vital theme in injury and infection. Acta Chir Scand (suppl) 498:20–25, 1980

78. Carpentier YA, Burr RE, Askanazi J, et al.: Effect of operative injury on rate of fat mobilization. Surg Forum 29:90–92, 1978

79. Carpentier YA, Nordenstrom J, Askanazi J, et al.: Relationship between rates of clearance and oxidation of ^{14}C-Intralipid in surgical patients. Surg Forum 30:72–74, 1979

80. Jeejeebhoy KN, Anderson GH, Sanderson I, et al.: Total parenteral nutrition: Nutrient needs and technical tips. Part I. Mod Med Canada 29:9, 1974

81. Askanazi J, Rosenbaum SH, Hyman AI, et al.: Respiratory changes induced by the large glucose loads of total parenteral nutrition. JAMA 243(14):1444–1447, 1980

82. Askanazi J, Weissman C, Rosenbaum SH, et al.: Nutrition and the respiratory system. Crit Care Med 10(3):163–172, 1982

83. Hunker F, Bruton CW, Hunker EM, et al.:

Metabolic and nutritional evaluation of patients supported with mechanical ventilation. Crit Care Med 8(11):628–633, 1980

84. Silberman H, Dixon N, Eisenberg D: The safety and efficacy of a lipid-based system of parenteral nutrition in acute pancreatitis. Am J Gastroenterol 77(7):494–497, 1982

85. Grundfest S, Steiger E, Selinkoff P, Fletcher J, et al.: The effect of intravenous fat emulsion in patients with pancreatic fistula. JPEN 4(1):27, 1980

86. Raasch RH, Hak LJ, Benaim V, et al.: Effect of intravenous fat emulsion on experimental acute pancreatitis. JPEN 7(3):254–257, 1983

87. Forget PP, Fernandes J, Bergemann PH: Enhancement of fat elimination during intravenous feeding. Acta Paediatr Scand 63:750, 1974

88. Gustafson A, Kjellmer I, Olegard R, et al.: Nutrition in low birthweight infants. Intravenous injection of fat emulsion. Acta Paediatr Scand 61:149–158, 1972

89. Paust H, Rating D, Park W, Helge H: Fat utilization in premature infants with and without heparin administration. Comparative examinations using ^{13}C-Triotein breath test. JPEN 6(6):574A, 1982

90. Coran AG, Edwards B, Zaleska R: The value of heparin in the hyperalimentation of infants and children with a fat emulsion. J Pediatr Surg 9:725–732, 1974

91. Hadfield JIH: Preoperative and postoperative fat therapy. Br J Surg 52:291–298, 1965

92. Waddell WR, Geyer RP, Olsen FR, et al.: Clinical observations on the use of non-phosphatide (pluronic) fat emulsions. Metabolism 6:815–821, 1957

93. Meng HC, Law DH, Zubowski CF: Studies on the nature of pathogenesis of fever in some patients given fat emulsion, Intralipid. In Symposium of the International Society of Parenteral Nutrition. Munchen, Lockhambec: Pallas, 1967, p 105

94. Meng HC: Fat emulsions in parenteral nutrition. In Fischer JE (ed): Total Parenteral Nutrition. Boston: Little, Brown, 1976, pp 305–334

95. Kapp JP, Duckert F, Hartmen G: Platelet adhesiveness and serum lipids during and after Intralipid infusions. Nutr Metab 13:92–99, 1972

96. Amiris CJ, Brockner J, Larsen V: Changes in coagulability of blood during infusion of Intralipid. Acta Chir Scand (suppl) 325:70, 1964

97. Bivins BA, Rapp RP, Record K, et al.: Parenteral safflower oil emulsion (Liposyn 10%). Safety and effectiveness in treating or preventing essential fatty acid deficiency in surgical patients. Ann Surg 191:307–316, 1980

98. Greene HL, Hazlett D, Herman RH, et al.: Effect of Intralipid on pulmonary membrane diffusing capacity and pulmonary capillary blood volume. Clin Res 19:677, 1971

99. Mayahara T, Fujiwara H, Yea Y, et al.: Abnormal lipoprotein appearing in plasma of patients who received a 10 percent soy bean oil emulsion infusion. Surgery 85:566–575, 1979

100. Bassler KH: The use and function of carbohydrates in parenteral nutrition. Acta Chir Scand (suppl) 498:115–119, 1980

101. Leutenegger AF, Göschke H, Stutz K, et al.: Comparison between glucose and a combination of glucose, fructose, and xylitol as carbohydrates for total parenteral nutrition of surgical intensive care patients. Amer J Surg 133:199–205, 1977

102. Metabolism and Safety of Glycerol. Technical Information Bulletin. American McGaw No. 3, 1982

103. Tao RC, Kelley RE, Yoshimura NN, Benjamin F: Glycerol: Its metabolism and use as an intravenous energy source. JPEN 7(5): 479–489, 1983

104. Fairfull-Smith RJ, Stoski D, Freeman JB: The addition of glycerol to postoperative protein sparing therapy. JPEN 5(6):578A, 1981

105. Chock E, Wolfe BM, Yamahata W, et al.: Comparison of glucose, fat emulsions, and glycerol in total parenteral nutrition. JPEN 5(6):578A, 1981

106. Fairfull-Smith R, Stoski D, Freeman JB: Use of glycerol in peripheral parenteral nutrition. Surgery 92(4):728–732, 1982

107. Freeman JB, Fairfull-Smith RJ, Rodman GH, et al.: Safety and efficacy of a new peripheral intravenously administered amino acid solution containing glycerol and electrolytes. Surg Gynecol Obstet 156:625–631, 1983

108. Bergström J, Hultman E, Roch-Norlund A: Lactic acid accumulation in connection with fructose infusion. Acta Med Scand 184:359–364, 1968

109. Bach AC, Babayan VK: Medium-chain tri-

glycerides: An update. Am J Clin Nutr 36:950–962, 1982

110. Grant JP: Handbook of Total Parenteral Nutrition. Philadelphia: W.B. Saunders, 1980

111. Trissel LA: Handbook on injectable drugs, 2 ed. Washington, D.C.: American Society of Hospital Pharmacists, 1980

112. Technical Information Bulletin. American McGaw No. 2, December 1982

113. King JC: Guide to parenteral admixtures. Updated quarterly. St. Louis, Mo: Doane Publishing Co. for Cutter Laboratories

114. Guidelines for essential trace element preparations for parenteral use: A statement by an expert panel. AMA Dept. of Foods and Nutrition. JAMA 241(19):2051–2054, 1979

115. Multivitamin preparation for parenteral use: A statement by the nutrition advisory group. AMA Dept of Foods and Nutrition. JAMA 3(4):258–262, 1979

116. Vitamin preparations for parenteral use. In White PL, Nagy ME, Fletcher DC (eds): Total Parenteral Nutrition. Acton, Mass: Publishing Sciences Group, 1974, Appendix A, pp 457–464

117. Ruggiero RP, Aisenstein TJ: Central catheter fibrin sleeve-heparin effect. JPEN 7(3):270–274, 1983

118. Fabri PJ, Mirtallo JM, Ruberg RL, et al.: Incidence and prevention of thrombosis of subclavian veins during total parenteral nutrition. Surg Gynecol Obstet 155:238–241, 1982

119. Baptista RJ: Medications compatible with hyperalimentation solutions. Nutr Supp Serv 3(5):18–22, 1983

120. Maki DG: Growth properties of microorganisms in lipid for infusion and implications for infection control. Proc 20th Interscience Conference on Antimicrobial Agents and Chemotherapy, New Orleans, La. September 1980

121. Melly MA, Meng, HC, Schaffner W: Microbial growth in lipid emulsions used in parenteral nutrition. Arch Surg 110:1479–1481, 1975

122. Crocker K, Noga R, Filibeck D, et al.: Microbial growth comparisons of five commerical lipid emulsions. JPEN 6(6):587A, 1982

123. Hardin T: Complex parenteral nutrition solutions. II. Addition of fat emulsions. Nutr Supp Serv 3(5):50–51, 1983

124. Pennington CR, Richards JM: Three-liter bags containing Intralipid for parenteral nutrition (letter to the editor). JPEN 7(3):304, 1983

125. Solassol CL, Joyeux H, Etco L, et al.: New techniques for long-term intravenous feeding: An artificial gut in 75 patients. Ann Surg 179:519–523, 1974

126. Jacobson S, Christenson I, Kager L, et al.: Utilization and metabolic effects of a conventional and a single-solution regimen in postoperative total parenteral nutrition. Am J Clin Nutr 34:1402–1409, 1981

127. Black CD, Popovich NG: Stability of intravenous fat emulsions (letter to the editor). Arch Surg 115:891, 1980

128. Black CD, Popovich NG: A study of intravenous emulsion compatibility. Effects of dextrose, amino acids, and selected electrolytes. Drug Intell Clin Pharm 15:184, 1981

129. Pamperl H, Kleinberger G: Stability of intravenous fat emulsions (letter to the editor). Arch Surg 117:859–860, 1982

130. Knutsen C, Miller P, Kaminski MV: Compatibility, stability, and effect of mixing fat emulsion in TPN solutions: A case report. JPEN 5:579A, 1981

131. Ang S, Muller R, Orlansky A, et al.: Clinical use of an admixture of amino acids, dextrose, and fat emulsion: Compatibility and stability. JPEN 6(6):586A, 1982

132. Epps DR, Kaminski MV, Abrahamian V, Huk I: Clinical results with total nutrient admixture for intravenous infusion. Clin Pharm 2:268–270, 1983

133. Kirkland WD, Wells PA, Lund LJ: Compatibility of Intralipid intravenous fat emulsion in nutrition admixtures. JPEN 6(6):586A, 1982

134. Hirsh J, Fratkin M, Wood J, Thomas R: Clinical significance of insulin adsorption by polyvinyl chloride infusion systems. Am J Hosp Pharm 34:583–588, 1977

135. Petrick RJ, Loucas SP, Cohl JK, Mehl B: Review of current knowledge of plastic intravenous fluid containers. Am J Hosp Pharm 34:357–362, 1977

136. Weisenfeld D, Podolsky S, Goldsmith L, Ziff L: Adsorption of insulin to infusion bottles and tubing. Diabetes 17:766–771, 1968

137. Peterson L, Caldwell J, Hoffman J: Insulin adsorbance to polyvinyl chloride surfaces with implications for constant-infusion therapy. Diabetes 25(1):72–74, 1976

138. Weber S, Wood W, Jackson E: Availability of insulin from parenteral solutions. Am J Hosp Pharm 34:353–357, 1977

139. Oh TE, Dyer H, Wall BP, et al.: Insulin loss in parenteral nutrition systems. Anaesth Intensive Care 4:342–346, 1976

140. Burke WA: In White PL, Nagy ME, Fletcher DC (eds): Total Parenteral Nutrition. Acton, Mass: Publishing Sciences Group, 1974, pp 329–349

141. Moore RA, Feldman S, Trenting J, et al.: Cimetidine and parenteral nutrition. JPEN 5(1):61–64, 1981

142. Rosenberg HA, Dougherty JT, Mayron D: Cimetidine hydrochloride compatibility. I. Chemical aspects and room temperature stability in intravenous infusion fluids. Am J Hosp Pharm 37:390–392, 1980

143. Leith JD: Trace element calculation (letter to the editor). Nutr Supp Serv 3(4):7, 1983

144. Athanikar N, Boyer B, Deamer R: Visual compatibility of 30 additives with a parenteral nutrient solution. Am J Hosp Pharm 36:511–513, 1979

145. Weinstein MM, Siegel FP, Blake MI: Formulation of a stable trace element solution for TPN. Am J Hosp Pharm 37:1620, 1980

146. Hardin TC, Clibon U, Page CP, Cruz AB: Compatibility of 5-fluorouracil and total parenteral nutrient solutions. JPEN 6(2):163–166, 1982

147. Turco SJ, Davis NM: Particulate matter in intravenous fluids—phase 3. Am J Hosp Pharm 30:611–613, 1973

148. Turco S, King RE: Sterile Dosage Forms. Philadelphia: Lea & Febiger, 1974, p 140

149. Chion WL, Moorhatch P: Interaction between vitamin A and plastic intravenous fluid bags (letter to the editor). JAMA 223:328, 1973

150. Deardorff DL: Osmotic strength, osmolality, and osmolarity. Am J Hosp Pharm 37:504–510, 1980

151. Gazitua R, Wilson K, Bistrian BR, Blackburn GL: Factors determining peripheral vein tolerance to amino acid infusions. Arch Surg 114:827–900, 1979

152. Duke JH (Course Director): Post-graduate Course II. Fluid, Electrolyte, and Acid-Base Balance. Washington, D.C.: ASPEN, 1981

153. Nutt RE: Fluid and electrolytes: Basic concepts. Nutr Supp Serv 2(10):44, 1982

154. Randall HT: Fluid, electrolyte, and acid-base balance. Surg Clin North Am 56(5):1019–1059, 1976

155. Rose DB: Clinical Physiology of Acid-Base and Electrolyte Disorders. New York: McGraw-Hill, 1977

156. O'Donnell J: Electrolytes in parenteral nutrition. Lyphomed Nutr Newsletter 3(2):Summer 1983

157. Recommended methods for compounding intravenous admixtures in hospitals. National Coordinating Committee on Large Volume Parenterals. Am J Hosp Pharm 32:261–270, 1975

158. Recommended guidelines for quality assurance in hospital centralized intravenous admixture services. National Coordinating Committee on Large Volume Parenterals. Am J Hosp Pharm 37:645–655, 1980

159. Recommended procedures for in-use testing of large volume parenterals suspected of contamination or of producing a reaction in a patient. National Coordinating Committee on Large Volume Parenterals. Am J Hosp Pharm 35:678–682, 1978

160. Recommendations to pharmacists for solving problems with large-volume parenterals. National Coordinating Committee on Large Volume Parenterals. Am J Hosp Pharm 37:663–667, 1979

161. Intralipid Admixture Manual. Berkeley, Calif: Cutter Medical, 1982

162. McClendon RR: A comparative evaluation of methods used to compound parenteral nutrition solutions. Nutr Supp Serv 3(12):46–49, 1983

19. Altering Parenteral Nutrition for Specific Disease States

Regina O'Shea

Since its advent in 1968,[1] parenteral nutrition (PN) has proven its potential as life-saving adjunctive therapy. The proponents of PN have observed and participated in the technical maturation of this nutrition support from the simple sugar/amino acid (AA) solutions infused into beagle puppies to the precisely formulated nutrient solutions designed to support patients with specific diseases. The recent marketing of specialized AA solutions for renal and hepatic failure and stress confirms this growth.

The development of PN has not proceeded without rebuttals regarding the efficacy of its use.[2] Nonetheless, specialization of parenteral nutrition support (NS) continues. PN advocates realized that just as one drug is not ubiquitous to treat all disease, one standard PN solution is not appropriate for all patients unable to utilize their gastrointestinal (GI) tract. Critically ill patients often require the professional tailoring of their NS regimens. The PN can be modulated to meet individual needs in accordance with nutrient requirements and tolerances. It is the purpose of this chapter to review and update the reader with the currently accepted methods of modulating total parenteral nutrition

(TPN) solutions to meet the needs imposed by specific disease states (See Table 19–1).

PANCREATITIS

Pathophysiology

Pancreatitis is an inflammation of the pancreas, which, depending upon the duration and/or recurrence, can present itself clinically as hyperamylasemia, severe abdominal pain, malabsorption, glucose intolerance, and protein–calorie malnutrition (PCM). The essential role of the pancreas in normal body function is the regulation of digestive enzyme and hormonal synthesis and secretion.

The etiology of pancreatitis has been related to chronic alcohol (ETOH) abuse, biliary tract disease, drug therapy especially with corticosteroids and thiazides, surgery, hypercalcemia, and hyperlipidemia.[3] Despite the multiple possible etiologies, investigators have found that 70 percent of patients with pancreatitis had a history of chronic ETOH abuse.[3,4]

The diagnosis and treatment of this dis-

TABLE 19–1. POTENTIAL MODULATION OF STANDARD TPN (4.25% AA/25% DEXTROSE) WITH STANDARD ELECTROLYTES, MULTIVITAMINS, AND TRACE MINERALS IN VARIOUS DISEASES[a]

	Dextrose	Amino Acids	Fat	Electrolyte	Vitamins	Trace Minerals
Pancreatitis	NM	↑(5%)	Daily if glucose intolerance Omit if ↑TG	↑NaCl if NG losses are excessive	↑B-vit, folate if ETOH ↑A,D,E,K if steatorrhea	NM
Renal failure	↑(35%) if fluid restriction	↓(2.1% mixed EAA and non-EAA) or (EAA only 1.35–2.7%) ↑(5%) if dialysis	Daily if glucose intolerance Omit if ↑TG	↓Na$^+$ ↓other electrolytes per labs and renal function	Provide ↑B-vits if dialysis	Omit
Cardiac disease	↑(35%) if fluid restriction	NM	Omit if ↑TG	↓Na ↑K$^+$, Mg^{++}, Ca^{++} if diuretic therapy ↑$\overline{PO_4}$	NM	Se supplementation ↑Zinc if diuresis
Pulmonary disease	↑(35%) if fluid restriction Carb should provide no > 50% calories	NM	Daily → Fat should provide 50% kcal	↓Na$^+$ if fluid balance is + ↑$\overline{PO_4}$	NM	NM
Liver disease	↑(35%) if fluid restriction	↑(5%) If encephalopathy ↓(2.1%) or ↓(4%– ↑BCAA/↓AAA)	Daily if glucose intolerance √TG level	↓Na$^+$ ↑K$^+$, Mg^{++}, Ca^{++} if lactulose therapy ↑bicarb if laculose therapy	↑A, D, E, K if steatorrhea ↑B$_1$ ↑folate	Omit Cu and Mn if cholestasis
Stress	In ebb/complicated stress ↓(15–20%)	↑(5–7%) or provide ↑BCAA Solution ↑(5%)	Daily if glucose intolerance Omit if ↑TG	↑Mg, K$^+$, $\overline{PO_4}$	NM	↑Zn
Gastrointestinal disease	NM	↑(5%)	NM	↑NaCl if ↑NG losses ↑bicarb, K$^+$, Mg^{++} if lower GI losses are excessive	↑Biotin, Vit K ↑Vitamin C	↑Zn with high fistula/ileostomy output/diarrhea

↑( ), increase concentration to; ↓( ), decrease concentration to; NM, no modulation necessary; ↑, increase; ↓, decrease; TG, triglyceride; EAA, essential amino acids; NEAA, nonessential amino acids.

[a]Standard electrolytes, multivitamins, and trace minerals: Na, 45 mEq/L; Ca, 4.5 mEq/L; Cl, 35 mEq/L; PO$_4$, 10 mEq/L; K, 20 mEq/L; Mg, 5 mEq/L; Acetate, 29.5 mEq/L; MVI-12, 1 amp; Trace minerals, 1 amp providing the 4 following minerals: Zinc, 3 mg; Copper, 1 mg; Manganese, 0.4 mg; Chromium, 0.001 mg.

ease depend on many factors, of which etiology is just one. The decision regarding the most appropriate mode of NS for the patient with pancreatitis is also multifaceted. For the purpose of this discussion, only PN will be reviewed in depth.

Indications for Parenteral Nutrition Support

The primary indication for the institution of PN therapy in a pancreatitic is a need to promote pancreatic rest. Such a condition may exist in the patient with (1) a pseudocyst causing persistent pain and failure to take food by mouth; (2) a pancreatic fistula; (3) concomitant malabsorption and PCM; and (4) a prolonged ileus after extensive pancreatic surgery.

Efficacy of Use of Parenteral Nutrition Support

Although clinical studies have demonstrated an overall reduction in the mortality of patients having severe pancreatitis treated with PN[5,6] the improvement is not primarily secondary to the PN per se. Malnutrition is well documented among patients with pancreatitis. Aggressive NS serves as adjunctive medical therapy in the reversal of malnutrition and optimization of nutrition status during the acute illness.

Early research by Dudrick et al.[7] and Hamilton et al.[8] demonstrated that the delivery of PN will not stimulate significantly GI/pancreatic/biliary secretion. Therefore in those patients who require pancreatic rest, PN can meet the nutrition requirements without further irritating the damaged organ.

In general, most pancreatitics remain strictly NPO until relatively pain free. The use of transpyloric feedings, i.e., into the jejunum, of elemental diets has been proposed as an alternative to TPN in the stable pancreatitic.[9]

Modulation of Parenteral Nutrition

Glucose. Perhaps the most anticipated complication observed in the pancreatitic receiving TPN and the one requiring the most aggressive modulation of nutrient components is glucose intolerance. This pancreatic diabetes[10] occurs secondary to the altered insulin production in the cells in response to a glucose load.[11]

Persistent and untreated hyperglycemia is a potentially fatal complication of TPN. Careful monitoring of the blood sugar and urinary sugars and acetones is critical to assure tolerance. Fundamental to the treatment of hyperglycemia and glucosuria exacerbated by TPN is the use of regular insulin, generally administered on a sliding scale, i.e., insulin dosage based on blood sugar. In general, insulin therapy is initially administered subcutaneously and if a consistent delivery is required, then the insulin can be added directly to the PN solution. One-half to two-thirds the amount of insulin administered to the patient subcutaneously is added to the next day's PN.

Fat. Often, the use of insulin alone is not sufficient. A reduction in the amount of dextrose and substitution with fat calories can be beneficial in improving TPN and glucose tolerance. Parenteral lipid solutions have been used safely in the pancreatitic population.[12–14] The primary contraindication to its use is hypertriglyceridemia. Triglycerides (TG) greater than 250 mg/100 ml,[15] may indicate an inherent difficulty clearing lipid and may provoke a worsening of the pancreatitis. TG levels should be checked before lipid infusion and 4 to 6 hours after the lipid infusion has stopped. If tolerated, lipid as a source of nondextrose, nonprotein calories should be delivered daily instead of biweekly as a source of essential fatty acids. If lipid is required as a calorie replacement, general recommendations include provision of 40 to 50 percent of calories from the fat and delivery of each 500 ml bottle of 10 percent solution over a 4- to 6-hour period.

Protein. Pancreatitic patients usually require a higher than normal protein intake. The reduced protein stores caused by malabsorption and/or inadequate intake contribute largely to the elevated needs. These patients are often extremely catabolic as a result of autodigestion of the inflamed pancreas.[4] A rough index of total protein requirements can be estimated with serial 24-hour urinary urea N. Utilization of a higher percentage of amino acid (AA) in the PN, i.e., 5 percent, is necessary to meet these increased needs.

Minerals/Vitamins. References have been made to the severely compromised nutrition status of many pancreatitics because of the effects of their disease as well as their ETOH abuse. Adequate provision of the major intracellular electrolytes, specifically potassium (K), magnesium (Mg), and phosphorous (PO_4), is basic to the successful nutritional repletion of these individuals. Failure to provide the appropriate amounts of any one of these electrolytes can inhibit the proper anabolic response.[16] Insulin therapy, necessary in the treatment of the glucose intolerance, hastens the movement of these electrolytes intracellularly. Without monitoring and repletion, this can facilitate the hypokalemia, hypomagnesemia, and hypophosphatemia often seen with aggressive refeeding. In addition, many alcoholics are Mg deficient from dietary deprivation[17] and/or secondary to the pancreatitis itself.[18] It is often necessary to initiate PN with higher dosages of Mg (0.45 mEq/kg/day).[20]

Pancreatitis complicated by a pancreatic–enteric fistula may precipitate excessive bicarbonate losses and lead to acidosis. It may be necessary to supply the electrolytes as acetate in a ratio of 1:1 rather than as chloride salts.[19]

Medical treatment can also incur electrolyte imbalances. For example, the use of continuous nasogastric suction may result in dehydration and metabolic alkalosis. This will require the appropriate alteration in PN electrolyte content, i.e., augmenting the sodium (Na), chloride (Cl), and hydrogen to compensate for upper GI losses.

Deficiencies of the B vitamins and folate are well documented in the alcoholic patient. Steatorrhea, caused by fatty malabsorption, may also induce vitamin A, D, E, and K losses. Close monitoring of vitamin status is essential to the success of this nutritional therapy.

RENAL DISEASE

The primary function of the kidneys is the excretion of metabolic waste products and the regulation of fluid and electrolyte balance. The medical and nutritional management of the individual with renal failure is often difficult since renal malfunction does not manifest itself in any singular aberration. Depending upon the nature, etiology, and degree of failure, kidney malfunction may present with any possible combination of fluid and electrolyte abnormalities. Fluid overload/hyponatremia secondary to oliguria and dehydration/hypernatremia secondary to obligatory solute diuresis[30] are only two examples of the extremes of fluid and electrolyte imbalances that can occur depending upon the nature of the renal failure.

In general, however, as functional kidney capacity decreases, the patients exhibit fluid and electrolyte retention. The excretion of toxic end products of metabolic degredation, especially urea, is also markedly reduced.

Goal of Nutrition Support

The parenteral NS of the patient with renal disease is neither simple nor straightforward. Because of the metabolic abnormalities associated with the disease, the quantity and quality of each nutrient delivered must be carefully scrutinized to assure tolerance and adequacy. Decisions regarding the optimal feeding modality are dependent upon the nature and stage of the renal disease. In this section, we will discuss the nutrition therapy of those patients exhibiting both acute and chronic failure. Acute renal failure occurs as a result of or in conjunction with trauma, injury, or drug treatment and is of short-term duration. Chronic renal failure is congenital or disease based and reflects a long-term malfunction of the kidney.

The goal of NS in the renal patient is two-fold. The NS regimen should not only meet the estimated energy and protein requirements to support protein synthesis, but do so without inducing uremia or other metabolic disorders.

Dialysis can ease the responsibility of this task since the toxic end products of nutrient metabolism are removed. Consequently, nutrient delivery, especially of AA, can be liberalized. It is important to note that dialysis can incur significant protein and AA losses. Hemodialysis is associated with AA losses up to 2 to 3 g/hour[21] and peritoneal dialysis promotes wastage of both individual AA (13 to 15 g/40 liter exchange) and proteins (20 to 40 g).[22] Protein must be delivered in amounts to account for these losses. Hemodialysis can also result in glucose losses if a glucose-free dialysate is used.[21]

Indication for Parenteral Nutrition Support

Although acute and chronic renal failure may vary in their etiology and duration, marked wasting is synonymous with both. Inadequate intake, impaired metabolic and endocrine function, and dialysis are all recognized as contributors to this cachexia. Perhaps more influential in the perpetuation of this wasting, however, is the catabolic nature of the kidney malfunction itself.[23]

Current nutritional therapy reflects the need for protein to promote renal repair, maintain the patient's circulating body proteins, and optimize immunocompetence during this catabolic state. In fact, the provision of parenteral NS has been shown, in some cases, to improve overall patient survival[24] and possibly even renal function in acute re-

nal failure.[25] Provision of adequate calories may reduce protein catabolism and the use of AA for energy. This will result in a reduction in the blood urea nitrogen (BUN).[24]

Although this research has been limited and has had its inadequacies,[26] one cannot avoid consideration of the implications of such results. Aggressive parenteral NS, when delivered and monitored properly, may enhance the overall recuperation of patients with renal failure.

Modulation of Parenteral Nutrition

Renal failure is characterized by a vast array of metabolic abnormalities, the existence of which necessitates the modulation of the parenteral solutions.

Glucose. Aberrations in glucose tolerance are well-known manifestations of renal failure. Possible instigators of this abnormality include stress, electrolyte imbalances (hypokalemia, hypocalcemia, and hypermagnesemia interfere with insulin release), pH, hormones (glucagon, catecholamines, and growth hormone promote peripheral insulin antagonism), and metabolic end products (urea and creatinine).[27] Close monitoring of blood sugars is necessary when adjusting glucose concentration of the PN solution and insulin therapy to facilitate tolerance to the high glucose PN.

Fat. Hypertriglyceridemia is another common phenomenon in renal failure. The exact etiology is not well identified. Researchers postulate that elevated triglycerides may result from a combination of metabolic events. These include augmented hepatic synthesis and secretion of very low density lipoprotein-triglycerides (VLDL-TG) secondary to hyperinsulinemia and decreased clearance of the VLDL-TG as a result of the azotemia. [28,29] Routine monitoring of the triglyceride level and clearance is warranted. As mentioned previously, triglyceride level should be checked prelipid infusion and 4 to 6 hours after the lipid infusion has stopped. Hypertriglyceridemia may contraindicate the use of parenteral lipid.

Although interest in glucose and fat is key in optimizing the nutrition management of the patient with renal failure, the issue of protein, its quality and quantity, deserves stricter attention.

Protein. The toxic accumulation of urea, the end product of protein degradation, in the blood necessitates the modulation of the protein content of the TPN solution. Protein tolerance is based on kidney fuction, clinically indicated by the BUN and creatinine clearance (CrCl). In the absence of dialysis, the more pronounced the kidney involvement, the more severe the protein restriction.

Steffee has made recommendations for protein requirements in both the stressed and unstressed patient with renal failure.[30,31] In the stressed patient, protein delivered in amounts of 0.5 to 1.2 g/kg are recommended, based on the degree of stress.[31] In unstressed man, the CrCl is used to more closely estimate protein tolerances.[30]

CrCl (ml/minute)	Recommended intake (g/kg)
30	Unrestricted
30–20	0.9–0.75
19–7	0.5
7	0.3–0.26

The utilization of urea kinetics and the calculation of urea nitrogen generation/appearance rates allow closer definition of protein requirements based on the patient's protein catabolism. Utilization of these urea kinetics has been shown to improve the protein delivery and, subsequently, the nutrition status of these protein-intolerant patients.[32,33]

The current controversy regarding protein concerns the type of AA appropriate for the parenteral NS of these renal failure patients. The debate focuses on the use of essential amino acids (EAA) versus nonessential amino acids (NEAA).

The use of only EAA in non-dialyzed patients with renal failure was based on the assumption that provision of only EAA would allow the recycling of the urea N and result in a reduction of the BUN. The currently available parenteral renal failure fluids were formulated with this concept in mind. They contain only EAA and histidine. Histidine has been identified as an EAA in renal failure;[35] 250 ml of this solution will meet EAA requirements for adults (See Table 18–1 in Chapter 18).

Recent research questions the ability of the stressed patient to appropriately recycle the urea,[34] and recommends the delivery of standard parenteral AA solutions containing both EAA and NEAA to assure optimal nutrient balance.

Vitamin/Mineral Requirements. Other macro- and micronutrient requirements are also altered with kidney malfunction. Fluid/ electrolyte and acid–base balances, as well as specific vitamin, mineral, and trace element tolerances, vary with kidney function.

Specific TPN Recommendations

In general, undialyzed individuals with renal failure would have TPN regimens manipulated as outlined below.

Protein is generally restricted if the patient is not dialyzed. Initially, a 2.1 percent AA solution should meet these requirements. The choice between the standard TPN solution (mixed EAA and NEAA) and the more expensive renal failure fluid (EAA plus histidine) is balanced against the need to prevent initiation of equally costly dialysis. Protein intake can be liberalized as renal function improves or stabilizes, or if dialysis is introduced.

A calorie to N ratio of 300:1 is recommended for the renal failure patient to promote protein turnover and synthesis in light of concomitant protein intolerance. The provision of a calorically dense formula, with a final concentration of 35 percent dextrose, will meet the calorie requirements. Additionally, since this patient population is usually fluid overloaded, a 35 percent solution will optimize nutrient delivery in reduced volume. If glucose intolerance presents a problem, it may be necessary to increase the percentage of total calories derived from parenteral lipid or begin insulin therapy.

If lipid is utilized on a daily basis, the patient should be monitored closely for hypertriglyceridemia. Parenteral lipid contains 400 mg PO_4/L and may not be tolerated if hyperphosphatemia is a problem.

The alterations of electrolytes are based on daily laboratory results. Metabolic acidosis is common in renal failure. The appropriate substitution of chloride with acetate in the TPN can improve the situation. To prevent fluid retention, Na is usally restricted. K, PO_4, and Mg are initially restricted. These electrolytes are subsequently supplemented as refeeding is initiated. The specific requirements for calcium (Ca) are unknown. Hypocalcemia may result from the hyperparathyroidism, hypoalbuminemia, and altered vitamin D status.

Alterations in vitamin content of the TPN are not extensive. The usual amounts of B complex and vitamin C are required. There may be increased losses of the B complex during dialysis that require supplementation. Because of the inability of the damaged kidney to activate the precursor, patients require the active form of vitamin D (1,25-dihydroxycholecalciferol). Blood levels of vitamin A are increased in renal failure and supplementation beyond standard doses of 3300 IU is avoided.

Trace minerals are eliminated. Their toxicity levels are not well defined with reduced renal clearance.

Because of the high dextrose concentration of the recommended solution, the fluid sensitivity, and possible glucose intolerance of these patients, conservative initiation and progression of the solution will optimize its tolerance. These solutions should be started at 30 to 40 cc/hour and advanced by 10 cc increments per day.

Peripheral solutions are not recommended for these patients because of their increased calorie needs and limited fluid tolerance.

CARDIAC DISEASE

Many investigators have recognized and documented the existence of a nutritional wasting in patients with severe cardiac disease.[63–66] Patients who are at an increased risk for developing this cardiac cachexia include those with chronic heart disease, especially congestive heart failure, and those with prolonged and complicated postoperative courses.[67]

PCM and Cardiac Function

Common clinical findings in these patients include a reduction in heart size, decreased heart weight in proportion to body weight loss, hypotension, reduced heart rate and cardiac output.[63–66] Heymsfield et al.[63] have postulated two mechanisms for the changes in heart size and volume induced by PCM. There may be a pathologic wasting of the heart muscle from reduced protein synthesis, or the heart size reduction may be an adaptive response to the decreased blood volume and cardiac output requirements of malnourished patients.

Potential Refeeding Complications

The nutritional repletion of these individuals using PN can exacerbate cardiac and other metabolic complications. Congestive heart failure, increased cardiac output, and elevated heart and pulse rates are documented side effects of refeeding the patient with cardiac cachexia.[63] Glucose intolerance may pose a problem. This is the result of a hypermetabolic state possibly induced by one or the combination of several factors, including stress and elevated catecholamine release, fever, increased metabolic demands of compromised respiratory and cardiac tissue, or the refeeding itself.[63,68] Hyperlipidemia, which is often an inherent condition in this patient population, may contraindicate the use of parenteral lipid infusions.

Adjunctive diuretic therapy may facilitate the depletion of K, Ca, and Mg. Since these three electrolytes are influential as stimulators of cardiac muscle activity, deficiency states induced by diuresis or PN could potentially complicate the cardiac patient's recovery. Assuring the adequacy of PO_4 levels is also an important consideration in the refeeding of this patient population. Dorsee et al.[69] have reported three cases of severe congestive cardiomyopathy secondary to hypophosphatemia. These patients had depleted PO_4 levels caused by the ingestion of large amounts of PO_4-binding antacids, e.g., Amphogel. Malnourished cardiac patients are at a similar risk for developing hypophosphatemia if aggressive refeeding is initiated without adequate PO_4 repletion.

A rare, but nonetheless deleterious, effect of TPN on cardiac function is congestive cardiomyopathy induced by selenium (Se) deficiency. Many standard PN regimens do not include Se supplementation. In short-term PN, the patient's Se stores and the Se contamination of the TPN solution, bottles, and tubing should meet basic Se requirements. Assurance of adequate Se nutriture assumes more clinical significance in those patients on long-term TPN. Case reports of individuals with Se deficiency-related cardiomyopathy indicate that the long-term delivery of non-Se-supplemented TPN promoted the deficiency.[71,72]

Goals of Nutrition Support of the Cardiac Patient

The goal of NS is to reverse the cachexia and improve myocardial strength without imposing unnecessary fluid or metabolic challenges in these individuals. Experience has shown that the use of concentrated PN solutions (1.3 to 1.4 kcal/cc) with 35 percent dextrose and 5 percent AA, as well as the re-

striction of Na, can prevent fluid overload.[63] Dilute peripheral PN solutions are not optimal feeding choice in these patients because of the large volume of solution required to meet basal requirements. Close monitoring of heart function, fluid balance, and serum electrolytes is warranted during refeeding to prevent complications.

The delivery of high dextrose formula requires conservative initiation and advancement, i.e., starting at 30 to 40 cc/hour and progressing in 10 cc/hour increments according to patient tolerance. This will minimize glucose intolerance. Insulin therapy may still be necessary, however. If hyperlipidemia precludes the use of parenteral lipid, the patient may require the topical administration of safflower oil to prevent essential fatty acid deficiency.[101]

Close monitoring of serum levels of K, Ca, Mg, and PO_4 is essential to prevent deficiency states induced by refeeding or medical therapy. Supplementation of K (80 to 90 mEq/d), Ca (8.0 to 9.0 mEq/d), Mg (12 to 16 mEq/d) and PO_4 (80 to 100 mEq/d) is recommended if the patient becomes deficient.[70] The actual amount of Se delivered to each patient will vary with requirements and losses. A general recommendation, however, is to provide 80 to 100 µg/d.[71]

PULMONARY DISEASE

The effect of PCM and the subsequent PN repletion on respiratory function has been well documented.[50]

PCM and Pulmonary Function

Chronic inanition results in a reduction of total body muscle mass, of which the respiratory musculature, i.e., diaphragm, and intercostal and accessory muscles are included.[51] The muscle atrophy, induced by the PCM or prolonged mechanical ventilation,[50] can severely compromise respiratory function, and has been linked with an increased incidence of pneumonia,[52] atelectasis,[51] and pulmonary infection.[53] It is therefore critical to provide NS to facilitate the reversal of the PCM and thus improve respiratory function.

Modulation of Parenteral Nutrition

Glucose. Although glucose is necessary as the major source of nonprotein calories in the nutritional repletion of most patients, an excessive carbohydrate load can be detrimental to patients with pulmonary failure.[54,55] Askanazi et al[56] have shown that the actual response to excessively infused glucose differs somewhat in stressed versus unstressed patients. In an unstressed, starved patient, excessive carbohydrate (6 to 7 mg/kg/min)[80] promotes increased lipogenesis, increased carbon dioxide (CO_2) production, and a shift of the respiratory quotient (RQ) from 0.7 to 1.0.[56] In the stressed patient, excessive carbohydrate stimulates elevated catecholamine release without a significant net increase in lipogenesis. There is an increase in both CO_2 and O_2 production and the RQ shifts from 0.7 to 0.9. Despite the different response, the net result in both situations is an augmentation in CO_2 production. More demand is placed on already compromised respiratory muscles to remove the excess CO_2.

To avoid PN-induced hypercarbia, Askanazi et al.[57] propose the substitution of 50 percent of dextrose calories with fat calories. This recommendation has limitations. There are potentially detrimental pulmonary effects of parenteral lipid infusion, i.e., decreased pulmonary diffusion capacity in adults[58] and pulmonary fat accumulation in preterm infants.[59] It is critical to monitor pulmonary function and lipid tolerance, to avoid a total carbohydrate intake in excess of 6 mg/kg, and to provide fat and carbohydrate calories in approximately a 1:1 ratio.

Protein. The AA required for anabolism can also alter pulmonary function by increasing ventilatory drive response to CO_2.[60] Although this may be beneficial in some pa-

tients, dyspnea can result in those individuals unable to increase their minute ventiliation.[50] These data do not contraindicate use of protein in these depleted patients but the potential side effects of nutritional therapy should be recognized.

Vitamins/Minerals. The requirements for the other macro- and micronutrients, with the exception of PO_4, are not respiratory-function dependent or specific. Changes in fluid (in pulmonary edema) or acid–base balance may necessitate the routine alterations in the TPN.

Hypophosphatemia has been associated with acute respiratory failure.[61] This pulmonary malfunction is caused by the inactivation of the PO_4-dependent ATP-producing enzyme system responsible for O_2 transport.[61,62]

Nutritional repletion in respiratory failure requires thorough evaluation and close monitoring of pulmonary parameters during refeeding. Inappropriate elevations of the pCO_2, pH, and RQ, as well as inability to wean a patient off the ventilator, are general indications of nutritionally related pulmonary malfunction. The goal of NS for these compromised patients is restoration of lean body mass without precipitation of further pulmonary distress. Standard TPN (4.25 percent AA/25 percent dextrose) with daily parenteral lipid, to provide 50 percent calories, should meet these requirements. Concentration of the dextrose to 35 percent or lipid to 20 percent will provide a more calorically dense solution if fluid restriction is necessary. PO_4 supplementation (80 to 100 mEq/d)[71] is recommended if hypophosphatemia becomes a problem.

LIVER DISEASE

The liver has a paramount role in nutrient synthesis, secretion, metabolism and detoxification. Liver disease can therefore have catastrophic effects on a patient's nutrition status.

The delivery of PN to the patient with hepatic disease presents a significant challenge to those responsible for the task. As with renal failure, the dilemma is one of high protein requirements to promote regeneration of a damaged organ, but with reduced protein tolerance secondary to primary organ failure.

Liver Disease Classification

Liver disease is complex and not simply characterized. The clinical manifestations, exclusive of the PCM often seen, pathophysiology, and altered liver function tests, vary with the classification, stage, and etiology of the disease.

Hepatitis is an inflammatory process characterized by hepatocellular necrosis. It presents as malaise, anorexia, jaundice, fluid retention, and immune abnormalities. ETOH hepatitis is characterized by fatty liver, hepatomegaly, obstructive jaundice, and portal hypertension. Exacerbation of this liver malfunction coincides with a recent bout of abusive ETOH intake. As ETOH is withdrawn, liver function usually improves.

The fatty liver syndrome is characterized by abnormal hepatic storage of fat and glycogen. Prolonged, continuous infusion of PN is a common cause.[37]

Cirrhosis represents a more chronic, clinically devastating form of liver disease. There is widespread fibrosis and nodule formation as bands of connective tissue replace necrosed parenchyma. Hepatic blood flow and function become significantly impaired.[36]

Encephalopathy occurs in severe or end stage hepatic failure. It is characterized by neurologic alterations such as mania, psychosis, loss of judgment, and asterixis.[36]

Metabolic Aberrations

The metabolic derangements instigated and potentiated by liver disease necessitate the modulation of parenteral NS. Alterations in all nutrient metabolism are pronounced and deserve strict attention.

Carbohydrate. Decreased glycogen storage and synthesis, elevated gluconeogenesis, and subsequent glucose intolerance characterize the potential alterations in carbohydrate metabolism. Intolerance to high concentrations of IV dextrose may pose a problem with PN repletion. Insulin therapy may be necessary to treat this hyperglycemia.

Some researchers recommend the substitution of dextrose calories with fat in these hyperglycemic patients (approximately 30 to 50 percent) as long as the triglyceride levels are monitored closely.[80] Other investigators dispute this recommendation, postulating that elevated blood levels of fat may displace tryptophan from its carrier, albumin. Unbound tryptophan may aggravate an encephalopathic state.[38]

Fat. Lipogenic ability is reduced in hepatic disease. In addition, the damaged liver is unable to adequately metabolize and absorb long chain triglycerides, potentially resulting in lymphatic vessel clogging. Circulating levels of nonesterified fatty acids also increase because of the inability of the liver to metabolize and clear them adequately from circulation. Enteral lipids are not utilized effectively as a result of reduced bile salt and lipoprotein synthesis, especially VLDL and high density lipoprotein (HDL). Despite this abnormal fat metabolism, parenteral lipid solution is usually well cleared if adequate lipoprotein lipase exists throughout the periphery.

Fluid. Hypoalbuminemia and lymphatic blockage contribute to the abnormalities in fluid status characterized by ascites and anasarca. The hypersecretion of aldosterone, stimulated by portal hypertension and edema, compounds this fluid retention by facilitating Na retention. Consequently, fluid allowances in most liver failure patients are restricted.

Vitamins/Minerals. The vitamin and mineral deficiencies observed with liver disease represent the cumulative effect of decreased liver synthesis and metabolism, as well as the PCM of the alcoholic patient.

Hepatic dysfunction itself interferes with the activation of the B vitamins. Alcoholism is associated with folate, and vitamin B_1 and C deficiencies. Steatorrhea as a result of fat malabsorption causes fat-soluble vitamin and calcium losses. Diarrhea induced by lactulose therapy may promoke K, Mg, and zinc deficiencies, as well as metabolic acidosis. Reduced hepatobiliary excretion of copper and manganese alters the metabolism and requirements of these trace minerals.

Protein. Despite the serious nature of these other nutrient alterations, the derangement in protein metabolism and AA patterns is potentially more clinically deleterious. Protein synthetic ability is reduced in liver failure. The synthesis of albumin, VLDL, HDL, transferrin, and clotting factors II, III, IX, and X is depressed. These reductions directly affect the evaluation of nutrition status, fluid balance, and blood-clotting ability.

Hepatic Encephalopathy. The effect of protein and AA on the etiology and course of encephalopathy has been the focus of extensive research. Investigators have proposed and debated two hypotheses.

The Toxin Theory. The toxin theory implies that the production and circulation of toxic substances, chiefly ammonia, promote encephalopathy.[39,40] Normally, ammonia is removed through hepatic ureagenesis. In liver failure, however, detoxification of ammonia is inadequate and elevated serum levels result. This is the classic theory of encephalopathy. Recent literature contests its validity.[41]

The False Neurotransmitter Theory. The second hypothesis involves the combined effect of hepatic failure-induced AA imbalances and their action as false neurotransmitters on the central nervous system. The nature of the AA imbalances include elevation of serum levels of the aromatic AA, tryptophan, tyrosine, and phenylalanine, as well as methionine, glutamate, aspartate, and ornithine, because of their reduced uptake and clearance by the liver. There is a concomitant decrease in the serum levels of the branch chain amino acids (BCAA) valine, leucine, and isoleucine as a result of continuous muscle metabolism.

The normal BCAA to aromatic AA ratio in man is 3:1 to 3.5:1.[42] In encephalopathy, this ratio approaches 1:1 to 1.5:1[42] apparently allowing greater influx of aromatic AA across the blood–brain barrier. The severity of these AA pattern imbalances depends upon the nature and extent of the liver malfunction.[43] The excess tyrosine and phenylalanine are converted to octopamine, a false neurotransmitter. Additionally, elevated circulating levels of unbound tryptophan, the AA precursor of serotonin, are implicated as a possible etiologic factor.[44]

Modulation of Parenteral Nutrition

The selection of the PN solution for the patient with liver disease relies heavily on the nature of the disease. In general, unless encephalopathy is present or anticipated, protein is delivered in sufficient amounts (1.0 to 1.5 g/kg) to facilitate hepatic cell healing and regeneration. Standard PN (4.25 percent AA, 25 percent dextrose) is appropriate unless the metabolic profile reflects abnormalities. Carbohydrate, fat, fluid, vitamin, and mineral requirements are specific to the patient's condition and medical therapy (Table 19–1).

Potential PN modulations include the substitution of dextrose with fat calories (30 to 50 percent) and the addition of insulin to the TPN if hyperglycemia exists. A positive fluid balance may require the elimination of Na as well as the reduction of dextrose in the PN solution to 35 percent. Conservative initiation and progression of the concentrated PN solution is recommended, i.e., starting the solution at 20 to 30 cc/hour and advancing by 10- to 20-cc increments. Additional Mg, K, PO_4, and zinc may be necessary when refeeding or when lactulose therapy is initiated as a result of increased needs or losses respectively. ETOH-related liver disease necessitates the close monitoring of the B complex vitamins, folate, and vitamin K. Additional supplementation may be required to optimize nutritional repletion. If cholestasis or biliary obstruction is present, copper and manganese should be eliminated.

Cyclic Hyperalimentation. If the liver disease has been exacerbated by the PN itself, i.e., the fatty liver syndrome, cycling the PN infusions is warranted. With cycling, the PN is delivered in two phases, a glucose and a glucose-free infusion. During the glucose-free phase, circulating levels of insulin drop, allowing for the mobilization of stored hepatic glycogen and fat. This results in improved liver function.[37]

Specialized Liver Failure Solutions. If protein intolerance exists or the patient is clinically encephalopathic, more extensive modulations in the form of specialized AA mixtures may be indicated. Before the FDA approval and marketing of the experimental hepatic failure formula F080, designed and studied by Fischer,[41] the PN solution utilized was a low protein (2.1 percent standard AA), high dextrose (35 percent) mix. Although this formula restricted protein, many researchers were not satisfied with its protein quality and efficacy of use. Pharmaceutical companies issued warnings regarding the use of standard AA mixtures in patients with abnormal AA profiles.[92]

The design of the newest feeding modality for the encephalopathic patient was based on the AA imbalance/false neurotransmitter hypothesis. Hepatamine (McGaw Laboratories) contains a high percentage of BCAA (36 percent) and a low percentage of aromatic AA. Tyrosine is absent. Methionine is reduced. In addition, arginine, the AA respon-

sible for the processing of ammonia in the urea cycle, is increased.

Researchers propose that Hepatamine is superior to standard AA solutions in that higher levels of protein (1 g/kg versus 0.5 g/kg) are tolerated by the encephalopathic patient, thus promoting improved N balance.[45,46] The 8 percent Hepatamine can be diluted with 50 percent dextrose or, if more stringent fluid restriction is necessary, with 70 percent dextrose. Conservative initiation and administration of the solution is again recommended to assure glucose tolerance.

Although Hepatamine can be delivered peripherally with 5 or 10 percent dextrose, this is not recommended because of the high calorie requirements and reduced fluid tolerance of the patient population.

In addition to the proposed nutritional benefits of utilizing this solution, some researchers have positively correlated the efficacy of use of Hepatamine with an improvement of the encephalopathy.[45, 47] Other investigators, however, dispute this claim. Their research indicates similar positive N balances and normalization of the plasma AA, but no significant alteration in the encephalopathy.[48,49]

This debate continues. Additional clinical trials are required to clarify each set of claims. The decision regarding the use of Hepatamine in the encephalopathic patient is an individual one. It is important to note that no serious complications of the use of Hepatamine, other than hypotyrosinemia and hypocystinemia, have been noted.[48]

STRESS/TRAUMA/SEPSIS

In response to a stressful insult, i.e., trauma, injury, or sepsis, the body undergoes hormonal changes that subsequently result in a cascade of metabolic alterations. They can be summarized as the following: elevated basal metabolic rate, abnormal protein catabolism, glucose intolerance with peripheral insulin resistance, Na and water retention, and lipolysis.[73,74] The degree of each alteration depends upon the extent of the injury. The more extensive the insult, the more exaggerated the metabolic response.[73,74]

In addition to the hormonal changes, the septic or immediately posttrauma state is accompanied by hemodynamic changes including increased cardiac output, reduced peripheral resistance, and increased oxygen uptake.[75]

Simplified, the metabolic and hemodynamic changes are actually the consequence of the body's compensatory response to stress. The body catabolizes its own stores and increases perfusion to provide the fuel and nutrients for wound healing, synthesis of acute phase proteins, and maintenance of host defense.

The interplay of various hormones results in derangements of substrate utilization. Modulation of standard PN is therefore necessary to optimize the patient's response and to support the individual throughout the crisis without exacerbating metabolic abnormalities or organ malfunction. The selection and utilization of the appropriate nutrition regimen during stress requires a complete understanding of a patient's metabolic status.

Hormonal Intermediaries: The Catecholamines

Catecholamines are the most prominent hormonal intermediaries in the sequence of metabolic alterations.[79] They stimulate glucagon secretion and inhibit insulin release. The combined effect promotes hyperglycemia secondary to hypoinsulinemia and increased peripheral insulin resistance. This defect in glucose uptake necessitates the provision of fuel from other sources.

Catecholamines stimulate lipolysis, which is indicated by elevated free fatty acid levels. Lipogenesis is simultaneously reduced as a result of the ineffective action of insulin. There is an increase in hepatic glycogenolysis and gluconeogenesis from muscle protein.[73]

This autodigestion results in significant losses of lean body mass and explains in part the extensive muscle wasting characteristic of these critically ill patients. Recent research postulates the influence of a circulating peptide, found in higher amounts in the septic/traumatized patient, on this proteolysis.[76] The implications of this new theory for nutrition are yet to be defined. Present information and subsequent research may lead to a better understanding of the stressed state and result in improved therapeutic measures.

Phases of the Metabolic Response to Stress

There are three phases of the metabolic response to stress. The nature of the NS in each phase is defined by the hormonal flux.

Initial Phase. During the initial 24 to 36 hours, sometimes termed "flow phase," fluid resuscitation, hemodynamic stabilization, and emergency life-saving measures are key. The role of NS here is undocumented.[77,81]

Ebb Phase. The provision of NS assumes more importance in the following ebb phase,[76] which may extend from 24 hours to 10 days after the initial insult. The hormonal responses are the most exaggerated in these two phases.

Because of the flux of hormonal activity, glucose intolerance, and peripheral insulin insensitivity, the delivery of hypercaloric, high dextrose PN is contraindicated during this phase. Excessive carbohydrate infusion, greater than 6 to 7 mg/kg/minute[80] in unstressed man, has been documented to result in reduced glucose oxidation,[80,83] increased fat synthesis, resultant elevated CO_2 and respiratory quotient,[54] respiratory failure,[54] and a fatty liver.[80] In stressed/septic patients these effects are magnified.[56] A carbohydrate intake of less than 3 to 5 mg/kg/minute is recommended.[80]

The administration, however, of exogenous AA may facilitate hepatic protein synthesis,[76] thus promoting the restoration of acute phase proteins and immunocompetence. Large dosages of AA are required (2.5 to 3.5 g/kg)[32,76] to meet the protein requirements incurred by the stressed state (see Chapter 10).

Branch Chain Amino Acid Therapy. The role of BCAA in the protein metabolism of the stressed patient has been investigated intensively in the past 3 to 4 years. Review of the literature reveals three proposed benefits of the administration of TPN solutions with a high dosage of BCAA: improved N retention,[84–87] improved hepatic protein synthesis,[87,88] and reduced muscle protein catabolism.[85] Standard parenteral crystalline AA solutions contain approximately 15.5 to 24 percent BCAA. The parenteral crystalline AA solution designed for the stressed patient contains 45 to 50 percent BCAA and will meet the recommended BCAA intake of 0.5 to 0.7 g/kg/day.[84]

Leucine has been singled out as the primary modulator of muscle protein turnover.[90] It is important that this BCAA is present in the appropriate concentrations to optimize the BCAA effect.

Although research on this topic has been extensive, clinical investigators reiterate the need for continued studies. More specific data regarding the mechanisms of protein turnover, synthesis, and degradation with the use of isotopes, and morbidity and mortality rates, as well as more specific classification of subjects in terms of stress, are warranted.[84]

Optimizing Nutrition Therapy. The goal of NS in this phase is to meet metabolic demands and compensate for nitrogen losses. Attempts at anabolism via vigorous feeding are futile.

Cerra[82] has recommended a calorie to nitrogen ratio of 100:1 to meet the dual requirements of high protein and reduced calories. The substitution of fat for carbohydrate may improve the calorie delivery without provoking glucose intolerance. The utiliza-

tion of high-density BCAA solutions as outlined above may also improve the nutritional response.

The protein catabolism associated with this metabolic response to stress also correlates with increased urinary losses of the intracellular electrolytes that co-exist with N in muscle tissue, i.e., K, PO_4, Mg, and zinc.[74,91] The close monitoring and appropriate repletion of these nutrients with refeeding are prerequisites to the success of future anabolic attempts.

Restorative Phase. As the patient moves out of the flow phase, he or she moves into a restorative phase. Hormonal stimulation subsides and catabolism changes into anabolism. The markers of this hormonal transition include normalization of blood sugar, fluid diuresis, and improved N balance.[82] Reduced plasma lactate and pyruvate levels, and normalization of the AA pattern can also be seen.

Once this occurs, a more aggressive feeding regimen, i.e., higher calories with continued high protein, can be instituted to promote healing and anabolism. A calorie to N ratio of 150:1 is more realistic in this phase. Overzealous feeding is still not recommended. Carbohydrate intakes of less than 5 mg/kg/minute are optimal.[80]

Repletion of the intracellular electrolytes and zinc is equally important in this phase.

Complicated Stress Phase. The above NS recommendations assume that the patient improves and progresses out of this metabolically abnormal state. If, however, the patient worsens and encounters additional stress, e.g., sepsis, the nutrition regimen may need to be redesigned further. Additional insults will magnify the metabolic response. As a result, further reduction in carbohydrate intake and more emphasis on protein, with a calorie to nitrogen ratio of 80:1, is recommended.[82] In addition, parenteral lipid is usually contraindicated in this highly stressed patient, secondary to hypertriglyceridemia and reduced lipid clearance.[102]

Specialized High BCAA PN Solutions During Stress

The research describing the preferential use of BCAA as a fuel source in the stressed individual, as well as their beneficial effect on N status, provided the impetus for the formulation and marketing of high BCAA PN solutions.

FreAmine HBC (McGaw Laboratories) is a 6.9 percent crystalline AA solution, of which 45 percent is BCAA. Other EAA and methionine are present in appropriate concentrations to prevent AA imbalances. The molar ratio of isoleucine:leucine:valine is 1:1.8:1.3. [92] This is the optimal ratio for utilization of the BCAA.

Dilution of the FreAmine HBC to a 5 percent solution and delivery of this with 15 to 25 percent dextrose should meet all the metabolic requirements of the stressed patient, while promoting a positive N balance.

Before the marketing of this stress solution, Hepatamine, another high BCAA solution was often used for the stressed patient. This practice is inappropriate.[92] Hepatamine was designed for use in liver failure. Although it is enriched with BCAA, it does not contain adequate amounts of the aromatic AA and methionine. Stressed patients require not only high BCAA, but also a full complement of other AA to ensure an appropriate AA profile.

General Recommendations

In summary, the NS of the stressed patient requires a comprehensive understanding of the body's metabolic response to stress. PN solutions of 5 to 7 percent AA and 15 to 20 percent dextrose are recommended for those patients in the flow/ebb or high stress phase. A 5 percent/25 percent solution will optimize anabolism in the restorative phase; 10 to 20 percent lipid may be used to augment non-carbohydrate calories unless containdicated by hypertriglyceridemia.

GASTROINTESTINAL DISEASE

TPN has been utilized as an important adjunctive therapy in the medical and surgical treatment of patients with GI disease, including inflammatory bowel disease, fistulas, and short gut syndrome. PN promotes bowel rest while simultaneously allowing nutritional repletion and GI mucosal healing. The modification of the PN solutions reflects an attempt at repleting protein, electrolyte, vitamin, and mineral losses, and correcting the generalized malnutrition often incurred by the chronicity of GI disease.[93]

GI Fistula

Numerous clinical studies have documented spontaneous closure of enterocutaneous fistulas with bowel rest and PN.[94,95] Even in the absence of spontaneous closure, requiring surgical intervention, PN can optimize nutrition status preoperatively and potentially reduce overall morbidity and mortality.[97,98]

The nutritional management of the patient with GI fistulas requires close monitoring of N, fluid, electrolyte, and acid–base balance. Fistulas of the upper GI tract and those requiring nasogastric suction can precipitate metabolic alkalosis resulting from abnormal losses of Na, chloride, and hydrogen. Lower GI fistulas may result in metabolic acidosis because of excessive loss of bicarbonate in the fistula drainage. Depressed levels of zinc, K, and Mg are other potential complications of lower GI fistulas. Wolman et al.[99] recommend up to 12 mg zinc/liter of ileostomy or fistula drainage to compensate for the loss of zinc-rich lower GI fluid. Drainage from the lower gut is also concentrated with Mg. Chernow et al.[20] recommend Mg supplementation of 0.45 mEq/kg/day to replace losses. Both zinc and Mg are also lost in the upper GI fluid but to a less significant degree.

Protein losses in the fistula fluid can be significant. Kjeldhal analysis for N content of this excrement quantifies the N losses and provides more specific information regarding protein requirements. In general, higher percentages of AA, i.e., 5 percent, are recommended in PN for the patient with draining GI fistula.

Inflammatory Bowel Disease/Short Gut Syndrome

The use of PN in inflammatory bowel disease depends upon the nature, severity, and extent of the bowel malfunction, as well as the degree of malnutrition. PN has been used successfully as an adjunct to medical therapy by promoting bowel rest and nutritional repletion.[98,100]

Severe or multiple bowel resections, resulting in greater than 50 percent loss of small bowel, lead to short gut syndrome. Initially, PN is utilized almost exclusively. The introduction and ultimate transition to an oral diet promoting GI mucosal hypertrophy depends upon the extent of the resection and the presence of the ileocecal valve. Most patients with significant resections and the loss of the ileocecal valve require long-term or home PN.

The malabsorptive or secretory diarrhea often associated with IBD and the short gut syndrome can result in electrolyte and mineral disturbances especially of K, Mg, zinc, and bicarbonate. Repletion is based on the losses quantitated in the stool and serum levels. Steatorrhea promotes Ca and fat losses. The parenteral administration of Ca, lipid, and the fat-soluble vitamins prevents the perpetuation of these deficiencies and can normalize essential fatty acid and fat-soluble vitamin status.

Modulation of Parenteral Nutrition

Generally, high protein PN solution (5 percent AA, 25 percent dextrose) with standard multivitamins is appropriate for the nutritional repletion of individuals with GI disease. Modulations of the electrolyte and trace mineral content of the solution rely solely on the individual losses as previously outlined.

The chronic malnutrition usually seen in these patients demands strict attention. The clinician should focus on the identification of potential deficiencies, especially of EFA, biotin, and vitamin K, and make corrections early in the course of the nutrition therapy. Overaggressive NS is contraindicated in these emaciated patients, since it may precipitate the refeeding syndrome of fatty liver, hypomagnesemia, hypokalemia, hypophosphatemia, and, potentially, congestive heart failure. PN solutions should be initiated and advanced conservatively to assure optimal tolerance.

REFERENCES

1. Dudrick SJ, Wilmore DW, Vars HM, Rhoads JE: Long term total parenteral nutrition with growth, development and positive nitrogen balance. Surgery 64:134, 1968
2. Goodgame JT: A critical assessment of the indications for total parenteral nutrition. Surg Gynec Obstet 151:433, 1980
3. Ranson J: Pancreatitis. Curr Prob Surg 16(11):7–11, 1979
4. Snodgrass PJ: Diseases of the pancreas. In Harrison's Principles of Internal Medicine. Thorn G, Adams R, Braunwald E et al. (eds): New York: McGraw-Hill, 1970, p 1636
5. Feller JH, Brown RA, MacLaren-Toussaint GP, Thompson AG: Changing methods in the treatment of severe pancreatitis. Am J Surg 127:196, 1974
6. Goodgame JT, Fischer JE: Parenteral nutrition in the treatment of acute pancreatitis. Effect on complications and mortality. Ann Surg 186:651, 1977
7. Dudrick SJ, Wilmore DW, Steiger E, et al.: Spontaneous closure of traumatic pancreatoduodenal fistulas with total intravenous nutrition. J Trauma 10(7):542, 1970
8. Hamilton RF, Davis WC, Stephenson DV, Magee DF: Effects of parenteral nutrition on upper gastrointestinal tract secretions. Arch Surg 102:348, 1971

9. Blackburn GL, Williams LF, Bistrian B, et al.: New approaches to the management of severe acute pancreatitis. Am J Surg 131:114, 1976

10. Taubin HL, Spiro HM: Nutritional aspects of chronic pancreatitis. Am J Clin Nutr 26:367, 1973

11. Peters NA: Exocrine and endocrine pancreatic function in diabetes mellitus and chronic pancreatitis. Gut 7:277, 1966

12. Raasch RH, Hak LJ, Benaim V, et al.: Effect of intravenous fat emulsions on experimental acute pancreatitis. JPEN 7(3):254, 1983

13. Eisenberg D, Dixon NP, Silberman H: Safety and efficacy of lipid infusions in pancreatitics (abst.). JPEN 4:599, 1980

14. Silberman H, Dixon NP, Eisenberg D: The safety and efficacy of a lipid based system of parenteral nutrition in acute pancreatitis. Am J Gastroenterol 77:494, 1982

15. Third J, Bremner W: Lipid and lipoprotein metabolism. In Fischer JE (ed): Surgical Nutrition. Boston: Little, Brown, 1983, p 297

16. Rudman D: Elemental balances during intravenous hyperalimentation of underweight adult subjects. J Clin Invest 55:94, 1975

17. Martin HE: Clinical magnesium deficiency. Ann NY Acad Sci 169:891, 1975

18. Edmondson HA, Berne CJ, Homann RE, Wertmann M: Calcium, potassium, magnesium and amylase disturbances in acute pancreatitis. Am J Med 12:34, 1952

19. Grant J: Handbook of Total Parenteral Nutrition. Philadelphia: W.B. Saunders, 1980

20. Chernow B, Smith J, Rainey TG, Finton C: Hypomagnesemia: Implications for the critical care specialist. Crit Care Med 10(3):193, 1982

21. Young GA, Parsons FM: Amino nitrogen loss during hemodialysis, its dietary significance and replacement. Clin Sci 31:299, 1966

22. Berlyne GM, Jones JH, Hewitt V, et al.: Protein loss in peritoneal dialysis. Lancet 1:738, 1964

23. Giordano C, DeSanto NG, Senatore R: Effects of catabolic stress in acute and chronic renal failure. Am J Clin Nutr 31:1561, 1978

24. Abel RM, Beck CH, Abbott WM, et al.: Improved survival from acute renal failure after treatment with intravenous essential amino acids and glucose: Results of a prospective, double-blind study. N Engl J Med 288:695, 1973

25. Toback FG: Amino acid enhancement of renal regeneration after acute tubular necrosis. Kidney Internat 12:193, 1977

26. Miller DA: Use of total parenteral nutrition in patients with renal failure. Nutr Supp Serv 1:14, 1981

27. Fröhlich J, Schollmeyer P, Gerok W: Carbohydrate metabolism in renal failure. Am J Clin Nutr 31:1541, 1978

28. Bagdade JD, Porte D, Bierman EL: Hypertriglyceridemia: A metabolic consequence of chronic renal failure. N Engl J Med 279:181, 1968

29. Reaven GM, Swenson RS, Sanfelippo M: An inquiry into the mechanism of hypertriglyceridemia in patients with renal failure. Am J Clin Nutr 33:1476, 1980

30. Steffee WP: Parenteral nutritional support in varying degrees of renal failure. In ASPEN Monograph, Progressive Nutritional Support in Renal Disease. Postgraduate Course 9, 1983

31. Geller R, Blackburn SA, Glendon D, et al.: Computerized optimization of enteral hyperalimentation. JPEN 3:79, 1979

32. Sargent JA, Gotch F, Borah M, et al.: Urea kinetics: A guide to nutritional management of renal failure. Am J Clin Nutr 31:1696, 1978

33. Kopple JD, Ganciaruso B: Nutritional management of acute renal failure. In Fischer JE (ed): Surgical Nutrition. Boston: Little, Brown, 1983, pp 576–577

34. Steffee WP: Nutritional support in renal failure. Surg Clin North Am 61(3):661, 1981

35. Kopple JD, Swendseid ME: Evidence that histidine is an essential amino acid in normal and chronically uremic man. J Clin Invest 55:881, 1975

36. Merck Manual of Diagnosis and Therapy. Berkow R, Talbott JM (eds). Rahway: Merck, Sharp and Dohme Research Laboratories, 1977, pp 836–837

37. Maini B, Blackburn GL, Bistrian B, et al.: Cyclic hyperalimentation: An optimal technique for preservation of visceral protein. J Surg Res 20:515, 1976

38. Fischer JE: Nutritional support in hepatic failure. In Fischer JE (ed): Surgical Nutrition. Boston: Little, Brown, 1983, p 561

39. Zieve FJ, Zieve L, Doizaki WM, Gilsdorf RB: Synergism between ammonia and fatty acids in the production of coma: Implications for hepatic coma. J Pharmacolog Exp Ther 191:10, 1974

40. Onstad GR, Zieve L: What determines blood ammonia. Gastroenterology 77(4):803, 1979

41. Fischer JE, Rosen HM, Ebeid AM, et al.: The effect of normal plasma amino acids on hepatic encephalopathy in man. Surgery 80:77, 1976

42. Fischer JE, Funovics JM, Aguirre A, et al.: The role of plasma amino acids in hepatic encephalopathy. Surgery 78:276, 1975

43. Rosen HM, Yoshimura N, Hodgman JM, Fischer JE: Plasma amino acid patterns in hepatic encephalopathy of differing etiology. Gastroenterology 72:483, 1977

44. James JH, Hodgman JM, Funovics JM, et al.: Brain tryptophan, plasma free tryptophan and distribution of plasma neutral amino acids. Metabolism 25:471, 1976

45. Cerra FB, McMillen M, Angelico R, et al.: Cirrhosis encephalopathy and improved results with metabolic support. Surgery 94(4):612, 1983

46. Freund H, Dienstag J, Lehrich J, et al.: Infusion of branched chain enriched amino acid solution in patients with hepatic encephalopathy. Ann Surg 196:209, 1982

47. Cerra FB, Cheung NK, Fischer JE, et al.: A multicenter trial of branched chain enriched amino acid infusion (F080) in hepatic encephalopathy. Hepatology 2:699, 1982

48. Millikan WJ, Henderson M, Warren WD, et al.: Total parenteral nutrition with F080 in cirrhotics with subclinical encephalopathy. Ann Surg 197(3):294, 1983

49. Wahren J, Denis J, Desurmont P, et al.: Is intravenous administration of branch chain amino acids effective in the treatment of hepatic encephalopathy? A multicenter trial. Hepatology 3(4):475, 1983

50. Askanazi J, Weissman C, Rosenbaum SH, et al.: Nutrition and the respiratory system. Crit Care Med 10(3):163, 1982

51. Arora NS, Rochester DF: Effect of general nutritional and muscular status on the human diaphragm. Am Rev Resp Dis 115(4 suppl):84, 1977

52. Rosenbaum SH, Askanazi J, Hyman AI, et al.: Respiratory patterns in profound nutritional depletion (abstract). Anesthesiology 51:366(suppl), 1979

53. Gibson GJ, Pride NB, Davis JN, Lon LC, et al.: Pulmonary mechanics in patients with respiratory muscle weakness. Am Rev Resp Dis 115:389, 1977

54. Askanazi J, Rosenbaum SH, Hyman AI, et al.: Respiratory changes induced by the large glucose loads of total parenteral nutrition. JAMA 243:1444, 1980

55. Robin AP, Askanazi J, Cooperman A, et al.: Influence of hypercaloric glucose infusions on fuel economy in surgical patients. Crit Care Med 9(9):680, 1981

56. Askanazi J, Carpenter YA, Elwyn DH, et al.: Influence of total parenteral nutrition on fuel utilization in injury and sepsis. Ann Surg 191:40, 1980

57. Askanazi J, Nordenstrom J, Rosenbaum SH, et al.: Nutrition for the patient with respiratory failure: Glucose versus fat. Anesthesiology 54:373, 1981

58. Greene HC, Hazlett D, Demaree R: Relationship between intralipid induced hyperlipidemia and pulmonary function. Am J Clin Nutr 29:127, 1976

59. Levene MI, Wigglesworth JS, Desai R: Pulmonary fat accumulation after intralipid infusion in the preterm infant. Lancet 2:815, 1980

60. Askanazi J, Rosenbaum SH, Hyman AI, et al.: Effects of parenteral nutrition on ventilatory drive (abstract). Anesthesiology 53:185 (suppl), 1980

61. Lichtman MA, Miller DR, Cohen J, Waterhouse C: Reduced red cell glycolysis, 2,3–diphosphoglycerate and adenotriphosphate concentration and increased hemoglobin oxygen affinity caused by hypophosphatemia. Ann Intern Med 74:562, 1971

62. Newman JH, Neff TA, Ziporin P: Acute respiratory failure associated with hypophosphatemia. N Engl J Med 296:1101, 1977

63. Heymsfield SB, Bethel RA, Ansley JD, et al.: Cardiac abnormalities in cachectic patients before and during nutritional repletion. Am Heart J 95(5):584, 1978

64. Smythe D, Swanpoel A, Campbell JAH: The heart in kwashiorkor. Brit Med J 1:67, 1962

65. Keys A, Henschel A, Taylor HL: The size and function of the human heart at rest, in semistarvation and in subsequent rehabilitation. Am J Physiol 50:153, 1947

66. Keys A, Brozak A, Wenschel O, et al.: Morphology of the heart and blood vessels. In Biology of Human Starvation, vol I. Minneapolis: University of Minnesota Press, 1950, pp 198–208

67. Heymsfield SB, Smith J, Redd S, Whitworth HB: Nutritional support in cardiac failure. Surg Clin North Am 61(3):635, 1981

68. Heymsfield SB, Chandler J, Nutter DO: Hyperalimentation causes a hyperdynamic hypermetabolic state. Clin Res 26:284A, 1978
69. Darsee JR, Nutter DO: Reversible severe congestive cardiomyopathy in three cases of hypophosphatemia. Ann Intern Med 89:867, 1978
70. Bumpus CP: Total parenteral nutrition in a community hospital. Am J IV Therapy Clin Nutr 6(4):23, 1979
71. Johnson RA, Baker SS, Fallon JT, et al.: An occidental case of cardiomyopathy and selenium deficiencies. N Engl J Med 304:1210, 1981
72. Fleming CR, Lie JT, McCall JT, et al.: Selenium deficiency and a fatal cardiomyopathy in a patient on home parenteral nutrition. Gastroenterology 83(3):689, 1982
73. Meguid MM, Brennan MF, Aoki TT, et al.: Hormone-substrate interrelationships following trauma. Arch Surg 109:776, 1974
74. Cuthbertson SD, Tilstone WJ: Metabolism during post injury period. Adv Clin Chem 12:1, 1969
75. Siegal JH, Cerra FB, Coleman B, et al.: Physiological and metabolic correlations in human sepsis. Surgery 86:163, 1979
76. Clowes GHA, Heideman M, Lindberg B, et al.: Effects of parenteral alimentation on amino acid metabolism in septic patients. Surgery 88:531, 1980
77. Kudsk KA, Stone J, Sheldon GF: Nutrition in trauma. Surg Clin North Am 61(3):671, 1981
78. Wilmore DW, Long JM, Mason AD, et al.: Catecholamines: Mediator of the hypermetabolic response to thermal injury. Ann Surg 180:653, 1974
79. Clowes GHA, George BC, Villee CA, Saravis CA: Muscle proteolysis induced by a circulating peptide in patients with sepsis and trauma. N Engl J Med 308(10):545, 1983
80. Blackburn GL, Wolfe RR: Clinical biochemistry and intravenous hyperalimentation. In Albert and Prince (eds): Recent Advances in Biochemistry. Edinburgh: Churchill and Livingstone, 1981, pp 197–228.
81. Elwyn DH, Kinney JM, Jeevanandam M, et al.: Influence of increasing carbohydrate intake on glucose kinetics in injured patients. Ann Surg 190:117, 1979
82. Cerra FB: Profiles in Nutritional Management: The Trauma Patient. Chicago: Monograph Medical Direction, 1982
83. Wolfe RR, Allsop JR, Burke JF: Glucose metabolism in man: Responses to intravenous glucose infusion. Metabolism 28(3):210, 1979
84. Cerra FB, Mazuski J, Teasley K, et al.: Nitrogen retention in critically ill patients is proportional to branched chain amino acid load. Crit Care Med 11(10):775, 1983
85. Cerra FB, Upson D, Angelico R, et al.: Branched chains support post-operative protein synthesis. Surgery 92(2):192, 1982
86. Blackburn GL, Moldawer LL, Usui S, et al.: Branch chain amino acid administration and metabolism during starvation, injury and infection. Surgery 86(2):307, 1979
87. Freund H, Hoover HC, Atamian S, Fischer JE: Infusion of the branched chain amino acids in post-operative patients. Anticatabolic properties. Ann Surg 190(1):18, 1979
88. Nuwer N, Cerra FB, Shronts EP, et al.: Does modified amino acid total parenteral nutrition alter immune response in high level surgical stress. JPEN 7(6):521, 1983
89. Freund H, Yoshimura N, Lunetta L, Fischer J: The role of branched chain amino acids in decreasing muscle catabolism in vivo. Surgery 83(6):611, 1978
90. Buse MG, Reid SS: Leucine—A possible regulator of protein turnover in muscle. J Clin Invest 56:1250, 1975
91. Fells GS, Fleck A, Cuthbertson DP, et al.: Urinary zinc levels as an indication of muscle catabolism. Lancet 1:280, 1973
92. Disease Specific Amino Acid Therapy: Hepatamine Compared to Freamine HBC. Technical Information Bulletin. American McGaw, No. 6, 1983
93. Driscoll RH, Rosenberg IH: Total parenteral nutrition in inflammatory bowel disease. Med Clin North Am 62:185, 1978
94. MacFayden BV Jr, Dudrick SJ, Ruberg R: Management of gastrointestinal fistulas with parenteral hyperalimentation. Surgery 74:100, 1973
95. Dietal M: Nutritional management of external small bowel fistulas. Can J Surgery 19:505, 1976
96. Aguirre A, Fischer JE, Welch CE: The role of surgery and hyperalimentation in the therapy of gastrointestinal-cutaneous fistulas. Ann Surg 180:393, 1974
97. Soeters PB, Ebeid AM, Fischer JE: Review of 404 patients with gastrointestinal fistulas: Impact of parenteral nutrition. Ann Surg 190:189, 1979

98. Mullen JL, Hargrove WC, Dudrick SJ, et al.: Ten years experience with intravenous hyperalimentation and inflammatory bowel disease. Ann Surg 187:523, 1978

99. Wolman SL, Anderson GH, Marliss EB, Jeejeebhoy KN: Zinc in total parenteral nutrition: Requirements and metabolic effects. Gastroenterology 76:458, 1979

100. Elson CO, Layden TJ, Nemchausky BA, et al.: An evaluation of total parenteral nutrition in the management of inflammatory bowel disease. Dig Dis Sci 25:42–48, 1980

101. Skolnik P, Eaglestein WH: Human essential fatty acid deficiency. Treatment by topical application of linoleic acid. Arch Dermatol 113:939, 1977

102. Robin AP, Askanazi J, Greenwood MRC, et al.: Lipoprotein lipase activity in surgical patients: Influence of trauma and infection. Surgery 90:401, 1981

20. Metabolic Complications of Parenteral Nutrition

Molly Aalyson

Total parenteral nutrition is well recognized today as a therapeutic modality for the treatment of individuals who are unable to obtain adequate nutrition enterally. Nutrition support teams, strict nursing protocols, improved nutrient solutions, and clinical research have all contributed to the reduced incidence of technical, septic, and metabolic complications that were associated with the early use of parenteral nutrition (PN). A recent study has suggested, however, that the frequency of metabolic abnormalities associated with PN remains undesirably high.[3] Proper monitoring and a good understanding of the causes and treatment of these metabolic alterations can significantly reduce their occurrence.

The purpose of this chapter is to review the various metabolic complications that may arise with PN. The text includes suggestions for monitoring patients, preventing and correcting metabolic abnormalities. Patients at risk for specific metabolic derangements are identified and the mechanism underlying the abnormality is reviewed.

METABOLIC COMPLICATIONS OF GLUCOSE INFUSIONS

Hyperglycemia

Causes of hyperglycemia during PN include excessive glucose infusion rate, impaired insulin secretion, and peripheral insulin resistance. The first can be avoided by initiating infusions of dextrose, amino acid (AA) solutions at a reduced rate, and then increasing slowly according to patient tolerance. Blood glucose levels should be monitored daily and urine fractionals done every 6 hours at the start of the hyperalimentation program.

More frequent and prolonged monitoring is necessary in patients suffering from conditions that predispose them to alterations in insulin secretion and metabolism. These patients may require exogenous insulin, which can be added to the PN solution. An acceptable target range for blood glucose is 130 to 140 mg/dl.[1]

Renal failure,[2] trauma,[4] sepsis,[5] pancreatitis,[9] and corticosteroid administration are all associated with glucose intolerance. In these instances, providing a portion of the nonprotein calories as lipid is an acceptable solution if hypertriglyceridemia does not prevail. It should be noted that chromium deficiency, a rare occurrence in individuals receiving long-term PN, results in insulin resistance.[6,7] Correction of this condition can restore glucose tolerance.

Hyperosmolar Hyperglycemic Nonketotic Coma

When elevated blood glucose levels exceed the renal threshold, glycosuria results. Two grams of glucose per 100 ml urine is accompanied by an osmotic diuresis, which if persistent, can lead to the development of hyperosmolar hyperglycemic nonketotic coma.[8] This syndrome is characterized by marked hyperglycemia (blood glucose levels are usually greater than 800 mg/dl), hypernatremia, polyuria, confusion, and, eventually, coma.[9] Conditions associated with the development of hyperosmolar hyperglycemic nonketotic coma include parenteral and nasogastric tube feedings, severe burns, dialysis, hypernatremia, and any condition predisposing to glucose intolerance.[9] The mortality rate associated with this condition is estimated to be as great as 50 percent; therefore, prompt diagnosis and treatment are essential.

Treatment consists of insulin administration and aggressive rehydration with hypotonic saline solutions.[9] Hyperglycemia resulting from PN can be avoided by gradually increasing the volume of infusate while monitoring blood glucose levels.

Respiratory Alterations

Askanazi et al. described respiratory changes induced by glucose infusions in patients receiving PN support.[10,11] Glucose oxidation requires relatively large amounts of oxygen, resulting in an equivalent amount of carbon dioxide production. When glucose is the primary source of calories in PN, carbon dioxide production increases markedly. Resultant increases in minute ventilation occur. This response could precipitate respiratory failure in susceptible patients. Others may experience difficulty in weaning from ventilators. The hypermetabolic patient exhibits a concomitant increase in oxygen consumption, which may pose a circulatory stress as well.

Substituting parenteral lipid emulsion for a portion of the carbohydrate calories is an effective solution to these problems. In one study in which fat provided 50 percent of the nonprotein calories, carbon dioxide production decreased by 20 percent while oxygen consumption remained at baseline levels.[11] These results suggest a role for parenteral

lipid emulsion as a caloric source in the nutrition support of hypermetabolic patients and those requiring mechanical ventilatory support. To date, however, no studies have been done regarding the optimal percentage of calories as fat for patients with pulmonary disease. A restriction may be indicated since a decrease in pulmonary diffusing capacity has been noted with lipid infusion.[38-40] Furthermore, when lipid administration exceeds lipolytic enzyme capacities, lipid deposition occurs in the lungs and other tissues.[2,25,39] Adult dosage should not exceed the general recommendation for a maximum of 2.5 g of fat/kg body weight.[12]

Hypoglycemia

Hypoglycemia may follow the abrupt termination of a concentrated dextrose infusion.[13] This is particularly true if the infusion rate has been increased for a short period of time before cessation.[14] Downward adjustments in the dosage of exogenous insulin will prevent hypoglycemia in previously insulin-resistant patients whose insulin response is improving.

Symptoms of hypoglycemia include headache, nausea, diaphoresis, tremors, confusion, and coma. When time permits, tapering the infusion rate prior to cessation or scheduling the termination point during a meal is an effective means of preventing hypoglycemia. In instances requiring immediate termination of the PN solution, 5 or 10 percent dextrose solutions should replace the hyperalimentation.

METABOLIC COMPLICATIONS OF LIPID INFUSIONS

Essential Fatty Acid Deficiency

Burr and Burr[15] originally produced essential fatty acid deficiency (EFAD) in rats in 1929. Although this deficiency is rarely seen in the healthy adult consuming conventional foods, its appearance has been well documented since the advent of PN. Subjects maintained on fat-free parenteral regimens have developed abnormal serum fatty acid profiles indicative of EFAD in as little as 1 day.[16] Complete manifestation of this deficiency depends on several factors, including the size of adipose depots, growth rate, and serum insulin levels. Infants and young animals are more likely to develop an EFAD, presumably because of increased needs during growth that cannot be met by their limited stores of linoleic acid. Helmkamp et al.[17] suggest that adequate adipose stores (a source of linoleic acid in the fasting state) are a factor in the prevention of EFAD.

Hyperinsulinemia, as occurs during hypertonic glucose infusions, prevents fatty acid mobilization from adipose tissues.[16] Thus, even in the presence of adequate body stores of linoleic acid, EFAD is possible with a fat-free parenteral regimen. Under these circumstances, a deficiency can develop within 2 weeks.[16,18]

Biochemical findings in EFAD are (1) a triene to tetraene ratio greater than 0.4,[19] (2) detectable serum levels of eicosatrienoic acid,[16] and (3) depressed serum and skin levels of linoleic acid.[20] Clinical manifestations include dry scaling skin or dermatitis, alopecia,[20] slow rate of healing, and, in infants, decreased growth rate and thrombocytopenia.[20]

Normal serum linoleic acid levels may be restored immediately with the intravenous (IV) administration of lipid emulsion.[18] Clinical manifestations usually resolve within 2 weeks after initiation of this therapy.[18] Goodgame et al.[18] suggest a minimum of 1 percent of total calories as essential fatty acids to prevent a deficiency. Most practitioners routinely provide 4 percent of the total calories as linoleic acid.[12,22] This can usually be accomplished by delivering 500 ml of 10 percent lipid emulsion two or three times a week.

If oral or IV sources of linoleic acid are contraindicated, topical application of linoleic acid-rich oils has reversed the skin lesion associated with EFAD.[20] The recommended dose is at least 2 to 3 mg/kg/day linoleic acid, or 10 to 15 ml of corn or safflower oil applied topically three times per day.[23] This therapy does not restore normal serum fatty acid ratios.[18,20] Linoleic acid, however, be it IV, enteral, or topical, should be provided to all patients receiving nutrition support.

Hyperlipidemia

Diabetes mellitus, hypothyroidism, familial hyperlipoproteinemias (types I–V), and acute pancreatitis are all associated with hyperlipidemia. This condition also occurs when IV lipid emulsion is infused too rapidly or in excessive amounts. Maximum recommended rates of infusion are 125 cc/hr for 10 percent lipid emulsion and 60 cc/hr for 20 percent lipid. Furthermore, lipid calories should not exceed 60 percent of the total calories provided by the PN regimen. Infants receiving greater than 4 g lipid/kg/day can develop a "fat overload syndrome" that is characterized by abnormal clotting studies and liver function tests, fever, easy bruisability, spontaneous bleeding, and jaundice.[25,26] Therefore, in this group of patients, 2 to 4 g/kg/day is the recommended dose, depending on metabolic needs.

Parenteral lipid emulsions are contraindicated in patients with abnormal fat metabolism that results in fasting hyperlipidemia. Individuals in this category include those with pathologic hyperlipidemia, lipoid nephrosis, and, in some instances, acute pancreatitis. Baseline triglyceride values should be obtained prior to the administration of fat emulsion. Weekly triglyceride levels are recommended by some authors to document ongoing tolerance to daily lipid infusions.[24,28,29] Although hypercholesterolemia has been noted with lipid infusions, atherogenesis has not been documented in patients receiving long-term TPN. Fischer[24] maintains that measures of serum cholesterol are not necessary for patient care; however, others recommend drawing weekly levels.[28,29]

Miscellaneous Complications of Lipid Infusions

Nausea and vomiting, back pain or "colloidal reactions," chills, flushing, and fever are some of the side effects associated with the early use of Lipomul, a cottonseed oil preparation that has since been withdrawn from parenteral use. These reactions are seen infrequently with emulsions of soybean and safflower oils; complications that do arise are frequently attributable to excessive dose or infusion rate.[25,27] Some clinically relevant complications that are associated with the use of the newer lipid preparations are addressed below.

Coagulopathy. Hypercoagulability secondary to enhanced platelet adhesiveness can be induced by long chain fatty acids in vivo, in vitro, in animals and in humans.[32–35] Bivins et al.,[36] however, found no significant changes in a variety of clotting factors when 30 to 50 percent of calories was administered as fat. These findings correlate with those of Cronberg and Nilson,[37] who included patients with prolonged bleeding times in their study population and demonstrated that Intralipid had no effect on bleeding times in these patients or in normal volunteers. Based on these findings, the authors concluded that increased platelet adhesiveness resulting from Intralipid infusion was of no clinical significance. Others recommend that caution be exercised when administering lipid emulsions to patients with bleeding abnormalities.[12]

Decreased Pulmonary-Diffusing Capacity. Lipid infusions in normal subjects are accompanied by alterations in pulmonary-diffusing capacity that may have implications for patients with pulmonary disorders. Decreases in pulmonary-diffusing capacity appear to follow serum triglyceride levels, returning to near baseline values 45 minutes to 3 hours after the lipid infusion ceases.[39,40]

The mechanism for this alteration is unclear. Greene et al.[40] suggest that lipid-induced changes in erythrocytes and blood viscosity may be responsible for the changes observed in oxygen diffusion. Attempts to keep serum triglyceride levels low with heparin or low infusion rates may prevent this complication.

METABOLIC COMPLICATIONS OF AMINO ACID INFUSIONS

Hyperchloremic Metabolic Acidosis

Patients suffering from pulmonary or renal dysfunction are particularly prone to acid–base disturbances secondary to a tendency to retain metabolic byproducts. Adults with renal or pulmonary dysfunction develop hyperalimentation-induced alterations in acid–base balance infrequently but neonates may be prone to these disturbances. In the latter, insufficiently developed kidneys may be unable to excrete the acid load presented to them during hyperalimentation.

The source of this acid load may be attributed to the infusate itself; amino acid (AA) solutions are by nature slightly acidic (pH 5.5 to 6.2). Although the titratable acidity of the currently used crystalline AA solutions is significantly lower than that of the protein hydrolysates,[42] AA that are precipitated as chloride salts yield chloride or hydrochloric acid when metabolized. If the dextrose, AA solution contains other cations as their chloride salts, an excessive chloride load is created. Dudrick et al.[13] report the development of hyperchloremic metabolic acidosis in virtually all patients who presented with a chloride load of this magnitude.

Metabolism of positively charged AA yields hydrogen ions.[42] This can also result in hyperchloremic acidosis if compounds that can accept hydrogen ion are lacking. Hyperchloremic metabolic acidosis can be prevented in adults with normal renal function through the addition of buffers such as phosphate, acetate or lactate to the infusate.[13,42] This can be accomplished by exchanging the chloride salts of the nonprotein anions (e.g., sodium and potassium) for the corresponding acetate, lactate, or phosphate derivative. Neonates may require yet a further reduction in the chloride load, which necessitates a reduction in the proportion of AA that exist as chloride salts.

Hyperammonemia

Premature infants and adult patients with liver disease seem particularly prone to hyperammonemia during PN therapy.[13] In infants, the etiology of this disorder is unknown, but researchers have suggested the ammonia content of the parenteral solution,[43] liver immaturity,[45,47] protein load,[13,45] and arginine deficiency[44] as possible causes. It is likely that the ammonia content of casein and fibrin hydrolysates contributed to hyperammonemia in infants receiving PN.[43] Heird et al.,[44] however, also found elevated serum ammonia levels in three infants receiving crystalline AA solutions containing only trace amounts of ammonia. These authors questioned the adequacy of arginine in the AA solution since arginine supplementation reversed hyperammonemia in these infants. As a rate-limiting substrate for the urea cycle, arginine could play an important role in the development of hyperammonemia. Consequently, the arginine content of all crystalline AA solutions has been increased and the incidence of hyperammonemia caused by these infusates has diminished.

While many hyperammonemic patients are asymptomatic, infants may develop grand mal seizures and cerebral atrophy.[45,47] Encephalopathy and coma have been attributed, at least in part, to the hyperammonemia that accompanies advanced liver disease and portal systemic shunting.[48–50] Serum ammonia, a byproduct of nitrogen (N) metabolism, is normally cleared by the liver and incorporated into urea.[50] As liver function declines and ammonia accumulates in the serum, skeletal muscle becomes a major homeostatic organ clearing up to 50 percent of serum ammonia as a substrate for glutamine synthesis.[50]

Therapeutic measures are aimed at reducing exogenous and endogenous substances that generate ammonia.[49] Neomycin or lactulose administration is an effective means of eliminating gastrointestinal sources of ammonia such as protein and bacteria. Restricting or modifying dietary protein sources can be beneficial; parenteral solutions rich in branch chain amino acids and decreased in aromatic amino acids effectively reduce serum ammonia concentrations in cirrhotic patients,[51] possibly by facilitating glutamine synthesis in skeletal muscle.[48] These infusates may offer additional benefits to hyperammonemic individuals with liver disease since leucine has been found to decrease muscle proteolysis.[52] Lockwood et al.[48] emphasize the importance of maintaining a normal skeletal muscle mass because it plays an integral role in regulating serum ammonia levels.

Azotemia

Blood urea N levels may climb during parenteral alimentation because of increased endogenous AA turnover rates and exogenous AA infusion. These levels usually do not exceed the normal range in patients with normal renal and hepatic function, though. This is particularly true if sufficient nonprotein calories are provided.[53] The optimal calorie to N ratio is a controversial subject; however, it is clearly dependent on clinical condition. In general 150 and 300 nonprotein calories per gram of N are acceptable ratios for stressed and for protein-intolerant patients, respectively.

AA solutions formulated specifically for patients with renal failure may be useful in moderating blood urea N levels and avoiding dialysis (for a complete discussion, see Chapter 19). Otherwise, decreasing the total amount of AA infused while increasing the nonprotein calorie to N ratio may be of benefit. (See Chapter 10 for a discussion of energy and N requirements in renal failure.)

ALTERATIONS IN MINERAL METABOLISM

Metabolic Bone Disease

Two separate groups of researchers, Shike et al.[55] and Klein et al.,[61] have reported the development of metabolic bone disease in patients receiving long-term PN. Both groups describe similar, but not identical features of the disorder. All patients present with severe bone pain and bone biopsies significant for osteomalacia. Biochemical features include hypercalciuria, hypercalcemia, normal or mild hyperphosphatemia, elevated alkaline phosphatase levels, and depressed serum levels of 1,25-dihydroxycholecalciferol. The etiology of this disorder is speculative at this point. Trace element toxicity, nutrient deficiency, or an unidentified component of the PN solution are among the causative factors suggested by Klein et al.[61] This group has investigated a role for aluminum, which was present in high concentrations in protein hydrolysate solutions. When these solutions were replaced by aluminum-free infusates, one patient demonstrated improved bone histology and reduced symptoms.[63] Further studies are needed to document the reversibility of aluminum toxicity.[62,63]

Shike and others[65] suspect that vitamin D may play a role in this disorder. The dosage of this vitamin correlated positively with the severity of the disease; in fact, other researchers have found that serum calcium levels increased proportionately to vitamin D supplementation.[64] When vitamin D was deleted from the PN solution, bone pain resolved and the osteomalacic process subsided.[65] Klein et al.[66] found that discontinuing hyperalimentation altogether effectively halted metabolic bone disease. This, however, was accompanied by the onset of malnutrition.[66] Withholding vitamin D as long as 14 months has not been associated with any ill effects.[65] Therefore, the latter would seem an appropriate mode of therapy pending discovery of the exact cause of metabolic bone disease.

Hypercalcemia

The etiology of hyperalimentation-related hypercalcemia is unknown. It has been reported in conjunction with metabolic bone disease (see above) and in patients receiving PN for short periods of time.[66,68–70] Although excessive administration of vitamin D and calcium can promote hypercalcemia, solutions devoid of these nutrients have also been associated with the disorder.[54,67,70] Izsak's group[68] found that hypercalcemia persisted after calcium was deleted from the parenteral solution. They suspected that vitamin D may play a role in this disorder, secondary to its ability to promote bone resorption in vitro.[71] When both calcium and vitamin D were withheld by another group of researchers, however, serum calcium levels became elevated in response to increases in the rate of infusion.[67]

Hypercalcemia is associated with a variety of symptoms including nausea, vomiting, anorexia, diarrhea, constipation, weakness, lethargy, confusion, and coma. Once other causes of hypercalcemia have been ruled out,[53] treatment may begin by deleting calcium and/or vitamin D from the parenteral solution. If this is ineffective, other therapies such as phosphate administration or calcitonin injections are indicated, especially in severe cases (serum calcium > 15 mg percent).

Hypocalcemia

Assays for serum calcium generally measure total calcium concentration, which comprises several forms of this mineral. While ionized calcium is the physiologically active variant, 40 percent of serum calcium is bound to albumin. Therefore, in instances of hypoalbuminemia, the total serum calcium value should be increased by 0.8 mg percent for each serum albumin decrement of 1 g per deciliter below normal.[53]

Iatrogenic causes of a low serum ionized calcium include inadequate magnesium or calcium administration. The latter is likely to induce acute hypocalcemia if phosphate supplementation continues. Severe hypomagnesemia leads to hypocalcemia by directly inhibiting secretion of parathyroid hormone.[53] Otherwise, because of tight hormonal control and substantial skeletal stores, serum calcium levels will be maintained for long periods in the face of insufficient calcium intake.[13]

Other clinical conditions characterized by hypocalcemia are pancreatitis, hypoparathyroidism, and vitamin D deficiency states.[73] Hospitalized patients receiving inadequate vitamin D via the parenteral route may be prone to vitamin D deficiency since exposure to sunlight may be limited. Lastly, patients with renal or hepatic disease may suffer a deficiency of 1,25-dihydroxycholecalciferol from altered vitamin D metabolism.[74]

Hypocalcemia related to PN requires adjustment of the micronutrient content of the solution to provide sufficient amounts of the aforementioned nutrients.

Hyperphosphatemia

Hyperalimentation-related hyperphosphatemia is most commonly associated with phosphorus administration during the deterioration of renal function.[53] Elevated serum levels of phosphorus in patients receiving PN have also been documented in metabolic bone disease.[55] Acute hypocalcemia and extravascular calcification are consequences of hyperphosphatemia that can be prevented with monitoring.

The deletion of phosphorus from the PN regimen (keeping in mind the phosphorus content of lipid emulsion: 7.5 mmol/500 cc) is usually adequate therapy for hyperphosphatemia. In some instances, however, antacid administration may be required. These compounds bind dietary and intestinally secreted phosphate, creating a negative phosphate balance and reducing serum levels. Acetazolamide, saline, and bicarbonate infusions can also be used to normalize elevated serum phosphorus concentrations by enhancing renal phosphate excretion. If renal function is compromised, and symptomatic hypocalcemia is present, the treatment of choice is hemodialysis, which can transiently reduce serum phosphorus levels.

Hypophosphatemia

The primary cause of hypophosphatemia during PN is an inadequate level of phosphorus in the solution itself. Profound hypophosphatemia (serum levels < 1 mg/dl) can occur in as little as 24 hours with aggressive refeeding of a severely malnourished individual.[56] In the latter instance, phosphorus moves intracellularly in response to an increased demand for phosphorus in multiple anabolic activities such as glycolysis.[57,58] Refeeding should therefore be initiated cautiously with careful monitoring of serum phosphorus levels. Other clinical conditions predisposing individuals to hypophosphatemia are alcohol abuse, diabetes mellitus, respiratory alkalosis, and those conditions requiring antacid therapy.[59]

Symptoms of severe hypophosphatemia are numerous. They include neuromuscular abnormalities that can lead to respiratory failure, hematologic abnormalities such as increased oxyhemoglobin affinity, bony deformities, and gastrointestinal disturbances resulting in anorexia, nausea, and vomiting.[58] Recommendations for phosphate supplementation in PN are dependent on calories provided as well as on individual requirements. Sheldon and Grzyb[60] suggest 20 to 25 mEq of potassium dihydrogen phosphate per 1000 calories. Individual needs can be determined and adjusted with careful monitoring of serum phosphorus levels.

Hypermagnesemia

Hypermagnesemia characteristically occurs in acute and chronic renal failure when the glomerular filtration rate drops below 30 ml/minute. Other causes of hypermagnesemia are chiefly iatrogenic; these comprise excessive magnesium administration via antacid therapy, enemas, or hyperalimentation.[75] Clinical symptoms of magnesium toxicity appear once serum levels have exceeded 4 mEq/liter. Patients with renal failure have experienced nausea, vomiting, hypotension, central nervous system depression, and cardiac arrest when serum magnesium levels were between 4 and 7.5 mEq/liter.[76] These levels are somewhat lower than other reports describing magnesium toxicity in normal subjects and animals. Randall et al.[76] attribute this to concurrent conditions such as hyperkalemia and hyperphosphatemia that they feel may contribute to the development of symptoms. In patients susceptible to hypermagnesemia, it may be necessary to delete this mineral from the PN solution, especially if serum levels are greater than normal. In general, once magnesium administration is interrupted, renal excretion will return serum levels to normal. Dialysis will hasten this process in patients with renal failure.

Hypomagnesemia

Failure to supplement parenteral solutions with adequate levels of magnesium leads to hypomagnesemia in the parenterally fed patient. Other clinical conditions predisposing individuals to hypomagnesemia are alcoholism, diuretic therapy, aminoglycosides, gastrointestinal anomalies, and diabetic ketoacidosis.[77] While magnesium deficiency may occur in the presence of normo- or hypermagnesemia, clinical symptoms and ECG changes are manifested when serum levels fall below 1.0 mEq/liter.[1,77] These symptoms include neuromuscular hyperactivity and gastrointestinal disturbances such as nausea, vomiting, and anorexia.[78] Magnesium deficiency is associated with hypocalcemia and hypokalemia, both of which correct with magnesium supplementation.[1,77] The development of magnesium deficiency can be prevented by adding 10 to 15 mEq of magnesium to each liter of PN solution.[77] This amount may vary in magnesium retention syndromes such as renal insufficiency, or in the presence of excessive losses such as those that occur with renal tubular acidosis.

ALTERATIONS IN SERUM POTASSIUM AND SODIUM DURING PARENTERAL NUTRITION

A complete review of electrolyte and fluid requirements during PN is included in Chapter 12. Therefore, alterations in serum sodium and potassium levels will only briefly be discussed here.

Hypokalemia

Potassium shifts intracellularly in response to increased serum glucose and insulin levels and the onset of anabolism. Hypokalemia can be prevented with adequate supplementation, usually 35 to 90 mEq/day. Requirements for potassium are greater in trauma, burns, diuretic and steroid therapy, and in the presence of excessive gastrointestinal losses. In these instances, requirements can increase to 80 to 120 mEq/day.

Symptoms of hypokalemia are nonspecific but include fatigue, muscle cramps, confusion, anorexia, and tachycardia. Paralytic ileus can result from hypokalemia.

Hyperkalemia

Hyperkalemia frequently accompanies renal failure as a result of reduced renal potassium clearance. Acidosis, insulin deficiency, and hemolysis are other common causes of hyperkalemia in the hospitalized patient. Pseudohyperkalemias, such as that caused by test tube hemolysis, pose no threat to patients; however, true hyperkalemia can be fatal. This, and other complications of hyperkalemia during PN, can be avoided by deleting potassium from the infusate once serum potassium has exceeded the normal range.

Hyponatremia

Dilutional hyponatremia commonly occurs after sodium-rich fluid losses are replaced with low sodium fluids. Salt-losing nephropathy, excessive gastrointestinal losses (e.g., vomiting, diarrhea, fistula drainage), and excessive insensible losses predispose patients to sodium depletion. In these instances, additional sodium should be provided in the parenteral solution.

Excessive sodium administration is not indicated in hyponatremia that results from excessive total body water or sequestration of plasma volume. Edema, ascites, tachycardia, elevated blood pressure, shortness of breath, and low hematocrit can result with fluid overload or "third spacing." In these instances, total body sodium is increased and the hyponatremia is dilutional. Patients in these categories include those suffering from renal, cardiac, or hepatic disorders in whom fluid and sodium restriction is advised. Hyperglycemia also precipitates dilutional hyponatremia by creating an osmotic gradient that facilitates the movement of sodium-free fluid into the vascular space. This can be a transient phenomenon, as the diuresis that accompanies hyperglycemia will normalize serum sodium levels. If hyperglycemia persists, progressive diuresis will eventually precipitate hypernatremia and dehydration.

Hypernatremia

Fever, burns, and hyperventilation can all contribute to excessive water losses through the skin and lungs. These large insensible losses will result in dehydration, the most common cause of hypernatremia, if appropriate fluid replacement is not instituted.

Normal serum sodium levels will be maintained if fluid replacement consists of fluids with a sodium concentration that is approximately equal to that of the body fluid lost. For instance, if normal saline (154 mEq/L) is used to replace half-normal urine (77 mEq/L), hypernatremia will result. Conversely, if half-normal saline is used to replace sodium-rich ileostomy output, hyponatremia will develop. Grant recommends a range of sodium supplementation from 60 to 150 mEq/day depending on sodium needs.[1]

Elevations in Serum Liver Enzymes

Alterations in the liver function tests of patients receiving PN have been well documented since Peden et al. first reported a case in 1971.[79] Liver biopsies from patients with elevated liver function tests have revealed fatty infiltration,[80–82,100] cholestasis,[80] and extensive glycogen deposition.[82] Various mechanisms have been proposed for the histologic changes that are associated with elevated enzymes, including nutrient deficiency, nutrient excess, or a relative imbalance among nutrients provided.

EFAD has been suggested as a factor in the development of hepatic steatosis. Langer et al.[83] described the development of fatty liver in a patient on a fat-free PN regimen, which resolved with the addition of parenteral lipid emulsion. Fatty infiltration of the liver is known to occur in animals deprived of a dietary source of essential fatty acids.[84] Specifically, EFAD in rats is characterized by changes in organ fatty acid composition and enhanced fatty acid deposition in liver triglycerides.[84] At this time, it is not clear that hepatic steatosis results from increased triglyceride synthesis alone. Studies by Fukazawa et al.[84] in rats with EFAD also demonstrated impaired lipid transport out of the liver. If one examines the mechanism for lipid transport from the liver, i.e., incorporation of fatty acids into plasma lipoproteins, possible mechanisms for altered transport are revealed. Phospholipids, such as phosphatidylcholine, are an integral part of plasma lipoproteins. Therefore, some authors have suggested that PN-induced choline deficiency would be responsible for hepatic steatosis. Though choline has not been identified as an essential nutrient for humans,[85] it is essential for various species of animals. One of the earliest signs of choline deficiency in these animals is the appearance of a fatty liver.[86,87]

It is clear that adequate PN must supply carbohydrate, protein, and fat, but the optimal contribution of these energy substrates to the total caloric intake has yet to be defined. Evidently, excessive amounts of glucose or fat induce fatty accumulation in the livers of humans and animals. Burke and associates[88] found hepatomegaly and fatty infiltration in patients when glucose infusion rates exceeded 5 mg/kg/minute. Chang and

Silvis[89] produced hepatic steatosis in rats when glucose was infused as the sole caloric source. The latter findings may reflect the development of an EFAD or a kwashiorkor-like state. Fatty liver, a common clinical finding in the latter condition, is thought to result from an inadequate supply of AA for lipoprotein synthesis.[90] Sheldon et al.[80] suggest an additional mechanism whereby acetyl co-enzyme A, in the absence of sufficient AA, is converted to a fatty acid; hence, increased fat production and deposition occurs within the liver. It appears that alterations in liver function tests that occur when parenteral lipid emulsion provides greater than 60 percent of the total daily calories are due to an entirely different mechanism, i.e., excessive exogenous lipid may be deposited within the hepatocyte.[91]

Grant et al.[92] have proposed hepatotoxic tryptophan metabolites as a possible cause of hepatic dysfunction during hyperalimentation. Rapid tryptophan degradation reportedly occurs in the presence of an antioxidant, sodium bisulfite, which is an additive in most commercially available PN formulas. In one study, however, use of a sodium bisulfite-free solution did not eliminate alterations in serum enzyme levels.[93]

Though the mechanism for hepatic dysfunction remains unclear, present studies indicate that it occurs (as characterized by elevated liver function tests) within 1 to 3 weeks after initiation of PN. In fact, Wagman et al.[94] state that initial elevations occurring after this time are probably not related to PN. Therefore, patients should be carefully evaluated for other causes of altered liver enzymes, including sepsis, underlying liver disease, hepatotoxic drug ingestion, anesthetics, and mechanical biliary obstruction.

Alkaline phosphatase has been cited by some authors as a "leading indicator" in PN-induced alterations in hepatic enzymes.[80,95] Elevations of any liver enzyme greater than 1.5 times normal are considered significant, though elevations greater than five times normal have been reported.[92] These altera-tions appear to be transient in nature even when the PN regimen is not altered.[96] The pathologic consequences are therefore unclear. In fact, Wagman et al.[94] imply that elevated liver function tests are not an indication to delay initiation of or to cease PN.

Cessation of PN usually returns liver function tests to baseline.[96–98] Continuing PN while reducing the total caloric load is frequently effective. However, this is clearly not an optimal solution if nutrient requirements are compromised.[96,99] Cyclic PN is another alternative. During cyclic PN, the dextrose component of the parenteral solution is infused for a limited number of hours each day. This allows a postabsorptive state to develop, during which hepatic lipid and glycogen stores are mobilized.[82] Lipid or AA solutions may be infused throughout the day, as desired, to meet energy or protein requirements. In most instances, however, nutrition needs can be met by increasing the rate of infusion of the dextrose, AA solution. Cyclic PN is presently the preferred method of treating PN-induced hepatic dysfunction.

REFERENCES

1. Grant JP: Handbook of Total Parenteral Nutrition. Philadelphia: W. B. Saunders, 1980
2. DeFronzo RA, Alvestand A, Smith D, et al.: Insulin resistance in uremia. J Clin Invest 67:563, 1981
3. Weinsier RL, Bacon J, Butterworth CE: Central venous alimentation: A prospective study of the frequency of metabolic abnormalities among medical and surgical patients. JPEN 6:421, 1982
4. Wieman TJ: Nutritional requirements of the trauma patient. Heart Lung 7:278, 1978
5. Clowes GHA Jr, Martin H, Walji S, et al.: Blood insulin responses to blood glucose levels in high output sepsis and septic shock. Am J Surg 135:577, 1978
6. Jeejeebhoy KN, Chu RC, Marliss EB, et al.: Chromium deficiency, glucose intolerance, and neuropathy reversed by chromium supplementation, in a patient receiving total parenteral nutrition. Am J Clin Nutr 30:531, 1977

7. Freund H, Atamian S, Fisher JE: Chromimum deficiency during total parenteral nutrition. JAMA 241:496, 1979

8. McCurdy DK: Hyperosmolar, hyperglycemic, nonketotic diabetic coma. Med Clin North Am 54:683, 1970

9. Flanigan WJ, Thompson BW, Casali RE, Caldwell FT: The surgical significance of hyperosmolar coma. Am J Surg 120:652, 1970

10. Askanazi J, Rosenbaum SH, Hyman AI, et al.: Respiratory changes induced by the large glucose loads of total parenteral nutrition. JAMA 243:1444, 1980

11. Askanazi J, Nordenstrom J, Rosenbaum SH, et al.: Nutrition for the patient with respiratory failure: Glucose versus fat. Anesthesiology 54:373, 1981

12. Pelham LD: Rational use of intravenous fat emulsions. Am J Hosp Pharm 38:198, 1981

13. Dudrick SJ, MacFayden BV, Van Buren CT, et al.: Parenteral hyperalimentation. Metabolic problems and solutions. Ann Surg 176:259, 1972

14. Sanderson I, Deitel M: Insulin response in patients receiving concentrated infusions of glucose and casein hydrolysate for complete parenteral nutrition. Ann Surg 179:387, 1974

15. Burr GO, Burr MM: A new deficiency disease produced by the rigid exclusion of fat from the diet. J Biol Chem 82:345, 1929

16. Wene JD, Connor WE, DenBesten L: The development of essential fatty acid deficiency in healthy men fed fat-free diets intravenously and orally. J Clin Invest 56:127, 1975

17. Helmkamp GM, Wilmore DW, Johnson AA, Pruitt BA: Essential fatty acid deficiency in red cells after thermal injury: Correction with intravenous fat therapy. Am J Clin Nutr 26:1331, 1973

18. Goodgame, JT, Lowry SF, Brennan MF: Essential fatty acid deficiency in total parenteral nutrition: Time course for development and suggestions for therapy. Surgery 84:271, 1978

19. Holman RT: The ratio of trienoic:tetraenoic acid in tissue lipids as a measure of essential fatty acid requirement. J Nutr 70:405, 1960

20. Skolnik P, Eaglstein WH, Ziboh VA: Human essential fatty acid deficiency: Treatment by topical application of linoleic acid. Arch Dermatol 113:939, 1977

21. Caldwell MD, Jonsson HT, Otherson HB: Essential fatty acid deficiency in an infant receiving prolonged parenteral alimentation. J Pediatr 81:894, 1972

22. Holman RT: Essential fatty acid deficiency. In Prog Chem Fats Other Lipids. Elmsford: Pergamon Press, 1968, p 275

23. Press M, Hartop PJ, Protty C: Correction of essential fatty acid deficiency in man by cutaneous application of sunflower seed oil. Lancet 1:597, 1974

24. Fischer JE: Total Parenteral Nutrition. Boston: Little Brown, 1976

25. Belin RP, Jona JZ: Fat overload with a 10% soybean oil emulsion. Arch Surg 111:1391, 1976

26. Heyman MB, Storch S, Ament ME: The fat overload syndrome. Am J Dis Child 135:628, 1981

27. Hansen, EM, Hardie MS, Hidalgo J: Fat emulsions for intravenous administration: Clinical experience with Intralipid 10%. Ann Surg 184:80, 1976

28. Englert DM: Rational use of fat emulsions. Nutr Supp Serv 2(9):35, 1982

29. Silberman H, Eisenberg D: Parenteral and Enteral Nutrition for the Hospitalized Patient. East Norwalk, Conn: Appleton-Century-Crofts, 1982

30. Geyer RP: Parenteral nutrition. Physiol Rev 40:150, 1960

31. Meng HC, Kaley JS: Effects of multiple infusions of a fat emulsion on blood coagulation, liver function and urinary excretion of steroids in schizophrenic patients. Am J Clin Nutr 16:156, 1965

32. Hoak JC, Warner ED, Connor WE: Platelets, fatty acids and thrombosis. Circ Res 20:11, 1967

33. Zbinden G: Modification of the fatty acid-induced thrombyocytopenia by anticoagulants and compounds which inhibit in vitro platelet aggregation. J Pharmacol Exp Ther 159:163, 1968

34. Connor WE, Hoak JC, Warner ED: The effects of fatty acids on blood coagulation and thrombosis. Thromb Haemost (suppl) 17:89, 1965

35. Doll VP, James AT, Webb JPW: The fatty acid patterns of plasma lipids during alimentary lipemia. J Clin Invest 38:1544, 1959

36. Bivins BA, Bryant PJ, Record KE, et al.: The effect of ten and twenty percent safflower oil emulsion given as thirty to fifty percent of total calories. Surg Gynecol Obstet 156:433, 1983

37. Cronberg S, Nilsson IM: Coagulation studies after administration of a fat emulsion, Intralipid.® Thromb Haemost 18:664, 1967

38. Greene HL, Hazlett D, Herman RH, et al.: Effect of Intralipid on pulmonary membrane diffusing capacity and pulmonary capillary blood volume. Clin Res 19:677, 1971

39. Sundström G, Zauner CW, Aborelius M: Decrease in pulmonary diffusing capacity during lipid infusion in healthy man. J Appl Physiol 34:816, 1973

40. Greene HL, Hazlett D, Demaree R: Relationship between Intralipid®-induced hyperlipemia and pulmonary function. Am J Clin Nutr 29:127, 1976

41. Chan JCM, Asch MJ, Lin S, Hays DM: Hyperalimentation with amino acid and casein hydrolysate solutions: Mechanisms of acidosis. JAMA 220:1700, 1972

42. Heird WC, Dell RB, Driscoll JM, et al.: Metabolic acidosis resulting from intravenous alimentation mixtures containing synthetic amino acids. N Engl J Med 287:943, 1972

43. Ghadimi H, Abaci F, Kumar S, Rathi M: Biochemical aspects of intravenous alimentation. Pediatrics 48:955, 1971

44. Heird WC, Nicholson JF, Driscoll JM, et al.: Hyperammonemia resulting from intravenous alimentation using a mixture of synthetic l-amino acids: A preliminary report. J Pediatr 81:162, 1972

45. Johnson JD, Albritton WL, Sunshine P: Hyperammonemia accompanying parenteral nutrition in newborn infants. J Pediatr 81:154, 1972

46. Räiha NCR, Suihkonen J: Development of urea-synthesizing enzymes in human liver. Acta Pediatr Scand 57:121, 1968

47. Seashore JH, Seashore MR, Riely C: Hyperammonemia during total parenteral nutrition in children. JPEN 6:114, 1982

48. Lockwood AH, McDonald JM, Reiman RE, et al.: The dynamics of ammonia metabolism in man: Effects of liver disease and hyperammonemia. J Clin Invest 63:449, 1979

49. Zieve L: The mechanism of hepatic coma. Hepatology 1:360, 1981

50. Crossley IR, Wardle EN, Williams R: Biochemical mechanisms of hepatic encephalopathy. Clin Sci 64:247, 1983

51. Fischer JE, Rosen HM, Ebeid AM, et al.: The effect of normalization of plasma amino acids on hepatic encephalopathy in man. Surgery 80:77, 1976

52. Lindberg BO, Clowes GHA Jr: The effects of hyperalimentation and infused leucine on the amino acid metabolism in sepsis: An experimental study in vivo. Surgery 90:278, 1981

53. Chen W, Ohaslu E, Kasai M: Amino acid metabolism in parenteral nutrition: With special reference to the calorie:nitrogen ratio and the blood urea nitrogen level. Metabolism 23:1117, 1974

54. Agus ZS, Goldfarb S: Clinical disorders of calcium and phosphate. Med Clin North Am. 65:385, 1981

55. Shike M, Harrison JD, Sturtridge WC, et al.: Metabolic bone disease in patients receiving long-term total parenteral nutrition. Ann Int Med 92:343, 1980

56. Weinsier RL, Krumdieck CL: Death resulting from overzealous total parenteral nutrition: The refeeding syndrome revisited. Am J Clin Nutr 34:393, 1980

57. Ritz E: Acute hypophosphatemia. Nephrol Forum 22:84, 1982

58. Stoff JS: Phosphate homeostasis and hypophosphatemia. Am J Med 72:489, 1982

59. Knochel JP: The pathophysiology and clinical characteristics of severe hypophosphatemia. Arch Int Med 137:203, 1977

60. Sheldon GF, Grzyb S: Phosphate depletion and repletion: Relation to parenteral nutrition and oxygen transport. Ann Surg 182:683, 1975

61. Klein GL, Ament ME, Bluestone R, et al.: Bone disease associated with total parenteral nutrition. Lancet 2:1041, 1980

62. Klein GL, Alfrey AC, Miller NL, et al.: Aluminum loading during total parenteral nutrition. Am J Clin Nutr 35:1425, 1982

63. Ott SM, Maloney NA, Klein GL, et al.: Aluminum is associated with low bone formation in patients receiving chronic parenteral nutrition. Ann Int Med 98:910, 1983

64. Sloan GM, White DE, Brennan MF: Calcium and phosphorous metabolism during total parenteral nutrition. Ann Surg 197:1, 1983

65. Shike M, Sturtridge WC, Tam CS, et al.: A possible role of vitamin D in the genesis of parenteral-nutrition-induced metabolic bone disease. Ann Int Med 95:560, 1981

66. Klein GL, Horst RL, Norman AW, et al.: Reduced serum levels of 1α, 25-dihydroxyvita-

min D during long-term total parenteral nutrition. Ann Int Med 94:638, 1981

67. Gilligan JE, Hagley S, Worthley LIG, et al.: Hypercalcemia associated with parenteral amino acid and dextrose infusion. Am J Clin Nutr 35:993, 1982

68. Izsak ME, Shike M, Roulet M, Jeejeebhoy KN: Pancreatitis in association with hypercalemia in patients receiving total parenteral nutrition. Gastroenterology 79:555, 1980

69. Manson RR: Acute pancreatitis secondary to iatrogenic hypercalcemia. Arch Surg 108:213, 1974

70. Ulstrom RA, Brown DM: Hypercalcemia as a complication of parenteral alimentation. J Pediatr 81:419, 1972

71. Raisz LG, Trummal CL, Holick MF, DeLuca HF: 1,25-dihydroxycholecalciferol: A potent stimulator of bone resorption in tissue culture. Science 175:768, 1972

72. Henley BR: Management of the parathyroid crisis. Am J Surg 108:183, 1964

73. Scriver CR: Rickets and the pathogenesis of impaired tubular transport of phosphate and other solutes. Am J Med 57:43, 1974

74. Favus MJ: Vitamin D physiology and some clinical aspects of the vitamin D endocrine system. Med Clin North Am 62:1291, 1978

75. Agus ZS, Wasserstein A, Goldfarb S: Disorders of calcium and magnesium homeostasis. Am J Med 72:473, 1982

76. Randall RE, Cohen MD, Spray CC, Rossmeisl EC: Hypermagnesemia in renal failure: Etiology and toxic manifestations. Ann Int Med 61:73, 1964

77. Juan D: Clinical review: The clinical importance of hypomagnesemia. Surgery 91:510, 1982

78. Shils ME: Experimental human magnesium depletion. Medicine 48:61, 1969

79. Peden VH, Witzleben CL, Skelton MA: Total parenteral nutrition. J Pediatr 78:180, 1981

80. Sheldon GF, Peterson SR, Sanders R: Hepatic dysfunction during hyperalimentation. Arch Surg 113:504, 1978

81. Lindor KD, Fleming CR, Abrams A, Hirschkorn MA: Liver function values in adults receiving total parenteral nutrition. JAMA 241:2398, 1979

82. Maini B, Blackburn GL, Bistrian BR, et al.: Cyclic hyperalimentation: An optimal technique for preservation of visceral protein. J Surg Res 20:515, 1976

83. Langer B, McHattie JD, Zohrab WJ, et al.: Prolonged survival after complete bowel resection using intravenous hyperalimentation at home. J Surg Res 15:226, 1973

84. Fukazawa T, Privett OS, Takahashi Y: Effects of essential fatty acid deficiency on lipid transport from liver. Lipids 6:388, 1971

85. Zeisel SH: Dietary choline: Biochemistry, physiology and pharmacology. Ann Rev Nutr 1:95, 1981

86. Lombardi B: Effects of choline deficiency on rat hepatocytes. Fed Proc 30:139, 1971

87. Kaminski DL, Adams A, Jellinek M: The effect of hyperalimentation on hepatic lipid content and lipogenic enzyme activity in rats and man. Surgery 88:93, 1980

88. Burke JF, Wolfe RR, Mullany CJ, et al.: Glucose requirements following burn injury. Ann Surg 190:274, 1979

89. Chang S, Silvis SE: Fatty liver produced by hyperalimentation of rats. Am J Gastroenterol 62:410, 1974

90. Stein TP, Buzby GP, Gertner MH, et al.: Effect of parenteral nutrition on protein synthesis and liver fat metabolism in man. Am J Physiol 239:280, 1980

91. Thompson SW: Hepatic toxicity of intravenous fat emulsions. In Meng HC, Wilmore DW (eds): Fat Emulsions in Parenteral Nutrition. American Medical Association, 1976

92. Grant JP, Cox CE, Kleinman LM, et al.: Serum hepatic enzyme and bilirubin elevations during parenteral nutrition. Surg Gynecol Obstet 145:573, 1977

93. Salvian AJ, Allardyce DB: Impaired bilirubin secretion during total parenteral nutrition. J Surg Res 28:547, 1980

94. Wagman LD, Burt ME, Brennan MF: The impact of total parenteral nutrition on liver function tests in patients with cancer. Cancer 49:1249, 1982

95. Allardyce DB: Cholestasis caused by lipid emulsions. Surg Gynecol Obstet 154:641, 1982

96. Lowry SF, Brennan MF: Abnormal liver function during parenteral nutrition: Relation to infusion excess. J Surg Res 26:300, 1979

97. Rodgers BM, Hollenbeck, JI, Donnelly WH, Talbert JL: Intrahepatic cholestasis with par-

enteral alimentation. Am J Surg 131:149, 1976

98. Postuma R, Trevenen CL: Liver disease in infants receiving total parenteral nutrition. Pediatrics 63:110, 1979

99. Buzby GP, Mullen JL, Stein TP, Rosato EF: Manipulation of total parenteral nutrition

caloric substrate and fatty infiltration of the liver. J Surg Res 31:46, 1981

100. Tulikoura I, Huikuri K: Morphological fatty changes and function of the liver, serum free fatty acids, and triglycerides during parenteral nutrition. Scand J Gastroent 17:177, 1982

21. Home Parenteral Nutrition
Lorraine See Young

Home parenteral nutrition (HPN) has proven to be a realistic form of support for patients requiring long-term (greater than 30 days) intravenous (IV) feeding to establish or maintain normal nutrition. Over the past decade many advances have been made in the field of parenteral nutrition (PN) to reduce significantly the mechanical, metabolic, and septic complications that can be associated with this technique. Because of the scientific and technical advances that have been made, the morbidity and mortality of many individuals with nonfunctional gastrointestinal tracts are greatly reduced.

The progress made in the field of PN as a life support system, coupled with efforts to contain rising health care costs and length of hospitalization, has resulted in the formation and implementation of HPN programs. Through the establishment of a multidisciplinary team of health care professionals, hospitalized patients and their families can be adequately prepared for HPN prior to discharge and successfully monitored on a regular basis after discharge from the hospital.

ASSESSMENT OF THE HPN CANDIDATE

Because of the high cost of inhospital parenteral nutrition, patients with stable disease processes precluding an adequate enteral intake are being successfully maintained at much less expense in the home. The psychological benefits of allowing an individual with a debilitating disease to return home can also not be understated. With the rationale for HPN clearly delineated, it is important next to decide who are appropriate candidates for HPN.

Table 21–1 lists a few of the general requirements for patient selection to a HPN program.[2] Selection criteria for individual patients can be further categorized into nutritional, medical, psychosocial, and financial concerns. The nutritional issues that need to be assessed include the presence of a nonfunctional gastrointestinal tract and the need for IV fluid and nutrients for survival. Once these requirements are met, the specifics of the formula design must be established.

The medical issues that must be addressed include evaluating the underlying disease process and its effects on the patient, plus any other debilitating chronic ailments, i.e., heart disease, arthritis, that may dictate how HPN is managed in the particular patient. Not only the nutrient prescription but also the patient's ability to care for him or herself may be affected. It is also important to assess any other medical therapies the patient may be receiving, as these may affect the administration of HPN. In addition, it is essential to know the patient's course of illness and ultimate prognosis because these may influence the medical, social and financial decisions necessary to embark on an HPN pro-

TABLE 21–1. REQUIREMENTS FOR PATIENT SELECTION

1. Intravenous administration required to maintain fluid and nutritional equilibrium
2. Capable of self-care: able to spend greater than 50 percent of time out of bed
3. Mentally, physically, and emotionally able to start, stop, and control infusion
4. Expected survival 3 or more months
5. Aware of diagnosis and desire for home treatment
6. Gastrointestinal condition precluding oral or enteric feeding and no alternative to parenteral feeding

gram, especially if suspected length of survival is less than 3 months. Each case must be individually assessed and decided upon in a thoughtful manner.

The psychosocial concerns that must be addressed are multifaceted. The patient must be aware of the diagnosis and must desire home care. The optimal patient is capable of self-care and should be mentally, physically, and emotionally able to understand and control the HPN infusion apparatus. If the patient is not, then additional support must be identified. Even when the patient will be responsible for self-care, support systems must be assessed and evaluated. Questions as— Are family and friends a help or a hindrance to the patient? Does the patient have storage space for infusion apparatus? Is the patient available for follow-up monitoring?—need to be answered.

Last, but certainly not least important, the prospective HPN patient's financial status and reimbursement potential must be determined. Does the patient have insurance coverage? Is the patient the primary breadwinner for the family? These concerns must be evaluated before patients are enrolled into an HPN program.

A recent review by Evans in *Nutritional Support Services* summarizes the major categories of patients who may qualify for HPN.[3]

In this paper, individuals who experience gastrointestinal dysfunction resulting in inadequate nutrient intake or absorption are considered candidates for HPN. These include patients with: short bowel syndrome, with and without the potential for bowel adaptation; motility disorders, such as pseudoobstruction; Crohn's disease and its resulting medical/surgical problems, such as enterocutaneous fistulas and growth failure; inflammatory bowel disease requiring bowel rest because of severe malabsorption; malabsorption syndromes such as nontropical sprue and celiac disease, which are refractory to dietary and medical treatment; and radiation enteritis.

The role of HPN in the cancer patient is the topic of much debate. HPN can be useful in some cancer patients who, because of their antineoplastic treatments, have lost bowel function for a period of time, but who are expected to recover and do not require hospitalization.[4] Issues involved in treating the terminal cancer patient, specifically the role of HPN in this population, are briefly summarized below.

Weiss et al.[5] have fed a carefully selected group of nine patients suffering from recurrent, incurable cancer and a gastrointestinal condition precluding an enteral intake. Their goal was to allow the patients to live their final months at home instead of confined to a hospital. In addition, a substantial cost savings has been realized compared to in-hospital care. Eight out of the nine patients have subsequently died (six of the deaths were from progressive cancer) with the range of time on HPN having been from ½ month to 19 months. Complications were few and in all cases the patients and families were pleased to be at home. The authors emphasize the importance of selecting appropriate patients in regard to physical, mental, and prognostic characteristics. Being adequately nourished and feeling stronger may serve to improve the quality of the limited life-span remaining to cancer patients and may help to assist the host in responding to antineoplastic treatment. In contrast to this belief, there is evidence from animal studies that nutrient infusions to meet energy requirements or infusion of amino acids alone will stimulate tumor growth at the expense of the host when given without antitumor therapy.[6,7] The decision to use HPN in cancer patients should be made on a case-by-case basis after clear discussions with the patient, family, and the patient's primary caretakers.

Another decision that must be made as part of the initial assessment of the HPN patient is whether the therapy will be permanent—as in the terminal phases of chronic disease or in those patients with a massive bowel resection precluding enteral intake in the foreseeable future—or temporary, where the patient will see daily improvement leading to the eventual cessation of PN altogether. When HPN is to be permanent, the patient will require much psychosocial support in learning to live without eating and usual food intake. The goals of HPN in all cases are to attempt to enhance the individual's quality of life, reduce hospitalization, and support the return to normal daily activities including family life and employment.

Individuals who would not be suitable candidates for HPN include the senile patient, as in the case of the elderly; a patient who lives alone, with no friends or family nearby to assist with care; psychiatrically disturbed patients; and possibly the patient with terminal disease who is known to have less than 2 to 3 months to live.

ESTABLISHING A HOME PARENTERAL NUTRITION PROGRAM

Once a patient has been selected as a candidate for HPN, a series of steps must be taken to ensure adequate training of the patient and organization of the program. One of the first decisions—whether a home care program is to be used or whether the individual institution will organize and implement the HPN program—should be made before pa-

tient selection. With the large number of home care companies available and the growing number of home care patients, it is rare that an individual institution can comfortably handle this responsibility. Table 21–2 lists some of the current home care companies. Although the specific responsibilities of the home care companies vary from company to company, generally they will provide supplies, program consultation, and financial management assistance, and serve as a professional liaison between the discharge hospital and the patient for continuing care. The services supply products, equipment, and trained personnel directly to the patient's home on a 24-hour basis. Supplies and equipment can, in fact, be sent to other locations when patients are traveling. These HPN services bill third-party agencies for supplies, relieving the hospital of the responsibility for collecting charges for the home patients.[8]

If an individual institution decides to manage its own HPN needs, there are certain questions that must be answered before the patient is discharged. The following are some of these questions: How and by whom will the solutions be prepared? How are prescriptions relayed to appropriate personnel, and is there a lag time before necessary changes in solution composition can be made? An assessment should be made of the quality assurance of solution preparation to ensure minimal mistakes and maximum sterility. Who is responsible for the training of the patient and family, and how much time is allotted for education? How often and by whom will supplies be delivered to the patient? Who is responsible for the clinical management of the patient—a physician in the patient's home area, the physician at the hospital from which the patient is discharged, or the HPN vendor nurse–clinician? And finally, the cost of the various programs must be evaluated and methods of reimbursement established. It is because of these many factors that most institutions choose a home care company to care for their HPN patients.

Once an HPN program suitable to a partic-

TABLE 21–2. HOME CARE COMPANIES[a]

Travacare	6301 Lincoln Avenue
	Morton Grove, IL 60053
Medical Electronics	335 Newbury Street
	Boston, MA 02115
Medical Marketing	Box 4456
	Portsmouth, NH 03801
New England Critical Care	45 New York Avenue
	Framingham, MA 01701
Home Health Care of America	1055 East Street
	Tewksbury, MA 01876
TPN Pharmacy	75 Blossom Court
	Boston, MA 02114
Home Nutritional Support	201 Bloomfield Avenue
	Verona, NJ 07044
Theranutrix	22 Paris Avenue
	Rockleigh, NJ 07647
Abbott Home Care	Abbott Laboratories—Home Care Division
	Abbott Park
	North Chicago, IL 60064

[a]Note: This list is not meant to be comprehensive.

ular institution and patient is selected, the patient can then be prepared for discharge.

THE TEAM APPROACH TO HPN

To facilitate the process of planning and implementing an HPN program and to ensure a smooth transition from hospital to home care, a multidisciplinary team approach is critical to the success of the program. Figure 21–1 illustrates the essential elements of an HPN team.

Each member of the team serves a distinct and important role in the management of the HPN patient. Unfortunately, not all institutions utilize this team approach and a dietitian may be the only person knowledgeable to facilitate the program. The dietitian should be prepared to seek out the necessary resources both within the hospital and locally to effectively implement an HPN program.

The dietitian is responsible for evaluating

the patient's initial and follow-up nutrition status, and for determining the patient's nutrient requirements in relation to what form and amounts they will be provided in the PN solution. The dietitian plays an important role in patient and family education. The nutrition assessment parameters that must be

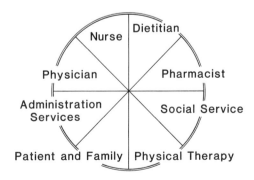

Figure 21–1. The multidisciplinary team for efficient implementation of a home parenteral nutrition program.

followed, the nutrient compounds of the PN solutions, and their essentiality for body functions must be explained simply and in an organized fashion to the patient and family before discharge. In addition, if the patient is eating, instruction is necessary regarding diet modifications and recommendations while the patient is receiving PN.[9]

Further responsibilities of the dietitian include coordination of the transition to home care, making logistic arrangements if necessary; inservice education to other hospital personal and professional education of other dietitians; research regarding optimal nutrient infusions and techniques in HPN; and administrative activities such as publications and budgeting.

If the dietitian is the sole person responsible for preparing the patient for discharge, he or she will need to instruct the patient as to solution storage, examining solutions for incompatibilities, using aseptic technique, e.g., when changing the dressing and tubing, and how to recognize complications or problems. Patient proficiency must be documented. Records must be kept of all care given the patient. The dietitian may also serve as the primary person assisting the patient in transfer to home care. These are all tasks for which other personnel (i.e., pharmacists, nurses) are responsible if a team approach is utilized.

TECHNIQUES OF HPN

Initial Preparation for Home

Once a patient has been favorably assessed as a candidate for HPN, it is imperative that the benefits and risks of HPN be clearly explained to the patient and family or significant others. It is important that the patient and supportive personnel understand the limitations and constraints imposed by the HPN program, plus the possible therapeutic alternatives and potential complications, before catheter placement and teaching begin.[1,10]

The next steps in preparation for home include catheter insertion, nutrition assessment and determination of nutrient needs, including infusion techniques, and patient education. To complete this process, a sufficient amount of time must be allotted before the patient is discharged, specifically to ensure adequate education. This will depend on the medical stability of the patient.

Central Venous Access

The first concerted efforts to nourish rehabilitative patients requiring IV hyperalimentation at home were made at the University of Washington. From experience in the renal dialysis unit, Broviac and Scribner[11] designed an implantable silicone rubber, central venous feeding catheter along with a delivery system consisting of a 2-liter bottle of nutrients suspended from a beam scale, which incorporated an alarm system that warned the patient when the IV infusion was close to completion.[11,12] Their nonthrombogenic catheter, composed of a thin intravascular portion and a Dacron-cuffed extravascular portion, could be used for prolonged periods of time. At about the same time in Toronto, Jeejeebhoy et al. reported on a patient surviving 25 months at home with a noncuffed silicone catheter placed in a central vein.[13,14]

The ideal characteristics of a venous access system include: a minimal number of parts for the patient to manipulate, understand, lose, or replace (easy availability and access for patient); the catheter should be durable and made from stable material that is compatible with a variety of infusates; it should be painless and comfortable and have minimal foreign body reaction.[15]

Of the two types of catheters most commonly used, Silastic and the polyethylene/polyvinyl/polyurethane types, the Silastic variety is the more popular. This is due to its flexibility, greater stability over time, retention of its original shape, and ability to "float" in the bloodstream, thus decreasing contact with the endothelium and possible problems with localized delivery of hyperosmolar solutions. The delivery of hyperosmolar solutions to a localized area may hasten the formation of fibrin sheaths and deposits.[15]

For long-term HPN, the current catheters of choice at most institutions include the original Broviac–Scribner catheter and a wider-bore modification, the Hickman catheter (1.6 mm inside diameter as opposed to 1 mm in the Broviac catheter).[16]

Before insertion of the central catheter, venograms are often performed to ensure patency of the central veins, especially in previously hospitalized patients who in the past received central lines.

Hickman and Broviac catheter insertions are accomplished in the operating room under general anesthesia, and insertion is made via any of the several tributary veins that provide access to the superior vena cava. The tip of the catheter should be just above or in the right atrium. The cephalic vein is generally used, but the internal or external jugular veins, or muscular branches of the subclavian vein can also be used.[14,15,17]

The extravascular portion of the catheter is tunneled under the skin and brought out at a point where the patient can easily see it and care for it. The area lateral to the sternum at about the fourth or fifth interspace is quite suitable. The Dacron cuff around the extravascular portion of the catheter allows the growth of fibrous tissue, which aids in fixing the catheter in place and acts as a barrier to bacteria. The catheter has a plastic cap that can be heparinized and sealed between nutrient infusions. (Fig. 21–2).[13]

Determining Nutrient Needs and Infusion Techniques

Once the catheter is securely in place, the patient should be assessed to determine nutrient and fluid requirements. Only then can the patient's HPN infusion schedule be established.

In general, the PN infusate is delivered continuously when total nutrient requirements are infused by vein or intermittently when PN is supplemented by oral nutrition. Most institutions utilize intermittent infusions or cyclic hyperalimentation in which the solution is administered in the evening so that the patient is allowed more freedom during the day. One of the delivery systems currently in use includes an ambulatory hyperalimentation vest capable of holding nutrient solutions in its pockets. This gives the patient more freedom of motion by avoiding the cumbersome volumetric infusion pumps. The vest is lightweight, comfortable, and custom-fitted to the patient, and there have

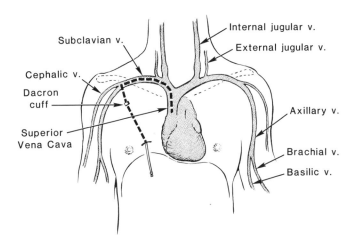

Figure 21–2. Catheter placement for long-term use.

TABLE 21-3. SAMPLE HPN SOLUTIONS

Composition		Volume	Dose	Other Characteristics
Crystalline amino acids	4.25%	500 cc	42.5 g	Nitrogen: 7.15 g/L
Dextrose	25%	500 cc	250 g	Total kcal: 1029
Sodium			35 mEq	Osmolarity: 1800
Potassium			30 mEq	Nonprotein kcal/N: 119
Magnesium			5 mEq	
Calcium			4.7 mEq	
Phosphate			15 mM	
Acetate			65 mEq	
Chloride			35 mEq	
Vitamins		5 ml		
Ascorbic acid			100 mg	
Vitamin A			3300 IU	
Vitamin D			200 IU	
Thiamine (B_1)			3.0 mg	
Riboflavin (B_2)			3.6 mg	
Pyridoxine (HCl) (B_6)			4.0 mg	
Niacinamide			40.0 mg	
Pantothenic acid			15.0 mg	
Vitamin E			10 IU	
Biotin			60 μg	
Folic acid			400 μg	
Vitamin B_{12}			5 μg	
Trace elements		5 ml		
Zinc			2.5 mg	
Copper			0.5 mg	
Manganese			0.8 mg	
Chromium			10 μg	

been no significant complications related to its use. This is just one example of how modifications in HPN technology and manufacture may prove both clinically efficacious to the professional and esthetically favorable to the patient.

After the patient's nutrient needs are assessed and the mechanical delivery system is decided upon, the PN formulations need to be designed and patterns of infusion determined. Oral nutrition is encouraged, for those patients who are able, to promote bowel adaptation. Allowing the patient to eat not only provides necessary stimulation to the bowel in an effort to prevent mucosal atrophy, it also allows the patient to interact socially at mealtime and may promote self-worth by letting the patient do something without outside assistance.

The majority of HPN patients require 1500 to 3000 milliliters of PN fluids/day. More intravenous crystalloid fluid supplementation is needed for patients with high-output stomas or fistulas.[9] Each liter of PN fluid routinely contains approximately 25 percent dextrose and 4.25 percent amino acids, vitamins, minerals, and trace elements. A typical HPN formula for 1 liter of fluid is shown in Table 21-3.

If the patient is not eating, exogenous essential fatty acid must be administered in the form of IV fat emulsion. The actual amount of fat required for optimal physiologic functioning is the subject of much debate. It is known that linoleic acid should supply at least 4 percent of the total energy requirements to prevent essential fatty acid deficiency.[19] One to two 500-ml bottles of 10 percent fat emulsion per week is sufficient in most cases. Jeejeebhoy, however, feels that there is strong metabolic and physiologic evidence supporting a glucose/fat regimen where 30 to 40 percent of the total calories are from fat.[20] He cites inappropriate calorie–protein mixtures or all-glucose solutions as possible causes of fatty liver. In addition, chronic infusions of hypertonic dextrose may cause hyperinsulinemia and a greater risk for hypoglycemia when a glucose/protein infusion is terminated abruptly. The more frequent use of fat emulsion in the HPN regime, however, is an added expense (as fat is more expensive than glucose) and requires additional manipulation of the central venous system on the part of the patient. Ideally, if the patient could ingest 60 ml daily of safflower, soybean, or any highly polyunsaturated vegetable oil, it would alleviate the problem of IV administration of essential fatty acids. In addition, the oral ingestion of fat stimulates bile acid and gastrointestinal enzyme secretion, thus reducing the risk of developing the intrahepatic cholestasis so prevalent in long-term PN patients.

The electrolyte and mineral requirements of patients will vary depending upon their individual gastrointestinal losses and underlying disease. Requirements should be set before the patient is discharged, and an outpatient monitoring system should be determined for the patient. It should be remembered that requirements for the intracellular ions (potassium, phosphorus, magnesium) will increase as the patient becomes anabolic. Specific care should also be taken for individuals with renal or hepatic disease.

The vitamin and trace mineral requirements of HPN patients can be met by standard IV supplements. With the exception of vitamin D, optimal dose and frequency of administration have not been studied in detail. The most recent studies are simple observations of plasma or blood levels during a given regimen.[20] Recently, many institutions have been deleting vitamin D from the preparations and increasing the calcium because of observations of an osteomalacia with bone pains and fractures that were reversed when vitamin D was withdrawn.[20] Exposure to the sun is encouraged to maintain normal vitamin D levels in these patients.

For the patient who is unable to take oral iron supplementation, intramuscular injections or slow IV infusions of iron dextran (Imferon) may be administered as required to maintain normal hematologic levels. Vitamin preparations and regimes should be carefully selected to ensure intake of folate, B_{12}, and vitamin K as well as the usual B complex and C vitamins.

In diabetic patients and in other patients where glucose intolerance may be a problem, short-acting crystalline zinc insulin can be added to the PN infusate to help control blood sugar. The patient will probably require more physiologic fine-tuning in the hospital before discharge, especially if cyclic feedings are to be attempted at home. For example, the diabetic patient may require 2 to 3 hours of tapering of HPN solution before stopping the infusion during cyclic feedings to prevent a marked hypoglycemia. An example of how to proceed with tapering solutions, to evolve into cyclic feedings, is as follows.

Before the patient is discharged there is usually an adaptive phase lasting anywhere from three to 21 days depending upon available hospitalization. During this time the volume infused over 24 hours is held constant while the duration of infusion is reduced by approximately 1 hour per day depending upon the home training time available. The rate of infusion is increased so that all solutions are infused at night, permitting the patient a more normal life during the day. During this adaptive phase the patient should be monitored closely for signs of hyper- or hypoglycemia or other metabolic complications that may occur, and solutions should be modified accordingly. It is preferable that the patient be stable on a certain parenteral regime for at least 1 week before being sent home.

Patient Education

Probably of greatest importance in assuring adequacy of the HPN patient's understanding and feeling of comfort with the system is the development of a good training program. Many excellent manuals have been written to assist the institution that is just starting a program. Some of these include the Mayo Clinic,[21] Cleveland Clinic Foundation,[22] and the University of Washington[23] manuals.

Any training program in HPN should include explanations of PN solution preparation and administration, catheter care, pump usage, heparin "lock" manipulation, and nutrient needs (Table 21–4).

HPN instruction begins soon after catheter placement. Typically the first procedure taught is change of the catheter dressing. The patient's learning experiences continue each consecutive day during preparation for home.[9] The rate of progress is geared to the individual. The training program includes typed instructions, simple visual aids, observation, progressive participation in solution preparation, frequent practice in correct handling of syringes, needles, ampules, and dressing changes,[24] and final demonstration performed by the patient to confirm understanding. Videotapes can demonstrate the procedural steps, and although complicated at first, the experience of most institutions is that the patient can satisfactorily learn the system in daily sessions over 1 to 2 weeks if necessary. Many institutions require the patient to take a written test and certainly to be able to satisfactorily perform all steps of technical care before discharge.[9,24] Depending on the system of infusion chosen (continuous or intermittent), the patient should have complete understanding of how to initiate and taper solution rates before stopping, as in the case of intermittent feedings, and

TABLE 21–4. CHARACTERISTICS OF HPN TRAINING PROGRAMS

1. Description of HPN, with a definition of the role of each nutrient in performing body functions
2. Details of the procedure of care of the catheter
3. Outlines of the aseptic preparation of the PN solution and discussion of aseptic technique, touch contamination, and the metric system
4. Delineation of the procedure for setting up, starting, and stopping the PN solution infusion, and fat emulsion if used
5. Description of the infusion pump, and how to use and care for it
6. Explanation of the complications that may occur related to the catheter or metabolic abnormalities with instructions for action to be taken
7. Lists of the personnel responsible for the patient's home care, and explanation of how to contact them
8. How to use syringes for flushing the catheter with heparin
9. Explanation of how and where to store solutions and supplies
10. Description of routine monitoring procedures and follow-up appointments with the HPN team

especially of what signs may be warnings for possible metabolic complications (i.e., rebound hypoglycemia).

Prior arrangements need to be made with either the local Visiting Nurse Association for home supervision or the institution's own PN nurses to make periodic visits to the patient at home. Initially, a nurse should make daily or weekly home visits. Logistic arrangements also need to be made regarding where the necessary material will be purchased or picked up. Some of the major materials necessary for HPN include:

1. Volumetric infusion pump or vest system
2. Refrigeration for PN solutions, additives, fat emulsions, heparin
3. Sterile catheter dressing kits, antiseptic solutions, IV tubing, catheter plugs, rubber cannula clamp, syringes

Finally, before the patient is ready for discharge, a monitoring system needs to be developed. This includes scheduling of outpatient clinic visits, written directions as to what medications need to be taken and other treatment orders, and instructions as to specific monitoring that the patient can do at home, precautions to take, and what steps to take in the event of an emergency (i.e., sudden onset fever, chills). The potential septic, metabolic, or mechanical complications of PN and treatment for each are discussed elsewhere in this book (see Chapter 20 for a more detailed explanation).

MONITORING THE PATIENTS ON HPN

Patients are seen weekly for the first month, depending on medical stability of the patient, and then visits can be lengthened to bimonthly and then monthly if no complications develop. At each visit the following are performed:

1. The patient is weighed to assess accuracy of nutritional input and hydration status.
2. Blood is drawn for complete blood count, electrolytes, blood urea nitrogen, creatinine, glucose, magnesium, phosphate, total protein, albumin, liver function tests, iron, total iron-binding capacity (only if CBC warrants), transferrin, copper, zinc, folate, B_{12} (monitored less frequently).
3. Urine is tested for sugar and acetone.
4. Physical examination by physician, including vital signs, evaluation of medications used, and reevaluation of psychosocial status.
5. At each visit the patient should be interviewed by a nutritionist, reassessed, and, if necessary, IV nutrient and/or oral diet modifications should be made. An assessment of nutritional status is performed.
6. Review of patient's skills and techniques to check for errors, oversights, or shortcuts that may cause problems. Table 21–5 lists the monitoring procedures that the HPN patient may be asked to perform at home.

A rehabilitative program is essential not only to restore and maintain the patient's physical conditions, but to improve his or her psychosocial situation as well. A program of physical activity to restore strength and stamina and to prepare the patient for activities of daily living is essential for the patient to effectively execute the HPN program. The patient should be encouraged to resume employment if this is deemed medically advisable by the physician. Of utmost importance is that the patient avoid becoming too dependent on the family or visiting nurse for care.[24]

The resumption of as normal a living situation as possible by the patient and family should be encouraged, and every effort should be made on the part of the HPN team to facilitate this.

Presently, completed studies examine the psychological impact, permanent or long-term, of HPN on the patient. Although a discussion of this is beyond the scope of this chapter, a recent psychosocial survey of patients on permanent HPN was performed to assess the quality of life in these patients. They were asked questions regarding their physical symptoms, social and leisure activities, interpersonal relationships, sexuality, psychological problems, and feelings about HPN. The interviews were repeated at

TABLE 21–5. HOME MONITORING FOR THE HPN PATIENT: POSSIBLE PARAMETERS

Weigh regularly—according to prescribed schedule

Check urine for sugar and acetone

Keep fluid intake and output records

Check daily temperature

Be aware of clinical symptoms: lethargy, edema, chills, sweat intervals of 6 to 10 months in certain patients, and revealed no systematic or significant improvement or deterioration of quality of life during HPN over time. In general, 46 percent of the 13 patients surveyed claimed they were psychologically affected by the HPN, but social and leisure activities were normal or only slightly impaired in most. The study demonstrates that in addition to the time commitment necessary for therapy, the patient's quality of life depended on restitution of physical health, the presence of an ostomy, personality, finances, and support from family and hospital.[25] Other reports have noted serious psychosocial problems may occur with HPN patients; these include depression, drug addiction, organic brain syndrome, and family stress.[26]

Cost

Unfortunately, the most devastating dilemma that most HPN patients face is the large financial burden of HPN and the difficulty in receiving reimbursement from many insurance companies. Naturally, the cost of HPN will vary depending upon the type and amounts of solution and infusion apparatus used. It has been estimated that the cost of HPN ranges from $3000 to $4000/month.[27] However, Burke et al. report, "A cost comparison for treating patients in the home TPN program versus similar therapy in the hospital indicates a reduction of about 60 percent in the per diem expenses."[28]

Table 21–6 lists the typical TPN expenses and compares inpatient to outpatient ex-

TABLE 21–6. TYPICAL TOTAL PARENTERAL NUTRITION EXPENSES[a]

Item	Inpatient Expenses		Outpatient Expenses	
	Unit Cost	Monthly Rate	Unit Cost	Monthly Rate
Room	$260.00/day	$ 7908.33	—	—
Solutions				
Standard IVH 2 liters/day and administration sets	$ 45.50	$ 2767.92	$35.00	$2129.17
Fat emulsion 10% 500 ml 2× weekly	52.65	456.30	30.00	260.00
Equipment				
Cassette	15.00/day	456.25	7.00	212.90
Pump	—	—	—	150.00
Pole	—	—	—	15.00
Central supply charge	10.00	304.17	—	—
Dressing kit (MWF and prn)	—	—	4.00	53.33
Laboratory fees Electrolytes: weekly Iron: monthly IBC: monthly CBC: weekly Glucose: weekly Mg: weekly SMA-12: biweekly BUN: weekly	—	500.41	—	102.83
Visiting nurse	—	—	25.00	325.00
Total		$12,393.45		3328.03

[a]Physician fees and catheter expenses excluded.

penses. Hospital room charges account for the major difference between inhospital costs of $12,400 per month and home care costs of $3300 per month.[5] Documentation of these substantial savings to cost-conscious medical administrators, insurance companies, and government insurers will help to acquire reimbursement of HPN for all patients.

The Reimbursement Process

The question of who pays for HPN is critical and needs addressing before an HPN program is chosen. Private insurance companies vary in coverage. Patients and their families face negotiating insurance coverage before discharge. At present, Medicare varies by state from complete coverage to none at all.

The social service department usually assists in solving funding problems for HPN. It also has the capability to solicit funds available from many community services to help financially support the HPN family.[8]

Complications of HPN

A discussion of HPN is not complete without addressing the issue of complications—those most common and how to avoid them. Most HPN complications are minor and only require adjustments in the HPN prescription to rectify the situation. More serious problems, however, can require hospitalization, i.e., sepsis, mechanical catheter problems, fluid and electrolyte imbalances, or longstanding metabolic problems.

The establishment of the Registry of Patients on HPN by the New York Academy of Medicine in 1977 has allowed health professionals to follow the course and progress of HPN on a national level. It demonstrated that between January 1, 1978 and December 31, 1979 there was a significant number of readmissions to the hospital for a variety of reasons (Table 21–7).[29]

The evidence suggests that a large percentage (40.8 percent) of rehospitalizations were due to sepsis and/or catheter-related problems. In addition, of the 34 patients ad-

TABLE 21–7. REASONS FOR READMISSIONS

Cause of Admission	Number of Admissions	Percent of Total Admissions
Sepsis	18	16.7
Catheter problems	26	24.1
Metabolic problems	17	15.7
Fluid and electro-lyte problems	9	8.3
Other	34	31.5
Unreported	4	3.7
Total	108	

mitted for other reasons, 17 were admitted for fever (presumably with negative cultures). These data stress the importance of adequate training prior to discharge regarding aseptic technique and care of the catheter, and also adequate follow-up at home to ensure that the patient continues to follow strict protocol and does not become lax in technique.

The most common mechanical complication is damage to the external segment of the catheter, which is easily repaired on an outpatient basis with a catheter repair kit. The patient is instructed how to use the kit to repair the catheter. Thrombophlebitis and thrombosis can also be significant problems if they effect the subclavian vein or superior vena cava. They are more likely to occur in patients whose primary disease is associated with a hypercoagulable state.[30]

Metabolic problems such as hyperglycemia, dehydration or hyponatremia may occur, especially when solutions are first started. These are corrected by modifying the solution, ideally before the patient is discharged from the hospital. Prolonged IV nutrition makes the HPN patient at risk for nutrient deficiencies. In short-term therapy, these are rarely encountered. Essential fatty acid deficiency,[31] zinc,[32,33] chromium,[34] biotin,[35] and selenium deficiencies[36] have all been reported. Efforts are necessary to ensure an adequate intake of these minerals and to monitor for symptoms of deficiency or excess in this patient population.

SUMMARY AND CONCLUSIONS

With the recent trend toward more comprehensive home health care programs partially resulting from rising hospital costs, HPN has become a very viable alternative for patients who otherwise would have to remain in the hospital solely for nutritional purposes. Because of the technical and physiologic advances made in PN in the last 10 years, HPN proves to be a relatively safe and cost-effective life support system for hundreds of patients.

The keys to a successful HPN program include adequate assessment—medical, nutritional, and psychosocial—of the possible HPN candidates and their families; a complete and organized training program for home care; and appropriate follow-up surveillance. HPN is best implemented as a team approach.

The utilization of professionals from various medical fields will facilitate the achievement of a sound HPN program. In addition, it is imperative that the HPN team members keep abreast of current research in the rapidly growing area of PN, and that they be prepared and receptive to change and progress for the benefit of the HPN patient.

REFERENCES

1. Dudrick SJ, Englert DM, Barroso AD, et al.: Update on ambulatory home hyperalimentation. Nutr Supp Serv 1:18–21, 1981
2. Wateska LP, Sattler LL, Steiger E: Cost of a home parenteral nutrition program. JAMA 244:2303–2304, 1980
3. Evans RW: Indications for home TPN. Nutr Supp Serv 3:33–34, 1983
4. Shils ME: Cancer and home parenteral nutrition. In Home Parenteral Nutrition. Proc Comprehensive Symposium on Total Parenteral Nutrition in the Home. February 17–18, 1980, pp 18–21
5. Weiss SM, Worthington PH, Prioleau M, Rosato FE: Home total parenteral nutrition in cancer patients. Cancer 50L1210–1213, 1982
6. Popp MB, Wagner SF, Brito OJ: Host and tumor responses to increasing levels of intravenous nutritional support. Surgery 94:300–308. 1983
7. Buzby GP, Mullen JL, Stein TP, et al.: Host-tumor interaction and nutrient supply. Cancer 45:2940–2948, 1980
8. Schneider PJ, Mirtallo JM: Home parenteral nutrition programs. JPEN 5:157–160, 1981
9. Srp F, Steiger E, Montague N, et al.: Patient preparation for cyclic home parenteral nutrition; a team approach. Nutr Supp Serv 1:30–34, 1981
10. Byrne WJ, Ament ME, Burke M, Fonkalsrud E: Home parenteral nutrition. Surg Gynecol Obstet 149:593–599, 1979
11. Broviac JW, Scribner BH: Prolonged parenteral nutrition in the home. Surg Gynecol Obstet 139:24–28, 1974
12. Dudrick SJ, Englert DM, Van Burne CT, et al.: New concepts of ambulatory home hyperalimentation. JPEN 3:72–76, 1979
13. Jeejeebhoy KN, Zohrad WJ, Langer B, et al.: Total parenteral nutrition at home for twenty-three months without complication and with good rehabilitation. Gastroenterology 65:811, 1973
14. Steiger E, Grundfest S: A review of home hyperalimentation. Contemp Surg 15:33–40, 1979
15. Mullen JL: Long-term venous access in home parenteral nutrition. Proc Comprehensive Symposium on Total Parenteral Nutrition in the Home. February 17–18, 1980, pp 22–26
16. Bjeletich J, Hickman RO: The Hickman indwelling catheter. Am J Nurs January 1980, 62–65
17. Englert DM, Dudrick SJ: Principles of ambulatory home hyperalimentation. Am J Intraven Ther August/September 1978, 11–28
18. Jeejeebhoy KN, Zohrad WJ, Langer B, et al.: Access and pumping systems. Gastroenterology 65:32–34, 1973
19. Elwyn DH: Nutritional requirements of adult surgical patients. Crit Care Med 8:9–19, 1980
20. Jeejeebhoy KN: Meeting nutrient requirements of the HPN patient in home parenteral nutrition. Proc Comprehensive Symposium on Total Parenteral Nutrition in the Home. February 17–18, 1980, pp 35–48
21. Berkner S, Fleming CR: Home Parenteral Nu-

trition: A Handbook. Rochester, Minnesota: Rochester Methodist Hospital, 1979

22. Sattler L, Wateska LP, Siska B, et al.: Cleveland Clinic Foundation Home TPN Manual. Cleveland, Ohio: Cleveland Clinic Foundation, 1978

23. Ivey MF, Scribner BM, Miller DG: Home Parenteral Nutrition Instruction Manual. Seattle, Washington: University of Washington Hospital, 1979

24. Shils ME: A program for total parenteral nutrition at home. Am J Clin Nutr 28:1429–1435, 1975

25. Ladefoged K: Quality of life in patients on permanent home parenteral nutrition. JPEN 5:132–137, 1981

26. Gulledge AD: Social and psychiatric implications of HPN in home parenteral nutrition. Proc Comprehensive Symposium on Total Parenteral Nutrition in the Home. February 17–18, 1980, pp 39–42

27. Ivey MA, Riella M, Meuller W, et al.: Long-term parenteral nutrition in the home. Am J Hosp Pharm 32:1032–1036, 1975

28. Burke WA, et al.: Total parenteral nutrition and the ambulatory patient at home. Am J Intraven Ther 3:53–66, 1976

29. Shils ME: Registry of patients on HPN. In Home Parenteral Nutrition. Proc Comprehensive Symposium on Total Parenteral Nutrition

in the Home. February 17–18, 1980, pp 42–44

30. Bothe A, Orr G, Bistrian B, and Blackburn GL: Home hyperalimentation. Comp Ther 5:54–61, 1979

31. Fleming GR, Smith LM, Hodges RE: Essential fatty acid deficiency in adults receiving total parenteral nutrition. Am J Clin Nutr 29:976–983 1976

32. Wolman SL, Anderson GH, Marks EB, et al.: Zinc in total parenteral nutrition. Requirements and metabolic effects. Gastroenterology 76:458–476, 1978

33. Fleming GR, Hodges RE, Hurley LH: A prospective study of serum copper and zinc levels in adult patients receiving total parenteral nutrition. Am J Clin Nutr 29:70–77, 1976

34. Jeejeebhoy KN, Chu RC, Marliss EB, et al.: Chromium deficiency, glucose intolerance and neuropathy reversed by chromium supplementation in a patient receiving long term parenteral nutrition. Am J Clin Nutr 30:531–538, 1977

35. McClain CJ, Baker H, Onstad GR: Biotin deficiency in an adult during home parenteral nutrition. JAMA 247:3116–3117, 1982

36. Fleming CR, Lie JT, McCall JT, et al.: Selenium deficiency and fatal cardiomyopathy in a patient on home parenteral nutrition. Gastroenterology 83:689–693, 1982.

Part VI. EVALUATION OF THE NUTRITION CARE PLAN

22. Reassessment and Determining an End Point of Therapy

Laura E. Matarese

Documentation of the efficacy of nutrition therapy at first glance appears relatively simple. Unfortunately, over the short term, this assessment can be quite difficult since the changes in nutrition status are often very subtle and the underlying disease state that interacts with nutrition is often complex. The thought process that leads to a decision to terminate aggressive nutrition intervention and therapy has more of the characteristics of an art than a science. Nevertheless, adequate reassessment will become more critical as the costs of therapy increase and economic resources become less available.

The goal of nutrition support is to maintain lean body mass and optimize nutrition status in order to accelerate healing and shorten hospital stay. Nutrition assessment is the tool by which malnutrition can be objectively identified. It provides evidence on which aggressive nutrient repletion regimens may be initiated and carefully monitored.

RESOLVING NUTRITION DEFICIENCIES

It is imperative that nutrients are delivered accurately, safely, and in amounts adequate to meet the patient's requirements. Thus, it is necessary to check that the patient receives both the type and amount of nutrient solution as ordered. The patient who does not receive 500 cc of a standard parenteral nutrition (PN) solution each day is denied approximately 500 kcal and 21 g of protein. Over the course of 1 week, this translates into approximately 3500 kcal, enough to increase weight by 1 pound.[1] Patients who are being nourished via the gastrointestinal (GI) tract should be routinely evaluated as to their ability to digest and absorb the nutrients they are provided. The patient who is receiving enteral feedings by tube who has intractable diarrhea may not gain any benefit from the therapy and may develop other complications; precious time in which the patient could be nourished is lost and hospital stay is lengthened. Aggressive monitoring and documentation of patient tolerance and nutritional gains help prevent this.

Malnutrition is rarely a condition that develops over short periods of time. Even kwashiorkor, which is considered to be a more acute process, takes weeks to months to develop.[2] Thus it is unrealistic to expect that patients can be repleted and returned to a normal nutritional status over a few days. Severely depleted patients will seldom achieve normal or premorbid nutritional status during their hospitalization and repletion usually continues in the home setting. The length of time for which nutrition therapy must be provided to improve nutritional status, surgical risk, and tolerance of medical treatment varies for each patient, depending on their initial nutritional states and medical conditions.

MONITORING RESULTS OF NUTRITION SUPPORT

As the clinical course progresses, therapy is withdrawn when the patient can be expected to meet nutrient requirements through diet and perhaps oral supplementation. Generally, this occurs before the patient returns to "normal" nutritional status.

Although patients may gain weight during nutrition therapy, apparently the majority of this initial weight gain represents increases in body water and fat rather than lean body mass. Thus, it is unlikely that a significant increase in creatinine–height index (CHI) will be apparent. Likewise, anthropometric measurements lack the specificity to show subtle changes and, therefore, the triceps skinfold and arm muscle circumference measurements may not reflect a significant change during patient hospitalization.[3]

Kilocalories need to be provided in amounts that will meet estimated expenditure and promote weight gain where indicated. Since the patient's energy expenditure may change often during hospitalization, a periodic reassessment of energy requirements is essential. Provision of adequate energy can be documented by weight gain, provided that the patient is in fluid balance. As the provision of kilocalories exceeds the demand, the patient will begin to increase adipose stores. Over time, this change in tissue composition may be apparent as an increase in the triceps skinfold measurement. (See Chapter 6, Anthropometric Evaluation.)

The provision of adequate protein can be evaluated by several techniques. Since nitrogen (N) is a primary constituent of protein, the N balance reflects changes in protein status. N balance is intimately related to energy balance since a relative imbalance of energy intake alters the effective utilization of N.[4–6] As a result, the N balance becomes more negative as caloric intake decreases and more positive as caloric intake approaches or surpasses the requirement for energy. Determination of N balance using a 24-hour urine urea N measurement is a most useful tool to assess whether anabolism has been achieved in response to nutrition therapy.[7,8] (See Chapter 10, Protein and Energy Requirements.) These test results can be skewed by kidney malfunction and by frequent practical problems of obtaining accurate urine collections.

Since anabolism and catabolism occur simultaneously, the body is in a constant state of N flux. During catabolism, muscle protein is broken down to provide a source of amino acids (AA) to the liver for gluconeogenesis.[9] The CHI provides an estimate of skeletal muscle mass because urinary levels of creatinine are dependent upon the extent of skeletal muscle catabolism. Both the creatinine excretion and CHI may increase initially, reflecting increased breakdown of muscle mass, then decrease as muscle mass is depleted. In the anabolic phase when gluconeogenesis has been halted, the patient may begin to increase lean muscle mass and over time, a modest improvement in the CHI will become apparent.

Urinary creatinine excretion has been significantly correlated with arm muscle circumference.[10,11] Serial determinations of arm muscle circumference are compared to indicate longitudinal changes in skeletal muscle during nutrition therapy, although the limitations of the anthropometric measurements should be noted.[3] The test does not reflect subtle changes in muscle protein.

As aggressive nutrition therapy is provided, certain laboratory studies improve while others seem to lag behind. As energy and protein are provided in sufficient quantities to promote anabolism, synthesis of serum proteins will occur in the liver. Because of its long half-life, serum albumin may not return to normal levels until well after the patient has been discharged from the hospital. Serum transferrin will return to normal levels much sooner because of its shorter half-life.[12,13] Thyroxine-binding prealbumin (TBPA) has a significantly smaller total body pool, a lower plasma concentration, and a short half-life of approximately 2 to 3 days.[12] Retinol-binding protein (RBP), which is sometimes bound with prealbumin, has a biologic half-life of 12 hours and a slightly smaller pool than TBPA. The concentration of the TBPA-RBP complex decreases in the acute stage of protein malnutrition and returns to normal during refeeding.[12,14–16] Both RBP and TBPA are much more sensitive to nutrition therapy than either transferrin or albumin. Thus, they may show a trend toward normalization of protein status much sooner. (See Chapter 5, Laboratory Values and Their Interpretation.)

Total lymphocyte count (TLC) is another laboratory test used to evaluate protein–calorie status. The depressed TLC has been correlated with increased morbidity and mortality in hospitalized patients.[17–22] But after refeeding, TLC may not return to normal due to a variety of clinical factors.

Patients may or may not return to normal skin test reactivity after nutrition therapy. Skin tests should be repeated every 2 weeks in an attempt to document a change. Like the TLC, however, there are many nonnutritional factors that affect skin test reactivity.[23] (See Chapter 7, Tests of Immune Function.)

Malnutrition may result in frank vitamin and mineral deficiencies. Most mineral deficiencies, especially electrolyte problems, can be corrected fairly rapidly. Clinical signs of deficiencies will reverse with therapeutic doses of the appropriate limiting vitamin or mineral. But patients' stores of these nutrients may take weeks to months to replenish. Thus, the micronutrient repletion process may also continue in the home setting. (See Chapters 4 and 11.)

Patients should be in fluid and electrolyte balance before withdrawing special nutrient solutions and before considering hospital discharge. Intake should equal output, allowing approximately 500 cc for insensible losses. Weights should be stable and increase at a steady rate. Weight gain greater than a half pound per day probably represents fluid accumulation and not tissue synthesis. Serum electrolytes and acid–base balance should be within normal limits before discontinuation of therapy. Because nutritional solutions are easily manipulated, correction of electrolyte and acid–base imbalances is far more difficult after therapy is withdrawn. Unless nutrition therapy is to be continued at home, the patient should be able to demonstrate oral intake adequate to maintain nutritional status before termination of support. (See Chapter 23 on transition techniques.)

Many patients will not return to "normal" or even premorbid nutritional status until well after discharge. Consequently, one cannot look for an absolute laboratory value or nutritional parameter to determine the end point of therapy. It is, however, important to look for general trends in the patient's condition, in laboratory values, and in weight changes. It is also important to consider the point at which the patient started therapy. Those patients who started in a severely depleted state complicated by a serious illness may only show slow, modest improvements in nutritional status. This is acceptable as long as the improvements are constant. It is likewise important to look at the patient's clinical course to see if there is an improvement. General signs of improvement in clinical condition include ability to sit up in a chair and then to walk with and without assistance, expressions of interest in eating, and a desire to be discharged from the hospital. These subjective signs of improvement must be considered along with the objective nutritional parameters. Judgment must be exercised in differentiating between the patient who has attained normal laboratory values but clinically is not ready to have therapy discontinued or to be discharged from the hospital, and the patient who shows dramatic clinical improvement without having normal laboratory tests.

Although many of the tests used to evaluate nutritional status lack the sensitivity to reveal short-term changes, it is important to establish a protocol for reassessment. Serial

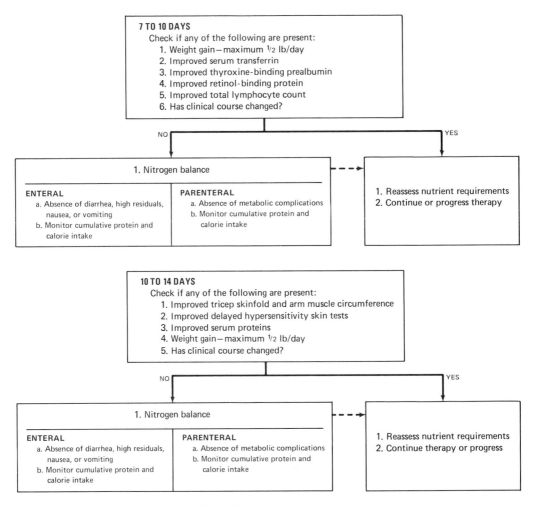

Figure 22–1. Algorithm for reassessment.

assessments are much more meaningful than the one-time static nutrition assessment. Follow-up assessments should be scheduled at regular intervals (see Fig. 22–1). The time period will vary depending on the type of institution and patient population. Patients who are stable enough to be transferred to an extended care facility may not require as frequent reevaluation as those patients who require the services of a tertiary care center. Also, the dietitian will have to select the parameters that would be most meaningful to his or her patient population. Thus, one may not choose to use skin tests on patients who are not likely to react (i.e., oncology patients). It is only through continuous reevaluation of the patient's condition and therapy provided that nutrition support can be effective.

TRANSITIONING NUTRITION SUPPORT

If the GI tract is functional and accessible, it is always the preferred method of nutrition support for several reasons. First, GI tract utilization maintains integrity of epithelial cell lining.[24–27] Absorption of nutrients by the portal system with subsequent delivery to the liver may better support visceral protein synthesis. Certain processes such as transamination that occur in the wall of the gut are bypassed when administering parenteral feedings. Fatty infiltration of the liver is uncommon, as are trace nutrient deficiencies. Lastly, it is generally much simpler and more cost effective to use the GI tract.[27]

After prolonged periods of illness or nil per os, return of GI function may be slow. PN should not be discontinued until the patient can be adequately nourished by tube feedings, diet, oral supplements, or a combination of these. There are several ways to determine the presence of adequate GI function. The best signs are normal upper GI and small bowel x-ray, and normal flatus or bowel movement. Other clinical signs include the presence of bowel sounds and hun-

ger. There should be no vomiting, uncontrolled diarrhea, or evidence of GI obstruction or ileus (see Fig. 22–2).

If the GI tract is functional and accessible but the patient remains anorexic or incapable of self-feeding, tube feedings should be initiated. At this point the patient still needs the close monitoring that was indicated for PN to document the safety and efficacy of enteral therapy. As with PN, tube feedings should not be discontinued until the patient can demonstrate the ability to take adequate nourishment and fluids by mouth.

If appetite is present, dietary support should be initiated. It is essential to determine the patient's ability to feed, chew, and swallow. The diet may have to be advanced slowly until ability to take nourishment by mouth improves. During the weaning process from PN to diet, it is necessary to document caloric and protein intake. Reevaluation of nutritional status should continue every 7 to 10 days to assure a sustained improvement of nutritional parameters and oral intake.

It should be noted that in most instances there must be resolution of the disease process to allow for maintenance of positive nutrient balance. If the patient is still in a state of metabolic stress, it will be extremely difficult, perhaps impossible, to achieve improved nutritional status.

PLANNING FOR DISCHARGE

Plans should be made early, in anticipation of the patient's discharge (see Fig. 22–3). In fact, discharge plans are frequently considered at the initiation of therapy, e.g., whether short-term or long-term venous access or enteral support is indicated. Medical social workers or discharge planners offer invaluable assistance with financial and logistic aspects of discharge planning. These plans will depend largely on the patient's ability to nourish him- or herself. Even the patient who is "independent" as to nourishment, i.e., without special devices or for-

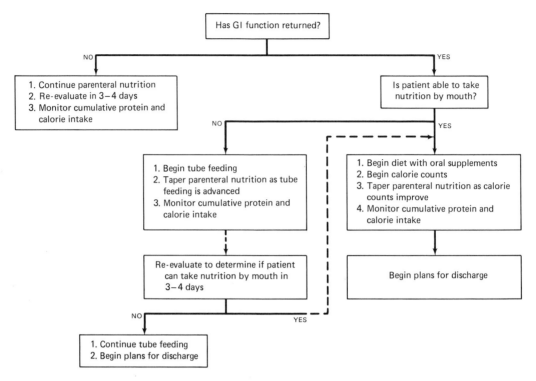

Figure 22–2. Algorithm for advancing nutrition support.

mulas, may have other factors that need to be considered. From a nutritional standpoint, the patient must be able to prepare nourishing meals. The problem may be resolved if there are other people living at home who can provide aid. Difficulties may arise, however, for those individuals who live alone, especially the elderly. The patient must also have sufficient funds to purchase food. It may be necessary to arrange for financial assistance. The patient must be ambulatory or have someone who can shop for and prepare the food.

Some patients may remain partially dependent on specialized nutrition support. If they cannot take in adequate nutrition from diet, it may be necessary to prescribe oral supplements. Commercial supplements must be palatable to the patient and readily accessible from a local pharmacy or home health care agency. Commercially available supplements may not be reimbursed by insurance companies because they are often considered to be self-administered drugs. In such cases, it may be necessary to give the patient and the family recipes for protein–calorie supplements, which they may prepare from standard foods, and instructions for use.

In some instances, patients may be totally dependent on specialized therapy for nutrition support. The patient with a functioning GI tract who cannot take adequate nutrition by mouth may be a candidate for home tube feeding. Patients without adequate GI function may require home parenteral feedings. Both of these therapies require careful planning and teaching so that nutrition support can be self-administered safely and effectively in the home setting. This is best accom-

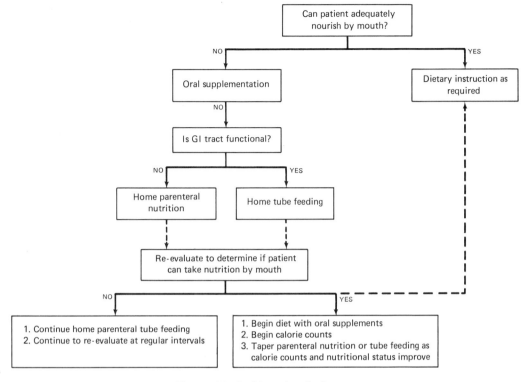

Figure 22–3. Plans for discharge.

plished inhouse through a multidisciplinary approach involving the dietitian, nurse, pharmacist, physician, psychiatrist, social worker, and, after discharge, by a reputable home health care provider who communicates regularly with the multidisciplinary support team. The amount of time required to train a patient will vary depending upon the patient's ability to learn and the learning objectives.

There are some patients who are not candidates for home nutrition support because the level of care required is greater than can be achieved by the patient or provided by family members. In these cases, it may become necessary to consider an extended care facility. The facility must be evaluated carefully. Many will not accept patients who require specialized nutrition therapy. Most extended care facilities will accept patients with tube

feedings, but may not be equipped to handle patients on continuous infusions. It may be necessary to adapt the patient to a bolus or timed intermittent tube feeding before transfer to the extended care facility. Most extended care facilities still do not accept home PN patients, although this is beginning to change.

There are times when one is faced with the decision to continue the nutrition support of a terminally ill patient for whom there is no remaining medical or surgical treatment. In such situations, it is best to attempt to nourish the patient with enteral feedings if at all possible. Enteral feedings have been reported to improve the quality of life remaining to terminal cancer patients.[28] Many believe that PN should not be utilized to nourish these patients.[29] PN is expensive relative to other forms of nutrition support and there is some question as to the benefit of providing PN to the terminal cancer patient. Cameron et al.[30] and Steiger et al.[31] suggested that nutrition support in tumor-bearing, malnourished rats stimulated tumor growth. It may be necessary to provide fluids and electrolytes by vein to maintain comfort and adequate hydration, but the use of amino acids, dextrose, and lipids is contraindicated.

DISCONTINUING NUTRITION THERAPY

Nutrition therapy should not be discontinued without alternate plans for nourishment. Patients receiving PN with high concentrations of dextrose, D_{25} or D_{35}, should have infusions tapered gradually to prevent hypoglycemic episodes. Catheter patency is maintained for continued venous access if it is anticipated that the catheter may be used again in the near future. For patients receiving peripheral PN, the IV may be stopped abruptly since the dextrose concentration is only 10 percent.

The rate of a tube-feeding is gradually reduced with concomitant increases in oral food intake until the latter is sufficient to allow discontinuation of the tube-feeding. However, tube-feedings may be stopped abruptly. Attention must be given to serum glucose concentrations of those patients who are insulin dependent or sensitive to sudden changes of sugar. In all cases, it is crucial that the patient be able to take in adequate fluid to maintain normal balance and urine output.

FOLLOW-UP AFTER DISCONTINUING THERAPY

Some patients require follow-up after hospital discharge. Those patients receiving home parenteral and enteral nutrition require regular periodic check-ups to assure adequacy and safety of nutrition therapy. The composition or rate of the solution may have to be altered as the patient's clinical condition changes, enabling the return to a normal mode of self-nourishment.

SUMMARY AND CONCLUSIONS

At first glance, documentation of the efficacy of nutrition support appears relatively simple. Over the short term, however, assessment and monitoring can be quite challenging because the changes in nutritional status are often subtle and the underlying disease states that interact with nutrition therapy are often complex. The art and science of adequately reassessing nutritional status to establish end points of therapy will become more critical as therapy costs continue to increase and economic resources become even more scarce. The challenge lies in developing clinically accessible, objective criteria to assess the nutritional status of the individual patient with a greater degree of reproducibility, sensitivity, and precision. Discrimination must be used in selecting the best parameters for the specific patient populations. The tools described in this chapter should be used as a guide to continually reevaluate patients and document the efficacy of therapy. The algorithms shown in Figures 22–1 through 22–3 outline suggested protocols for patient reassessment and decision making with respect to weaning from nutrition support.

REFERENCES

1. Guthrie AH: Energy balance. In Introductory Nutrition. St. Louis: C. V. Mosby, 1975, p 101
2. Silberman H, Eisenberg D: Parenteral and Enteral Nutrition for the Hospitalized Patient. Norwalk, Conn: Appleton-Century-Crofts, 1982, p 46
3. Jensen TG, Englert DM, Dudrick SJ: Nutritional Assessment. Norwalk, Conn: Appleton-Century-Crofts, 1983
4. Benditt EP, Humphreys EM, Wissler RW, et al.: The dynamics of protein metabolism. 1.

The interrelationship between protein and caloric intakes and their influence upon the utilization of ingested protein for tissue synthesis by the adult protein-depleted rat. J Lab Clin Med 33:257, 1948

5. Oldham H, Sheft BB: Effect of caloric intake on nitrogen utilization during pregnancy. J Am Dietet Assoc 27:847, 1951

6. Rosenthal HL, Allison JB: Some effects of caloric intake on nitrogen balance in dogs. J Nutr 44:423, 1951

7. Munro HN, Crum MC: The proteins and amino acids. In Goodhart RS, Shils ME (eds): Modern Nutrition in Health and Disease, ed. 6. Philadelphia: Lea & Febiger, 1980

8. Wilmore D: The Metabolic Management of the Critically Ill. New York: Plenum Medical Book, 1977

9. Meguid M, Brennan MF, Aoki T, et al.: Hormone-substrate interrelationships following trauma. Arch Surg 109:776, 1974

10. Standard KL, Willis VG, Waterlow JC: Indirect indicators of muscle mass in malnourished infants. Am J Clin Nutr 7:271, 1959

11. Reindorp S, Whitehead RG: Changes in serum creatinine kinase and other biological measurements associated with musculature in children recovering from kwashiorkor. Br J Nutr 25:273, 1973

12. Ingelbleek Y, Van Den Schrieck HG, DeNayer P, et al.: Albumin, transferrin and the thyroxine-binding prealbumin/retinol-binding protein (TBPA-RBP) complex in assessment of malnutrition. Clin Chem Acta 63:61, 1975

13. Reeds PJ, Laditan AAO: Serum albumin and transferrin in protein-energy malnutrition: Their use in the assessment of marginal undernutrition and the prognosis of severe undernutrition. Br J Nutr 36:255, 1976

14. Ingenbleek Y, De Visser M, DeNayer P: Measurement of prealbumin as index of protein–calorie malnutrition. Lancet 2:106, 1972

15. Ingenbleek Y, Van Den Schrieck HG, DeNayer P, et al.: The role of retinol binding protein in protein-calorie malnutrition. Metabolism 24:633, 1975

16. Smith FR, Goodman DS, Zaklama MS: Serum vitamin A, retinol binding protein and prealbumin concentrations in protein calorie malnutrition: Functional defect in hepatic retinol release. Am J Clin Nutr 26:973, 1973

17. Bistrian BR, Blackburn GL, Scrimshaw NS, et al.: Cellular immunity in sensitized states in hospitalized adults. Am J Clin Nutr 28:1148, 1975

18. Law DK, Dudrick SJ, Abdow NI: Immunocompetence in patients with protein-calorie malnutrition. Ann Int Med 79:545, 1973

19. Lewis RT, Klein H: Risk factors in postoperative sepsis: Significance of preoperative lymphocytopenia. J Surg Res 26:365, 1975

20. Harvey KB, Bothe A, Blackburn GL: Nutritional assessment and outcome during oncologic therapy. Cancer 43:2065, 1975

21. Morath MA, Miller SF, Finley RK: Nutritional indicators of postburn bacteremic sepsis. JPEN 5:488, 1981

22. Seltzer MH, Fletcher HS, Slocum BA, et al.: Instant nutritional assessment in an intensive care unit. JPEN 5:70, 1981

23. Twomey P, Ziegler D, Rombeau J: Utility of skin testing in nutritional assessment: A critical review. JPEN 6(1):50, 1982

24. Feldman EJ, Dowling RH, McNaughton J, Peters TJ: Effects of oral versus intravenous nutrition on intestinal adaptation after small bowel resection in the dog. Gastroenterology 70:712, 1976

25. Johnson LR, Copeland EM: Structural and hormonal alterations in the gastrointestinal tract of parenterally fed rats. Gastroenterology 68:1177, 1975

26. Levine GM, Deren JJ, Steiger E, Einno R: Role of oral intake in maintenance of gut mass and disaccharide activity. Gastroenterology 67:975, 1974

27. Matarese LE: Enteral alimentation. In Fischer JE (ed): Surgical Nutrition. Boston: Little Brown, 1983, pp 719–755

28. Pareira MD, Conrad EJ, Hicks W, Elman R: Clinical response and changes in nitrogen balance, body weight, plasma proteins, and hemoglobin following tube feeding in cancer cachexia. Cancer 8:803, 1955

29. Copeland EM, Dudrick SJ, Daly JM, Ota DM: Nutritional Changes in neoplasia. In Fischer JE (ed): Surgical Nutrition. Boston: Little Brown, 1983, pp 515–534

30. Cameron IL, Pavlat WA: Stimulation of growth of a transplantable hepatoma in rats by parenteral nutrition. J Natl Cancer Inst 56:597, 1976

31. Steiger E, Oram-Smith J, Miller E, et al.: Effects of nutrition on tumor growth and tolerance to chemotherapy. J Surg Res 18:455, 1975

23. Parenteral and Enteral Transition Techniques

Joanne Wade

Advances in the techniques of parenteral and enteral alimentation[1-5] have allowed the nutrition support of patients who otherwise may have received limited nutrient/metabolic support or inappropriate amounts of individual nutrients for prolonged periods. Transitional feeding[3,6] programs bridge the gap between the termination of parenteral nutrition (PN) and the initiation of complete enteral nutrition. As patients are weaned from parenteral alimentation, optimal transition programs aid them in maintaining adequate, sustained nutrition until they can be fed totally by enteral means.

PATIENT ASSESSMENT

Prior to the administration of enteral nutrients, the functional capacity of the gastrointestinal (GI) tract must be evaluated.[7] The presence of bowel sounds is usually the first indication that the GI tract is ready to accept enteral nutrients. The length of time the GI tract has not received enteral nutrition, the length of GI surface area available for digestion and absorption, the concurrent use of certain medical therapies, i.e., antibiotics, chemotherapy, radiation therapy, and the underlying cause of illness may dictate which enteral administration techniques are employed and in what form the nutrient sources are consumed or delivered.[8]

Patients whose GI function may be limited from the outset by surgery, disease, age, or effects of medical treatment, i.e., short bowel syndrome, severe Crohn's disease, elderly malnourished, radiation enteritis, may require a conservative approach to the reintroduction of enteral nutrition. For such patients, the rate-limiting steps to digestion and absorption of nutrients include the structural form of the nutrient source and the length of bowel available to digest and absorb simple versus complex sources of nutrients, i.e., monosaccharides versus oligosaccharides, amino acids versus hydrolyzed or whole proteins, medium chain triglycerides versus long chain triglycerides; the ability of the bowel to process increasing osmotic loads; the rate and the concentration of the nutrients provided; and concurrent medical and surgical treatment modalities.

Establishment of the goals of enteral feeding is necessary in defining how and what to feed. Consideration must be given to the individual patient's current clinical status and prognosis. Enteral feeding, especially by tube, can be used to provide access for fluids, electrolytes, and certain medications, or to provide nutrients to replete or maintain a patient's current nutritional status. Methods and goals of enteral feeding differ for chronic (≥ 3 months) tube feeding patients versus patients with a limited prognosis. In each situation, clarification of goals will ease the transition process.

Once the degree of GI function and the goals of enteral nutrition have been established, the selection of the mode of nutrient delivery and the appropriate enteral solution (see Chapter 13) may be made. In making these decisions, consideration is given to (1) the use of oral or tube feeding, (2) the degree of GI function available for digestion and absorption, (3) the individual patient's nutrient requirement, (4) the selection of an appropriate enteral formula to satisfy both the nutrient requirements and the degree of GI function, (5) the fluid allotment, and (6) the goals of enteral feeding as related to the overall clinical status and prognosis of the patient.

TECHNIQUES OF TRANSITIONAL FEEDING

A variety of enteral feeding techniques may be employed to assist the patient in making the transition from (1) PN to tube feeding, (2) PN to an oral formula, (3) PN to an oral diet, (4) tube feeding to an oral formula, or (5) tube feeding to oral food diet. Determination of the appropriate method is made after consideration of the aforementioned assessment criteria.

PN to Tube Feeding

Perhaps the simplest method of transitional feeding is that which is initiated by tube (see Chapter 13). By this method, the clinician is able to control both the type and concentration of solution infused, the method of infusion, and the rate at which the formula is delivered. Obviously, assessment of the clinical status of the patient and the type(s) of concurrent medical–surgical therapies administered will influence individual patient tolerance. However, a gradual progression in

the amount of the infusate or the rate of delivery will improve GI adaptation.[9]

For those patients who have received nothing by mouth for greater than 2 weeks and who have mechanically intact GI tracts, i.e., head and neck patients, patients with central nervous system dysfunction, initiation of tube feeding may begin with the administration of a meal replacement formula at full concentration, delivered at a rate of 40 to 50 ml/hour. Patients with head and neck or neurologic impairment tend to have a mechanical inability to consume nutrients orally. The remaining portion of their GI tract, however, remains functional for adequate digestion and absorption of complex nutrients.

Initially, patients are maintained on PN support at the individual's current rate and concentration to ensure adequate nutrition is provided during the early phases of the transition. As the rate of the tube feeding is increased (by 10 to 15 ml/hour every 24 hours), the rate or concentration of the parenteral solution is decreased accordingly. Abrupt cessation of the parenteral support is avoided to ensure reasonable GI tolerance to the enteral nutrition and to maintain adequate fluid and macronutrient–micronutrient balance.

In general, the transition to enteral feeding by tube may be accomplished in 4 to 7 days depending on the patient's requirements for fluid and macronutrients, and the ability of the GI tract to digest and absorb the enteral nutrients. However, for patients who have been nil per os for extensive periods, i.e., 3 weeks or more, who are fed transpylorically, or who may have mild maldigestion or malabsorption, a more cautious approach to the initiation of enteral feeding may be required. It may be necessary to reduce the concentration of the meal replacement formula by one half and to reduce the rate of administration to 20 ml/hour. The GI tract's capacity to readapt to the influx of enteral nutrients and to gradually adapt to the volume and osmotic concentrations of the infusate is thus promoted.[9] Progression of the tube feeding may continue by increments of 10 to 15 ml/hour/24 hours with an equally appropriate decrease in the parenteral nutrients.

Throughout the administration of any enteral nutrients (orally or by tube), symptoms of GI intolerance (nausea, vomiting, distention, diarrhea) may be indications to maintain enteral feeding at a particular stage of transition, to reduce the concentration or rate of the infusion, or, if required, to discontinue enteral feeding. Therefore, continuation of PN ensures adequate nutrient and metabolic support in the interim until enteral nutrition can progress or be reinstituted.

Patients exhibiting limited capacity to digest or absorb complex nutrients may benefit from a formula diet in which the nutrient sources are more refined (see Chapter 13). These formulations, usually of increased osmolality, require a gradual progression of both their concentration and their rate of infusion to prevent osmotically induced GI dysfunction, i.e., diarrhea.

The portion of the GI tract, i.e., stomach, duodenum, or jejunum, into which chemically defined formula diets are infused will dictate the choice of administration technique to be employed and the rate at which both the concentration and volume are increased. Patients receiving nil per os, in whom a defined formula diet will be infused via the stomach or small bowel, will generally have less complicating effects (diarrhea, distention) as a result of osmolality when tube feeding is initiated at slow infusion rates, i.e., 20 to 30 ml/hour, and dilute concentrations, i.e., half concentration.

Bolus or meal feedings by syringe should be avoided during the early stages of transitional feeding. Patients who have received limited enteral nutrition may be unable to tolerate the volume load i.e., 150 to 300 ml every 2 to 3 hours while awake, and the increased infusion time, usually 10 to 15 minutes, required by bolus methods.[9] Symptoms of nausea, distention, or diarrhea may become evident. Positioning of the patient (especially those with central nervous system dysfunction or a poor gag reflex) with the head elevated at a minimum of 30 degrees is mandated in this method of feeding to prevent the incidence of aspiration.

Perhaps the most conservative means of initiating transitional tube feeding is to administer isotonic parenteral amino acid solutions, or an enteral protein feeding module (see Chapter 13), diluted to an isomolar level, via the feeding tube. Although both of these solutions provide limited nutrition, they do aid in reintroducing the GI tract to exogenous fluid intake. More specifically, when amino acid solutions or enteral protein modules are used, the administration of protein stimulates gut hypertrophy and function.[10–13] Enteral formulas of increasing nutrient complexity may then be gradually introduced, completing the weaning process to full enteral nutrition with the gradual decline of intravenous (IV) support.

PN to Oral Formula Diets

The administration of oral formula diets to the patient shifting from parenteral nutrition is initiated slowly. After assessment of the individual patient's clinical status and nutritional requirements is made, an appropriate formula (see Chapter 13) is selected.

Administration of the oral formula, depending on its nutrient complexity and the functional capacity of the GI tract, will begin with small volumes (30 to 60 ml/hour) sipped over a 20- to 30-minute period during waking hours. IV nutrition is continued at full concentration and rate during the first 24 to 48 hours of oral intake to maintain adequate hydration and nutrition. This ensures that an established support system is not discontinued in the event the GI tract is intolerant, i.e., manifested by nausea, vomiting, diarrhea, to enteral nutrition.

The volume of the oral formula is increased daily, i.e., by 30- to 60-ml increments, with the time span between oral feedings increasing. The concentration of the formula, if it has been diluted, may increase by 25 to 50 percent, once the desired volume is achieved. Simultaneous increases in volume and concentration should be avoided to prevent symptoms of diarrhea, nausea, and distention.

The transition from PN to an oral formula diet is more difficult to manage than the transition by feeding tube. Several factors are responsible. First, the subjective tolerance of an individual patient's taste[14] may dictate early in the transition whether or not adequate consumption of a particular formula will be possible. Often, the bland, sweet, or metallic tastes associated with a variety of formulas, and the monotony of a liquid consistency, prevent a patient's compliance. Under these circumstances, the ingenuity of the clinical dietitian to circumvent these taste and consistency problems, and the supportive assistance of the food service system to prepare and deliver alternative flavor and consistency choices, is paramount in gaining patient acceptance.

Second, the rate of consumption of an oral formula diet is less well controlled than by the use of devices, i.e., pumps or manual control devices, in tube feeding. Patients may be asked to sip formulas slowly, i.e., over 20 to 30 minutes, several times, i.e., every hour or 2 hours, daily. If consumed more rapidly, diarrhea, distention, or nausea may occur.

Third, the volume of fluid (formula and free water) necessary to provide adequate sustained nutrition, although variable for each patient, may range from 1 to 3 liters daily. Depending on the goals of enteral support and the estimated length of time required for the patient to be on formula diet alone, compliance may again be limited.

PN is decreased by half when the patient is able to maintain half of the nutrient requirements (fluids and macronutrients) orally. Oftentimes, cycling, i.e., nighttime infusion of the PN, is beneficial in encouraging an increased oral intake. Patients may view discontinuance of the daytime infusion of IV support as a positive step in their recovery. Also, by removing the infusion apparatus, patients are more apt to increase their mobility.

Discontinuance of the PN is indicated when oral consumption of the formula is adequate and sustained, GI tolerance is maintained, and positive results in nutritional status are documented.

PN to Oral Food Diet

Food diets are initiated in a similar manner as that of oral formula diets, beginning with fluids or foods that are the least stimulatory in promoting symptoms of maldigestion and/or malabsorption, and gradually increasing nutrient complexity and quantity. The use of a food diet versus a formula diet is usually indicated when the progression to full enteral nutrition is anticipated to move rapidly; when there is little evidence of maldigestion or malabsorption; or when, as in the case of home hyperalimentation patients, the progression to a food diet, rather than formula diet, is psychologically important to the patient.

When properly planned, modified diets designed to meet the individual clinical needs of the patient can be implemented. The length of time required for transition to an oral food diet will be variable. Factors that will influence the transition are the length of time a patient has received nil per os, the prognosis for improvement in the clinical status, the patient's subjective food preferences in relation to the dietary modification(s), the ingenuity of the clinical dietitian in designing the nutrition prescription, and the supportive assistance of the food service in the preparation and delivery of foods to meet the requirements of the prescription.[15]

Standard clear liquid diets are implemented in the initial phases of the transition process. Volumes are low, i.e., 30 to 60 ml/hour, given while the patient is awake, and gradually (every 24 hours) progressed to ad libitum within 48 to 72 hours. During this phase of transition, IV nutrition is maintained to ensure adequate volume and nutrient input.

Within the following 72 hours, the diet is

advanced in consistency (full liquids to soft solids to regular), thereby increasing the nutrient density. Foods and fluids are provided as small (1 to 2 ounce portions, 2 to 5 items per tray), frequent (6 to 8) meals daily. Nutrient-dense foods and fluids, rich in protein and energy, are emphasized within the constraints of the overall dietary modification. Low kilocalorie fluids and foods are avoided or limited until adequate oral intake is established.

Psychologically, the provision of small meal trays is far more acceptable to patients than the standard three daily meals served to the majority of hospitalized patients. The appearance and consumption of these "mini" meals are seen as positive reinforcement by the patient. Presentation of three standard size trays often overwhelms the patient, thereby preventing adequate consumption.

Calorie counts, calculated records of actual patient nutrient consumption (both parenteral and enteral) are computed daily for close approximations of protein, energy and electrolyte intake. IV nutrition is reduced or cycled according to the adequacy of the oral intake and GI function as related to the enteral diet. Once a patient has sustained and tolerated an oral intake of approximately 1000 to 2000 kilocalories and 50 to 60 g protein for 3 to 5 consecutive days, IV support may be discontinued.

Fluctuation in oral intake because of diagnostic tests and procedures, the psychological state of the patient, and individual food preferences or tolerances are variables that may inhibit a rapid transition from parenteral nutrition to an oral food diet. Also, patients may have a strong desire to eat even though the GI tract may not be fully functional. Overzealous progression of oral diets may lead to symptoms of maldigestion and malabsorption. The other extreme is the patient with limited appetite whose GI tract is, through objective assessment, fully functional, but who nevertheless remains anorectic. In both situations, the clinical dietetics staff can be instrumental in designing and implementing alternative meal selections and in educating patients, family, and the health care team as to reasonable progressions of oral intake.

Tube Feeding to Oral Formula or Oral Diets

The actual progression from tube feeding to an oral formula or food diet is similar to that from PN. More attention, however, is given to methods of decreasing the enteral tube feeding, to GI symptomatology, and to the mechanisms of optimizing spontaneous oral intake.

Patients transitioning from tube feeding are obviously being fed into a portion (stomach, duodenum, jejunum) of the GI tract. Because the patient realizes that some source of "food" is constantly being infused, he or she may refuse additional oral intake. Several methods of handling this situation may be employed. First, during the first 24 to 48 hours, it is usually necessary to continue the tube feeding at full rate and concentration simply to assess the patient's capacity, subjectively and objectively, to consume oral nutrients. Explaining to the patient that the tube feeding is to be maintained temporarily, until calorie counts indicate a gradual improvement, may be all that is necessary to encourage an increased consumption. As calorie counts indicate, tube feeding may be (1) maintained if oral intake does not improve, (2) decreased in total volume but maintained on a 24-hour infusion, or (3) cycled during the evening and night. This latter method is often preferable in encouraging increased consumption. The patient is freed from the daytime infusion of tube feeding, thus allowing the opportunity for increased oral intake and physical activity.

Cyclic tube feeding, i.e., infusion of a formula for an 8- to 20-hour period, is usually indicated for patients who are transitioning to an oral diet, food or formula, or for patients on home tube feeding programs. The length of the cycle will be dependent on (1) the patient's ability to tolerate large fluid volumes infused at increased rates (patients with congestive heart failure, impaired renal function, or the elderly may not be candidates for these reasons); and (2) the functional capacity of the GI tract to tolerate increased fluid volumes, to digest and absorb increased quantities of nutrients over a shortened time span, and to process the increased osmotic load.

Tube feeding may be discontinued when an oral intake of approximately 1000 to 1200 kilocalories, a protein intake of approximately 50 to 60 g and an adequate fluid intake, i.e., 30 ml/kg body weight, are established and sustained. Further increases in consumption are expected as the patient's clinical status progresses from the acute stages of illness to convalescence.

Modular Feeding

In any one technique of transitional feeding, either formula feeding (by tube or by mouth) or solid food by mouth, the induction of feeding may require a slow, deliberate approach. Patients exhibiting symptoms of severe radiation enteritis, short bowel syndrome, or chronic pancreatitis, and those patients having received nil per os for lengthy periods, i.e., for more than 1 month, may benefit from the gradual reintroduction of specific nutrient sources and the elimination of others. In this manner, the GI tract, especially the small bowel,[11,12] develops a progressive readaptation to the influx of enteral nutrition. In addition, subsets of patients exhibiting renal dysfunction, cardiac decompensation, hepatic dysfunction, and the like may require the deliberate limitation of certain nutrients, particularly protein, potassium, sodium, or fluid. Thus, individually designed formulas versus premixed formulas may be of benefit. For these reasons, feeding modules (see Chapter 13) have been developed to allow greater flexibility in the design of individualized specialty formulas for this small patient population.

The incorporation of feeding modules into a transition program usually begins with the administration of a protein module. The amount of protein provided is usually calculated to meet approximately 30 to 50 percent of the patient's need. The protein or amino acid powder is diluted to an appropriate volume to meet the initial fluid demands of the patient. While continuing full IV support, this protein-rich solution initiates the enteral transition program. As tolerance to fluid and protein administration is established, additional modules, i.e., carbohydrate or fat, vitamins, and minerals, can be added according to the individual's requirements. The individualized prescription incorporating both macro- and micronutrients is gradually increased both in nutrient density and volume as indicated by the patient's overall clinical status.

The increased clinical flexibility of modular feeding, however, is not without difficulty. Personnel trained in the design, preparation, and monitoring of such formulas, are necessary in both clinical and food services. The preparation of specialized modular formulas is currently labor intensive. Additional clinical trials are needed to establish the clinical benefits in relationship to their economic feasibility.

Combined Feeding Modalities

A final mode of transitional feeding may incorporate several methods of enteral feeding at various stages to assist in a more rapid progression to the enteral route. Patients may be initiated on the enteral feeding by tube. The initial formula may be a single feeding module (usually protein), later combined with a premixed formula, thus increasing the nutrient density.

Patients progressing to an oral food diet may have a limited volume capacity. It may, therefore, be advantageous to incorporate either (1) a feeding module directly mixed into a variety of foods or fluids or (2) a nutrient-dense supplement providing protein, energy, vitamins, and minerals in addition to small frequent meals.

The method(s) of combined feeding will be chosen according to (1) the clinical status of the patient, (2) the patient's nutrient requirements, (3) the patient's compliance, (4) the capacity of the clinical dietetics staff to recommend and the food service staff to provide appropriate enteral prescription components, and (5) daily monitoring of nutrient intake in relationship to changes in the patient's clinical and nutritional status.

Clinical Monitoring of Transitional Feeding Programs

Standard methods of nutrition assessment are necessary to determine how and what to feed patients either enterally or parenterally. The major considerations for transitional feeding programs include: (1) Assessment of protein and energy consumption via calculation of estimated parenteral and enteral nutrition intakes on a daily or three times per week basis (based on this objective assessment, PN is either maintained or decreased in preference to enteral nutrition); (2) GI function as related to digestion and absorption (the presence or absence of nausea, vomiting, distention, diarrhea, cramping may dictate the degree to which enteral nutrition is maintained or progressed); (3) The biochemical assessment of protein–calorie utilization, as evidenced by albumin and transferrin synthesis, may be assessed biweekly. Gross nitrogen balance studies performed twice weekly provide an estimate of the body's ability to synthesize lean tissue with regard to the amount of substrate (energy and protein) provided and the patient's clinical status. (4) Serum electrolytes, vitamins, iron, urea, glucose, creatinine, and liver enzyme activity may be monitored weekly or as clinically indicated. These parameters, other than selected electrolytes, i.e., potassium and sodium, need not be monitored more often than indicated.

SUMMARY

Scientific, medical, and technologic advances have improved the quality of nutritional care provided to patients. Approaches to both enteral and PN support techniques have proliferated. The current techniques of transitional feeding are easily employed and ensure adequate nutrition and metabolic support between the parenteral phase of nutrient support and that of complete enteral feeding.

REFERENCES

1. Bistrian BR, Wade JE: Feeding the hospitalized patient. In Garry PS (ed): Human Nutrition, Clinical and Biochemical Aspects. Washington, DC: The American Association for Clinical Chemistry, 1981, pp 352–370
2. Grant J: Handbook of Total Parenteral Nutrition. Philadelphia: W.B. Saunders, 1980
3. Bothe A, Wade JE, Blackburn GL: Enteral nutrition—an overview. In Hill G (ed): Nutrition and the Surgical Patient. Edinburgh: Churchill Livingston, 1981, pp 76–103
4. Heymsfield SB, Horowitz J, Lawson DH: Enteral hyperalimentation. In Burke E (ed): Developments in Digestive Diseases. Philadelphia: Lea & Febiger, 1980, pp 59–83
5. Torosian MH, Rombeau JL: Feeding by tube enterostomy. Surg Gynecol Obstet 150:918, 1980
6. Skipper A: Transitional feeding and the dietitian. Nutr Supp Serv 2:45, 1982
7. Woodward ER: The stomach and duodenum. In Kinney JM, Egdahl RH, Zuidema GD (eds): Manual of Preoperative and Postoperative Care, ed 2. Philadelphia: W. B. Saunders, 1971, pp 336–344
8. Young EA, Cioletti LA, Traylor JB, Baldaros L: Gastrointestinal response to nutrient variation of defined formula diets. JPEN 5:478, 1981
9. Hostetler CA, Lipman TO: Techniques of providing enteral nutrition. Drug Therapy, September 1982, pp 31–40
10. Spector MH, Levine GM, Deren JJ: Direct and

indirect effects of dextrose and amino acids on gut mass. Gastroenterology 72:706, 1977

11. Weser E: Nutritional aspects of malabsorption. Am J Med 67:1014, 1979

12. Feldman EJ, Dowling RH, McNaughton J, Peters TJ: Effects of oral versus intravenous nutrition on intestinal adaptation after small bowel resection in the dog. Gastroenterology 70:712, 1976

13. Sheldon GF: Role of parenteral nutrition in patients with short bowel syndrome. Am J Med 67:1021, 1979

14. Bayless E: Taste tray increases acceptance of nutritional supplements. J Am Dietet Assoc 73:542, 1978

15. Blackburn GL, Tower JB, Clark NG, et al.: Optimizing spontaneous intake: A challenge for the hospital food service. In Hospital Patient Feeding Systems. Washington, DC: National Academy Press, 1982, pp 346–357

Index

497